UPPER AND LOWER RESPIRATORY DISEASE

LUNG BIOLOGY IN HEALTH AND DISEASE

Executive Editor

Claude Lenfant
Director, National Heart, Lung, and Blood Institute
National Institutes of Health
Bethesda, Maryland

ADDITIONAL VOLUMES IN PREPARATION

The opinions expressed in these volumes do not necessarily represent the views of the National Institutes of Health.

UPPER AND LOWER RESPIRATORY DISEASE

Edited by

Jonathan Corren
Allergy Research Foundation, Inc.
Los Angeles, California, U.S.A.

Alkis Togias
Johns Hopkins Asthma and Allergy Center
Baltimore, Maryland, U.S.A.

Jean Bousquet
Hôpital Arnaud de Villeneuve
Montpellier, France

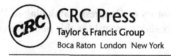

CRC Press
Taylor & Francis Group
Boca Raton London New York

CRC Press is an imprint of the
Taylor & Francis Group, an **informa** business

First published 2003 by Marcel Dekker, Inc.

Published 2019 by CRC Press
Taylor & Francis Group
6000 Broken Sound Parkway NW, Suite 300
Boca Raton, FL 33487-2742

© 2003 by Taylor & Francis Group, LLC
CRC Press is an imprint of Taylor & Francis Group, an Informa business

No claim to original U.S. Government works

ISBN-13: 978-0-8247-0723-1 (hbk)

Visit the Taylor & Francis Web site at
http://www.taylorandfrancis.com

and the CRC Press Web site at
http://www.crcpress.com

Library of Congress Cataloging-in-Publication Data
A catalog record for this book is available from the Library of Congress.

INTRODUCTION

In the second century, Claudius Galen—certainly one of the fathers of modern respiratory physiology—defined the nose as a "respiratory instrument." This pronouncement was made in his work *De usu partium* (on the usefulness of the [body] parts). Yet, it is interesting that Galen failed to recognized the usefulness, or role of respiration. In fact, he went so far as to say that because the air we inhale is immediately removed and discarded, we have proof that "it is not the substance (we breathe) that is needed."

On the other hand, Galen clearly indicated that the release of the breath is tied to the production of the voice. This indeed is not an inconsequential consideration, as "one of the first products of the human mind is human language. In fact, it is the very first of these products, and that the human brain and the human mind evolved in interaction with language."*

However, today the importance of the air we breathe is very well recognized, and we know that the nose—the uppermost part of the respiratory tract—serves as an essential filter that protects the lower airways. From this, it is evident that there is a functional, as well as a structural, interrelationship between the nose and the lungs. Furthermore, this interrelationship is as important in health as it is in disease. In disease, it has been the object of many studies and debates. Critical questions have been raised; for instance, are rhinitis and asthma related? . . . interdependent?

---

*Popper KR, and Eccles JC. The Self and its Brain. Springer-Verlag, Berlin-Heidelberg-New York: Springer-Verlag, 1997.

Ever since its initiation, the series the monographs *Lung Biology in Health and Disease* has presented many volumes to its readership in which allergic disease of the lower airway or of the upper airway (the nose) has been explored and discussed. However, this new volume is a unique contribution to the series in the sense that it does not examine only the upper or the lower airway, but rather, the totality of the respiratory tract.

The editors of this volume, Drs. Jonathan Corren, Alkis Togias, and Jean Bousquet, as well as the authors they selected, bring years of clinical and investigative experience, as well as an international dimension.

I am thankful to them for this contribution.

Claude Lenfant, M.D.
Bethesda, Maryland

PREFACE

Over the past decade, our understanding of allergic airway diseases has evolved tremendously. In particular, the scientific community has gained a growing appreciation for the connection between the upper and lower airways. While there are a great number of outstanding books dealing with allergic rhinitis, sinusitis, and asthma, as well as allergy in general, none has focused specifically on the interrelationship between the nose and lungs. Therefore, we sought to create a new textbook that would examine all aspects of this relationship, including both basic and clinical science.

We have divided the book into four parts. The first deals with structural relationships between the upper and lower airways, looking specifically at both the microscopic and gross anatomy of the respiratory tract. The second part emphasizes functional relationships, utilizing both human and animal models of disease. In the third portion, we delve into the very important connection between allergic rhinitis and sinusitis and asthma, and include chapters on pathophysiology, epidemiology, diagnosis, and treatment. The final part reviews systemic diseases characterized by involvement of both the upper and lower respiratory tracts. Using this comprehensive approach, we hope our new book will serve the needs of both clinicians and investigators in the fields of allergy, immunology, pulmonology, otorhinolaryngology, and physiology.

Most of the chapters can be read as free-standing monographs on that particular subject. Some of the chapters in this book represent the most up-to-date and comprehensive reviews of the subject available from any source. It is our hope that *Upper and Lower Airways Disease* will act as a valuable reference for all readers interested in this topic.

We were very fortunate to work with a truly outstanding collection of authors to help us write the book. An international group of experts from the United States, United Kingdom, France, and Japan—all distinguished in their respective fields—participated and collaborated in the preparation of this book. We thank them for their diligent efforts and are especially appreciative of the updating that was required as the project came to fruition.

In addition to our contributors, we are also indebted to a number of other individuals, without whose help this book would not have been completed. These include Sandra Beberman and Paige Force of Marcel Dekker, Inc., whose unflagging support and encouragement were invaluable.

We hope this book will provide physicians and scientists with a new and unique reference on a topic of great importance.

Jonathan Corren
Alkis Togias
Jean Bousquet

CONTRIBUTORS

Daniel C. Adelman, M.D., F.A.C.P., F.A.A.A.A.I. Adjunct Professor, Division of Allergy/Immunology, Department of Medicine, University of California, San Francisco, California, U.S.A.

Isabella Annesi-Maesano, M.D. Respiratory Epidemiologist, Institut National de la Sante et de la Recherche Medicale, Villejuif, France

Robert D. Ballard, M.D. Director, Sleep Disorders Center, National Jewish Medical and Research Center, and University of Colorado Health Sciences Center, Denver, Colorado, U.S.A.

Fuad M. Baroody, M.D. Associate Professor, Otolaryngology—Head and Neck Surgery–and Pediatrics, University of Chicago, Chicago, Illinois, U.S.A.

Robert Bocian, M.D., Ph.D., F.A.A.A.A.I. Assistant Clinical Professor, Department of Pediatrics, Stanford University, Stanford, and Head, Department of Allergy, Palo Alto Medical Foundation, Palo Alto, California, U.S.A.

Larry Borish, M.D. Asthma and Allergic Disease Center, University of Virginia, Charlottesville, Virginia, U.S.A.

Jean Bousquet, M.D. Professor, Department of Pulmonary Medicine, Montpellier University, Montpellier, France

vii

Brendan J. Canning, M.D. Associate Professor, Department of Clinical Immunology, Johns Hopkins University, Baltimore, Maryland, U.S.A.

Jonathan Corren, M.D. Medical Director, Allergy Research Foundation, Los Angeles, California, U.S.A.

Pascal Demoly, M.D. Service de Maladies Respiratoires, Hôpital Arnaud de Villeneuve, Montpellier, France

Michael Diament, M.D. Associate Professor, Center for the Health Sciences, University of California, Los Angeles, California, U.S.A.

William K. Dolen, M.D. Professor, Department of Pediatrics, Section of Allergy and Immunology, Medical College of Georgia, Augusta, Georgia, U.S.A.

Stephen R. Durham, M.D., F.R.C.P. Professor, Department of Upper Respiratory Medicine, National Heart and Lung Institute, London, United Kingdom

Ronald Eccles, B.S., Ph.D., D.Sc. Professor, Common Cold Center, Cardiff University, Cardiff, United Kingdom

David B. Hellmann, M.D. Professor and Chairman, Department of Medicine, Bayview Medical Center, Johns Hopkins University, Baltimore, Maryland, U.S.A.

Imran R. Hussain, MB. BS., M.R.C.P. Consultant, Department of Respiratory Medicine, North Staffordshire Hospital, Stoke-on-Trent, Staffordshire, United Kingdom

Charles G. Irvin, Ph.D. Professor, Department of Physiology and Biophysics, University of Vermont, Burlington, Vermont, U.S.A.

R. Jankowski, M.D. Professor, Department of Otorhinolaryngology—Head and Neck Surgery, Henri Poincaré University, Nancy, France

Sebastian L. Johnston, M.D., Ph.D., F.R.C.P. Professor, Department of Respiratory Medicine, National Heart and Lung Institute, London, United Kingdom

Jeffrey L. Kishiyama, M.D. Assistant Clinical Professor, Department of Medicine, University of California, San Francisco, California, U.S.A.

Shoji Kudoh, M.D. Professor and Director, Department of Internal Medicine, Nihon Medical School, Tokyo, Japan

Peter Maguire, M.D. Allergy Department, Palo Alto Medical Clinic, Palo Alto, California, U.S.A.

David R. Moller, M.D. Associate Professor, School of Medicine, Johns Hopkins University, Baltimore, Maryland, U.S.A.

Kenneth B. Newman, M.D. Forest Laboratories, New York, New York, U.S.A.

Judy Palmer, M.D. Stanford University, Stanford, California, U.S.A.

Irina Petrache, M.D. Instructor, Division of Pulmonary and Critical Care Medicine, Johns Hopkins University, Baltimore, Maryland, U.S.A.

K. Rajakulasingam, D.M., F.R.C.P., F.A.C.P. Consultant Physician and Honorary Senior Lecturer, Department of Respiratory Medicine and Allergy, Homerton University Hospital, London, United Kingdom

Dale Rice, M.D. Professor and Chair, Otolaryngology—Head and Neck Surgery, University of Southern California, Los Angeles, California, U.S.A.

Ray Slavin, M.D., M.S. Professor and Director, Division of Allergy and Immunology, St. Louis University, St. Louis, Missouri, U.S.A.

Sheldon Spector, M.D. Clinical Professor, School of Medicine, University of California, Los Angeles, California, U.S.A.

Chester Stafford, M.D. Professor Emeritus, Section of Allergy and Immunology, Medical College of Georgia, Augusta, Georgia, U.S.A.

Donald D. Stevenson, M.D. Senior Consultant, Scripps Clinic, Adjunct Member, Department of Molecular and Experimental Medicine, Scripps Research Institute, La Jolla, California, U.S.A.

Yukihiko Sugiyama, M.D., Ph.D., F.C.C.P. Professor, Division of Pulmonary Medicine, Jichi Medical School, Minamikawachi, Iochigi, Japan

Alkis Togias, M.D. Associate Professor, Divisions of Clinical Immunology and Respiratory and Critical Care Medicine, Johns Hopkins Asthma and Allergy Center, Baltimore, Maryland, U.S.A.

Dale T. Umetsu, M.D., Ph.D.   Professor and Director, Center for Asthma and Allergic Immunological Diseases, Stanford University, Stanford, California, U.S.A.

A. Maurizio Vignola, M.D.   Instituto di Fisiopatologia Respiratoria, Palermo, Italy

James A. Wilde, M.D., F.A.A.P.   Associate Professor, Departments of Emergency Medicine and Pediatrics, Medical College of Georgia, Augusta, Georgia, U.S.A.

Hugh Windom, M.D.   Associate Clinical Professor, Department of Medicine, University of South Florida, Tampa, Florida, U.S.A.

CONTENTS

UPPER AND LOWER
RESPIRATORY DISEASE

1

Comparative Anatomy of the Nasal and Tracheal/Bronchial Airways

FUAD M. BAROODY

University of Chicago
Chicago, Illinois, U.S.A.

BRENDAN J. CANNING

The Johns Hopkins University
Baltimore, Maryland, U.S.A.

Introduction

The relationship between the upper and lower airways in man has long been recognized. This relationship stems, in part, from similarities between the anatomy and physiology of these airways. This chapter addresses these components of the upper and lower airways, stressing the similarities and differences between the two organs and complementing other chapters that detail the interactions between the upper and lower airways in health and disease.

I. Gross Anatomy of the Airways

A. Nasal Airways

External Framework

The external bony framework of the nose consists of two oblong, paired nasal bones located on either side of the midline that merge to form a pyramid (Fig. 1). Lateral to each nasal bone is the frontal process of the

1

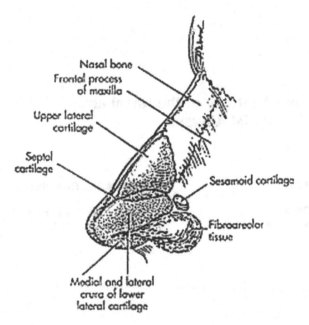

Nasal bone
Frontal process
of maxilla

Upper lateral
cartilage

Septal
cartilage

Sesamoid cartilage

Fibroareolar
tissue

Medial and lateral
crura of lower
lateral cartilage

Figure 1   External nasal framework. (From Drumheller GW. Anat Rec 1973;176: 321, with permission of Wiley-Liss.)

maxilla, which contributes to the base of the nasal pyramid. The pyriform aperture is the bony opening that leads to the external nose.

The cartilaginous framework of the nose consists of the paired upper lateral, the lower lateral, and the sesamoid cartilages (Fig. 1). The upper lateral cartilages are attached to the undersurface of the nasal bones and frontal processes superiorly, and their inferior ends lie under the upper margin of the lower lateral cartilages. Medially, they blend with the cartilaginous septum. Each lower lateral cartilage consists of a medial crus that extends along the free caudal edge of the cartilaginous septum and a lateral crus that provides the framework of the nasal ala, the entrance to the nose (Fig. 1). Laterally, between the upper and lower lateral cartilages, are one or more sesamoid cartilages and fibroadipose tissue.

Nasal Septum

The nasal septum divides the nasal cavity into two sides and is composed of cartilage and bone. The bone receives contributions from the vomer, the perpendicular plate of the ethmoid bone, the maxillary crest, the palatine bone, and the anterior spine of the maxillary bone. The main supporting framework of the septum is the septal cartilage, which forms the most anterior part of the septum and articulates posteriorly with the vomer and the perpendicular plate of the ethmoid bone. Inferiorly, the cartilage rests in the crest of the maxilla, whereas anteriorly it has a free border when it approaches the membranous septum. The latter separates the medial crura of the lower lateral cartilages from the septal cartilage. The perpendicular plate of the ethmoid bone forms the posterosuperior portion of the septum, and the vomer contributes to its posteroinferior portion. In a study of cadaveric specimens, Van Loosen and colleagues showed that the cartilaginous septum increases rapidly in size during the first years of life, with the total area remaining constant after the age of 2 years (1). In contrast, endochondral ossification of the cartilaginous septum resulting in the formation of the perpendicular plate of the ethmoid bone starts after the first 6 months of life and continues until the age of 36 years. The continuous, albeit slow, growth of the nasal septum until the third decade might explain frequently encountered septal deviations in adults. Other causes for septal deviations may be spontaneous, or they may result from previous trauma. Deviations can involve any of the individual components of the nasal septum and can lead to nasal obstruction because of impairment to airflow within the nasal cavities. In addition to reduction of nasal airflow, some septal deviations obstruct the middle meatal areas and can lead to impairment of drainage from the sinuses, with resultant sinusitis. Severe anterior deviations can also prevent the introduction of intranasal medications to the rest of the nasal cavity and therefore interfere with the medical treatment of rhinitis (2). It is important to examine the nose in a patient with complaints of nasal congestion to rule out such deviations. It is also important to realize that not all deviations lead to symptoms and that surgery should be reserved for deviations that are thought to contribute to the patient's symptomatology.

Nasal Vestibule

The nasal vestibule, located immediately posterior to the external nasal opening, is lined with stratified squamous epithelium and numerous hairs (or vibrissae) that filter out large particulate matter. The vestibule funnels air toward the nasal valve, which is a slit-shaped passage formed by the junction of the upper lateral cartilages, the nasal septum, and the inferior turbinate. The nasal valve accounts for approximately 50% of the total resistance to respiratory airflow from the anterior nostril to the alveoli. The surface area of this valve, and consequently resistance to airflow, is modified by the action of the alar muscles. An increase in the tone of the dilator naris muscle, innervated by the facial nerve, dilates the nares, increases the cross-sectional area of the nasal valve, and thus decreases resistance to airflow.

This occurs in labored breathing, such as during exercise, and is a physiological mechanism to increase nasal airflow. On the other hand, collapse of the nasal valve and the vestibule depends on the pressure gradient between ambient and respired air. As negative pressure in the nose increases to increase airflow, the cartilages collapse in spite of the opposing action of the dilator muscles. An example of these paradoxical actions occurs during sniffing, when resistance to airflow increases across the vestibule–nasal valve complex. Aging results in loss of strength of the nasal cartilages, with secondary weakening of nasal tip support and the nasal valve, with resultant airflow compromise (2).

Lateral Nasal Wall

The lateral nasal wall commonly has three turbinates, or conchae: inferior, middle, and superior (Fig. 2). The turbinates are elongated laminae of bone

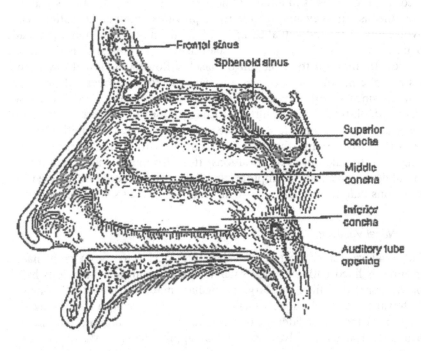

Figure 2 A sagittal section of the lateral nasal wall showing the three turbinates or conchae, the frontal and sphenoid sinuses, and the opening of the eustachian tube in the nasopharynx. (From Cummings CW, Fredrickson JM, Harker LA et al. Otolaryngology—Head and Neck Surgery. 2nd ed. St. Louis: Mosby-Year Book, 1993.)

attached along their superior borders to the lateral nasal wall. Their unattached inferior portions curve inward toward the lateral nasal wall, resulting in a convex surface that faces the nasal septum medially. They not only increase the mucosal surface of the nasal cavity to about 100 to 200 cm^2 but regulate airflow by alternating their vascular content, hence thickness, through the state of their capacitance vessels (3). The large surface area of the turbinates and the nasal septum allows intimate contact between respired air and the mucosal surfaces, thus facilitating humidification, filtration, and temperature regulation of inspired air. Under and lateral to each of the turbinates are horizontal passages or meati. The inferior meatus receives the opening of the nasolacrimal duct, whereas the middle meatus receives drainage originating from the frontal, anterior ethmoid, and maxillary sinuses (Fig. 3). The sphenoid and posterior ethmoid sinuses drain into the sphenoethmoid recess, located below and posterior to the superior turbinate.

The middle meatus is an important anatomical area in the pathophysiology of sinus disease. It has a complex anatomy of bones and mucosal folds, often referred to as the osteomeatal unit, between which drain the frontal, anterior ethmoid, and maxillary sinuses. Anatomical abnormalities or inflammatory mucosal changes in the area of the osteomeatal complex

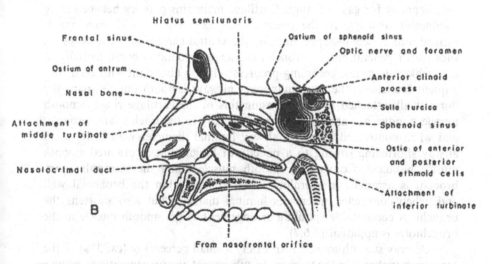

Figure 3 A detailed view of the lateral nasal wall. Parts of the inferior and middle turbinates have been removed to allow visualization of the various openings into the inferior, middle, and superior meati. (From Montgomery WW. Surgery of the Upper Respiratory System. Philadelphia: Lea Febiger, 1979, with permission.)

can lead to impaired drainage from these sinuses which can, at least in part, be responsible for acute and chronic sinus disease. Endoscopic sinus surgery is targeted at restoring the functionality of this drainage system in patients with chronic sinus disease that is refractory to medical management.

B. Tracheal/Bronchial Airways

By convention, the larynx marks the boundary between the upper and lower airways. Comprising an asymmetrical branching structure, the lower airways extend from the trachea to the alveoli. The trachea branches into right and left mainstem bronchi, which branch 7 to 22 times further in an asymmetrical pattern in the right and left lungs. Bronchi are defined structurally as the intrathoracic and primarily intrapulmonary airways lined with cartilage. Bronchi branch terminally into bronchioles, which lack cartilage, and ultimately form terminal bronchioli. Bronchioli are the last and thus the smallest of the conducting airways. Thereafter, one to three orders of respiratory bronchioles appear with associated alveolar ducts and alveolar sacs. The terminal bronchioli, respiratory bronchioles, alveolar ducts, and alveolar sacs comprise the basic respiratory unit or acinus. Gas movement in the acini occurs by diffusion, not conductance (4,5).

The primary function of the lower airways is to act as a conduit for gas exchange. The structure of the airways thus serves to facilitate and preserve lung capacity for gas exchange. Cartilage maintains patency between large conducting airways. In the trachea and mainstem bronchi, cartilage is formed into crescent-shaped rings on the ventral surface of the airways. In subsequent generations of bronchi, cartilage is found circumferentially in plaquelike structures, becoming progressively less abundant with each subsequent branch. In the extrapulmonary airways, smooth muscle spans the dorsal wall, attached to the opposing tips of the cartilage rings. Smooth muscle bundles are arranged circumferentially in the trachea and bronchi, and when contracted, decrease airway luminal diameter with little or no airway shortening (owing to a paucity of longitudinally oriented smooth muscle bundles). Conversely, smooth muscle lining the intrapulmonary bronchi is arranged in spiraling bands that envelop the bronchial wall and, when contracted, decreases luminal diameter but also shortens the bronchi. A comparable spiraling arrangement of the smooth muscle in the bronchioles is apparent (4,6,7).

Airway smooth muscle forms only a small percentage (ca. 3%) of the cross-sectional area in the trachea. In subsequent airway generations, airway smooth muscle assumes a progressively larger proportion of the airway wall, comprising about 20% of the bronchiolar walls. The comparatively small amount of smooth muscle along with the cartilage lining the tracheal and bronchial wall limits airways narrowing evoked by tracheal and bronchial smooth muscle contraction, thereby preventing airway closure. By contrast, the large muscle mass and the absence of cartilage in the bronchioles permits complete airways closure upon bronchiolar smooth muscle contraction (8,9).

Luminal diameters decrease progressively and predictably from the trachea to the terminal bronchioli. Concurrently, the number of each successive airway generation increases exponentially. This marked increase in airway number renders the cross-sectional area of the peripheral airways far greater than that in the central conducting airways. Resistance to airflow in the healthy lung thus resides primarily in the larger conducting bronchi. In asthma, however, where mucus plugging and excessive constriction of the musculature lining the peripheral airways occurs, resistance to airflow is primarily attributable to resistance in the small airways. This manifests clinically as a fall in vital capacity (5,10).

Smooth muscle contraction and the transpulmonary pressures associated with expiration tend to force collapse or closure of the intrapulmonary airways. These forces are opposed by the interdependence of the lung, whereby the elastic tethering properties associated with adjacent airways serves to pull open closed adjacent airways during inspiration and resist closure during expiration (5,9). In both asthma and chronic obstructive pulmonary disease (COPD), the bronchoprotective effects of deep inspiration are dysfunctional (11,12). Whether this phenomenon in asthma and COPD is due in part or in whole to the loss of an active dilating process, the appearance of an aberrant constricting process, or a loss of airway interdependence has not been firmly established. Pathological studies indicate that a loss of interdependence is likely in emphysema and α_1-antitrypsin deficiency but far less common or likely in asthma (9,13–15).

Airway closure in the peripheral lung may occur despite the forces of interdependence. This may create areas of inadequate ventilation. The lung counteracts this physiologically by diverting blood flow away from hypoxic alveolar capillary beds (through pulmonary vascular constriction) (5). Structurally, the lung counteracts airway closure by diverting airflow into collateral airways between adjacent alveolar sacs (pores of Kohn) or between bronchioles (communications of Lambert) (16).

II. Histology of the Airways

A. Nasal Airways

Nasal Epithelium

A thin, moderately keratinized, stratified squamous epithelium lines the vestibular region. The anterior tips of the turbinates provide a transition from squamous to transitional and finally to pseudostratified columnar ciliated epithelium, which lines the remainder of the nasal cavity except for the roof, which is lined with olfactory epithelium (Fig. 4) (3). All cells of the pseudostratified columnar ciliated epithelium contact the basement membrane, but not all reach the epithelial surface. The basement membrane separates the epithelium from the lamina propria, or submucosa. Within the epithelium, three types of cells are identified: basal, goblet, and columnar, which are either ciliated or nonciliated.

Basal Cells

Basal cells lie on the basement membrane and do not reach the airway lumen. They have an electron-dense cytoplasm and bundles of tonofilaments. Among their morphological specializations are desmosomes, which mediate adhesion between adjacent cells, and hemidesmosomes, which help anchor

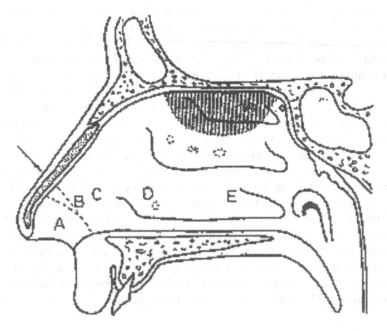

Figure 4   Distribution of types of epithelium along the lateral nasal wall. The hatched region represents the olfactory epithelium. The arrow represents the area of the nasal valve: (A) Skin. (B) Squamous epithelium without microvilli. (C) Transitional epithelium. (D) Pseudostratified columnar epithelium with few ciliated cells. (E) Pseudostratified columnar epithelium with many ciliated cells. (From Proctor DF, Andersen IB. The Nose—Upper Airway Physiology and the Atmospheric Environment. Amsterdam: Elsevier Biomedical Press, 1982.)

the cells to the basement membrane (17). These cells have long been thought to be progenitors of the columnar and goblet cells of the airway epithelium, but experiments in rat bronchial epithelium suggest that the primary progenitor cell of airway epithelium might be the nonciliated columnar cell population (18). Currently, basal cells are believed to help in the adhesion of columnar cells to the basement membrane, and indeed, columnar cells do not have hemidesmosomes; rather, they attach to the basement membrane only by cell adhesion molecules (e.g., laminin).

Goblet Cells

The goblet cells are secretory cells that are named based on their unique profile in cross section. They arrange themselves perpendicular to the epithelial surface (19). The mucous granules give the mature cell its characteristic goblet shape, in which only a narrow part of the tapering basal cytoplasm touches the basement membrane. The nucleus is situated basally, with the organelles and secretory granules that contain mucin toward the lumen. The luminal surface, covered by microvilli, has a small opening, or stoma, through which the granules secrete their content. There are no goblet cells in the squamous, transitional, or olfactory epithelia of adults, and they are irregularly distributed but present in all areas of pseudostratified columnar epithelium (19).

Columnar Cells

The columnar cells are related to neighboring cells by tight junctions apically and, in the uppermost part, by interdigitations of the cell membrane. The cytoplasm contains numerous mitochondria in the apical part. Every columnar cell, whether ciliated or nonciliated, is covered by 300 to 400 microvilli, uniformly distributed over the entire apical surface. These are not precursors of cilia. Rather, they are short and slender fingerlike cytoplasmic expansions that increase the surface area of the epithelial cells, thus promoting exchange processes across the epithelium. The microvilli also prevent drying of the surface by retaining moisture essential for ciliary function (3). In man, ciliated epithelium lines the majority of the airway from the nose to the respiratory bronchioles, as well as the paranasal sinuses, the eustachian tube, and parts of the middle ear.

Inflammatory Cells

Different types of inflammatory cell have been described in the nasal epithelium obtained from normal, nonallergic subjects. Using immunohistochemical staining, Winther and colleagues identified consistent anti-HLA-DR staining in the upper portion of the nasal epithelium as well as occasional lymphocytes interspersed between the epithelial cells (20). There appeared to be more T (Leu 4$^+$) than B (Leu 14$^+$) lymphocytes and more T helper (Leu 3$^+$) than Leu 2$^+$ cells. The detection of HLA-DR antigens on the epithelium suggests that the airway epithelium may be potentially participating in antigen recognition and processing. Bradding and colleagues observed rare mast cells within the epithelial layer and no activated eosinophils (21).

The nasal epithelium functions as more than just a barrier, and epithelial cells have been shown to contribute actively to nasal inflammatory processes by expressing various adhesion molecules such as intercellular adhesion molecule 1 (ICAM-1) and secreting various cytokines and chemokines. Many of these functions are upregulated in allergic inflammation.

Ion and Water Transport

An important function of the epithelium is ion and water transport. Water movement across epithelia, including the epithelium of the submucosal glands, is thought to follow passively after active ion transport (mainly Na$^+$ and Cl$^-$) as well as through molecular water channels called aquaporins (AQPs). Active ion transport of Na$^+$ occurs via a sodium channel at the apical surface of the epithelium and by a Na$^+$/K$^+$ ATPase at the basolateral membrane. Chloride ion transport is primarily regulated by the cystic fibrosis transmembrane regulator (CFTR) protein, which is impaired in cystic fibrosis. In recent work, Wioland and colleagues used immunohistochemistry to determine the differential localization of CFTR transmembrane protein in respiratory epithelium and glands in samples of surgically resected inferior turbinates (22). CFTR was detected, though inconsistently, in ciliated nasal epithelial cells either on the apical surface or with an intracytoplasmic distribution. In contrast, detection was much more consistent in nasal glands occurring in all serous cells, with intense labeling of the apical membrane, on the apical surface of ciliated cells and inside the lumen of collecting ducts. No staining was detected in glandular mucous cells. As for the AQPs, Kreda and colleagues used in situ hybridization and immunofluorescence to examine the tissue distribution and cellular localization of AQP3, AQP4, and AQP5 in the nasal mucosa (23). Although other AQPs have been described, these researchers chose to investigate those that have been previously detected in lower airways epithelium. Robust AQP5 mRNA expression was detected in the nasal epithelium and the glands by means of in situ hybridization. The presence of this protein was further substantiated by using immunofluorescence, which showed strong signals at the apical membrane of all columnar cells facing the luminal surface of the superficial epithelium and also at the apical membranes of serous cells in all submucosal glandular acini. Strong expression of AQP3 was also detected in the superficial nasal epithelium and was localized to the plasma membrane of all basal cells. AQP3 was also seen in basal cells of some serous gland acini. AQP4 was not detected in nasal epithelia. In the lower airways, by contrast, all three AQPs have been detected in various distributions (23).

Basement Membrane

The epithelium of the nasal mucosa rests on a basement membrane that has not been extensively studied. Agha-Mir-Salim and colleagues, who obtained biopsy samples from the inferior turbinates of normal controls and of subjects with turbinate hypertrophy or immotile cilia syndrome, observed that the basement membrane was relatively thick, measuring 10 to 12 μm by light microscopy irrespective of disease or patient's age (24). The basement membrane that looked homogeneous under light microscopy had a two-layered arrangement when examined by electron microscopy. The layer closest to the basal side of the epithelial cells, termed the basal lamina, consisted of a lamina densa and a lamina rara, which was closest to the epithelial cell basal membrane. The lamina densa was followed, toward the connective tissue, by a thick layer that covered, except for the basal lamina, the entire width of the basement membrane as seen by light microscopy. This layer contains densely packed, irregularly running, isolated 25 nm collagenous fibrils and is often referred to as the lamina reticularis. Contents of the basal lamina (lamina densa and lamina rara) include collagen type IV, laminin, nidogen, and heparan sulfate proteoglycan, in the lamina reticularis were found collagen types I, III, V, and VI. To address the effects of allergy and asthma on basement membrane thickness, Chanez and colleagues obtained nasal and bronchial biopsy samples from 6 healthy controls, 15 subjects with untreated asthma and perennial allergic rhinitis, and 6 patients with severe corticosteroid-dependent asthma and perennial allergic rhinitis (25). The authors used light microscopy to examine sections stained by hematoxylin–eosin and measured the thickness of the basement membrane from the base of the epithelium to the outer limit of the reticular layer. The thickness of the membrane was not significantly different between the nose and the bronchi in normal controls, and median thickness was 5 μm in the nose and 6 μm in the lung. In contrast, the subjects with asthma (both untreated and corticosteroid dependent) had significantly thicker basement membranes in the lung than in the nasal mucosa. Of interest to this section of the chapter is that the basement membrane in the nasal mucosa of the asthmatics (who also had perennial allergic rhinitis) was significantly thicker than that of the normal controls. These data suggest that allergic rhinitis, like asthma, results in an increase in the thickness of the nasal basement membrane, albeit to a lesser extent than the increase caused by the asthmatic state in the basement membrane of the bronchial epithelium. In another study, Sanai and colleagues obtained inferior turbinates from 13 subjects with perennial allergic rhinitis and 13 nonallergic controls and examined the thickness of the basement membrane by light microscopy and the types of collagen in the membrane by means of immunohistochemical staining (26). They reported that the subepithelial basement membrane was significantly thicker in the allergic group (average 17.2 μm) than in the nonallergic controls (average 8.9 μm). There was strong immunoreactivity in the sub-epithelial region for types I and III collagen in the allergic turbinates but a weaker intensity of staining for the same types of collagen in the nonallergic specimens. Electron microscopy of the specimens suggested that the differences between the allergic and nonallergic specimens were concentrated in the region of the lamina reticularis of the basement membrane. Finally, Shaida and colleagues examined nasal mucosal biopsy samples from control and allergic subjects for mRNA and protein expression of metalloproteinases (MMPs) and tissue inhibitors of MMPs (TIMPs) (27). These endopeptidases and their tissue inhibitors are thought to be important in degrading various components of the basement membrane and thus might be important in remodeling of the membrane in health and disease. The investigators found only small amounts of MMP-1,-2, -3, and -9 mRNA with no significant differences between the groups. In contrast, TIMP-1 and -2 mRNA were found in higher levels in the nasal mucosa, and so were protein levels of the same, but there were also no significant differences between groups. This study thus demonstrates a potential role for the endopeptidases and their tissue inhibitors in the nasal mucosa, but research is required to further elucidate their exact role.

Nasal Submucosa

The nasal submucosa lies beneath the basement membrane and contains a host of cellular components in addition to nasal glands, nerves, and blood vessels. The striking difference from the submucosa of the lower airways is the absence of airway smooth muscle in the nose. In a light microscopy study of nasal biopsy samples from normal individuals, the predominant cell in the submucosa was the mononuclear cell, which includes lymphocytes and monocytes (28). Much less numerous were neutrophils and eosinophils (28). Mast cells were also found in appreciable numbers in the nasal submucosa, as identified by immunohistochemical staining with a monoclonal antibody against mast cell tryptase (21).

Winther and colleagues evaluated lymhocyte subsets in the nasal mucosa of normal subjects using immunohistochemistry (20). They found T (Leu 4[+]) lymphocytes to be the predominant cell type, with fewer scattered B (Leu 14[+]) cells. The ratio of T-helper (Leu 3[+]) cells to Leu 2[+] cells in the lamina propria averaged 3:1 in the subepithelial area and

2:1 in the deeper vascular stroma, with the overall ratio being 2.5:1, similar to the average ratio in peripheral blood. Natural killer cells were very rare, constituting less than 2% of the lymphocytes.

Recent interest in inflammatory cytokines prompted Bradding and colleagues to investigate cells containing four interleukins (IL-4, IL-5, IL-6, IL-8) in the nasal mucosa of patients with perennial rhinitis and normal subjects (21). The normal nasal mucosa was found to contain cells with positive IL-4 immunoreactivity, with 90% of these cells also staining positive for mast cell tryptase, suggesting that they were mast cells. Immunoreactivity for IL-5 and IL-6 was present in 75% of the normal nasal biopsy samples, and IL-8 positive cells were found in all the normal nasal tissue samples. A median 50% of IL-5$^+$ cells and 100% of the IL-6$^+$ cells were mast cells. In contrast to the other cytokines, IL-8 was largely confined to the cytoplasm of epithelial cells.

From the foregoing studies, it is clear that the normal nasal mucosa contains a host of inflammatory cells the role of which is unclear. In allergic rhinitis, most of these inflammatory cells increase in number (29), and eosinophils are also recruited into the nasal mucosa (21). Furthermore, cells positive for IL-4 increase significantly in patients with allergic rhinitis in comparison to normal subjects (21).

Nasal Glands

The anterior nasal, seromucous, and intraepithelial nasal glands are located in the submucosa and epithelium.

Anterior Nasal Glands

The anterior nasal glands are serous glands with ducts (2–20 mm in length) that open into small crypts located in the nasal vestibule. The ducts are lined by one layer of cuboidal epithelium. Bojsen-Mueller found 50 to 80 crypts anteriorly on the septum and another 50 to 80 anteriorly on the lateral nasal wall (30). He suggested that these glands play an important role in keeping the nose moist by spreading their serous secretions backward, thus moistening the entire mucosa. Tos, however, was able to find only 20 to 30 anterior nasal glands on the septum and an equal number on the lateral wall (19). He deduced that the contribution of these glands to the total production of secretions is minimal and that they represent a phylogenetic rudiment.

Seromucous Glands

The main duct of the seromucous glands is lined with simple cuboidal epithelium. It divides into two side ducts that collect secretions from several tubules lined either with serous or mucous cells. At the ends of the tubules are acini, which may similarly be serous or mucous. Submucosal serous glands predominate over mucinous glands by a ratio of about 8:1. The glands first laid down during development grow deep into the lamina propria before dividing and thus develop their mass in the deepest layers of the mucosa with relatively long ducts. The glands that develop later divide before growing down into the mucosa and thus form a more superficial mass with short ducts. Vessels, nerves, and fibers develop in between, giving rise to two glandular layers: superficial and deep. The mass of the deep glands is larger than that of the superficial ones, and the total number of these glands is approximately 90,000.

Intraepithelial Glands

As the name implies, the intraepithelial glands are located in the epithelium and consist of 20 to 50 mucous cells arranged radially around a small lumen. Many intraepithelial glands exist in nasal polyps. In comparison to sero-mucous glands, intraepithelial glands produce only a small amount of mucus and thus play a minor role in the physiology of nasal secretions.

B. Tracheal/Bronchial Airways

Although the cellular composition of the airways differs in the central and peripheral conducting airways, the basic structure of the airway wall is well preserved: its cross section comprises five discrete layers: epithelium, basement membrane, subepithelial layer, submucosa, and adventitia (4).

Epithelium

The epithelium from the trachea through the small bronchi is pseudostratified and columnar. Multiple cell types comprise the epithelium of the trachea and bronchi (Fig. 5). *Ciliated epithelial cells* are the most readily identifiable cells in cross sections through the conducting airway wall. These structural cells have about 200 cilia each that extend into the liquid phase on the epithelial surface where they beat approximately 1000 times a minute and play an essential role in clearance. *Goblet cells* comprise 20 to 30% of the epithelial cells in the large airways, becoming progressively rarer in smaller bronchi and all but absent in bronchioles. Goblet cells secrete mucus. Goblet cell hyperplasia/metaplasia and enhanced goblet cell secretion may contribute to the mucus plugging associated with asthma and COPD (31–35). *Serous cells* and *Clara cells* are the other secretory cells that line the epithelium. In most species (including humans), Clara cells are confined to the peripheral airways, where they are thought to secrete surfactant but may also play a role in lung defense (4,36). Serous cells may be precursor epithelial cells able to differentiate into any of several

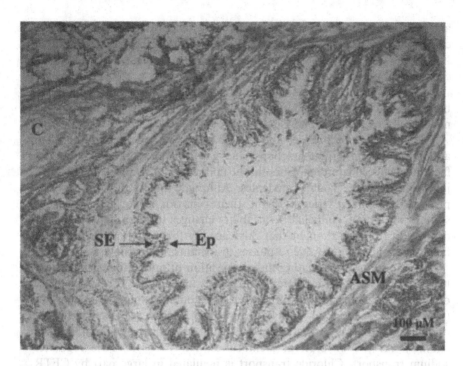

Figure 5 Cross section of a small intrapulmonary bronchi of a nonasthmatic human lung. Epithelium (Ep) is pseudostratified and columnar in structure. Epithelial cells are attached to the reticular basement membrane (not visible), below which lies the highly vascularized subepithelium (SE). The epithelium, basement membrane, and subepithelium comprise the airway mucosa, which as shown here has a characteristic folding apparent in cross section. Airway smooth muscle (ASM) envelops the bronchial wall in a spiraling structure. Airway smooth muscle and glands are found in the submucosa. Plaques of cartilage (C) are found in the adventitia of the airways, which also contains nerve bundles and vessels. (Slide kindly provided by Dr. Allen C. Myers, Johns Hopkins Asthma and Allergy Center, Baltimore.)

epithelial cell types (goblet cells, ciliated cells) during disease or following immunological or nonimmunological (toxic) insults (4). As in the nasal mucosa, *basal cells* were long thought to be epithelial precursor cells. This role for basal cells has been questioned recently, however, and it is unclear what if any homeostatic role basal cells play in the normal airway epithelium (37). It is also unclear what if any role *neuroendocrine cells* (also known as K cells) play in lung homeostasis (38). These excitable secretory cells are prevalent in fetal lungs but are sparse in the airways (both upper and lower) of adults. Neuroendocrine cells may cluster into groups of 10 to 30 cells to form neuroepithelial bodies (NEBs). Neuroendocrine cells in NEBs store and release a number of neurally active substances [serotonin, bombesin, calcitonin gene-related peptide (CGRP)]. Afferent nerve fibers terminate in NEBs and it has thus been suggested these structures may subserve a chemosensing role in the airways.

As mentioned, bronchiolar epithelial cells become nonciliated and cuboidal in structure. Clara cells far outnumber goblet cells in bronchioles, while mucus cells are rare or nonexistent.

Epithelial cells interact and interconnect with one another through adhering junctions, tight junctions, and gap junctions (4). Gap junctions facilitate cell–cell communication in the epithelium. The adhering and tight junctions form the zona occludentes. Although these structures serve to preserve epithelial barrier function, their behavior is not static. Various stimuli can initiate epithelial permeability changes through the zona occludentes (39,40). It is thought that this capacity for regulating permeability facilitates mucosal defensive responses to irritants and pathogens.

In addition to regulating the composition of mucus lining the airway lumen, epithelial cells regulate solute and water content of the sol phase of the airway lining fluid. Epithelial cells accomplish this by moving ions (primarily Na^+ and Cl^-) (41–44). Transport of sodium at the apical surface of the epithelium is regulated by the amiloride-sensitive sodium channel (ENaC). At the basolateral membranes, Na^+/K^+-ATPase regulates sodium transport. Chloride transport is regulated in large part by CFTR (cystic fibrosis transmembrane conductance regulator), a cAMP-regulated ion channel. Water moves either through the epithelium passively in response to solute gradients or through the water channels, or aquaporins. Aquaporin 3 (AQP3), AQP4, and AQP5 are expressed by tracheal and bronchial epithelial cells; bronchiolar epithelial cells and type II alveolar pneumocytes express only AQP3, while type I alveolar pneumocytes express only AQP5. Capillaries and fibroblasts of the airways and lungs express only AQP1. AQP4 and AQP5 are localized to airway glands (45).

The epithelium regulates immune cell trafficking by producing a variety of proinflammatory mediators, cytokines, and chemokines, either constitutively or upon challenge (46–49). Epithelial cells in the nose and lung also express a variety of cell adhesion molecules (ICAM-1, catenins, E-cadherins), which likely coordinate movement of inflammatory cells into the epithelium and in some instances into the airway lumen (50). Airway epithelial cells also express a wide variety of integrins, cell surface receptors comprising an α and a β subunit through which they interact with the basement membrane proteins (51).

The epithelium lining the lower airways is continually renewing itself (Fig. 6). This process can be dramatically accelerated following damage secondary to inflammation, infection or noxious insult (4,34,37,52).

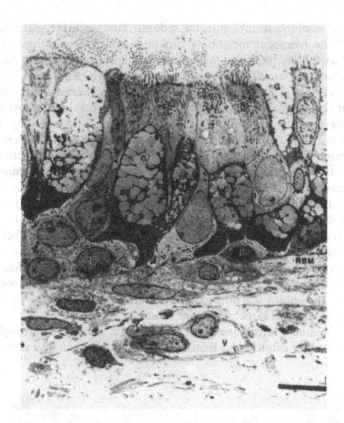

Figure 6 Electron micrograph showing the structure and cell types found in the mucosa of nonasthmatic human bronchi. Tracheal/bronchial epithelium is pseudo-stratified and columnar in structure. Cells typically found in the epithelium of the lower airways include ciliated epithelial cells (C), mucus-secreting goblet cells (G), and basal cells (B). Epithelial cells adhere to the matrix proteins of the reticular basement membrane (RBM). Below the basement membrane, the highly vascularized (V) subepithelium is the primary site of inflammatory cell recruitment in the airways and the primary location of mast cells in the airway wall. (Micrograph reproduced with permission from Ref. 31.)

Basement Membrane

The basement membrane is an acellular, extracellular matrix structure, only 200 nm thick in the healthy lung and thus not visible with conventional light microscopic techniques (4,9,34,52). Airway epithelial cells attach to the basement membrane, which, like all basement membranes throughout the body, is composed of proteins including type IV collagen, fibronectin (both soluble and insoluble forms), entactin, nidogen, laminin, proteoglycans, and tenascin. The basement membrane can be subdivided into three layers, arranged as follows luminally to serosally: lamina rara (or lamina lucida), lamina densa (or basal lamina), and lamina reticularis (Fig. 7).

Thickening of the basement membrane is a defining pathological feature of the asthmatic lung (4,52). This thickening may not be correlated to asthma severity or duration and is seemingly unaffected by most currently available therapeutic interventions including steroids. Thickening occurs primarily in the lamina reticularis and involves deposition of collagens types I, III, V, and VII, as well as glycoproteins, fibronectin, and tenascin. The characteristic thickening of the lamina reticularis has been called subepithelial fibrosis by some investigators (4,34,52,53).

The basement membrane plays an important role in regulating epithelial cell attachment and in regulating migratory cell movements between subepithelial vessels and the epithelium. The cellular source of the extracellular matrix proteins that make up the basement membrane has not been firmly established. It has been hypothesized, however, that myofibroblasts residing on the serosal side of the basement membrane may be the source of the thickened basement membrane in asthma (4,34,52,53).

The basement membrane undergoes constant remodeling through the formation of new extracellular matrix proteins and through degradation of

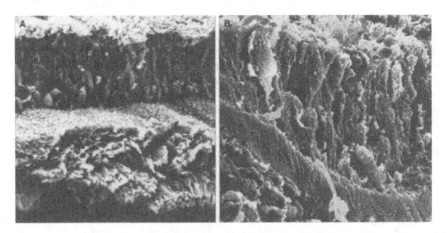

Figure 7 Electron micrographs showing the reticular basement membrane of the bronchial mucosa of (A) a nonasthmatic and (B) an asthmatic. Thickening of the basement membrane is a characteristic pathological finding in the airways of asthmatics but not patients with COPD. (Micrograph reproduced with permission from Ref. 52.)

existing proteins by matrix metalloproteinases (MMPs). The actions of MMPs are inhibited by locally released inhibitors, TIMPs (tissue inhibitors of matrix metalloproteinases). It has been suggested that thickening of the basement membrane in asthma is due to an imbalance in the formation of MMPs and TIMPs (54).

Subepithelium

The subepithelium lies below the basement membrane and can be distinguished from the basement membrane by the presence of an extensive vascular and capillary network. Deposition of fibrillar collagen fibers (type VII) and elastin fibers also defines the transition from basement membrane (lamina reticularis) to the subepithelium (4,9).

Inflammatory cells recruited to the airway mucosa (epithelium, basement membrane, and subepithelium) exit the postcapillary venules residing in the subepithelial compartment of the airway wall. The subepithelium is also a primary site for plasma exudation (again from postcapillary venules) and the primary location of resident mast cells in the airway wall.

Subepithelial blood flow is increased in asthma (52,55,56). Airway edema may also occur in the subepithelium of the airway mucosa. Sinusoid-like vessels are found in the subepithelium, and direct and indirect evidence indicates that vascular engorgement of subepithelial vessels may affect airways resistance to airflow. These vessels may become leaky in response to mediators (e.g., histamine, LTD4, thromboxanes) derived from mast cells and during axonal reflex-mediated neurogenic inflammation (mediated by neuropeptides; see later).

It has been suggested that vascular engorgement and edema in the subepithelium may be a primary cause of late phase airways obstruction in experimental allergen-induced asthma and may contribute to chronic airways obstruction (56). Available evidence indicates that such processes are unlikely to play a major role in the human lower airways (57,58). Thus, late phase airways obstruction can be rapidly reversed by intravenous β-adrenergic agonists (59). Edema is not amenable to such rapid reversal. Likewise, if vascular engorgement was mediating late phase airways obstruction, vasodilators such as β-adrenergic agonists would likely worsen airflow limitation (Fig. 8) (60).

Submucosa

Smooth Muscle

There has been much debate about the homeostatic role of airway smooth muscle. It has been argued that smooth muscle serves no role whatsoever in maintaining homeostasis in the mammalian lung, being merely a vestigial

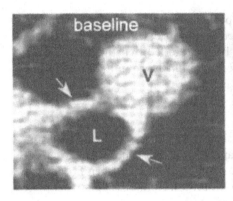 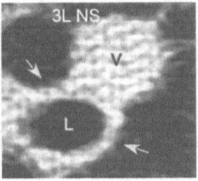

Figure 8 High resolution computed tomographic scan of the bronchi of a patient before (baseline) and after intravenous infusion of 3 L of normal saline (NS). Note the marked thickening of the airway wall, attributed to edema formation in the subepithelium. Also note that airway luminal diameter did not change considerably despite the pronounced edema. (Scan reproduced with permission from Ref. 60.)

feature of the lungs of amphibian species that do not respire passively through diaphragm contraction but, rather, move air into and out of their lungs through active, peristaltic smooth muscle contractions. Conversely, it has been argued that neural regulation of airway smooth muscle tone serves to optimize the work of breathing and optimizes airway clearance of particulate matter and secretions during coughing. Whatever its role, it is clear that the primary function of smooth muscle is to regulate airway caliber and length, and consequently smooth muscle is a primary structural determinant of airflow resistance (6,7,61–63).

Smooth muscle cells are not homogeneous. Subpopulations have been identified based on length, shortening capacity, and contractile protein expression. The relative proportion of these cell subtypes varies at different levels of the airway tree and may be altered during inflammation (64). The amount of smooth muscle in any given airway can also be altered, particularly in asthma (Fig. 9). With inflammation, smooth muscle hyperplasia is often noted. This may be precipitated by the mechanical stress put on the lung but may also be initiated by stimuli such as epidermal growth factor, insulin-like growth factor, platelet-derived growth factor, fibroblast growth factor, thrombin, tryptase, endothelins, neurokinins, and various eicosanoids (52,65).

Smooth muscle contraction is facilitated in part by electromechanical coupling of smooth muscle through structures such as gap junctions. The amount of electrical coupling of smooth muscle is limited, however, and thus coordination of smooth muscle contraction and relaxation must be

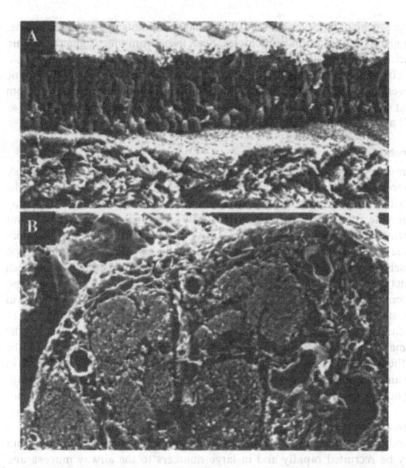

Figure 9 Electron micrographs of (A) the mucosa of a nonasthmatic and (B) the mucosa and submucosa of the bronchi from a patient who had died of asthma. Smooth muscle mass is greatly increased in asthma, and vascular engorgement and increased blood flow are characteristic of the asthmatic airway. Also note thickening of the basement membrane and the loss of covering epithelium in fatal asthma. See text for further details. (Micrographs reproduced with permission from Ref. 52.)

regulated extracellularly, likely through the coordinated actions of autonomic nerves (64,66).

Glands

Mucus glands of the lower airways are anatomically and physio- logically similar to the seromucous glands of the upper airways (67). Mucus cells outnumber serous cells in the glands of the lower airways. Mucus glands are most prevalent in larger airways, particularly at points of airway branching. No glands are found in bronchioles. Secretions from mucus glands contain mucins but may also contain lactoferrin, lysozyme, albumin, and IgA. Mucus gland secretion is regulated primarily by airway parasympathetic nerves but may also be initiated by inflammatory mediators derived from mast cells, basophils, and eosinophils (histamine, cysteinyl-leukotrienes), as well as elastase derived from neutrophils (4,67–69).

Lymphoid Tissue

Immune cells including mast cells, lymphocytes (both T and B cells), monocytes, macrophages, and dendritic cells are found throughout the airways and throughout the airway wall (4,34,52). Immune cells may aggregate in the airway wall, particularly at branch points in the lower airways, to form structures known as BALT (bronchus-associated lymphoid tissue) (70). These structures are not actually associated with the lymph vessels but are found in the subepithelium with a distinguishing epithelial cell structure above. Lymph nodes are localized primarily in the submucosa and adventitia of the extrapulmonary airways. Mast cells are found primarily in the subepithelium and occasionally in the submucosa. The number of submucosal mast cells may increase in asthma (71). Dendritic cells, the primary antigen-presenting cells of the airways, are associated with the epithelium (72). Monocytes, macrophages, and lymphocytes are found in the airway wall as well as in the airway spaces. CD8$^+$ T cells predominate in the normal airways (4,34,52). In asthma, however, TH2-like CD4$^+$ lymphocytes are more prominent (73). Plasma cells, thought to be IgA-secreting cells, can be localized to glands. Eosinophils, neutrophils, and basophils are found sparingly in the airway wall and in airway spaces of healthy lungs but may be recruited rapidly and in large numbers to the airway mucosa and adventitia and to air spaces upon inflammatory challenge (74).

III. Vascular and Lymphatic Supplies

A. Nasal Airways

The nose receives its blood supply from both the internal and external carotid circulations via the ophthalmic and internal maxillary arteries, respectively (Fig. 10). The ophthalmic artery gives rise to the anterior and posterior ethmoid arteries, which supply the anterosuperior portion of the septum, the lateral nasal walls, the olfactory region, and a small part of the posterosuperior region. The external carotid artery gives rise to the internal maxillary artery, which ends as the sphenopalatine artery. This enters the nasal cavity through the sphenopalatine foramen behind the posterior end

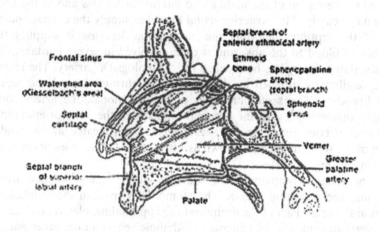

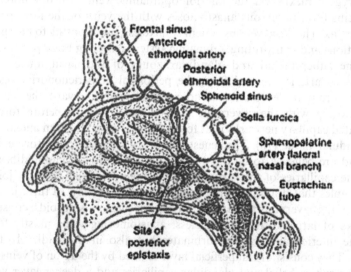

Figure 10 Nasal blood supply. The top panel represents the supply to the nasal septum and the bottom panel, that to the lateral nasal wall. (From Cummings CW, Fredrickson JM, Harker LA et al. Otolaryngology-Head and Neck Surgery. Vol. 1. St. Louis: CV Mosby, 1986.)

of the middle turbinate. The sphenopalatine artery gives origin to a number of posterior lateral and septal nasal branches. The posterolateral branches proceed to the region of the middle and inferior turbinates and to the floor of the nasal cavity. The posterior septal branches supply the corresponding area of the septum, including the nasal floor. Because it supplies the majority of blood to the nose and is often involved in severe epistaxis, the sphenopalatine artery has been called the "rhinologist's" artery. The region of the vestibule is supplied by the facial artery through lateral and septal nasal branches. The septal branches of the sphenopalatine artery form multiple anastomoses with the terminal branches of the anterior ethmoidal and facial arteries giving rise to Kiesselbach's area, located at the caudal aspect of the septum and also known as Little's area. Most cases of epistaxis occur in this region (75).

The veins accompanying the branches of the sphenopalatine artery drain into the pterygoid plexus. The ethmoidal veins join the ophthalmic plexus in the orbit. Part of the drainage to the ophthalmic plexus proceeds to the cavernous sinus via the superior ophthalmic veins and the other part to the pterygoid plexus via the inferior ophthalmic veins. Furthermore, the nasal veins form numerous anastomoses with the veins of the face, palate, and pharynx. The nasal venous system is valveless, predisposing to the spread of infections and constituting a dynamic system reflecting body position.

The subepithelial and glandular zones of the nasal mucosa are supplied by arteries derived from the periosteal or perichondrial vessels. Branches from these vessels ascend perpendicularly toward the surface, anastomosing with the cavernous plexi (venous system) before forming fenestrated capillary networks next to the respiratory epithelium and around the glandular tissue (76). The fenestrae always face the respiratory epithelium and are believed to be one of the sources of fluid for humidification (77). The capillaries of the subepithelial and periglandular network join to form venules that drain into larger superficial veins. They, in turn, join the sinuses of the cavernous plexus. The cavernous plexi, or sinusoids, consist of networks of large, tortuous, valveless, anastomosing veins mostly found over the inferior and middle turbinates but also in the midlevel of the septum. They consist of a superficial layer formed by the union of veins that drain the subepithelial and glandular capillaries and a deeper layer where the sinuses acquire thicker walls and assume a course parallel to the periosteum or perichondrium. They receive venous blood from the subepithelial and glandular capillaries and arterial blood from arteriovenous anastomoses. The arterial segments of the anastomoses are surrounded by a longitudinal smooth muscle layer that controls their blood flow. When the muscular layer contracts, the artery occludes; when it relaxes, the anastomosis opens, allowing the sinuses to fill rapidly with blood. Because of this function, the sinusoids are physiologically referred to as capacitance vessels. Only endothelium interposes between the longitudinal muscles and the bloodstream, making them sensitive to circulating agents. The cavernous plexi change their blood volume in response to neural, mechanical, thermal, psychological, or chemical stimulation. They expand and shrink, altering the caliber of the air passages and, consequently, the speed and volume of airflow. This alteration of the caliber of the nasal passages results in changes in airflow resulting in changes in the subjective feeling of nasal congestion, which is often mirrored by objective changes of nasal patency as measured by various tools such as nasal peak inspiratory flow, anterior rhinometry, posterior rhinometry, or acoustic rhinometry.

Lymphatic vessels from the nasal vestibule drain toward the external nose, whereas the nasal fossa drains posteriorly. The first-order lymph nodes for posterior drainage are the lateral retropharyngeal nodes, whereas the subdigastric nodes serve that function for anterior drainage.

B. Tracheal/Bronchial Vasculature

Blood supply to the lower airways and lungs comprises a bronchial and a pulmonary vasculature (4). The bronchial vessels originate in the aorta and intercostal arteries and provide blood supply to the airways from the trachea to the terminal bronchioles. Blood entering the bronchial circulation empties primarily in postcapillary vessels of the pulmonary vasculature (78). In the airways, the bronchial vasculature forms an intricate arbor that includes an extensive subepithelial plexus and an adventitial plexus comprising of larger arterioles and venules. The vasculature of the subepithelial plexus has an extensive capillary network and forms sinusoid-like vessels that drain into venules that connect the subepithelial and adventitial plexus. Blood flow through the mucosal and adventitial plexus is roughly equal, favoring slightly (60 vs 40%) the mucosal plexus (79). This may be altered by altering bronchial vascular pressure. Both sympathetic and parasympathetic nerves innervate the arterioles of the bronchial circulation (80).

Inflammation and infection can dramatically alter the structure of the airway vasculature and may alter mucosal blood flow (Fig. 11). The mechanisms by which these changes occur in disease are poorly understood (81).

The pulmonary vasculature originates in the right ventricle of the heart, forming the pulmonary artery. The pulmonary artery branches to provide venous blood to the right and left lungs. Pulmonary arterioles empty into an alveolar capillary plexus from which the blood flows into venules and veins. Pulmonary veins converge to return oxygenated blood to the left atria.

Lymphatics are also found in the lower airways and lungs where they may play an important role in resolution of airway and pulmonary edema.

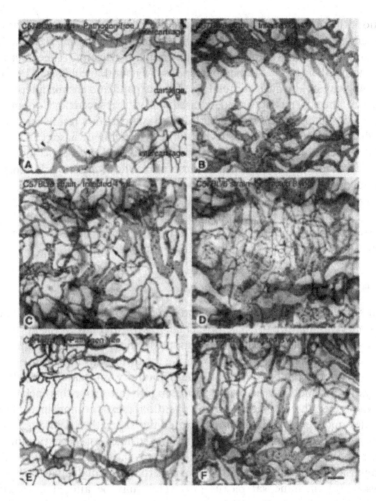

Figure 11 Tracheal vasculature in *Mycoplasma pulmonis*–infected C57BL/6 and C3H mice visualized in whole mounts. (A) Mucosal vasculature in trachea of pathogen-free C57BL/6 mouse, with capillaries crossing a cartilaginous ring, fed from arterioles (arrows) and drained by venules (arrowheads) in intercartilaginous regions. (B) Enlarged vessels in trachea of C57BL/6 mouse 2 weeks after infection. (C) Enlarged vessels and regions with increased numbers of capillaries (arrow) in trachea of C57BL/6 mouse 4 weeks after infection. (D) Numerous capillary-sized vessels and enlarged vessels in trachea of C57BL/6 mouse at 8 weeks after infection. (E) Tracheal vasculature of pathogen-free C3H mouse. (F) Enlarged vessels in trachea of C3H mouse at 8 weeks after infection. All segments of the vasculature appear enlarged. Comparable alterations in airway vasculature are thought to occur in asthma (52). Scale bars: 100 μm. (Reproduced with permission from Ref. 81.)

Not all airways have a lymphatic vasculature, however, and it is clear that edema clearance occurs primarily through vascular reabsorption. Lymphatic vasculature may, however, be altered with disease and may thus play a more prominent role during inflammation or infection (82–85).

A rich vascular supply characterizes both the nasal and the lower airways. The proximity of these vessels to nasal and bronchial end organs probably contributes to a strong interface between circulating cells and substances and these respective end organs. This interaction is even more pronounced in inflammatory states such as allergic rhinitis and asthma during which upregulation of vascular endothelial adhesion molecules has been documented in both the nose and the lung. A significant difference between the upper and the lower airways, however, lies in control of airway lumina. Whereas changes in the blood volume of the cavernous plexi is a major factor in controlling the caliber of the nasal airway and affecting nasal congestion, the same does not apply to the lower airway, where the larger contribution to the control of bronchial diameter is influenced by smooth muscles.

IV. Neural Supply to the Airways

The nervous system plays an essential role in regulating respiration. Airway nerves also play an important defensive role in preserving lung capacity for gas exchange and in facilitating clearance of inhaled pathogens and irritants. Central terminations of upper and lower airway sensory nerves are localized to discrete regions in the brain stem. The proximity of these termination sites to one another facilitates coordination of respiratory reflexes. This coordination is made possible by many projections between the nuclei regulating nasal reflexes (e.g., trigeminal nucleus) and those regulating pulmonary reflexes (e.g., nucleus tractus solitarius). However, these interactions may also facilitate transmission of inappropriate signals between the upper and lower airways in disease. Autonomic regulation of effector tissues is essentially identical in the upper and lower airways.

A. Nasal Airways

The nasal neural supply is overwhelmingly sensory and autonomic (sympathetic, parasympathetic, and nonadrenergic noncholinergic) (Fig. 12). The sensory nasal innervation comes via both the ophthalmic and maxillary divisions of the trigeminal nerve and supplies the septum, the lateral walls, the anterior part of the nasal floor, and the inferior meatus. The structure of afferent nerve endings in the nasal mucosa is poorly described. The parasympathetic nasal fibers travel from their origin in the superior salivary

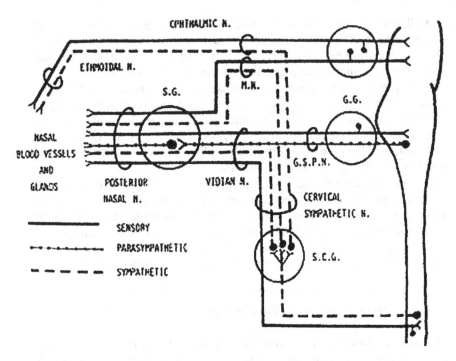

Figure 12 Sensory, sympathetic, and parasympathetic nasal neural supply: SG, sphenopalatine ganglion; MN, maxillary nerve; GG, geniculate ganglion; GSPN, greater superficial petrosal nerve; SCG, superior cervical ganglion. (From Proctor DF, Andersen IB. The Nose—Upper Airway Physiology and the Atmospheric Environment. Amsterdam: Elsevier Biomedical Press, 1982.)

nucleus of the midbrain via the nervus intermedius of the facial nerve to the geniculate ganglion, where they join the greater superficial petrosal nerve which, in turn, joins the deep petrosal nerve to form the vidian nerve. This nerve travels to the sphenopalatine ganglion where the preganglionic parasympathetic fibers synapse and postganglionic fibers supply the nasal mucosa. The sympathetic input originates as preganglionic fibers in the thoracolumbar region of the spinal cord, which pass into the vagosympathetic trunk and relay in the superior cervical ganglion. The postganglionic fibers end as the deep petrosal nerve, which joins the greater superficial nerve to form the vidian nerve. They traverse the sphenopalatine ganglion without synapsing and are distributed to the nasal mucosa.

Nasal glands receive direct parasympathetic nerve supply, and electrical stimulation of parasympathetic nerves in animals induces glandular secretions that are blocked by atropine. Furthermore, stimulation of the human nasal mucosa with methacholine, a cholinomimetic, produces an atropine-sensitive increase in nasal secretions (86). Parasympathetic nerves also provide innervation to the nasal vasculature, and stimulation of these fibers causes vasodilatation. Sympathetic fibers supply the nasal vasculature but do not establish a close relationship with nasal glands, and their exact role in the control of nasal secretions is not clear. Stimulation of these fibers in cats causes vasoconstriction and a decrease in nasal airway resistance. Adrenergic agonists are commonly used in man, both topically and orally, to decrease nasal congestion.

The presence of sympathetic and parasympathetic nerves and their transmitters in the nasal mucosa has been known for decades, but immunohistochemical studies have also established the presence of additional neuropeptides. These are secreted by unmyelinated nociceptive C fibers [tachykinins, calcitonin gene-related peptide (CGRP), neurokinin A (NKA), gastrin-releasing peptide], parasympathetic nerve endings [vasoactive intestinal peptide (VIP), peptide histidine methionine), and sympathetic nerve endings (neuropeptide Y). Substance P (SP), a member of the tachykinin family, is often found as a cotransmitter with NKA and CGRP and has been found in high density in arterial vessels, and to some extent in veins, gland acini, and epithelium of the nasal mucosa (87). SP receptors (NK1 receptors) are located in epithelium, glands, and vessels (87). CGRP receptors are found in high concentration on small muscular arteries and arterioles in the nasal mucosa (88). The distribution of VIP fibers in human airways corresponds closely to that of cholinergic nerves (89). In the human nasal mucosa, VIP is abundant, and its receptors are located on arterial vessels, submucosal glands, and epithelial cells (90).

B. Tracheal/Bronchial Airways

Extrinsic Innervation of the Lower Airways

The lower airways and lungs are innervated bilaterally by the vagus nerves. The majority of vagal fibers projecting to the airways are afferent (or sensory). The remaining vagal nerve fibers projecting to the airways are preganglionic parasympathetic nerve fibers innervating parasympathetic ganglia, and motor nerve fibers innervating the striated muscle of the larynx and upper airways (91).

Vagal afferent nerve fibers terminate centrally in integrative centers in the brain stem, primarily the nucleus tractus solitarius (nTS). The parasympathetic nerves and the vagal laryngeal motor nerve fibers arise from discrete brain stem nuclei, including the dorsal motor nucleus of the vagus nerve (dmnX) and the nucleus ambiguus (nA). Although these brain stem structures have viscerotopic organization, considerable overlap among the sites of afferent nerve subtype termination and of efferent projection is apparent. This overlap accounts in part for the clustering of autonomic reflexes (e.g., effects on heart rate, respiratory pattern, airway caliber) initiated by selective activation of specific afferent nerve subtypes. Moreover, the convergence of afferent nerves innervating multiple organs in nTS may facilitate organ–organ interactions, including interactions between the upper and lower airways (92,93).

Postganglionic sympathetic nerves projecting to the airways arise bilaterally, primarily from the superior cervical and thoracic sympathetic ganglia. Although there is evidence for spinal afferent innervation of the lung, its function is poorly understood. The superior laryngeal nerves, recurrent laryngeal nerves, and the bronchial branches of the vagus nerves carry the vagal and spinal nerve fibers projecting to the airways. Both afferent and efferent vagal nerves project bilaterally, although ipsilateral innervation is far more extensive (91–93).

Intrinsic Innervation of the Lower Airways

Afferent and efferent nerve fibers occupy multiple nerve plexuses in the lower airway wall from the larynx to the terminal bronchioles (94). Afferent nerve fibers surround epithelial cells in an epithelial nerve plexus. Efferent innervation of the epithelium has also been described. Both afferent and efferent nerves are found in the plexus below the basement membrane (subepithelium, submucosa), where most effectors of the airways (airway smooth muscle, mucus glands, arterioles) are located. Airway parasympathetic ganglia are localized primarily to an adventitial nerve plexus of the extrapulmonary airways, which merges with the submucosal plexus in the intrapulmonary airways (Fig. 13). Parasympathetic ganglia containing as few as one neuron to over 100 neurons are randomly and sparsely dispersed in the adventitial nerve plexus and are associated primarily with the extrapulmonary airways.

Except for afferent nerve endings terminating in neuroepithelial bodies of the epithelium (38), airway afferent nerves form apparently nonspecialized (based on appearance) receptive fields in the epithelium and basement membrane, and in and around various structures of the airway wall (96). Swellings associated with airway afferent nerve terminals in the epithelium contain synaptic vesicles with neurotransmitters that may be released during axonal reflexes. Afferent nerve fibers may also innervate other effector tissues in the airway wall, including glands, airway smooth muscle, blood vessels, and airway parasympathetic ganglia (94).

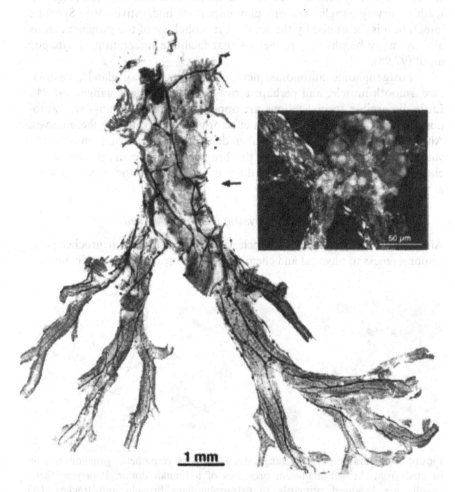

Figure 13 Montage revealing the adventitial nerve plexus innervating the trachea, bronchi, and bronchioles of human fetal lung (week 18 of gestation). Ganglia (inset shows higher powered magnification of a single ganglion) appear as swelling along the nerve trunks (stained black), particularly at nerve branches, and are more numerous in the plexus associated with the larger airways. (Figure reproduced with permission from Ref. 95.)

Airway ganglia neurons do not simply relay information between the central nervous system and the effector tissues of the airway wall (Fig. 14). Rather, airway ganglia neurons play important integrative roles. Synaptic integration is facilitated by the complex morphology of the ganglia neurons and by many biophysical properties that facilitate integration of synaptic input (97,98).

Postganglionic autonomic nerves innervate airway glands, vasculature, smooth muscle, and perhaps airway parasympathetic ganglia (91,94). Little discernible specializations are apparent on the postganglionic autonomic nerves of the airways or on effector cells innervated by these nerves. Although little change in nerve fiber densities in the smooth muscle and vasculature from the trachea to the bronchioles is apparent, the neurochemistry of the nerve fibers may differ considerably in the large and small airways (91,99,100).

Afferent Nerve Subtypes Innervating the Lower Airways

Airway afferent nerves can be subclassified based on their neurochemistry, responsiveness to physical and chemical stimuli, myelination, conduction ve-

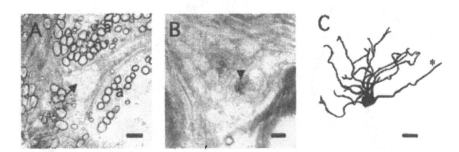

Figure 14 Parasympathetic ganglion and a parasympathetic ganglion neuron isolated from the left mainstem bronchus of a human donor. Parasympathetic ganglia are localized primarily to extrapulmonary bronchi and trachea. (A) Containing as few as 1 to as many as 100 neurons, ganglia are found primarily in an adventitial nerve plexus. (B) Nerve cell bodies are grouped tightly in clusters and receive synaptic input from vagal preganglionic parasympathetic nerves, from collateral axon branches from afferent nerves, and from adjacent parasympathetic ganglia. (C) Camera lucida drawing of a neuron impaled on a microelectrode and filled with neurobiotin for visualization. The complex dendritic arbor of these neurons suggests their important role in integrating synaptic input, a property confirmed in electrophysiological studies of these neurons isolated from human airways. Bars: 100 μm in (A) and 20 μm (B) and (C). (Figure reproduced with permission from Ref. 98.)

locity, sites of termination in the central nervous system, and ganglionic origin. Airway mechanoreceptors respond to the dynamic and/or sustained physical effects of lung inflation. Some mechanoreceptors can also be activated indirectly by bronchoconstrictors such as histamine, acetylcholine, and leukotrienes. When activated, airway mechanoreceptors initiate alterations in autonomic nerve activity and cough, and play an essential role in controlling respiratory rate and tidal volume. Not surprisingly, airway mechanoreceptors are sporadically active during the respiratory cycle. The continuous activation of airway mechanoreceptors may be of fundamental importance to the maintenance of baseline autonomic tone, and respiratory pattern, and it may influence evoked reflexes (91,101).

Afferent nerves that are similar to the nociceptors of the somatic nervous system also innervate the airways. Most airway nociceptors are unmyelinated C fibers and are generally unresponsive to mechanical stimuli and are thus essentially quiescent during tidal breathing (94,102–104). Airway nociceptors are activated by inflammatory mediators such as bradykinin and 5-HT, but may also be activated by low pH, hypertonic saline, or the vanilloid capsaicin. Other endogenous activators of airway nociceptors include 12- and 15-lipoxygenase products and anandamide (105–107). When activated, airway nociceptors may also initiate alterations in autonomic nerve activity and cough, perhaps with unique effects on respiratory pattern.

Nociceptive afferent nerves innervating the airway mucosa of most species including humans express the anatomical attributes of the sensory nerves mediating axon reflexes described in somatic tissues (92,94,96,103, 108). Many of these afferent nerve endings contain potent, proinflammatory peptides such as substance P, neurokinin A, and CGRP. When administered exogenously, these putative neurotransmitters have profound effects in the airways, initiating bronchospasm, mucus secretion, vasodilatation, plasma exudation, and inflammatory cell recruitment. These observations led to the intriguing hypothesis that axonal reflexes contribute to the pathogenesis of inflammatory airways disease. Many studies provide clear evidence for axonal reflexes in the lower airways of some animals (rats and guinea pigs) and compelling albeit circumstantial evidence for axonal reflexes in the human upper airways. The role of axon reflexes in the lower airways of humans is less clear (93,94,108).

Autonomic (Efferent) Nerve Subtypes Innervating the Lower Airways

The sympathetic and parasympathetic nervous systems innervate the airways (Fig. 15). Sympathetic nerves primarily innervate the bronchial vasculature, while airway parasympathetic nerves innervate the vasculature but also the glands, and of course the airway smooth muscle (80,91). In

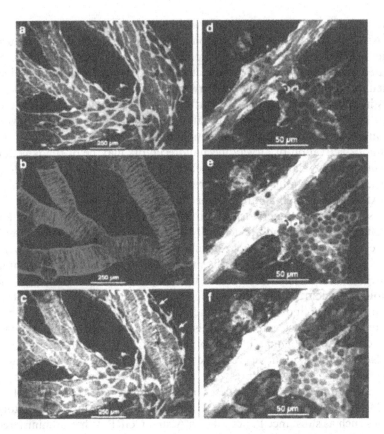

Figure 15 Innervation of airway smooth muscle in fetal human lung (day 58 of gestation) revealed through immunohistochemistry and confocal microscopy. In panel a, nerves are stained for the panneuronal marker protein gene product 9.5 (PGP 9.5). Airway smooth muscle is stained in panel b using an antibody to α-actin. Images in a and b are transposed onto one another in panel c. Parasympathetic ganglia appear as swellings in the neuronal plexus. Note the location of this nerve plexus in the adventitia of the intrapulmonary airways. These figures illustrate the complex and extensive neuronal innervation of the intrapulmonary airways. Postganglionic autonomic nerves (both sympathetic and parasympathetic), not visible at this low magnification, project from ganglia to innervate virtually every cell in the submucosa and many cells in the mucosa of the trachea and bronchi. Panels d–f show optical sections through a large nerve trunk and adjacent ganglia. Tissues are stained for Schwann cells and nerves. Schwann cells provide myelination, support, and excess neurotransmitter uptake to large extrinsic nerve fibers and ganglia. (Figure reproduced in black and white with permission from Ref. 95.)

addition to acetylcholine in parasympathetic nerves and norepinephrine in sympathetic nerves, a wide variety of nonadrenergic, noncholinergic neurotransmitters have been localized to autonomic nerve endings innervating the airways (Table 1). These neurotransmitters have multiple effects on the end organs in the airways, and their role as bona fide neurotransmitters and/or neuromodulators has been confirmed in many instances (109).

Postganglionic parasympathetic nerves innervate airway smooth muscle, mucus glands, and vessels throughout the airway tree. When activated, airway parasympathetic–cholinergic nerves initiate contractions of airway smooth muscle, mucus secretion, and vasodilatation. Sympathetic innervation of human airway smooth muscle is either sparse or nonexistent (109). Thus, even though human airway smooth muscle expresses abundant β-adrenoceptors (primarily β₂-adrenoceptors), direct functional evidence of sympathetic (adrenergic) innervation of human airway smooth muscle is lacking. Hormonal catecholamines are likely the primary endogenous ligand for the α-adrenoceptors expressed on human airway smooth muscle. Sympathetic nerves appear to play little or no role in regulating mucus secretion, either. Sympathetic nerves do, however, innervate the airway vasculature, mediating vasoconstriction.

Table 1 Effects of Various Neurotransmitters Synthesized by Airway Nerves

Neurotransmitters	Airway smooth muscle	Vasculature	Mucus glands	Leukocyte adhesion?	Plasma extravasation?
Acetylcholine	Constriction	Dilatation	Secretion	No	No
Norepinephrine	Dilatation	Constriction	?	No	Inhibition
Substance P	Constriction	Dilatation	Secretion	Yes	Yes
Neurokinin A	Constriction	Dilatation	Secretion	Yes	Yes
Neuropeptide Y	No effect	Constriction	?	?	Inhibition
VIP[a]	Dilatation	Dilatation	Secretion	?	?
Nitric Oxide[b]	Dilatation	Dilatation	?	Inhibition	Yes
CGRP[c]	Dilatation	Dilatation	?	?	No
Carbon Monoxide[d]	Dilatation	Dilatation	?	?	?
Neuromodulators					
Galanin					
Nociceptin					
γ Aminobutyric acid					
Met-enkephalin-Arg⁶-Gly⁷-Leu⁸					

[a] Vasoactive intestinal peptide and related peptides (e.g., PHI, PHM, PACAP).
[b] Synthesized from arginine by nitric oxide synthase.
[c] Calcitonin gene-related peptide.
[d] Synthesized from heme by heme oxygenase-2.

Noncholinergic parasympathetic nerves are the only functional relaxant nerves innervating the human lower airways (109). The neurotransmitters associated with noncholinergic parasympathetic nerves include the peptides VIP, PACAP, and PHI (or PHM), as well as the gaseous transmitter nitric oxide (NO, synthesized from arginine by the neuronal isoform of NO synthase). Nonadrenergic, noncholinergic parasympathetic relaxations of airway smooth muscle can be evoked in airways from the trachea to the small bronchi (99,109). Noncholinergic parasympathetic nerves also likely mediate mucus secretion and vasodilatation.

Studies in animals provide conclusive evidence that noncholinergic parasympathetic neurotransmitters are not coreleased with acetylcholine from postganglionic parasympathetic nerves. Rather, an entirely distinct parasympathetic pathway regulates noncholinergic nerve activity in the airways (109). Reflexes also differentially regulate cholinergic and non-cholinergic parasympathetic responses (110). Circumstantial evidence indicates a similar arrangement of the parasympathetic innervation of human airways. Recent studies suggest that noncholinergic parasympathetic nerves may be dysfunctional and/or dysregulated in asthma (109,111–113).

Reflexes initiating alterations in airway sympathetic nerve activity are poorly described. Adrenoceptors and thus the endogenous catecholamines do, however, play an important role in regulating airway caliber and airway responsiveness. It seems likely that in humans the hormonal catecholamines are more important in regulating airway function than the sparse sympathetic–adrenergic innervation of the airways.

V. Mucociliary Transport

A. Nasal Airways

A layer of mucus 10 to 15 μm deep covers the entire nasal cavity (114). It is slightly acidic, with a pH between 5.5 and 6.5. The mucous blanket consists of two layers: a thin, low viscosity, periciliary layer (sol phase) that envelops the shafts of the cilia, and a thick, more viscous layer (gel phase) riding on the periciliary layer. The gel phase can also be envisioned as discontinuous plaques of mucus. The distal tips of the ciliary shafts contact these plaques when they are fully extended. Insoluble particles caught on the mucous plaques move with them as a consequence of ciliary beating. Soluble materials like droplets, formaldehyde, and CO_2 dissolve in the periciliary layer. Thus nasal mucus effectively filters and removes nearly 100% of particles greater than 4 μm in diameter (115–117). An estimated 1 to 2 L of nasal mucus, composed of 2.5 to 3% glycoproteins, 1 to 2% salts, and 95% water, is produced per day. Mucin, one of the glycoproteins, gives mucus its unique attributes of protection and lubrication of mucosal surfaces.

The sources of nasal secretions are multiple and include anterior nasal glands, seromucous submucosal glands, epithelial secretory cells (of both mucous and serous types), tears, and transudation from blood vessels. Transudation increases in pathological conditions as a result of the effects of inflammatory mediators that increase vascular permeability. A good example is the increased vascular permeability seen in response to allergen challenge of subjects with allergic rhinitis as measured by increasing levels of albumin in nasal lavages after provocation (118). In contrast to serum, immunoglobulins make up the bulk of the protein in mucus; other substances in nasal secretions include lactoferrin, lysozyme, antitrypsin, transferrin, lipids, histamine and other mediators, cytokines, antioxidants, ions (Cl^-, Na^+, Ca^{2+}, K^+), cells, and bacteria.

Mucus functions in mucociliary transport, and substances will not be cleared from the nose without it, despite adequate ciliary function. Furthermore, mucus provides immune and mechanical mucosal protection, and its high water content plays a significant role in humidifying inspired air.

Mucociliary transport is unidirectional based on the unique characteristics of cilia. Cilia in mammals beat in a biphasic, or to-and-fro, manner. The beat consists of a rapid effective stroke during which the cilium straightens, bringing it in contact with the gel phase of the mucus, and a slow recovery phase during which the bent cilium returns in the periciliary or sol layer of the mucus, thus propelling it in one direction (Fig. 16).

Metachrony is the coordination of the beat of individual cilia, which prevents collision between cilia in different phases of motion and results in the unidirectional flow of mucus. Ciliary beating produces a current in the

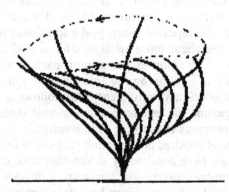

Figure 16 Schematic diagram of motion of a single cilium during the rapid forward beat and the slower recovery phase. (From Proctor DF, Andersen IB. The Nose—Upper Airway Physiology and the Atmospheric Environment. Amsterdam: Elsevier Biomedical Press, 1982.)

superficial layer of the periciliary fluid in the direction of the effective stroke. The mucous plaques move as a result of motion of the periciliary fluid layer and the movement of the extended tips of the cilia into the plaques. Thus, the depth of the periciliary fluid is the key factor in mucociliary transport. If excessive, the extended ciliary tips fail to contact mucous plaques, and the current of the periciliary fluid provides the only means of movement.

Mucociliary transport moves mucus and its contents toward the nasopharynx, except for the anterior portion of the inferior turbinates, where transport is anterior. This anterior current prevents many of the particles deposited in this area from progressing further into the nasal cavity. The particles transported posteriorly toward the nasopharynx are periodically swallowed. Mucociliary transport, however, is not the only mechanism by which particles and secretions are cleared from the nose. Sniffing and nose blowing help in moving airway secretions backward and forward, respectively. Sneezing results in a burst of air, accompanied by an increase in watery nasal secretions that are then cleared by nose blowing and sniffing.

Respiratory cilia beat about 1000 times a minute, which translates to surface materials being moved at a rate of 3 to 25 mm/min. Both the beat rate and propelling speed vary. Several substances have been used to measure nasal mucociliary clearance, and the most utilized are sodium saccharin, dyes, or tagged particles. The dye and saccharin methods are similar, consisting of placing a strong dye or saccharin sodium on the nasal mucosa just behind the internal ostium and recording the time it takes to reach the pharyngeal cavity; this interval is termed nasal mucociliary transport time. With saccharin, the time is recorded when the subject reports a sweet taste, whereas a dye appearance in the pharyngeal cavity triggers recording. Combining the two methods reduces the disadvantages of both—namely, variable taste thresholds in different subjects when saccharin is used and the repeated pharyngeal inspections needed to observe the dye— and makes them more reliable. The use of tagged particles involves placement of an anion exchange resin particle about 0.5 mm in diameter tagged with a ^{99}Tc ion on the anterior nasal mucosa, behind the area of anterior mucociliary movement, and following its subsequent clearance with a gamma camera or multicollimated detectors. This last method permits continuous monitoring of movement.

Studies of several hundred healthy adult subjects by the tagged-particle or saccharin methods have consistently shown that 80% exhibit clearance rates of 3 to 25 mm/min (average 6 mm/min), with slower rates in the remaining 20% (119). The latter subjects have been termed "slow clearers." The findings of a greater proportion of slow clearers in one group of subjects living in an extremely cold climate raises the possibility that the differences in clearance may be related to an effect of inspired air (119). In diseased

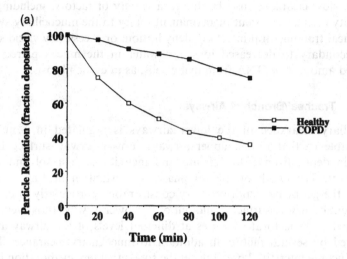

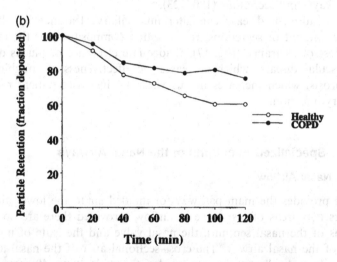

Figure 17 Mucociliary clearance is compromised in COPD patients in (a) central and (b) peripheral airways. Clearance is measured by monitoring (through whole-body scanning) retention time of an insoluble radiolabeled marker. Airways were partitioned into large and small airways, with small airways comprising 70% of the airway tree. Data are mean from 9 healthy controls (open symbols) and 10 patients with COPD (solid symbols). Coughing accelerates clearance, while therapeutics that reduce parasympathetic nerve effects (e.g., ipratroprium bromide) slows clearance (not shown). (Data modified from Ref. 123.)

subjects, slow clearance may be due to a variety of factors, including the immotility of cilia, transient or permanent injury to the mucociliary system by physical trauma, viral infection, dehydration, or excessively viscid secretions secondary to decreased ions and water in the mucus paired with increased amounts of DNA from dying cells, as in cystic fibrosis.

B. Tracheal/Bronchial Airways

Mucociliary clearance in the lower airways is regulated in a manner comparable to that in the upper airways. Lower airway surface liquid ranges in depth from 5 to 100 μm and includes both a sol and a gel component. The depth of the sol phase is constant in healthy airways, whereas the gel phase depth can vary considerably, particularly in disease. Movement of airway surface liquid out of the lower airways (it is eventually swallowed or expectorated) varies at different levels of the airway and is influenced by several factors in addition to mucociliary clearance. These factors include interstitial pressures in the subepithelium, evaporation in the larger airways, and secretions (120–123).

As mentioned, disease can alter mucociliary clearance by altering either the amount of secretions, the secretion composition, or the rate or effectiveness of clearance (Fig. 17). Inadequate clearance of mucus due to neuromuscular disease, which decreases the effectiveness of coughing, or cystic fibrosis, which increases mucus viscosity, increases patient risk for pulmonary infection.

VI. Specialized Functions of the Nasal Airways

A. Nasal Airflow

The nose provides the main pathway for inhaled air to the lower airways and offers two areas of resistance to airflow (provided there are no gross deviations of the nasal septum): the nasal valve and the state of mucosal swelling of the nasal airway. The cross-sectional area of the nasal airway decreases dramatically at the nasal valve to reach 30 to 40 mm^2. This narrowed area separates the vestibules from the main airway and accounts for approximately half of the total resistance to respiratory airflow from ambient air to the alveoli. After bypassing this narrow area, inspired air flows in the main nasal airway, which is a broader tube bounded by the septal surface medially, and by the irregular inferior and middle turbinates laterally. The caliber of the lumen of this portion of the airway is variable, being governed by changes in the blood content of the capillaries, capacitance vessels, and arteriovenous shunts of the lining mucosa and constituting the second resistive segment that inspired air encounters on its way to the lungs. Changes in the blood content of these structures occur spontaneously and rhythmically, resulting in alternating volume reductions in the lumina of the two nasal cavities, a phenomenon referred to as the nasal cycle. This occurs in approximately 80% of normal individuals and the reciprocity of changes between the two sides of the nasal cavity maintains total nasal airway resistance unchanged (124). The duration of one cycle varies between 50 min and 4 h and is interrupted by vasoconstrictive medications or exercise, leading is turn to a marked reduction of total nasal airway resistance. Kennedy and colleagues used T2-weighted magnetic resonance imaging to observe the nasal passages and demonstrated an alternating increase and decrease in signal intensity and turbinate size over time in a fashion consistent with the nasal cycle (125). The nasal cycle can be exacerbated by the increase in nasal airway resistance caused by exposure to allergic stimuli, and this explains why some allergic individuals complain of alternating exacerbations of their nasal obstructive symptoms.

Swift and Proctor presented a detailed description of nasal airflow and its characteristics (Fig. 18) (126). Upon inspiration, air first passes upward into the vestibules in a vertical direction at a velocity of 2 to 3 m/s, then converges and changes its direction from vertical to horizontal just prior to the nasal valve, where, owing to the narrowing of the airway, velocities reach their highest levels (≤12–18 m/s). After passing the nasal valve, the cross-sectional area increases, and velocity decreases concomitantly to about 2 to 3 m/s. The nature of flow changes from laminar before and at the nasal

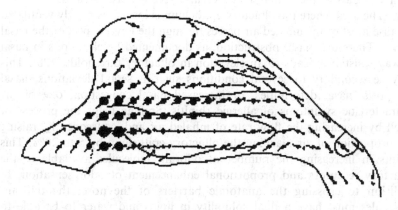

Figure 18 Schematic diagram of the direction and velocity of inspired air. The size of the dots is directly proportional to velocity, and the arrows depict direction of airflow. (From Proctor DF, Andersen IB. The Nose—Upper Airway Physiology and the Atmospheric Environment. Amsterdam: Elsevier Biomedical Press, 1982.)

valve to more turbulent posteriorly. As inspiratory flow increases beyond resting levels, turbulent characteristics commence at an increasingly anterior position and, with mild exercise, are found as early as the anterior ends of the turbinates. The airstream increases in velocity to 3 m/s to 4 m/s in the nasopharynx, where the direction again changes from horizontal to vertical as air moves down through the pharynx and larynx to reach the trachea. Turbulence of nasal airflow minimizes the presence of a boundary layer of air that would exist with laminar flow and maximizes interaction between the airstream and the nasal mucosa. This, in turn, allows the nose to perform its functions of heat and moisture exchange and of cleaning inspired air of suspended or soluble particles.

B. Olfaction

One of the important sensory functions of the nose is olfaction. The olfactory airway is 1 to 2 mm wide and lies above the middle turbinate just inferior to the cribriform plate between the septum and the lateral wall of the nose. The olfactory mucosa has a surface area of 200 to 400 mm^2 and contains numerous odor receptor cells with thin cilia that project into the covering mucous layer and increase the surface area of the epithelium (127). The olfactory mucosa also contains small, tubular, serous Bowman's glands situated immediately below the epithelium. Each receptor cell is connected to the olfactory bulb by a thin nonmyelinated nerve fiber that is slow conducting but short, making the conduction time as low as 50 m/s. The impulses from the olfactory bulb are conveyed to the olfactory cortex, which in man is part of the thalamus, which also receives taste signals.

The area where the olfactory epithelium is located is poorly ventilated because most of the inhaled air passes through the lower aspect of the nasal cavity. Therefore, nasal obstruction, as documented by elevations in nasal airway resistance, leads to an elevation in olfactory thresholds (128). This may be secondary to several conditions such as septal deviations, nasal polyposis, nasal deformities, or increased nasal congestion, one of the characteristic symptoms of allergic rhinitis. Sniffing helps the process of smell by increasing the flow rate of inhaled air and, consequently, raising the proportion of air reaching the olfactory epithelium by 5 to 20%. This results in increasing the number of odorant molecules available to the olfactory receptors and proportional enhancement of odor sensation. In addition to crossing the anatomic barriers of the nose, the odorant molecules must have a dual solubility in lipids and water to be able to reach the olfactory receptors. To penetrate the mucus covering the olfactory mucosa, they solubilize to a certain extent in water. Lipid solubility, on the other hand, enhances their interaction with the receptor membrane of the olfactory epithelial cilia. Finally, it is to be mentioned that olfactory sensitivity normally decreases with age, as evidenced by a recent longitudinal study of men and women between the ages of 19 and 95 followed over a 3-year period (129).

C. Vomeronasal Organ

Many vertebrate species, including many mammals, have a small chemosensory structure in the nose called the vomeronasal organ (VNO), dedicated to detecting chemical signals that mediate sexual and territorial behaviors. A similar structure appears to exist in the human nose and is described as two small sacs about 2 mm deep that open into shallow pits on either side of the nasal septum. In vertebrates, the pair of small sacs is lined by sensory neurons, tucked inside the vomer bone where the hard palate and nasal septum meet. In mice and rats, the VNO is connected to the brain through a neural pathway that is independent of the olfactory pathway, but it is not clear whether the human VNO is connected to the brain. There is recent renewed interest in researching the anatomy and function of this organ in man, an effort primarily funded by the perfume industry (130).

VII. Conclusion

As detailed in this chapter, the nose is an intricate organ with important functions that include filtration, humidification, and temperature control of inspired air in preparation for transit to the lower airways. It is also important in providing the sense of olfaction. It has an intricate network of nerves, vessels, glands, and inflammatory cells, all of which help to modulate its function. Chronic inflammation affects multiple end organs within the nasal cavity and will lead to diseases such as rhinitis (allergic and nonallergic) and sinusitis. The lower airways share many of the physiological and anatomical attributes of the nasal airways. The overview of the anatomy and function of the airways provided in this chapter should serve as a useful prelude to the coming chapters, which discuss different diseases of the respiratory system in the context of their simultaneous manifestations in the nose and the bronchi.

References

1. Van Loosen J, Van Zanten GA, Howard CV, et al. Growth characteristics of the human nasal septum. Rhinology 1996;34:78.
2. Gray L. Deviated nasal septum. III. Its influence on the physiology and disease of the nose and ears. J Laryngol 1967;81:953.

3. Mygind N, Pedersen M, Nielsen M. Morphology of the upper airway epithelium. In Proctor DF, Andersen IB, eds. The Nose. Upper Airway Physiology and the Atmospheric Environment. Amsterdam: Elsevier Biomedical Press; 1982.

4. Jeffery, P. K. Structural, immunological and neural elements of the normal human airway wall. In: Busse WW, Holgate ST, eds. Asthma and Rhinitis. Blackwell Science, Oxford UK, 2000, Chapter 14, 164–190.

5. West, J. B. (2000). Respiratory Physiology—The Essentials. Baltimore, Lippincott, Williams & Wilkins.

6. Miller WS. The musculature of the finer divisions of the bronchial tree and its relation to certain pathological conditions. Am Rev Tuber 1921; 5:689–704.

7. Macklin, CC. The musculature of the bronchi and lungs. Physiol Rev 1929; 9:1–60.

8. Cabezas GA, Graf PD, Nadel JA. Sympathetic versus parasympathetic nervous regulation of airways in dogs. J Appl Physiol 1971; 31(5):651-655

9. Hogg JC., Hegele RG. Postmortem pathology. In Barnes PJ, Grunstein MM, Leff AR, Woolcock AJ, eds. Asthma, Lippincott-Raven, Philadelphia, 1997, Chapter 16, 201–208.

10. Permutt. S. Nitric oxide in asthma is like insulin in type II diabetes. In Mechanics of Breathing, Aliverti A, ed. Springer-Verlag, Milan, In press.

11. Skloot G, Permutt S, Togias A. Airway hyperresponsiveness in asthma: a problem of limited smooth muscle relaxation with inspiration. J Clin Invest 1995; 96(5):2393–2403.

12. N Scichilone, personal communication.

13. Carrell RW, Lomas DA. Alpha$_1$-antitrypsin deficiency—a model for conformational diseases. N Engl J Med 2002;346(1): 45-53.

14. Gelb AF, Zamel N. Unsuspected pseudophysiologic emphysema in chronic persistent asthma. Am J Respir Crit Care Med 2000; 162(5):1778–1782.

15. Global initiative for chronic obstructive lung disease (GOLD), World Health Organization (WHO)/ National Heart, Lung and Blood Institute, National Institutes of Health (Bethesda, MD), NIH Publication No. 2701, 2001.

16. Mitzner W. Collateral ventilation. In: Crystal RG, West JB et al, eds. The Lung: Scientific Foundations. New York, Raven Press, 1991, Chapter 5.

17. Evans MJ, Plopper GG. The role of basal cells in adhesion of columnar epithelium to airway basement membrane. Am Rev Respir Dis 1988;138: 481.

18. Evans MJ, Shami S, Cabral-Anderson LJ, et al. Role of nonciliated cells in renewal of the bronchial epithelium of rats exposed to NO_2. Am J Pathol 1986;123:126.

19. Tos M. Goblet cells and glands in the nose and paranasal sinuses. In: Proctor DF, Andersen IB, eds. The Nose. Upper Airway Physiology and the Atmospheric Environment. Amsterdam: Elsevier Biomedical Press; 1982.

20. Winther B, Innes DJ, Mills SE, et al. Lymphocyte subsets in normal airway mucosa of the human nose Arch Otolaryngol Head Neck Surg 1987;113:59.

21. Bradding P, Feather IH, Wilson S, et al. Immunolocalization of cytokines in

the nasal mucosa of normal and perennial rhinitic subjects. J Immunol 1993; 151:3853.

22. Wioland M-A, Fleury-Feith J, Corlieu P, Commo F, Monceaux G, Lacau-St-Guily J, Bernaudin J-F. CFTR, MDR1, and MRP1 immunolocalization in normal human nasal respiratory mucosa. J Histochem Cytochem 2000;48: 1215-22.

23. Kreda SM, Gynn MC, Fenstermacher DA, Boucher RC, Gabriel SE. Expression and localization of epithelial aquaporins in the adult human lung. Am J Respir Cell Mol Biol 2001;24:224–34.

24. Agha-Mir-Salim P, Rauhut O, Merker H-J. Electron and fluorescence microscopic investigations on composition and structure of the epithelial basement membrane of the human inferior nasal concha. Eur Arch Otorhinolaryngol 1993; 250:401–407.

25. Chanez P, Vignola AM, Vic P, Guddo F, Bonsignore G, Godard P, Bousquet J. Comparison between nasal and bronchial inflammation in asthmatic and control subjects. Am J Resp Crit Care Med 1999;159:588–95.

26. Sanai A, Nagata H, Konno A. Extensive interstitial collagen deposition on the basement membrane zone in allergic nasal mucosa. Acta Otolaryngol (Stockh) 1999;119:473–478.

27. Shaida A, Kenyon G, Devalia J, Davies RJ, MacDonald TT, Pender SLF. Matrix metalloproteinases and their inhibitors in the nasal mucosa of patients with perennial allergic rhinitis. J Allergy Clin Immunol 2001;108:791–6.

28. Lim MC, Taylor RM, Naclerio RM. The histology of allergic rhinitis and its comparison to cellular changes in nasal lavage. Am J Respir Crit Care Med 1995;151:136.

29. Varney VA, Jacobson MR, Sudderick RM, et al. Immunohistology of the nasal mucosa following allergen-induced rhinitis. Am Rev Respir Dis 1992; 146:170.

30. Bojsen-Moller F. Glandulae nasales anteriores in the human nose. Ann Otol Rhinol Laryngol 1965;74:363.

31. Bousquet J, Jeffery PK, Busse WW, Johnson M, Vignola AM. Asthma. From bronchoconstriction to airways inflammation and remodeling. Am J Respir Crit Care Med. 2000; 161(5):1720–1745.

32. Thurlbeck WM, Malaka D, Murphy K. Goblet cells in the peripheral airways in chronic bronchitis. Am Rev Respir Dis 1975; 112(1):65–69.

33. Aikawa T, Shimura S, Sasaki H, Ebina M, Takishima T. Marked goblet cell hyperplasia with mucus accumulation in the airways of patients who died of severe acute asthma attack. Chest 1992; 101(4):916–921.

34. Jeffery PK. Comparison of the structural and inflammatory features of COPD and asthma. Giles F. Filley Lecture. Chest 2000; 117(5 suppl 1):251S-260S.

35. Rogers DF. Airway goblet cells: responsive and adaptable front-line defenders. Eur Respir J 1994; 7(9):1690-1706.

36. Crouch EC. Collectins and pulmonary host defense. Am J Respir Cell Mol Biol 1998; 19(2):177–201.

37. Evans MJ, Van Winkle LS, Fanucchi MV, Plopper CG. Cellular and

molecular characteristics of basal cells in airway epithelium. Exp Lung Res 2001;27(5):401–415.

38. Cutz E, Jackson A. Neuroepithelial bodies as airway oxygen sensors. Respir Physiol 1999; 115(2):201–214.

39. Persson CG, Andersson M, Greiff L, Svensson C, Erjefalt JS, Sundler F, Wollmer P, Alkner U, Erjefalt I, Gustafsson B, et al. Airway permeability. Clin Exp Allergy 1995; 25(9):807–814.

40. Fu L, Kaneko T, Ikeda H, Nishiyama H, Suzuki S, Okubo T, Trevisani M, Geppetti P, Ishigatsubo Y. Tachykinins via tachykinin NK(2) receptor activation mediate ozone-induced increase in the permeability of the tracheal mucosa in guinea-pigs. Br J Pharmacol 2002; 135(5):1331–1335.

41. Widdicombe JH, Widdicombe JG. Regulation of human airway surface liquid. Respir Physiol 1995; 99(1):3–12.

42. Landry JS, Eidelman DH. Airway surface liquid: end of the controversy? J Gen Physiol 2001; 117(5):419–422.

43. Boucher RC. Molecular insights into the physiology of the "thin film" of airway surface liquid. J Physiol 1999; 516 (pt 3):631-638.

44. Verkman AS, Matthay MA, Song Y. Aquaporin water channels and lung physiology. Am J Physiol Lung Cell Mol Physiol 2000; 278(5):L867–L879.

45. Matthay MA, Folkesson HG, Clerici C. Lung epithelial fluid transport and the resolution of pulmonary edema. Physiol Rev 2002; 82(3):569-600.

46. Hunter JA, Finkbeiner WE, Nadel JA, Goetzl EJ, Holtzman MJ. Predominant generation of 15-lipoxygenase metabolites of arachidonic acid by epithelial cells from human trachea. Proc Natl Acad Sci U S A 1985; 82(14): 4633–4637.

47. Adler KB, Fischer BM, Wright DT, Cohn LA, Becker S. Interactions between respiratory epithelial cells and cytokines: relationships to lung inflammation. Ann N Y Acad Sci 1994; 725:128–145.

48. Nickel R, Beck LA, Stellato C, Schleimer RP. Chemokines and allergic disease. J Allergy Clin Immunol 1999;104(4 pt 1):723-742.

49. Redington AE, Meng QH, Springall DR, Evans TJ, Creminon C, Maclouf J, Holgate ST, Howarth PH, Polak JM. Increased expression of inducible nitric oxide synthase and cyclooxygenase-2 in the airway epithelium of asthmatic subjects and regulation by corticosteroid treatment. Thorax 2001; 56(5):351–357.

50. Atsuta J, Sterbinsky SA, Plitt J, Schwiebert LM, Bochner BS, Schleimer RP. Phenotyping and cytokine regulation of the BEAS-2B human bronchial epithelial cell: demonstration of inducible expression of the adhesion molecules VCAM-1 and ICAM-1. Am J Respir Cell Mol Biol 1997;17(5): 571–582.

51. Sheppard D, Yokosaki Y. Roles of airway epithelial integrins in health and disease. The Parker B. Francis Lectureship. Chest 1996; 109(3 suppl):29S–33S.

52. Jeffery PK. Remodeling in asthma and chronic obstructive lung disease. Am J Respir Crit Care Med 2001; 164(10 pt 2):S28–38.

53. Roche WR, Beasley R, Williams JH, Holgate ST. Subepithelial fibrosis in the bronchi of asthmatics. Lancet 1989; 1(8637):520–524.

54. Mautino G, Capony F, Bousquet J, Vignola AM. Balance in asthma between matrix metalloproteinases and their inhibitors. J Allergy Clin Immunol 1999; 104(3 pt 1):530–533.

55. Kumar SD, Emery MJ, Atkins ND, Danta I, Wanner A. Airway mucosal blood flow in bronchial asthma. Am J Respir Crit Care Med 1998; 158(1):153–156.

56. Lemanske RF Jr. The late phase response: clinical implications. Adv Intern Med 1991; 36:171–193.

57. Brown RH, Mitzner W, Wagner EM. Interaction between airway edema and lung inflation on responsiveness of individual airways in vivo. J Appl Physiol 1997; 83(2):366–370.

58. Brown RH, Zerhouni EA, Mitzner W. Airway edema potentiates airway reactivity. J Appl Physiol 1995; 79(4):1242–1248.

59. Peebles RS Jr, Permutt S, Togias A. Rapid reversibility of the allergen-induced pulmonary late-phase reaction by an intravenous beta$_2$-agonist. J Appl Physiol 1998; 84(5):1500–1505.

60. King LS, Nielsen S, Agre P, Brown RH. Decreased pulmonary vascular permeability in aquaporin-1-null humans. Proc Natl Acad Sci U S A 2002; 99(2):1059–1063.

61. Otis AB. A perspective of respiratory mechanics. J Appl Physiol 1983; 54(5): 1183–1187.

62. Widdicombe JG, Nadel JA. Airway volume, airway resistance, and work and force of breathing: theory. J Appl Physiol 1963; 18:863–868.

63. Coleridge HM, Coleridge JC, Schultz HD. Afferent pathways involved in reflex regulation of airway smooth muscle. Pharmacol Ther 1989; 42(1):1–63.

64. Stephens NL, Li W, Wang Y, Ma X. The contractile apparatus of airway smooth muscle. Biophysics and biochemistry. Am J Respir Crit Care Med 1998; 158(5 pt 3):S80–S94.

65. Ammit AJ, Panettieri RA Jr. Invited review: the circle of life: cell cycle regulation in airway smooth muscle. J Appl Physiol 2001; 91(3):1431–1437

66. Dixon JS, Small RC. Evidence of poor conduction of muscle excitation in the longitudinal axis of guinea-pig isolated trachea. Br J Pharmacol 1983; 79(1): 75–83.

67. Nadel JA, Davis B, Phipps RJ. Control of mucus secretion and ion transport in airways. Annu Rev Physiol 1979; 41:369–381.

68. Liu YC, Khawaja AM, Rogers DF. Effects of the cysteinyl leukotriene receptor antagonists pranlukast and zafirlukast on tracheal mucus secretion in ovalbumin-sensitized guinea-pigs in vitro. Br J Pharmacol 1998; 124(3):563–571.

69. Nadel JA. Role of neutrophil elastase in hypersecretion during COPD exacerbations, and proposed therapies. Chest 2000; 117(5 suppl 2):386S–389S.

70. Sminia T, van der Brugge-Gamelkoorn GJ, Jeurissen SH. Structure and

function of bronchus-associated lymphoid tissue (BALT). Crit Rev Immunol 1989; 9(2):119–150.

71. Brightling CE, Bradding P, Symon FA, Holgate ST, Wardlaw AJ, Pavord ID. Mast-cell infiltration of airway smooth muscle in asthma. N Engl J Med 2002; 346(22):1699–1705.

72. Holt PG, Stumbles PA. Regulation of immunologic homeostasis in peripheral tissues by dendritic cells: the respiratory tract as a paradigm. J Allergy Clin Immunol 2000; 105(3):421–429.

73. Robinson DS, Hamid Q, Ying S, Tsicopoulos A, Barkans J, Bentley AM, Corrigan C, Durham SR, Kay AB. Predominant TH2-like bronchoalveolar T-lymphocyte population in atopic asthma. N Engl J Med 1992; 326(5):298–304.

74. Liu MC, Proud D, Lichtenstein LM, Hubbard WC, Bochner BS, Stealey BA, Breslin L, Xiao H, Freidhoff LR, Schroeder JT, Schleimer RP. Effects of prednisone on the cellular responses and release of cytokines and mediators after segmental allergen challenge of asthmatic subjects. J Allergy Clin Immunol 2001; 108(1):29–38.

75. Cauna N. Blood and nerve supply of the nasal lining. In Proctor DF, Andersen IB, eds. The Nose.Upper Airway Physiology and the Atmospheric Environment. Amsterdam: Elsevier Biomedical Press; 1982.

76. Dawes JDK, Prichard M. Studies of the vascular arrangement of the nose. J Anat 1953;87:311.

77. Cauna N, Hinderer KH. Fine structure of blood vessels of the human respiratory mucosa. Ann Otol Rhinol Laryngol 1969;78:865.

78. Wagner EM, Mitzner W, Brown RH. Site of functional bronchopulmonary anastomoses in sheep. Anat Rec 1999; 254(3):360–366.

79. Wagner EM, Brown RH. Blood flow distribution within the airway wall. J Appl Physiol 2002; 92(5):1964–1969.

80. Coleridge HM, Coleridge JC. Neural regulation of bronchial blood flow. Respir Physiol 1994; 98(1):1–13.

81. Thurston G, Murphy TJ, Baluk P, Lindsey JR, McDonald DM. Angiogenesis in mice with chronic airway inflammation: strain-dependent differences. Am J Pathol 1998; 153(4):1099–1112.

82. Pearse DB, Wagner EM, Sylvester JT. Edema clearance in isolated sheep lungs. J Appl Physiol 1993; 74(1):126–132.

83. Hainis KD, Sznajder JI, Schraufnagel DE. Lung lymphatics cast from the airspace. Am J Physiol 1994; 267(2 Pt 1):L199–L205.

84. Wagner EM, Blosser S, Mitzner W. Bronchial vascular contribution to lung lymph flow. J Appl Physiol 1998; 85(6):2190–2195.

85. Miserocchi G, Negrini D, Passi A, De Luca G. Development of lung edema: interstitial fluid dynamics and molecular structure. News Physiol Sci 2001; 16:66–71.

86. Baroody FM, Wagenmann M, Naclerio RM. A comparison of the secretory response of the nasal mucosa to histamine and methacholine. J Appl Physiol 1993; 74(6): 2661.

87. Baraniuk JN, Lundgren JD, Mullol J, et al. Substance P and neurokinin A in human nasal mucosa. Am J Respir Cell Mol Biol 1991;4:228.
88. Baraniuk JN, Castellino S, Merida M, et al. Calcitonin gene related peptide in human nasal mucosa. Am J Physiol 1990;258:L81.
89. Laitinen A, Partanen M, Hervonen A, et al. VIP-like immunoreactive nerves in human respiratory tract. Light and electron microscopic study. Histochemistry 1985;82:313.
90. Baraniuk JN, Okayama M, Lundgren JD et al. Vasoactive intestinal peptide (VIP) in human nasal mucosa. J Clin Invest 1990;86:825.
91. Canning BJ, and Widdicombe JG, eds. Innervation of the airways. Respir Physiol 2001;125(1-2):1–154.
92. Mazzone SB, Canning BJ. Central nervous system control of the airways: pharmacological implications. Curr Opin Pharmacol 2002;2(3):220–228.
93. Canning BJ. Neurology of allergic inflammation and rhinitis. Curr Allergy Asthma Rep 2002; 2(3):210–215.
94. Undem, BJ, Canning BJ. Neuronal control of airway function in allergy. In Middleton's Allergy, NF Adkinson, JW Yunginger, WW Busse, BS Bochner, ST Holgate, and FER Simons, eds., Elsevier Sciences, St. Louis, MO. In press.
95. Sparrow MP, Weichselbaum M, McCray PB. Development of the innervation and airway smooth muscle in human fetal lung. Am J Respir Cell Mol Biol 1999; 20:550–560.
96. Widdicombe J. Airway receptors. Respir Physiol 2001; 125(1-2):3–15.
97. Myers AC. Transmission in autonomic ganglia. Respir Physiol 2001; 125(1-2): 99–111.
98. Kajekar R, Rohde HK, Myers AC. The integrative membrane properties of human bronchial parasympathetic ganglia neurons. Am J Respir Crit Care Med 2001; 164(10 pt 1):1927–1932.
99. Ward JK, Barnes PJ, Springall DR, Abelli L, Tadjkarimi S, Yacoub MH, Polak JM, Belvisi MG. Distribution of human i-NANC bronchodilator and nitric oxide–immunoreactive nerves. Am J Respir Cell Mol Biol 1995; 13(2): 175–184.
100. Haberberger R, Schemann M, Sann H, Kummer W. Innervation pattern of guinea pig pulmonary vasculature depends on vascular diameter. J Appl Physiol 1997; 82(2):426–434.
101. Canning BJ. Interactions between vagal afferent nerve subtypes mediating cough. Pulm Pharmacol Ther 2002; 15(3):187–192.
102. Coleridge JC, Coleridge HM. Afferent vagal C fibre innervation of the lungs and airways and its functional significance. Rev Physiol Biochem Pharmacol 1984; 99:1–110.
103. Lee LY, Pisarri TE. Afferent properties and reflex functions of bronchopulmonary C-fibers. Respir Physiol 2001; 125(1-2):47–65.
104. Ho CY, Gu Q, Lin YS, Lee LY. Sensitivity of vagal afferent endings to chemical irritants in the rat lung. Respir Physiol 2001;127(2-3):113–124.
105. Hwang SW, Cho H, Kwak J, Lee SY, Kang CJ, Jung J, Cho S, Min KH, Suh YG, Kim D, Oh U. Direct activation of capsaicin receptors by products of

lipoxygenases: endogenous capsaicin-like substances. Proc Natl Acad Sci U S A 2000; 97(11):6155–6160.

106. Hwang SW, Oh U. Hot channels in airways: pharmacology of the vanilloid receptor. Curr Opin Pharmacol 2002; 2(3):235–242.

107. Kagaya M, Lamb J, Robbins J, Page CP, Spina D. Characterization of the anandamide-induced depolarization of guinea-pig isolated vagus nerve. Br J Pharmacol 2002; 137(1):39–48.

108. Barnes PJ. Neurogenic inflammation in the airways. Respir Physiol 2001; 125(1-2):145–154.

109. Canning BJ, Fischer A. Neural regulation of airway smooth muscle tone. Respir Physiol 2001; 125(1-2):113–127.

110. Mazzone SB, Canning BJ. Evidence for differential reflex regulation of cholinergic and noncholinergic parasympathetic nerves innervating the airways. Am J Respir Crit Care Med 2002; 165(8):1076–1083.

111. Silkoff PE, Sylvester JT, Zamel N, Permutt S. Airway nitric oxide diffusion in asthma: role in pulmonary function and bronchial responsiveness. Am J Respir Crit Care Med 2000; 161(4 Pt 1):1218–1228.

112. Grasemann H, Yandava CN, Storm van's Gravesande K, Deykin A, Pillari A, Ma J, Sonna LA, Lilly C, Stampfer MJ, Israel E, Silverman EK, Drazen JM. A neuronal NO synthase (NOS1) gene polymorphism is associated with asthma. Biochem Biophys Res Commun 2000; 272(2):391–394.

113. Ricciardolo FL, Geppetti P, Mistretta A, Nadel JA, Sapienza MA, Bellofiore S, Di Maria GU. Randomised double-blind placebo-controlled study of the effect of inhibition of nitric oxide synthesis in bradykinin-induced asthma. Lancet 1996; 348(9024):374–377.

114. Wilson WR, Allansmith MR. Rapid, atraumatic method for obtaining nasal mucus samples. Ann Otol Rhinol Laryngol 1976;85:391.

115. Andersen I, Lundqvist G, Proctor DF. Human nasal mucosal function under four controlled humidities. Am Rev Respir Dis 1979;119:619.

116. Fry FA, Black A. Regional deposition and clearance of particles in the human nose. Aerosol Sci 1973;4:113.

117. Lippmann M. Deposition and clearance of inhaled particles in the human nose. Ann Otol Rhinol Laryngol 1970;79:519.

118. Baumgarten C, Togias AG, Naclerio RM, et al. Influx of kininogens into nasal secretions after antigen challenge of allergic individuals. J Clin Invest 1985;76:191.

119. Proctor DF. The mucociliary system. Proctor DF, Andersen IB eds. The Nose: Upper Airway Physiology and the Atmospheric Environment. Amsterdam: Elsevier Biomedical Press 1982.

120. Mosconi P, Langer M, Cigada M, Mandelli M. Epidemiology and risk factors of pneumonia in critically ill patients. Intensive Care Unit Group for Infection Control. Eur J Epidemiol 1991; 7(4):320–327.

121. Adler KB, Li Y. Airway epithelium and mucus: intracellular signaling pathways for gene expression and secretion. Am J Respir Cell Mol Biol. 2001 Oct;25(4):397–400.

122. Robinson M, Bye PT. Mucociliary clearance in cystic fibrosis. Pediatr Pulmonol 2002; 33(4):293–306.
123. Michael Foster W. Mucociliary transport and cough in humans. Pulm Pharmacol Ther 2002; 15(3):277–282.
124. Hasegawa M, Kern EB. The human cycle. Mayo Clin Proc 1977;52:28.
125. Kennedy DW, Zinreich SJ, Kumar AJ et al. Physiologic mucosal changes within the nose and the ethmoid sinus: Imaging of the nasal cycle by MRI. Laryngoscope 1988;98:928.
126. Swift DL, Proctor DF. Access of air to the respiratory tract. In: Brain JD, Proctor DF, Reid LM, eds. Respiratory Defense Mechanisms. New York: Marcel Dekker; 1977.
127. Berglund B, Lindvall T. Olfaction. In Proctor DF, Andersen IB, eds. The Nose. Amsterdam: Elsevier Biomedical Press B; 1982.
128. Rous J, Kober F. Influence of one-sided nasal respiratory occlusion of the olfactory threshold values. Arch Klin Ohren Nasen Kehlkopfheiklk 1970; 196(2):374.
129. Ship JA, Pearson JD, Cruise LJ, et al. Longitudinal changes in smell identification. J Gerontol 1996;51(2):M86.
130. Taylor R. Brave new nose: sniffing out human sexual chemistry. J NIH Res 1994;6:47.

2

The Impact of Nasal Function and Dysfunction on the Lower Airways

ALKIS TOGIAS

Johns Hopkins Asthma
and Allergy Center
Baltimore, Maryland, U.S.A.

HUGH WINDOM

University of South Florida
Tampa, Florida, U.S.A.

Introduction

The nasal airways and their closely associated paranasal sinuses are an integral part of the respiratory tract. This notion was clearly documented by Galen, the great Greek physician of the second century A.D., who wrote:

> The apertures of the nose, how marvelously they come next after the sponge-like (ethmoid)... bone and how the connection was cut through into the mouth at the palate in order that inspiration may not begin in a straight line with the trachea and that the air entering it may first be bent and convoluted, so to speak. For I think this should be doubly advantageous: the parts of the lung will never be chilled when oftentimes the air surrounding us is very cold, and the particles of dust... will not penetrate as far as the trachea (1).

The most important concept regarding nose–lung integration is not the common embryological origin of the airways or the anatomical similarities, particularly with respect to the mucosa, but the functional complementarity that assigns to the nose the role of the protector of the lungs. This role is achieved through a variety of functional characteristics of the nose, which we review in this chapter.

The significance of nasal function for the lower airways is consistently and clearly emphasized in any treatise or textbook describing the physiology of the respiratory system. Yet, this fundamental concept has been absent from the minds of many clinicians, who regard the nose and the lungs as two distinct anatomic entities, subjected to distinct pathological conditions. This distorted view reflects our unfortunate consideration of medicine as a compartmentalized vocation, a trend that began in the midtwentieth century and has dominated ever since. Its impact is that physicians who are trained to treat respiratory diseases do not consider rhinitis or sinusitis as such and will often fail to diagnose or rule out these conditions. Inversely, physicians specialized in diseases of the upper airways tend to avoid any involvement in lower airways disease. The result is, of course, that many patients with respiratory illnesses, who, as should become evident from this book, frequently suffer from involvement of their entire respiratory tract, are not offered appropriate treatment opportunities. The same compartmentalization problem is observed in the research arena. With little or no information from the "producers of knowledge," the problem becomes legitimized and is perpetuated.

Despite our knowledge of the capabilities and the physiological roles of the nasal airways, we still lack an in-depth understanding of the importance of nasal function on the health of the lower respiratory tract. This is in part secondary to the failure to develop methodologies for evaluating nasal function in conjunction with the function of the lower airways. Yet, various experimental approaches have been used and are currently being employed in increasing frequency to address these problems. From these approaches, several speculations have been made about the mechanisms of the functional interaction between the nasal and the lower airways. This chapter presents the basis and discusses the validity of these speculations in some detail.

In attempting to conceptualize how the nasal airways affect the lower respiratory tract, one can differentiate their physiological functions into those that originate and manifest in the nose but are relevant to the lower airways and those that originate in the nose and manifest in the lower airways. A similar categorization could be also applied for pathological phenomena that originate in the nasal airways. Examples of local functions with impact on the lower airways are the air conditioning capacity of the nose and the elements of innate immunity that the nasal mucosa can provide. On the other hand, the nasobronchial reflex and the development of inflammation in the lower airways following an allergic reaction in the nose represent examples of phenomena that originate in the nose but manifest in the lower airways. To study the latter phenomena, the methodology of nasal provocation accompanied by lower airway assessment has been used with success. The data that have derived from such studies are described in more detail later in this chapter.

I. Conditioning of Inhaled Air

A. Warming and Humidification

Most of the conditioning of inhaled air takes place in the nasal passages (2–4). By the time inspired air at 20°C reaches the oropharynx, the average temperature is approximately 31 to 33°C and the air is water saturated (5,6). At extreme conditions, the capabilities of the nasal passages become even more evident: when air is inhaled with high (26 L/min), continuous, and unidirectional flow (inhalation through the nose, exhalation through the mouth) and temperature near the freezing point, the temperature in the nasopharynx can reach as high as 30°C in some individuals (7). Cole also showed that the absolute humidity (water content) of air samples from the oropharynx consistently reads around 32 mg/L during nasal breathing of room air at flows ranging from 7 to 42 L/min (8). For the above-mentioned temperatures, this is fully saturated air. In Ingelstedt's work, a wet/dry thermocouple psychrometer introduced in the larynx by puncturing the cricothyroid membrane showed that the relative humidity of inhaled air remained around 99%, even when subjects were exposed to a cold chamber (0 to −4°C) for 12 min (4).

The nasal mucosa constantly provides water and heat to inhaled air. At inspiration, mucosal surface cooling occurs (9), and theoretically, transient increases in the osmolarity of the epithelial lining fluid should take place, but there is no experimental evidence to support this postulate. A substantial portion of the water and heat supplied to the air by the mucosa at inspiration passively returns at expiration (4–6). The heat and water recovered from expiratory air in a temperate environment, at rest, are about one-third of what was transferred into the air during inspiration. Under these conditions, the nose of an adult human has a net loss of 300 to 400 mL of water and 250 to 350 kcal/24 h (6). Based on an estimate that, at any given time, the volume of the nasal airway surface liquid is approximately 150 μL [nasal surface = 150 cm^2, depth of mucus layer = 10 μm (10,11)], this liquid must be replaced every 1.5 min.

The mechanisms through which the nose humidifies and warms inhaled air are not clear. The anatomy of the nasal mucosa (reviewed in detail in Chapter 1) is of major importance. Perhaps one of the most pivotal structures is the dense, subepithelial capillary network that is equipped with fenestrae polarized toward the luminal surface (12). Blood flow through this network probably provides adequate heat for the warming of inhaled air. In addition, the fenestrae may facilitate water transportation into the interstitium and, eventually, the surface and the glandular epithelia. The venous sinusoids, lying below the subepithelial capillary network, are another important structural component of the nasal lining tissue. Pooling of large volumes of blood can occur very rapidly because the sinusoids are supplied by multiple arteriovenous anastomoses with draining vessels (cushion veins) capable of constricting in response to neural or chemical stimuli (13). When the sinusoids enlarge, the nasal submucosa engorges, and this results in increased contact surface with the airstream. This is probably the major mechanism through which heating (i.e., convective heat transfer from the mucosal surface to the airstream) takes place. Application of vasoconstrictors decreases the temperature of inspired air at the oropharynx (9). Humidification per se should also improve the heating function of the nasal mucosa. There is no agreement about which structural element is the primary contributor to air humidification. The abundance of seromucous submucosal glands [approximately 45,000 per nasal cavity (14)] and goblet cells supports the possibility that their secretions provide most of the required water for air humidification. Ingelstedt has shown that subcutaneous injection of 1 mg of atropine decreases (but does not eliminate) the ability of the nose to humidify air (3). In other studies, however, application of homatropine or ipratropium bromide to the nasal surface did not impair air humidification (15,16). In fact, Assanasen and colleagues have indicated that nasal ipratropium, if anything, increases the humidification capacity of the nose (17). Cauna believes that the role of humidification belongs to water from the fenestrated subepithelial capillaries, which diffuses through the paracellular epithelial space (18). However, Ingelstedt, who injected fluorescein intravenously in normal humans, was not subsequently able to detect it in their nasal secretions (19). It is possible that fluorescein is not able to cross the nasal basement membrane or that its dilution in nasal secretions is so high that the dye cannot be detected.

These arguments aside, the possible mechanisms through which water is supplied to the airstream can be summarized as follows: (1) within the short time frame of an inspiratory phase, during which water is passively lost into the airstream, a small osmotic drive is generated, moving water from the intraepithelial spaces into the airway lumen (20), (2) water from glandular secretions [close to 95% water content (21)] can move into the gas phase even though the highly charged mucous glycoproteins tend to retain it (21); and (3) although no osmotic drive for water to reach the lumen is spontaneously generated by the apical surface of nasal epithelium, which predominantly absorbs sodium ions under basal conditions (22), this could occur if the epithelial cells were exposed to hypertonicity or to chloride-secreting agents. Increased osmolarity of the periciliary fluid may lead to reduction of sodium absorption, followed by induction of chloride secretion (22). Agents that increase cAMP also increase chloride secretion. These include α_2- and β-adrenergic agonists and prostaglandins E_2 and $F_{2\alpha}$. Inflammatory mediators such as bradykinin, adenosine, eosinophil major basic protein, substance P, and mast cell products have shown similar effects (23,24). Methacholine-induced human nasal secretions are somewhat hyperosmolar (ca. 340 mosm/kg H_2O) (25) and, in vitro, acetylcholine induces a large secretory flow of both sodium and chloride (22), suggesting that cholinergic stimulation also results in the generation of an osmotic drive to provide water to the airway surface. Therefore, neural activation, as well as allergic or nonallergic inflammatory conditions, can lead to osmotically driven passive water transfer into the airway lumen. In support of this hypothesis, Assanasen et al. have recently demonstrated that after an allergic reaction takes place in the nose, its air-conditioning ability (including humidification) is improved (26).

B. Filtering and Mucociliary Clearance

Filtering of inhaled particles and gaseous materials takes place constantly in the nasal passages. The great majority of inhaled, naturally occurring dusts are either taken out of the air during inspiratory nasal passage or are breathed in and out without being deposited at any site in the respiratory tract. The factors that determine particle trapping are numerous and quite complicated (27). These include size, gravity, inertia, Brownian movement (for very small particles), hygroscopicity, and electric charge. For example, with nasal breathing, most particles having an aerodynamic diameter of 5 to 10 μm are deposited in the nasal mucosa. A significant proportion of even smaller particles are also deposited in the nose, although many particles smaller than 2 μm pass into the lower airways (28). Hygroscopic inhaled particles will absorb water from nasal air, and their aerodynamic diameter will rapidly increase. This will then precipitate nasal trapping. As expected, nasal factors will influence trapping, as well. The anatomy of the nasal passages is characterized by narrow cross sections, resulting in high linear velocities. In addition, sharp bends and nasal hairs promote particle impaction. Hounam and associates have shown a strong relationship between the percentage of particles trapped in the nose and nasal airway resistance (29). Similarly, one can deduce that high inspiratory flow rates will increase linear velocities and will promote turbulent flow, thus increasing the chance for particle trapping.

Inspired gases can also be removed from air during inspiratory passage from the nose. Many factors operating on particles apply to gases, as well. There are two major differences: gas absorption will primarily occur in the main nasal passages (as opposed to the anterior entrance segments), and solubility or reactivity of the involved gas is a strong determinant of absorption. Assuming that a gas is soluble in water (e.g., SO_2), nearly all of it will be removed by the nasal passages, as long as the amount of epithelial lining fluid is adequate. An irritant gas may be removed even more efficiently because, by irritating the mucosa, it could lead to increased secretory rate and, therefore, to increased rate of absorption.

The fate of trapped particles and chemicals is, to a large extent, determined by mucociliary clearance, the anatomical basis of which is described in Chapter 1. In addition to this consititutive function, the nose, by initiating the powerful sneezing reflex, utilizes its nervous system to expel materials that have strong irritant effects. Most inhaled particles are deposited in the anterior region of the nose, and it is in that region that the mucociliary clearance current moves forward. Thus, owing to this current, a large part of these particles never gain further access to the body. The particles that are deposited more posteriorly are moved by the mucociliary system toward the oropharynx, at which point they are swallowed and further handled by the gastrointestinal tract.

C.   Does Nasal Air Conditioning Impact the Lower Airways?

In agreement with Galen (1), we make the assumption that the air-conditioning functions of the nose are important for the health of the lower airways. The evidence supporting this concept is based on clinical situations or experiments that involve bypassing of the nasal passages. Unfortunately, the value of monitoring nasal function to identify individuals with impairment or to establish pharmacological means of manipulating the air-conditioning functions of the nose has not been established. However, as discussed below some data have been generated.

The most dramatic example of the contribution of the upper airways to the health of the lungs is seen in patients who have undergone laryngectomy and have chronic tracheostomy. In the absence of an upper airway in series with the lungs, these individuals frequently develop chronic bronchitis, squamous metaplasia of the trachea and major bronchi, and grossly impaired mucociliary clearance of the major airways (30,31). Bacterial colonization is frequently present and is related to the presence of the tracheostomy, not to the underlying disease that led to the chronic tracheostomized condition (32). Ultrastructural evaluations of the mucosa reveal the presence of giant cilia, compound cilia, and microplicae (33). The most impressive finding is the abundance of giant cilia, which seem to be outgrowths of normal cilia, and it is unlikely that they can produce a transport function coordinated in direction and time (34). Mucus aspirated from tracheostomies contains epithelial glycoprotein that accounts for 25% of all dialyzable material; this is virtually absent in normal tracheobronchial mucus (35).

A number of studies have demonstrated significantly increased lower airway resistance during oral breathing resulting from pathological nasal obstruction (36–38). Similarly, artificial nasal obstruction produced with nasal packing for 96 h resulted in increased pulmonary resistance in a group of five healthy subjects (39). When obstructing nasal pathology was relieved by means of a nasal vasoconstrictor, surgery, or nasal crust removal, lower airway resistance diminished (36). Also, nasal obstruction leads to a decrease in lung compliance and an increase in functional residual capacity (FRC), while resolution of nasal obstruction results in an increase in compliance associated with a decrease in FRC. The mechanism of these phenomena is not understood. One could speculate that poorly conditioned air reaching the lower airways can generate such functional changes, or that the lack of airflow through the nose or the increased airflow through the mouth can alter the state of the lower airways through a neural reflex. An alternative explanation could be that the nasal passages supply inhaled air with a product that modifies lower airways caliber and/or the dynamic properties of the lung. Some investigators have proposed a role for nitric oxide in this context (see later) (40,41).

The importance of nasal air conditioning is emphasized by exercise studies of asthmatic children and young adults, which show that nasal breathing prevents the bronchial obstruction seen with oral or spontaneous breathing (Fig. 1) (42–44). These observations are in agreement with clinical experience, which indicates that athletes with asthma benefit from nasal breathing whenever possible during exercise, to minimize the bypassing of nasal air conditioning that occurs with mouth breathing. Consistently with these observations, studies have shown that less airway obstruction occurs when exercise is conducted under warm and humid air conditions (45,46).

The role of nasal air filtration (contaminating gases dissolving in nasal secretions or particles being trapped by the mucus layer) on the function of the lower airways is less studied. Yet, most investigators in the field would agree that, by bypassing the nose, mouth breathers deposit more particles in the lungs and may increase the risk of pulmonary damage (47). In the case of chronic tracheostomy, this is manifested in the observation that the tracheobronchial mucus is highly colonized by various bacteria that are absent in the normal state (32). In work by Speizer and Frank, human subjects inhaled sulfur dioxide for 10 min, either through the nose or the mouth, while lower respiratory function was monitored (48). Pulmonary resistance increased more during oral than nasal sulfur dioxide administration, suggesting that nasal filtration of sulfur dioxide reduces lung deposition.

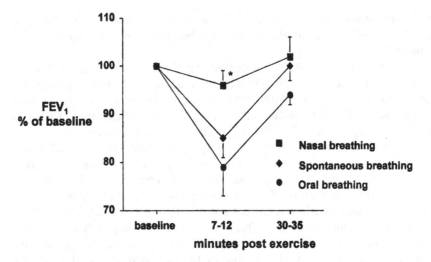

Figure 1 The effect of nasal breathing on exercise-induced bronchospasm in 12 children with mild to moderate non-steroid-dependent asthma. Three exercise (treadmill walking with a moderate workload achieving 75–80% of maximal heart rate) tests were performed in random order, utilizing different routes of breathing: oropharyngeal (spontaneous) breathing, oral breathing, and nasal breathing. Minute ventilation and heart rate tracings were not different among the three trials. The reduction in FEV_1 from baseline at the 7 to 12 min period was significantly lower with nasal breathing than with either spontaneous or oral breathing. (Modified with permission from Ref. 42.)

The matter of filtration of allergens by the nose is complicated. A simplistic thought would be to expect that allergic asthmatics should protect themselves by using the nasal passages as a filter to reduce allergen penetration into the lower airways. However, the only existing evidence in this regard argues against a protective role of nasal breathing. This evidence comes from a small group of asthma patients exposed to cat allergen for one hour, with and without a nose clip (49). In that study, the impact of allergen on the lower airways was the same with or without the use of the nasal passages. Since the vast majority of allergic asthmatics suffer from rhinitis (50,51), when allergenic particles are trapped by the nasal mucosa, one can expect local allergic reactions to occur. It is possible, as will be discussed shortly, that these nasal reactions affect the lower airways by causing bronchoconstriction through some form of nose–lung interaction. If so, any benefit that may have been obtained by nasal particle trapping and by reduction of direct deposit of allergen in the lower airways may be canceled by the detrimental effect of the allergic reaction in the nose.

D. Does Impaired Nasal Mucosal Air Conditioning Exist? How Does it Impact the Lower Airways?

Based on our understanding of nasal physiology and pathology, one would predict that several nosological entities may be associated with impaired nasal mucosal air-conditioning function. These entities are diseases that affect the structure and function of the nasal epithelium, as they pertain to water transportation and mucus production. Also, illnesses that reduce the ability of the mucosa to engorge (i.e., conditions impairing vascular function) would be expected to have similar effects. In theory, such conditions could include cystic fibrosis, atrophic rhinitis (ozena or excessive surgery), changes that occur in the nasal mucosa during aging, extensive squamous metaplasia of the nasal epithelium (perhaps as a result of a long history of smoking or exposure to high concentrations of industrial dust), and even Sjögren's syndrome, in which there is extensive reduction of the number of nasal submucosal glands (52). Except for some early work regarding nasal particle trapping in industrial workers, these conditions have not been investigated with respect to the presence of impaired nasal air conditioning. Such work needs to be conducted in the future. However, indirect evidence has started to emerge identifying potential abnormalities in various other populations.

Impaired Air Filtration

In the early part of the twentieth century, work by Lehman raised the possibility that impaired nasal clearance was associated with lung disease (53). Lehman devised a method through which air containing dust particles was insufflated under various flow rates in the nose of breath-holding humans. Since no breathing was taking place, the air exited through the mouth, where it was collected and analyzed for dust content. The difference in dust content between the air administered into the nose and the air captured at the oral orifice represented the particle-trapping capability of the nose and perhaps the nasopharyngeal, oropharyngeal, and oral mucosa. With these studies, Lehman was impressed by the wide variation in particle retention that he could observe consistently among healthy humans. He was further able to associate a disease state with reduced particle-trapping capability of the upper airway. He performed this test in a large population ($n = 426$) of miners, of whom 241 had the diagnosis of silicosis and 185 were considered healthy. Of the healthy workers, 63% had retention efficiencies over 40% and 18% of them were below a 30% efficiency limit. In the miners with established diagnosis of silicosis, only 20% had retention rates exceeding 40% (Fig. 2). These findings raised two possibilities: perhaps low retention rates were predisposing to silicosis as a result of larger numbers

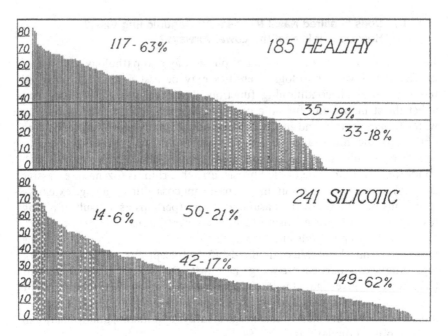

Figure 2 Decreased particle trapping efficiency by the nasal passages of miners with silicosis, compared with healthy miners. Every vertical line represents a single individual. The vertical axis represent retention efficiencies. Most healthy miners (63%) show retention efficiency above 40%; only 18% of this group had retention efficiency less than 30%. In the miners with silicosis, 21% show retention efficiency above 40% and 62% below 30%. (Reproduced with permission from Ref. 53.)

of particles reaching the lower airways; alternatively, the development of silicosis might have been associated with epithelial alterations along the entire respiratory tract, including the upper airways. Unfortunately, no prospective trials have been conducted in which workers exposed to high content of particles in inhaled air would undergo nasal testing before employment begins and longitudinally, during the time of exposure.

Decreased nasal mucociliary clearance has been observed in approximately 20% of healthy adults (47,54). The factors that determine this variability are not known. According to Andersen, Proctor, and their colleagues, who examined monozygotic twins (55), mucociliary clearance shows little evidence of heritability; these investigators claim that environmental history plays a significant role in this physiological function of the nasal mucosa. There is also evidence that individuals with chronic nasal disease suffer from decreased mucociliary clearance. In the work by Stanley and colleagues (56), all individuals with perennial rhinitis (allergic and nonallergic) as well as those with "chronic infected rhinosinusitis" had longer mucociliary clearance times, as assessed by the saccharin test, in comparison to healthy controls. When subjects with nasal/sinus involvement but no history of asthma were compared with those with asthma, and mean values were examined, mucociliary clearances did not differ. However, grossly prolonged clearance (>60 min) occurred in significantly more subjects diagnosed with "chronic infected rhinosinusitis" and, even more so, in those with "chronic infected rhinosinusitis and bronchiectasis" in comparison to all other tested groups. Microscopic evaluation of nasal cilia failed to demonstrate an intrinsic ciliary defect; it was concluded that the in vivo observations were secondary to factors associated with the consistency of mucus. The question of whether chronic bronchiectasis in these individuals could be a consequence of severe problems of nasal function remains unanswered. The sinobronchial syndrome (purulent rhinosinusitis and chronic bronchitis/bronchiectasis) is extensively discussed in Chapter 17.

Nasal Secretory Hyporesponsiveness

Recently, we have come across an interesting observation: individuals with refractory rhinosinusitis appear to have decreased secretory responsiveness to nasal histamine stimulation, compared with healthy controls (57). This finding is impressive because the nasal mucosa of these individuals is also characterized by a high level of mucosal inflammation. In other inflammatory conditions, such as perennial allergic rhinitis, nasal responsiveness is increased (58). In the refractory rhinosinusitis group, the degree of hyporesponsiveness to histamine correlates well with other nasal abnormalities such as the reduction in olfactory ability, suggesting that hyporesponsiveness is related to the severity of this condition. We have observed the same degree of secretory hyporesponsiveness in elderly individuals (> 70 years of age) who are devoid of chronic nasal or sinus disease (59). In this group, we also found that the secretory response to nasal methacholine provocation was diminished. Furthermore, when hyperosmolar mannitol was placed in the nose of elderly subjects and was allowed to dwell for 10 s, the osmolarity of the returned solution was reduced to a lesser extent than the reduction (correction) we observed in the control "young" group. This observation indicates that the difference between the younger and the older subjects may lie at the level of the nasal epithelium, the source of water for air humidification (and, in our case, for diluting the hyperosmolar mannitol). Since the secretions induced by histamine and methacholine probably derive from nasal glands, and since glands are made of specialized epithelium, epithelial function may be implicated in these observations. It is important to note that the secretory hyporesponsiveness phenomenon does not involve the sensory nerves of the nose: the sneezing response to histamine in both refractory rhinosinusitis and the elderly was not reduced, compared with the control groups. In contrast, in the hyperresponsive state of the nose associated with perennial allergic rhinitis, it is primarily the sensorineural apparatus that appears to be affected (58,60).

Impaired Air Warming and Humidification

Almost two decades ago, we identified a population of otherwise healthy adults who developed strong nasal reactions (rhinorrhea, congestion, burning), when inhaling cold, dry air (CDA) (61). The reaction to CDA is not secondary to nonspecific nasal hyperresponsiveness because the nasal response to histamine was not different between subjects with CDA sensitivity and those without (62). By a number of observations, however, individuals sensitive to nasal CDA could be clearly differentiated from those who had no nasal complaints upon exposure to the same stimulus. First, a reaction to CDA was associated with increased inflammatory mediators in nasal lavage fluids, their pattern identifying mast cells as the most logical source (61,63,64). Second, the nasal secretions of these individuals, after exposure to CDA, became hyperosmolar (65). This was in striking contrast with the CDA nonresponders, in whom no increase in the osmolarity was observed. Third, when the nasal mucosa of CDA-sensitive subjects was exposed to another hyperosmolar stimulus (high concentration mannitol solution), the response observed was stronger than that in the CDA nonresponders (62). Finally, we have recently found that when CDA-sensitive subjects are exposed to CDA, large numbers of epithelial cells are shed in nasal secretions, in contrast, again, to the CDA-nonresponder group (66). Our interpretation of these findings is that individuals who are sensitive to the effects of CDA have a defect in their ability to condition inhaled air, when a large amount of water needs to be given up. As a result of the exposure to CDA, water is lost into inhaled air faster than it can be replaced. The surface epithelium reaches a state of desiccation, and cells are shed. The hyperosmolar environment triggers sensory nerves, as well as mast cells, leading to the generation of a compensatory glandular response, expressed with the excessive rhinorrhea that eventually develops. Although this hypothesis is based on circumstantial evidence, it raises a good possibility that the phenomenon of nasal CDA reactivity is a manifestation of impairment in nasal air conditioning.

Recently, a methodology to assess the air-conditioning ability of the human nasal mucosa has been developed (67). A nasopharyngeal probe carrying sensors for temperature and for relative humidity is inserted through one nostril and positioned in the posterior nasopharynx in a manner that exposes the sensors to the airstream, but does not permit them to contact the airway mucosa. Air at different temperatures, flow rates, and relative humidities is passed through the nose, and measurements of its condition are made in the nasopharynx, at steady state. Knowing the temperature and the relative humidity of the air prior to its entry in the nasal passage and at the nasopharynx allows for calculation of the absolute water gradient along the nasal airways and, therefore, of the amount of water and heat given up by the nasal passages. Attempts to develop similar systems to assess the nasal air-conditioning capacity have been made in the past (3,4,6,8), but the new methodology appears to be the most promising from the perspective of standardization, thus allowing for physiological or pharmacological manipulation (17,68).

The investigators who developed the probe methodology have reported several interesting observations. First, patients with seasonal allergic rhinitis, when asymptomatic, have diminished ability to humidify and warm inhaled air (67). Second, this diminished ability is corrected after a nasal allergen challenge; also, it is absent in patients with active, perennial allergic rhinitis (26,69). These data raise the possibility that the allergic state is associated with impairment of the nasal air-conditioning capacity, but the development or presence of allergic inflammation corrects this problem, perhaps because of increased ease of plasma transudation into the lumina of the airways. Alternatively, mucosal inflammation may upregulate Cl^- ion fluxes from the epithelium into the lumina of the airways, thus facilitating water transportation and increasing the air-conditioning capacity of the nose (23,24). The most interesting observation that has been generated by these investigators is that the nasal mucosa of asthmatic subjects has reduced ability to condition inhaled air (Fig. 3) (69). The impairment in asthmatics was positively associated with the severity status of their airways disease, whether this was assessed through the Aas score or the guidelines of the National Heart, Lung, and Blood Institute–National Asthma Education Program (NHLBI/NAEP). Unfortunately, the work presented so far has not elucidated whether the detected problem in asthmatics is independent of the degree of nasal mucosal inflammation. Therefore, it is impossible to assess whether these data support the possibility that impaired nasal mucosal function (specifically with respect to air conditioning) is associated with rhinitis and asthma in a stepwise progressive fashion. However, in relation to this hypothesis, it is worth pointing out two additional, perhaps circumstantial, findings: (1) in an epidemiological study, Annesi and co-workers showed that subjects reporting nasal sensitivity to cold, dry air had a more rapid decline in forced expiratory volume in one second (FEV_1) over 5 years than did those without such sensitivity (70), and (2) in our hands,

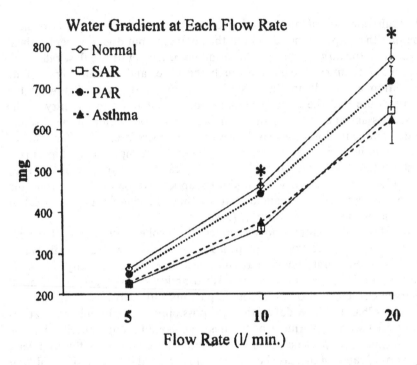

Figure 3 Differences (gradient) in the water content of air between the entrance of the nostril and the nasopharynx, determined by a nasopharyngeal probe equipped with temperature and relative humidity sensors. Cold, dry air at various flows (horizontal axis) is administered in four groups of volunteers: healthy individuals (Normal, $n = 15$), subjects with seasonal allergic rhinitis tested out of their respective pollen season (SAR, $n = 15$), subjects with perennial allergic rhinitis (PAR, $n = 15$), and individuals with asthma ($n = 15$). At flows of 10 and 20 L/min, the SAR and the asthma groups show lower water gradients than the normal subjects. This indicates that the amount of water delivered to the inhaled air by the nasal mucosa of the SAR and asthma subjects was reduced. (Reproduced with permission from Ref. 69.)

nasal provocation with CDA produces a stronger symptomatic response in individuals with allergic rhinitis and asthma than in those with allergic rhinitis alone (71).

Theoretical Considerations on the Impact of Nasal Dysfunction on the Lower Airways

In individuals with healthy lungs at resting breathing conditions, the impact of impaired or even absent nasal function is not known. In a comprehensive review of nasal physiology and its impact on the lower airways, Proctor posed the following question: "Might only a relative failure of nasal function over a period of years lead either to an increased susceptibility to disease or to a gradual deleterious change in the pulmonary airways?" (47). The same question should be asked for individuals who already suffer from a lower airways ailment. In the absence of direct evidence, which will require prospective evaluations, these questions cannot be answered. Yet, one can envision the impact on the lower airways of failed nasal function, especially in individuals who may be chronically exposed to extreme environmental conditions such as cold, dry climates. The large airways beyond those of the nose are not adequately equipped to compensate for defective nasal air conditioning. Their diameter is large, the air moves relatively rapidly through them and their mucosa does not have the vascular apparatus that can rapidly adjust to thermal/water demands. On the other hand, the small airways, which are characterized by a huge surface area, and in which the air moves at much lower speed, seem ideal for completion of the air-conditioning task. However, small airways lack mucus-secreting cells, have sparse cilia, and are covered by thin, serous epithelial lining fluid. Even small water losses may lead to desiccation and cellular damage. Also, chronic deposition of unwanted particles may lead to increased numbers of goblet cells, producing thicker secretions. The ciliary apparatus may not be able to handle increased mucus production, and clearance may come to a halt, leading to obstruction. Such a theory, if proven correct, could explain the increasing evidence that the earliest changes in a variety of airway conditions, including asthma, occur in the small airways (72,73).

II. Neural Responses of the Nose

The nasal mucosa has an abundance of sensory nerve endings, all of which have simple arborizations and appear to belong to the slow-conducting, C-fiber group. These fibers act as nociceptors; that is, they respond to environmental irritants. The molecular basis of these responses is not understood. The nasal sensory fibers travel through the trigeminal nerve to the central nervous system, and the efferent pathways include para-sympathetic and sympathetic fibers (see Chapter 1 for detailed discussion of nasal airway innervation).

Sensory nerves generate defensive responses that are of importance for the respiratory tract. These responses are primarily of central reflex nature and can result in typical rhinitis symptoms such as sneezing, glandular activation, and nasal congestion, which aim at expelling unwanted materials that enter the respiratory tree. From this perspective, the neural function of the nose can be quite important for the health of the lower airways. These responses are exaggerated in the presence of chronic allergic inflammation. In individuals with perennial allergic rhinitis, the sneezing response to histamine is about four to five times more potent than that of healthy subjects (74). Also, an induced allergic reaction in the nose results in a significant increase in the sneezing responsiveness to histamine, a phenomenon that is fully inhibitable by glucocorticosteroid treatment (75). The secretory responses to neural stimuli are also upregulated in chronic allergic inflammatory states. Capsaicin, for example, when delivered onto the nasal mucosa in only one nostril, generates secretory responses in both nostrils, ipsilateral and contralateral to its application site (74). Both the ipsilateral and the contralateral responses to capsaicin are approximately 100-fold stronger in subjects with perennial allergic rhinitis, than in healthy controls. Similarly, unilateral application of a hyperosmolar stimulus can induce bilateral secretory responses that are stronger in subjects with active allergic rhinitis than in controls (58). Analogous data with bradykinin have been published by Riccio and colleagues (76). In our hands, secretory hyperresponsiveness to methacholine, a direct stimulus to the nasal glands, is not present (58), supporting the notion that the hyperresponsiveness to capsaicin and to hyperosmolarity is secondary to neural and not glandular upregulation. Other investigators have reported conflicting data in this respect (77,78).

In addition, nasal sensory nerves may play an effector role through which they may generate even more mucosal secretions than through a central reflex and may induce local inflammation. This function manifests itself through the phenomenon of antidromic stimulation or axon reflex. Axon reflexes are produced when the action potentials generated at a nerve ending by a stimulus travel antidromically, through a collateral sensory nerve arborization, and activate other nerve endings to release inflammatory neuropeptides prestored in small granules (79–81). The human nasal mucosa has an abundance of such neuropeptides, including the tachykinins substance P and neurokinin A, as well as calcitonin gene-related peptide (CGRP), gastrin-releasing peptide (GRP) and others (82–85). It is presumed that most of these peptides are carried by C fibers. Neuropeptides can cause glandular secretion, plasma extravasation, and leukocyte recruitment (86–88). Neuropeptides can be also released by direct activation of the vanilloid receptor by capsaicin or its analogues (89,90). Stimulation of the human nose by capsaicin causes pain and nasal secretions. At higher concentrations, acute plasma extravasation and a late (peaking at 4 h) influx of leukocytes can be observed (91–93), supporting the notion that neuropeptides are released by the sensorineural endings. Although the release of neuropeptides has not been demonstrated in humans with nasal capsaicin challenge, these substances have been detected in human nasal secretions after allergen and after hyperosmolar nasal stimulation (94,95).

Neural reflexes generated at the level of the nasal mucosa may also affect the lower airways. In general, such a phenomenon manifests itself with transient bronchoconstriction resulting from irritant stimulation of nasal afferent nerves and has been termed "nasobronchial reflex." Significant debate still exists as to the existence of such a reflex in humans. This matter is examined in detail in Chapter 3, and some aspects are also discussed in the next section of this chapter. Teleologically, the existence of nasobronchial reflexes makes a lot of sense. Since the nasal mucosa is the first part of the respiratory tract to come in contact with an irritant, it should not only generate a local response to block this irritant's penetration into the remaining airways, but should "prepare" the lower airways to defend themselves, as well. The observed pattern of a transient bronchoconstrictive response fits such a function.

III. The Nose and Nitric Oxide

In 1994 Lundberg and colleagues reported that the levels of nitric oxide (NO) in nasally exhaled air are higher than the levels in orally exhaled air, indicating that the upper airways are a significant source of NO production (96). This work was supported by later studies from other groups (97). Most importantly, Lundberg demonstrated that the levels of NO in the human paranasal sinuses are very high (98) and argued that most NO in nasally exhaled air derives from the sinuses (40). In 1999 Haight et al. argued that 88% of nasal NO was derived from the nose itself, but this study was performed on only one individual, in whom the paranasal sinus ostia had been endoscopically obstructed (99). Even more recently, Weitzberg and Lundberg demonstrated that compared with quiet breathing, humming results in 15-fold elevated concentrations of NO in nasally exhaled air. In contrast, phonation during oral exhalation does not affect the levels of NO in orally exhaled air (100). This finding argues that air oscillations generated in the nasal cavities can increase the exchange of air between the sinuses and the nasal cavity and can enrich nasal air with high concentrations of NO.

Immunohistochemistry and in situ hybridization have demonstrated that inducible NO synthase (iNOS or NOS2) is constitutively expressed and produced by the apical portion of paranasal sinus epithelium, in the absence of an inflammatory condition; it was also shown that the NO synthase (NOS) activity in sinus epithelium is calcium independent, another characteristic of NOS2, but resistant to glucocorticosteroids, uncharacteristic of NOS2 (98,101). In other words, there is evidence to suggest that the production of NO by the paranasal sinuses is under the control of a unique enzymatic activity that has many, but not all, characteristics of NOS2. This could be interpreted as a sign that paranasal sinus NO has a distinct physiological role. In the nasal mucosa, almost all constitutive NOS activity appears to be calcium dependent (102).

The role of NO produced in the upper airways is not understood. Yet, there is enough evidence to raise the hypothesis that it plays a protective role for the entire respiratory tree. This is not only because upper airway NO may regulate aspects of upper airway function (e.g., nasal vascular tone) but because it may be continuously inhaled into the lower airways to exert various beneficial effects (103,104). Several researchers have shown that NO has antiviral and bacteriostatic activity, which would make it a prime candidate of innate immunity in the respiratory tract (105–109). It is also worth mentioning the study by Lundberg and colleagues in which air was collected from the nasal passages of intubated adults and injected back into the endotracheal tube, with immediate improvement in blood oxygenation (41).

Högman et al. have shown that NO introduced into the ventilatory circuit of intubated rabbits has a bronchodilatory effect against methacholine (110). In humans, the same authors showed a slight bronchodilatory effect, evident only in the course of bronchoprovocation with methacholine (111). Kacmarek et al. demonstrated that inhaled NO leads to bronchodilation in subjects with asthma and mild airways hyperresponsiveness to methacholine (112). Individuals with severe hyperresponsiveness ($PC_{20} < 1$ mg/mL) did not show improvement in lung function with NO. In both animals and humans, inhibition of NO synthesis results in increased airways responsiveness against a variety of stimuli (113–116). In the case of bradykinin-induced airway obstruction, for example, not only does NO synthesis inhibition increase airways responsiveness in humans (116), but after inhibition of NO synthesis, an allergen provocation cannot further increase airways responsiveness (117). This indicates that allergen-induced increases in airways responsiveness are also mediated by inhibition of protective NO pathways.

It is not clear whether the source of NO plays a role in the apparent protective effect of this molecule. However, since most NO in exhaled air probably derives from the upper airways, it is reasonable to hypothesize that NO generated from the paranasal sinuses and the nose is important. As an example, it is worth reporting an observation we have made in examining the bronchoprotective effects of deep inspiration, the loss of which appears to be crucial in the development of bronchial hyperresponsiveness (118,119). Deep inspirations have better bronchoprotective effect in healthy subjects when they are taken through the nose, with mouth closed, than through the mouth, with the nose clip in place.

Several chronic inflammatory conditions of the nose and sinuses have been associated with reduced or absent NO production. These include cystic fibrosis (120–123), diffuse panbronchiolitis (sinobronchial syndrome) (124), Kartagener's syndrome (96), and chronic sinusitis with or without polyposis (125,126). Most of these conditions are associated with lower airways disease.

IV. Impact of Nasal Stimulation on the Lower Airways

The coexistence of asthma and rhinitis [the vast majority of patients with asthma also have rhinitis (50,51)], most frequently with the rhinitis predating asthma, raises the hypothesis that nasal abnormalities initiate and perpetuate lower airway disease. This hypothesis was first put forward by Sluder, who, in 1919, suggested that nasal reflexes can initiate asthma (127). The overall concept that nasal abnormalities may impact on the lower airways is very logical, given our understanding of nasal airway physiology and the potential impact this may have on the function of the lungs (see earlier). While the epidemiological data are provocative, it is only through controlled laboratory experimentation that a true cause-and-effect relationship can be established. A rational approach to test the hypothesis of a nose–lung interaction is to stimulate or inflame the nose using an in vivo laboratory challenge procedure while monitoring the lower airways.

A. Irritant Nasal Challenge

Application of irritants in the nasal mucosa of animals consistently produces increases in tracheobronchial airway resistance. Human studies have used silica particles (128,129), white pepper powder (130,131), histamine (132–134), and methacholine (135) to stimulate the nasal mucosa and monitor the lower airways. Unlike the work in animals, these human studies have not consistently demonstrated the presence of nose–lung interactions.

In the work of Kaufman, all 10 healthy subjects undergoing a blinded nasal challenge with aerosolized crystalline silica experienced within 10 min a significant elevation of lower airway resistance measured by body plethysmography (128). Pretreatment with subcutaneous atropine blocked the increase in resistance, presumably by inhibiting a vagal efferent pathway. A follow-up study by this group used subjects who were status post–unilateral interruption of the second division of the trigeminal nerve as models of afferent impulse blockade (129). Exposure of the denervated side with aerosolized silica had no effect on pulmonary resistance. On the other hand, silica challenge of the neurologically intact side resulted in significant elevation of resistance in all subjects.

Sato dusted white pepper powder into both nasal cavities of healthy subjects, causing a significant increase in lower airway resistance (130). In a group of laryngectomized subjects, the same stimulation resulted in diminished lung resistance, raising the possibility that the findings in healthy subjects may have been secondary to inadvertent passing of pepper powder through to the larynx, causing laryngeal constriction. Yet, Konno and colleagues, in a subsequent study, demonstrated a statistically significant increase in pulmonary resistance after applying pepper powder in the nose of laryngectomized subjects (131).

Yan and Salome published the results of an uncontrolled study in which histamine nasal challenge led to a greater than 15% fall in FEV_1 in 7 of 12 subjects with asthma (132). More recent work by other investigators did not reproduce these findings (133,134). The positive study by Yan and Salome, although not incorporating a sham challenge, used subjects with perennial rather than seasonal rhinitis studied out of season. This feature of the study design may have taken advantage of the ongoing inflammation of the nasal mucosa. Littell et al. (135) challenged their subjects with intranasal methacholine and found an increase in lower airway resistance. The increased resistance was associated with flushing and salivation, suggestive of systemic absorption of the cholinergic stimulus. In fact, the pulmonary response was blocked by a nasal vasoconstrictor given prior to the nasal methacholine challenge.

B. Physical Stimulation of the Upper Airway

In 1973 Rodriguez-Martinez and colleagues demonstrated that nasal pretreatment with 4% lidocaine prevented the fall in FEV_1 provoked by environmental exposure to cold air in children with asthma (136). In 1983 Nolte and Berger reported that cold air in the nose resulted in immediate bronchoconstriction in 25 of 27 asthmatics, but none of 7 healthy subjects (137). Nolte and Berger also detected bronchoconstriction in laryngectomized asthmatics, consistent with the notion of a neural reflex mechanism initiated in the nose. In agreement with the foregoing studies, Fontanari and colleagues used a model in which bursts of cold, dry air or dry air alone were insufflated through the nose, eliciting significant increases in lower airways resistance (138,139). Local anesthesia to the nose or inhaled atropine blocked the nasal cold air stimulation effect on the lower airways, supporting the concept of a central reflex mediated through the trigeminal (afferent arm) and the vagus (efferent arm) nerves. These investigators could not differentiate asthmatics from healthy subjects with respect to the response to nasal cold air irritation (139). Koskela and colleagues have suggested that the lower airways responses to nasal cold air inhalation originate from sensory nerves of the facial skin, not the nasal mucosa (140). The possibility that oropharyngeal stimulation with cold air can initiate lower airways responses has been tested and has not been supported by most studies (43,138,141).

C. Allergen Nasal Challenge

Seasonal increases in bronchial responsiveness have been reported in patients with allergic rhinitis (142,143). Experimental models using allergen nasal provocation in asthmatics with seasonal allergic rhinitis have looked at changes in both airway caliber and lung responsiveness. From the start, such studies had to devise a way of ensuring that allergen is deposited only in the nasal passages, without passing into the lower airways. The methodology that Corren and his colleagues employed in their study was validated with the use of radioisotope tracings, which demonstrated lack of deposition into the lower airways (144).

Initial studies failed to show changes in pulmonary function despite profound upper airway stimulation with allergen (133,145,146). Subsequently, subjects with asthma and perennial rhinitis, rather than seasonal rhinitis, were evaluated on the assumption that nasal priming or simply more chronic nasal inflammation in these individuals would predispose them to a nose–lung interaction effect (147). Fifteen subjects were challenged with intranasally insufflated allergen. Pulmonary function tests were performed 30 min after nasal challenge. Although there was no overall group effect, 4 subjects had a fall in FEV_1 or FEF_{25-75} exceeding 15%. In another study performed by our group, a statistically significant reduction in both FEV_1 and forced vital capacity (FVC) was observed in a group of 12 asthmatics, 6 h after nasal allergen provocation. In some subjects, the nasal allergen–induced reduction in lung function was very impressive (Fig. 4). In that study, spirometry that was performed every 15 min for the first hour after the challenge showed no evidence of lower airway obstruction (148).

Investigators have also examined whether nasal allergen provocation has any effects on bronchial responsiveness. The original work in this area was performed by Corren and colleagues (144). Subjects in this study were required to have a history of worsening asthma symptoms during seasonal exacerbations of their rhinitis. The group of 10 asthmatics who participated in this study experienced a diurnal increase in methacholine PC_{20} over the course of the day following placebo nasal challenge. After nasal antigen challenge, no change in methacholine PC_{20} was observed. The conclusion was that nasal antigen challenge negatively affected bronchial responsiveness by eliminating the diurnal improvement in methacholine reactivity. Other groups also demonstrated increases in bronchial reactivity after nasal

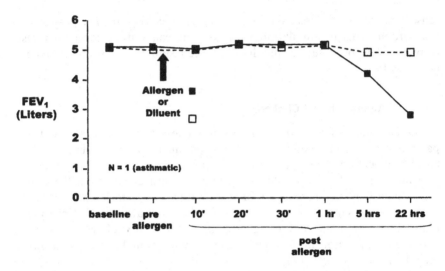

Figure 4 Nasal allergen provocation can cause substantial reductions in lung function that occur in the form of a late phase reaction, several hours after the provocation, as demonstrated by these FEV_1 data from a single individual with mild intermittent asthma and rhinitis. During the first hour after the nasal allergen provocation, no changes in lung function were observed. At 5 and 22 hs, lung function was markedly decreased. No fluctuations in FEV_1 were observed when a nasal provocation with the diluent was performed. No more than 30% of allergic asthmatics with rhinitis generate such responses after nasal allergen challenge. (Reproduced with permission from Ref. 155.)

antigen challenge (149,150). We have also attempted to assess the effects of nasal antigen challenge on lower airways responsiveness: in an unscreened population of 15 mild asthmatics with concomitant allergic rhinitis, we performed methacholine bronchoprovocation 2 h before antigen challenge, as well as at 1, 5, and 22 h after the nasal challenge (151). We found no effect of nasal allergen challenge on methacholine reactivity. However, the same subjects did not show changes in airways reactivity even with a whole-lung inhaled allergen provocation. When we selected asthmatics who had previously, on two consecutive occasions, demonstrated significant increases in airways responsiveness to methacholine 24 h after inhaled allergen provocation, we found that lower airways reactivity in these subjects could also be increased by a nasal allergen challenge.

The mechanisms through which the induction of allergic inflammation in the nasal passages may affect the lower airways within a few hours are not known. Some of the mechanisms through which the function of the nose may affect the function of the lower airways, as discussed in the early parts of this chapter, should be considered. These mechanisms include the loss of nasal air conditioning as a result of oral breathing or the generation of neural impulses initiated in the nasal passages with their efferent arm affecting the lower airway smooth muscle. In addition, one should not dismiss the possibility that inflammatory material secreted by the nasal mucosa drains into the lower airways, perhaps as a result of aspiration, primarily during nighttime (152). In humans, the aspiration hypothesis has been challenged (153).

Over the past few years, much interest has been generated around the hypothesis that allergic inflammation propagates from the upper to the lower airways via the systemic circulation. There is no question that various changes in peripheral blood can be documented following nasal allergen provocation. The changes include increases in peripheral blood eosinophilia (154,155). Recently, we have been able to demonstrate increased spontaneous expression of tumor necrosis factor α (TNF-α) mRNA, in basophil-depleted, peripheral blood leukocyte preparations, as well as increased spontaneous release of interleukin 13 in basophil-enriched preparations, between 3 and 24 h after three consecutive-day nasal allergen provocations, in subjects with seasonal allergic rhinitis, challenged out of the pollen season (156). Whole-lung allergen provocation also results in several peripheral

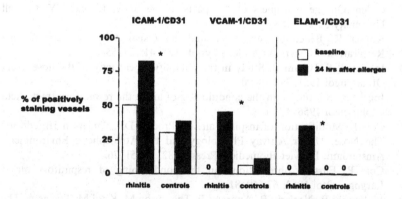

Figure 5 Nasal allergen provocation results in increased expression of vascular adhesion molecules in bronchial mucosa. Double immunohistochemistry for adhesion molecules and CD31 (endothelial marker) on bronchial biopsy samples obtained at baseline and 24 h after nasal allergen challenge in nine subjects with allergic rhinitis and in nine healthy, nonallergic controls. Bars represent median values, and asterisks indicate statistical significance over baseline. (Created from data presented in table form in Ref. 154.)

blood changes and, importantly, in changes that can be detected in the subjects' bone marrow (157,158). Studies of bone marrow aspirates following nasal allergen provocation have not been reported.

The most convincing evidence for systemic propagation of allergic inflammation, from the nose to the lung, derives from the work of Braunstahl and colleagues (154). In an elegant study, these investigators performed a nasal allergen provocation on subjects with allergic rhinitis and obtained both nasal and bronchial biopsy tissue prior to and 24 h after the allergen exposure. Their primary finding was that after the nasal provocation, the number of eosinophils was increased in the bronchial mucosa, concomitantly with an increase in the expression of various vascular adhesion molecules (Fig. 5). In another protocol, the same investigators demonstrated that if the allergen is to be directly placed in the lower airways through the wedged bronchoscope approach, eosinophil infiltration and other inflammatory changes will be detected not only in the bronchi, but in the nose, as well (159,160). These findings implicate the systemic route as a means through which allergic reactions can affect remote sites in a non-anaphylactic manner.

References

1. Galen. On the usefulness of the parts of the body. Ithaca, NY: Cornell University Press; 1968.
2. Kayser R. Bedeutung der Nase und der ersten Athmungswege für die Respiration. Pflugers Arch Ges Physiol 1887; 41:127–55.
3. Ingelstedt S, Ivstam B. Study in the humidifying capacity of the nose. Acta Otolaryngol 1951; 39:286–90.
4. Ingelstedt S. Studies on the conditioning of air in the respiratory tract. Acta Otolaryngol 1956; 131:1–80.
5. Cole P. Modification of inspired air. In: Proctor DF, Andersen IB, editors. The Nose. Upper Airway Physiology and the Atmospheric Environment. Amsterdam: Elsevier Biomedical Press; 1982. p. 351–76.
6. Cole P. Further observations on the conditioning of respiratory air. J Laryngol Otol 1953; 67:669–81.
7. Jankowski R, Naclerio R, Andrews B, Thompson M, Knol M, Togias A. The ability of the nose to warm inhaled air is unrelated to its reactivity to cold dry air (CDA). J Allergy Clin Immunol 1993; 91:182 (abstract).
8. Cole P. Some aspects of temperature, moisture and heat relationships in the upper respiratory tract. J Laryngol Otol 1953; 67:449–56.
9. Cole P. Respiratory mucosal vascular responses, air conditioning and thermo regulation. J Laryngol Otol 1954; 68:613–22.

10. Baroody F, Naclerio R. A review of anatomy and physiology of the nose. A self-instructional package from the Committee on Continuing Education in Otolaryngology. Alexandria, VA: American Academy of Otolaryngology– Head and Neck Surgery Foundation, Inc; 1990.

11. Dudley J, Cherry J. Scanning electron microscopic demonstration of goblet cell discharge and mucous layer on nasal ciliated respiratory epithelium. Otolaryngol Head Neck Surg 1980; 88:439–41.

12. Cauna N. Fine structure of the arteriovenous anastomosis and its nerve supply in the human nasal respiratory mucosa. Anat Rec 1970; 168:9–22.

13. Cauna N, Cauna D. The fine structure and innervation of the cushion veins of the human nasal respiratory mucosa. Anat Rec 1975; 181:1–16.

14. Tos M. Goblet cells and glands in the nose and paranasal sinuses. In: Proctor DF, Andersen IB, editors. The Nose. Upper Airway Physiology and the Atmospheric Environment. Amsterdam: Elsevier Biomedical Press; 1982, p. 99–144.

15. Drettner B, Falck B, Simon H. Measurements of the air conditioning capacity of the nose during normal and pathological conditions and pharmacological influence. Acta Otolaryngol 1977; 84:266–77.

16. Kumlien J, Drettner B. The effect of ipratropium bromide (Atrovent) on the air conditioning capacity of the nose. Clin Otolaryngol 1985; 10:165–8.

17. Assanasen P, Baroody F, Rouadi P, Naureckas E, Solway J, Naclerio R. Ipratropium bromide increases the ability of the nose to warm and humidify air. Am J Respir Crit Care Med 2000; 162:1031–7.

18. Cauna N. Blood and nerve supply of the nasal lining. In: Proctor DF, Andersen IB, editors. The Nose. Upper Airway Physiology and the Atmospheric Environment. Amsterdam: Elsevier Biomedical Press; 1982. p. 44–69.

19. Ingelstedt S, Ivstam B. The source of nasal secretion in infectious, allergic, and experimental conditions. Acta Otolaryngol 1949; 37:451–5.

20. Yankaskas J, Gatzy J, Boucher R. Effects of raised osmolarity on canine tracheal epithelial ion transport function. J Appl Physiol 1987; 62:2241–5.

21. Kaliner M, Marom Z, Patow C, Shelhamer J. Human respiratory mucus. J Allergy Clin Immunol 1984; 73:318–23.

22. Knowles M, Clark C, Fischer N, Fisher S, Kenan P, Pillsbury H, et al. Nasal secretions: role of epithelial ion transport. In: Mygind N, Pipkorn U, editors. Allergic and Vasomotor Rhinitis: Pathophysiological Aspects. Copenhagen: Munksgaard; 1983. p. 77–90.

23. Welsh M. Electrolyte transport by airway epithelia. Physiol Rev 1987; 67: 1143–84.

24. Boucher R, Chang E, Paradiso A, Strutts M, Knowles M, Earp H. Chloride secretory response of cystic fibrosis human airway epithelia. J Clin Invest 1989; 84:1424–31.

25. Cruz A, Naclerio R, Lichtenstein L, Togias A. Further support for the role of hypertonicity on mast cell activation during nasal dry air reactions. Clin Research 1990; 38:484A (abstract).

26. Assanasen P, Baroody F, Abbott D, Naureckas E, Solway J, Naclerio R. Natural and induced allergic responses increase the ability of the nose to warm and humidify air. J Allergy Clin Immunol 2000; 106:1045–52.

27. Brain JD, Valberg PA. Deposition of aerosol in the respiratory tract. Am Rev Respir Dis 1979; 120:1325–73.

28. Andersen I, Lundqvist G, Proctor D, Swift D. Human response to controlled levels of inert dust. Am Rev Respir Dis 1979; 119:619–27.

29. Hounam RF, Black A, Walsh M. Deposition of aerosol particles in the naso-pharyngeal region of the human respiratory tract. Nature 1969; 221:1254–5.

30. Matthews L, Spector S, Lemm J, Potter J. Studies on pulmonary secretions. 1. The over-all chemical composition of pulmonary secretions from patients with cystic fibrosis, bronchiectasis, and laryngectomy. Am Rev Respir Dis 1963; 88:199–204.

31. Potter J, LeRoy W, Spector S, Lemm J. Studies on pulmonary secretions. II. Osmolality and the ionic environment of pulmonary secretions from patients with cystic fibrosis, bronchiectasis, and laryngectomy. Am Rev Respir Dis 1967; 96:83–7.

32. Lusuardi M, Capelli A, Cerutti CG, Gnemmi I, Zaccaria S, Donner CF. Influence of clinical history on airways bacterial colonization in subjects with chronic tracheostomy. Respir Med 2000; 94:436–40.

33. Roessler F, Grossenbacher R, Walt H. Effects of tracheostomy on human tracheobronchial mucosa: a scanning electron microscopic study. Laryngo-scope 1988; 98:1261–7.

34. Roessler F, Grossenbacher R, Stanisic M, Walt H. Correlative histological and ultrastructural study of unusual changes in human tracheobronchial epithelium. Laryngoscope 1991; 101:473–9.

35. Bhaskar KR, O'Sullivan DD, Seltzer J, Rossing TH, Drazen JM, Reid LM. Density gradient study of bronchial mucous aspirates from healthy volunteers (smokers and nonsmokers) and from patients with tracheostomy. Exp Lung Res 1985; 9:289–308.

36. Ogura J, Nelson J, Dammkoehler R, Kawasaki M, Togawa K. Experimental observations of the relationships between upper airway obstruction and pulmonary function. Ann Otolaryngol 1964; 73:381–403.

37. Togawa K, Ogura J. Physiologic relationships between nasal breathing and pulmonary function. Laryngoscope 1966; 76:30–62.

38. Unno T, Nelson JR, Ogura JH. The effect of nasal obstruction on pulmonary, airway and tissue resistance. Laryngoscope 1968; 78:1119–39.

39. Wyllie JW, Kern EB, O' Brien PC, Hyatt RE. Alteration of pulmonary function associated with artificial nasal obstruction. Surg Forum 1976; 27:535–7.

40. Lundberg J, Rinder J, Weitzberg E, Lundberg J, Alving K. Nasally exhaled nitric oxide in humans originates mainly in the paranasal sinuses. Acta Physiol Scand 1994; 152:431–2.

41. Lundberg JO, Lundberg JM, Settergren G, Alving K, Weitzberg E. Nitric oxide, produced in the upper airways, may act in an "aerocrine" fashion to

enhance pulmonary oxygen uptake in humans. Acta Physiol Scand 1995; 155:467–8.

42. Shturman-Ellstein R, Zeballos R, Buckley J, Souhrada J. The beneficial effect of nasal breathing on exercise-induced bronchoconstriction. Am Rev Respir Dis 1978; 118:65–73.

43. Griffin M, McFadden E, Ingram R. Airway cooling in asthmatic and nonasthmatic subjects during nasal and oral breathing. J Allergy Clin Immunol 1982; 69:354–9.

44. Mangla PK, Menon MP. Effect of nasal and oral breathing on exercise-induced asthma. Clin Allergy 1981; 11:433–9.

45. Chen W, Horton D. Heat and water loss from the airways and exercise-induced asthma. Respiration 1977; 34:305–13.

46. Strauss R, McFadden E, Ingram R, Deal E, Jaeger J. Influence of heat and humidity in the airway obstruction induced by exercise in asthma. J Clin Invest 1978; 61:433–40.

47. Proctor D. The upper airways I. Nasal physiology and defense of the lungs. Am Rev Respir Dis 1977; 115:97–130.

48. Speizer R, Frank N. A comparison of changes in pulmonary flow resistance in healthy volunteers acutely exposed to SO_2 by mouth and by nose. Br J Ind Med 1966; 23:75–9.

49. Wood R, Eggleston P. The effects of intranasal steroids on nasal and pulmonary responses to cat exposure. Am J Respir Crit Care Med 1995; 151:315–20.

50. Kapsali T, Horowitz E, Togias A. Rhinitis is ubiquitous in allergic asthmatics. J Allergy Clin Immunol 1997; 99:S138 (abstract).

51. Horowitz E, Diemer FB, Poyser J, Rice V, Jean LG, Britt V, et al. Asthma and rhinosinusitis prevalence in a Baltimore city public housing complex. J Allergy Clin Immunol 2001; 107:S280 (abstract).

52. Jonsson R, Haga H-J, Gordon T. Current concepts on diagnosis, autoantibodies and therapy in Sjogren's syndrome. Scand J Rheumatol 2000; 29: 341–8.

53. Lehmann G. The dust filtering efficiency of the human nose and its significance in the causation of silicosis. J Ind Hyg 1935; 17:37–40.

54. Proctor D. The mucociliary system. In: Proctor DF, Andersen I, editors. The Nose. Upper Airway Physiology and the Atmospheric Environment. Amsterdam: Elsevier Biomedical Press; 1982. p. 245–78.

55. Andersen I, Camner P, Jensen P, Philipson K, Proctor D. Nasal clearance in monozygotic twins. Am Rev Respir Dis 1974; 110:301–5.

56. Stanley P, Wilson R, Greenstone M, Mackay I, Cole P. Abnormal nasal mucociliary clearance in patients with rhinitis and its relationship to concomitant chest disease. Br J Dis Chest 1985; 79:77–82.

57. Sampaio F, Leopold D, Proud D, Moylan B, Togias A. Determinants of the nasal secretory response to histamine (H) in refractory rhinosinusitis (RS). J Allergy Clin Immunol 1998; 101:S46 (abstract).

58. Sanico AM, Philip G, Lai G, Togias A. Hyperosmolar saline induces reflex

nasal secretions, evincing neural hyperresponsiveness in allergic rhinitis. J Appl Physiol 1999; 86:1202–10.

59. Togias A, Baroody F, Majchel A, Thompson M, Kagey-Sobotka A, Naclerio R. Aging is associated with decreased nasal mucosal secretory response. J Allergy Clin Immunol 1992; 89:302 (abstract).

60. Sanico A, Philip G, Proud D, Naclerio R, Togias A. Comparison of nasal mucosal responsiveness to neuronal stimulation in nonallergic and allergic rhinitis: effects of capsaicin nasal challenge. Clin Exp Allergy 1998; 28: 92–100.

61. Togias A, Naclerio R, Proud D, Fish J, Adkinson N, Kagey-Sobotka A, et al. Nasal challenge with cold, dry air results in the production of inflammatory mediators: possible mast cell involvement. J Clin Invest 1985; 76:1375–81.

62. Togias A, Eggleston P, A. K-S, Proud D, Lichtenstein L, Naclerio R. Hyperosmolar and histamine (H) nasal challenge of individuals with and without cold, dry air (CDA) sensitivity. J Allergy Clin Immunol 1989; 83:247.

63. Togias AG, Naclerio RM, Peters SP, Nimmagadda I, Proud D, Kagey-Sobotka A, et al. Local generation of sulfidopeptide leukotrienes upon nasal provocation with cold, dry air. Am Rev Respir Dis 1986; 133:1133–7.

64. Proud D, Bailey G, Naclerio R, Reynolds C, Cruz A, Eggleston P, et al. Tryptase and histamine as markers to evaluate mast cell activation during the responses to nasal challenge with allergen, cold, dry air, and hyperosmolar solutions. J Allergy Clin Immunol 1992; 89:1098–110.

65. Togias A, Proud D, Kagey-Sobotka A, Adams G, Norman P, Lichtenstein L, et al. The osmolality of nasal secretions increases when inflammatory mediators are released in response to inhalation of cold, dry air. Am Rev Respir Dis 1988; 137:625–9.

66. Cruz AA, Naclerio RM, Kagey-Sobotka A, Proud D, Togias A. Epithelial shedding, a feature of cold, dry air-induced rhinitis. Am J Respir Crit Care Med 2003; (In press).

67. Rouadi P, Barooody F, Abbott D, Naureckas E, Solway J, Naclerio R. A technique to measure the ability of the human nose to warm and humidify air. J Appl Physiol 1999; 87:400–6.

68. Abbott D, Baroody F, Naureckas E, Naclerio R. Elevation of nasal mucosal temperature increases the ability of the nose to warm and humidify air. Am J Rhinol 2001; 15:41–5.

69. Assanasen P, Baroody F, Naureckas E, Solway J, Naclerio R. The nasal passage of subjects with asthma has a decreased ability to warm and humidify inspired air. Am J Resp Crit Care Med 2001; 164:1640–6.

70. Annesi I, Neukirch F, Onoven-Friga E, Oryszcyn M, Korobaeff M, Dore M, et al. The relevance of hyperresponsiveness but not of atopy to FEV decline: Preliminary results in a working population. Bull Eur Physiopathol Resp 1987; 23:397–400.

71. Stephens L, Proud D, Togias A. Nasal cold, dry air (CDA) challenge results in stronger nasal and pulmonary responses in asthmatics compared to patients with rhinitis. J Allergy Clin Immunol 1996; 97:A315 (abstract).

72. Wagner E, Liu M, Weinmann G, Permutt S, Bleecker E. Peripheral lung resistance in normal and asthmatic subjects. Am Rev Respir Dis 1990; 141:584–8.

73. Carroll N, Elliot J, Morton A, James A. The structure of large and small airways in nonfatal and fatal asthma. Am Rev Respir Dis 1993; 147:405–10.

74. Sanico AM, Koliatsos VE, Stanisz AM, Bienenstock J, Togias A. Neural hyperresponsiveness and nerve growth factor in allergic rhinitis. Int Arch Allergy Immunol 1999; 118:153–8.

75. Baroody F, Cruz A, Lichtenstein L, Kagey-Sobotka A, Proud D, Naclerio R. Intranasal beclomethasone inhibits antigen-induced nasal hyperresponsiveness to histamine. J Allergy Clin Immunol 1992; 90:373–6.

76. Riccio M, Proud D. Evidence that enhanced nasal reactivity to bradykinin in patients with symptomatic allergy is mediated by neural reflexes. J Allergy Clin Immunol 1996; 97:1252–63.

77. Druce H, Wright R, Kossoff D, Kaliner M. Cholinergic nasal hyperreactivity in atopic subjects. J Allergy Clin Immunol 1985; 76:445–52.

78. van Wijk R. Perennial allergic rhinitis and nasal hyperreactivity. Am J Rhinol 1998; 12:33–5.

79. Pernow B. Role of tachykinins in neurogenic inflammation. J Immunology 1985; 135:812–5.

80. Barnes P. Neurogenic inflammation in airways. Int Arch Allergy Appl Immunol 1991; 94:303–9.

81. Meggs W. Neurogenic inflammation and sensitivity to environmental chemicals. Environ Health Perspect 1993; 101:234–8.

82. Lundberg J, Hokfelt T, Martling C, Saria A, Cuello C. Substance P–immunoreactive sensory nerves in the lower respiratory tract of various mammals including man. Cell Tissue Res 1984; 235:251–61.

83. Baraniuk J, Lundgren J, Goff J, Peden D, Merida M, Shelhamer J, et al. Gastrin-releasing peptide in human nasal mucosa. J Clin Invest 1990; 85:998–1005.

84. Baraniuk J, Lundgren J, Goff J, Mullol J, Castellino S, Merida M, et al. Calcitonin gene-related peptide in human nasal mucosa. Am J Physiol (Lung Mol Cell Physiol) 1990; 258:L81–L88.

85. Baraniuk J, Lundgren J, Okayama M, Goff J, Mullol J, Merida M, et al. Substance P and neurokinin A in human nasal mucosa. Am J Respir Cell Mol Biol 1991; 4:228–36.

86. Payan D. The role of neuropeptides in inflammation. In: Snyderman JI, editor. Inflammation: Basic Principles and Clinical Correlates. Second ed. New York: Raven Press; 1992. p. 177–91.

87. Carolan E, Casale T. Effects of neuropeptides on neutrophil migration through noncellular and endothelial barriers. J Allergy Clin Immunol 1993; 92:589–98.

88. Baluk P, Bertrand C, Geppetti P, McDonald D, Nadel J. NK1 receptors mediate leukocyte adhesion in neurogenic inflammation in the rat trachea. Am J Physiol 1995; 268:L263–9.

89. Szallasi A, Blumberg P. Vanilloid receptors: new insights enhance potential as a therapeutic target. Pain 1996; 68:195–208.
90. Caterina M, Schumachert M, Tominaga M, Rosen T, Levine J, Julius D. The capsaicin receptor: a heat-activated ion channel in the pain pathway. Nature 1997; 389:816–24.
91. Roche N, Lurie S, Authier S, Dusser D. Nasal response to capsaicin in patients with allergic rhinitis and in healthy volunteers: effect of colchicine. Am J Respir Crit Care Med 1995; 151:1151–8.
92. Philip G, Sanico A, Togias A. Inflammatory cellular influx follows capsaicin nasal challenge. Am J Respir Crit Care Med 1996; 153:1222–9.
93. Sanico A, Atsuta S, Proud D, Togias A. Dose-dependent effects of capsaicin nasal challenge: in vivo evidence of human airway neurogenic inflammation. J Allergy Clin Immunol 1997; 100:632–41.
94. Mosimann B, White M, Hohman R, Goldrich M, Kaulbach H, Kaliner M. Substance P, calcitonin gene-related peptide, and vasoactive intestinal peptide increase in nasal secretions after allergen challenge in atopic patients. J Allergy Clin Immunol 1993; 92:95–104.
95. Baraniuk J, Ali M, Yuta A, Fang S-Y, Naranch K. Hypertonic saline nasal provocation stimulates nociceptive nerves, substance P release, and glanduar mucous exocytosis in normal humans. Am J Respir Crit Care Med 1999; 160:655–62.
96. Lundberg JON, Weitzberg E, Nordvall SL, Kuylenstierna R, Lundberg JM, Alving K. Primarily nasal origin of exhaled nitric oxide and absence in Kartagener's syndrome. Eur Respir J 1994; 7:1501–4.
97. Kimberly B, Nejadnik B, Giraud G, Holden W. Nasal contribution to exhaled nitric oxide at rest and during breathholding in humans. Am J Respir Crit Care Med 1996; 153:829–36.
98. Lundberg J, Farkas-Szallasi T, Wetzberg E, Rinder J, Lidholm J, Anggard A, et al. High nitric oxide production in human paranasal sinuses. Nat Med 1995; 1:370–3.
99. Haight J, Djupesland P, Qjan W, Chatkin J, Furlott H, Irish J, et al. Does nasal nitric oxide come from the sinuses? J Otolaryngol 1999; 28:197–204.
100. Weitzberg E, Lundberg J. Humming greatly increases nasal nitric oxide. Am J Resp Crit Care Med 2002; 166:144–5.
101. Lundberg J, Weitzberg E, Rinder J, Rudehill A, Jansson O, Wiklund N, et al. Calcium-independent and steroid-resistant nitric oxide synthase activity in human paranasal sinus mucosa. Eur Respir J 1996; 9:1344–7.
102. Ramis I, Lorente J, Rosello-Catafau J, Quesada P, Gelpi E, Bulbena O. Differential activity of nitric oxide synthase in human nasal mucosa polyps. Eur Respir J 1996; 9:202–6.
103. Gerlach H, Rossaint R, Pappert D, Knorr M, Falke K. Autoinhalation of nitric oxide after endogenous synthesis in nasophyarynx. Lancet 1994; 343: 518–9.
104. Tornberg D, H. M, Schedin U, Alving K, Lundberg J, Weitzberg E. Nasal and oral contribution to inhaled and exhaled nitric oxide: a study in tracheotomized patients. Eur Respir J 2002; 19:859–64.

105. Mancinelli R, McKay C. Effects of nitric oxide and nitrogen dioxide on bacterial growth. Appl Environ Microbiol 1983; 46:198–202.
106. Croen K. Evidence for an antiviral effect of nitric oxide. J Clin Invest 1993; 91:2446–52.
107. Meng O, Springall D, Bishop A, Morgan K, Evans T, Habib S, et al. Lack of inducible nitric oxide synthase in bronchial epithelium: a possible mechanism of susceptibility to infection in cystic fibrosis. J. Pathol 1998; 184:323–31.
108. Sanders SP, Siekierski ES, Porter JD, Richards SM, Proud D. Nitric oxide inhibits rhinovirus-induced cytokine production and viral replication in a human respiratory epithelial cell line. J Virol 1998; 72:934–42.
109. Sanders S, Kim J, Connolly K, Porter J, Sierkierski E, Proud D. Nitric oxide inhibits rhinovirus-induced granulocyte macrophage colony-stimulating factor production in bronchial epithelial cells. Am J Respir Cell Mol Biol 2001; 24:317–25.
110. Högman M, Frostell C, Arnberg H, Hedenstierna G. Inhalation of nitric oxide modulates methacholine-induced bronchoconstriction in the rabbit. Eur Respir J 1993; 6:177–80.
111. Högman M, Frostell C, Hedenstrom H, Hedenstierna G. Inhalation of nitric oxide modulates adult human bronchial tone. Am Rev Respir Dis 1993; 148: 1474–8.
112. Kacmarek R, Ripple R, Cockrill B, Bloch K, Zapol W, Johnson D. Inhaled nitric oxide; a bronchodilator in mild asthmatics with methacholine-induced bronchospasm. Am J Respir Crit Care Med 1996; 153:128–35.
113. Nijkamp F, Van Der Linde H, Folkerts G. Nitric oxide synthesis inhibitors induce airway hyperresponsiveness in the guinea pig in vivo and in vitro: the role of the epithelium. Am Rev Respir Dis 1993; 148:727–34.
114. Aizawa H, Takata S, Inoue H, Matsumoto K, Koto H, Hara N. Role of nitric oxide released from iNANC neurons in airway responsiveness in cats. Eur Respir J 1999; 13:775–80.
115. De Sanctis G, MacLean J, Hamada K, Mehta S, Scott J, Jiao A, et al. Contribution of nitric oxide synthases 1, 2, and 3 to airway hyperresponsiveness and inflammation in a murine model of asthma. J. Exp. Med. 1999; 189: 1621–9.
116. Ricciardolo F, Geppetti P, Mistretta A, Nadel J, Sapienza M, Bellofiore S, et al. Randomised double-blind placebo-controlled study of the effect of inhibition of nitric oxide synthesis in bradykinin-induced asthma. Lancet 1996; 348:374–7.
117. Ricciardolo F, Timmers M, Geppetti P, van Schadewijk A, Brahim J, Sont J, et al. Allergen-induced impairment of bronchoprotective nitric oxide synthesis in asthma. J Allergy Clin Immunol 2001; 108:198–204.
118. Kapsali T, Permutt S, Laube B, Scichilone N, Togias A. The potent bronchoprotective effect of deep inspiration and its absence in asthma. J Appl Physiol 2000; 89:711–20.
119. Scichilone N, Permutt S, Togias A. The lack of the bronchoprotective and not the bronchodilatory ability of deep inspiration is associated with airways hyperresponsiveness. Am J Respir Crit Care Med 2001; 163:413–9.

120. Lundberg J, Nordvall S, Weitzberg E, Kollberg H, Alving K. Exhaled nitric oxide in paediatric asthma and cystic fibrosis. Arch Dis Child 1996; 75:323–6.

121. Kelley T, Drumm M. Inducible nitric oxide synthase expression is reduced in cystic fibrosis murine and human airway epithelial cells. J Clin Invest 1998; 102:1200–7.

122. Steagall W, Elmer H, Brady K, Kelley T. Cystic fibrosis transmembrane conductance regulator-dependent regulation of epithelial inducible nitric oxide synthase expression. Am J Respir Cell Mol Biol 2000; 22:45–50.

123. Mhanna M, Ferkol T, Martin R, Dreshaj I, van Heeckeren A, Kelley T, et al. Nitric oxide deficiency contributes to impairment of airway relaxation in cystic fibrosis mice. Am J Respir Cell Mol Biol 2001; 24:621–6.

124. Nakano H, Ide H, Imada M, Osanai S, Takahashi T, Kikuchi K, et al. Reduced nasal nitric oxide in diffuse panbronchiolitis. Am J Respir Crit Care Med 2000; 162:2218–20.

125. Lindberg S, Cervin A, Runer T. Nitric oxide (NO) production in the upper airways is decreased in chronic sinusitis. Acta Otolaryngol 1997; 117:113–7.

126. Colantonio D, Brouillette L, Parikh A, Scadding G. Paradoxical low nasal nitric oxide in nasal polyposis. Clin Exp Allergy 2002; 32:698–701.

127. Sluder G. Asthma as a nasal reflex. J Am Med Assoc 1919; 73:589–91.

128. Kaufman J, Wright G. The effect of nasal and nasopharyngeal irritation on airway resistance in man. Am Rev Respir Dis 1969; 100:626–30.

129. Kaufman J, Chen J, Wright G. The effect of trigeminal resection on reflex bronchoconstriction after nasal and nasopharyngeal irritation in man. Am Rev Respir Dis 1970; 101:768–9.

130. Sato T. Effect of nasal mucosa irritation on airway resistance. Auris, Nasus, Larynx (Tokyo) 1980; 7:39–50.

131. Konno A, Togawa K, Itasake Y, Hoshiino T. Computer analysis of changes in pulmonary resistance induced by nasal stimulation in man. Eur J Respir Dis 1983; 64:97–104.

132. Yan K, Salome C. The response of the airways to nasal stimulation in asthmatics with rhinitis. Eur J Respir Dis 1982; 64 (suppl 128):105–9.

133. Schumacher M, Cota K, Taussig L. Pulmonary response to nasal-challenge testing of atopic subjects with stable asthma. J Allergy Clin Immunol 1986; 78:30–5.

134. Levi C, Tyler G, Olson L, Saunders N. Lack of airway response to nasal irritation In normal and asthmatic subjects. Aust N Z J Med 1990; 20: 578–82.

135. Littell N, Carlisle C, Millman R, Braman S. Changes in airway resistance following nasal provocation. Am Rev Respir Dis 1990; 141:580–3.

136. Rodriguez-Martinez F, Mascia AV, Mellins RB. The effect of environmental temperature on airway resistance in the asthmatic child. Pediatr Res 1973; 7: 627–31.

137. Nolte D, Berger D. On vagal bronchoconstriction in asthmatic patients by nasal irritation. Eur J Respir Dis 1983; 64:110–4.

138. Fontanari P, Burneet H, Zattara-Hartman M, Jammes Y. Changes in airway resistance induced by nasal inhalation of cold dry, or moist air in normal individuals. J Appl Physiol 1996; 81:1739–43.

139. Fontanari P, Zattara-Hartmann M-C, Burnet H, Jammes Y. Nasal eupnoeic inhalation of cold, dry air increases airway resistance in asthmatic patients. Eur Respir J 1997; 10:2250–4.

140. Koskela H, Tukiainen H. Facial cooling, but not nasal breathing of cold air, induces bronchoconstriction: a study in asthmatic and healthy subjects. Eur Respir J 1995; 8:2088–93.

141. Fanta C, Ingram R, McFadden EJ. A reassessment of the effects of oropharyneal anesthesia in exercise-induced asthma. Am Rev Respir Dis 1980; 122:381–6.

142. Madonini E, Briatico-Vanagosa G, Pappacoda A, Maccagni G, Cardani A, Saporiti F. Seasonal increase of bronchial reactivity in allergic rhinitis. J Allergy Clin Immunol 1987; 79:358–63.

143. Sotomayor H, Badier M, Vervloet D, Orehek J. Seasonal increase of carbachol airway responsiveness in patients allergic to grass pollen. Am Rev Respir Dis 1984; 130:56–8.

144. Corren J, Adinoff A, Irvin C. Changes in bronchial responsiveness following nasal provocation with allergen. J Allergy Clin Immunol 1992; 89:611–8.

145. Hoehne JH, Reed CE. Where is the allergic reaction in ragweed asthma? J Allergy Clin Immunol 1971; 48:36–9.

146. Rosenberg GL, Rosenthal RR, Norman PS. Inhalation challenge with ragweed pollen in ragweed-sensitive asthmatics. J Allergy Clin Immunol 1983; 71:302–10.

147. Small P, Biskin N. The effects of allergen-induced nasal provocation on pulmonary function in patients with perennial allergic rhinitis. Am J Rhinol 1989; 3:17–20.

148. Noureddine G, Thompson M, Brennan F, Proud D, Kagey-Sobotka A, Lichtenstein L, et al. Nasal antigen challenge in asthmatics: effects of cetirizine on nasal and pulmonary responses. J Allergy Clin Immunol 1994; 93:177 (abstract).

149. Plotkowski L, Dessanges J, Lavaud F, Hanhhart F, Lockhart A. Nasal pollen challenge causes bronchial hyperresponsiveness to methacholine in patients with allergic rhinitis. Am Rev Respir Dis 1990; 141:A652 (abstract).

150. Incorvaia C, Guidoboni A, Pravettoni V, Mauro M, Pastorello EA. Bronchial hyperreactivity before and after nasal challenge in patients with mite-induced perennial rhinitis. J Allergy Clin Immunol 1990; 85:167 (abstract).

151. Windom H, Lim-Mombay M, Thompson M, Naclerio R, Togias A. The effect of nasal versus bronchial antigen (Ag) challenge on the asthmatic airways. J Allergy Clin Immunol 1992; 89:334 (abstract).

152. Huxley EJ, Viroslav J, Gray WR, Pierce AK. Pharyngeal aspiration in normal adults and patients with depressed consciousness. Am J Med 1978; 64:564–8.

153. Bardin P, VanHeerden B, Joubert J. Absence of pulmonary aspiration of sinus

contents in patients with asthma and sinusitis. J Allergy Clin Immunol 1990; 86:82–8.

154. Braunstahl G-J, Overbeek S, KleinJan A, Prins J-B, Hoogsteden H, Fokkens W. Nasal allergen provocation induces adhesion molecules expression and tissue eosinophilia in upper and lower airways. J Allergy Clin Immunol 2001; 107:469–76.

155. Togias A. Systemic immunologic and inflammatory aspects of allergic rhinitis. J Allergy Clin Immunol 2000; 106:S247–50.

156. Togias A, Bieneman A, Bloom D, Schleimer R, Iezzoni D, Harris A, et al. Changes in blood leukocyte cytokine expression following repeated nasal allergen provocation: evidence for systemic manifestations. J Allergy Clin Immunol 2002; 109:S262 (abstract).

157. Denburg J, Sehmi R, Saito H, Pil-Seob J, Inman M, O'Byrne P. Systemic aspects of allergic disease: bone marrow responses. J Allergy Clin Immunol (suppl) 2000; 106:S242–S246.

158. Wood L, Sehmi R, Dorman S, Hamid Q, Tulic M, Watson M, et al. Allergen-induced increases in bone marrow T lymphocytes and interleukin-5 expression in subjects with asthma. Am J Respir Crit Care Med 2002; 166:883–9.

159. Braunstahl G-J, Kleinjan A, Overbeek S, Prins J-B, Hoogsteden H, Fokkens W. Segmental bronchial provocation induces nasal inflammation in allergic rhinitis patients. Am J Respir Crit Care Med 2000; 161:2051–7.

160. Braunstal G-J, Overbeek SE, Fokkens W, KleinJan A, McEuen A, Walls A, et al. Segmental bronchoprovocation in allergic rhinitis patients affects mast cell and basophil numbers in nasal and bronchial mucosa. Am J Respir Crit Care Med 2001; 164:858–65.

3

Upper Airway Reflexes and Involvement of the Lower Airway

RONALD ECCLES

Cardiff University
Cardiff, United Kingdom

Introduction

The use of the terms "upper airways" and "lower airways" (to indicate regions above and below the larynx) is arbitrary because the airway acts as a single unified conduit. The functions of this airway may be broken down into sections, with the nasal passages acting as both chemosensor and air conditioner, the pharynx acting as a crossroads between the digestive and respiratory systems, the larynx acting as a sensitive protective valve, and the lungs acting as the gas exchange area. The sensory nerve supply to the upper airway has the capacity to detect potentially damaging gases, particulate matter, and the presence of food and fluid. Stimulation of upper airway sensory nerves can initiate reflex responses that either expel the source of the stimulus by sneeze or cough or close off the airway and inhibit breathing.

There is evidence from animal experiments, and from clinical observations in diseases such as nasal allergy and asthma, that there may be a reflex link between the upper and lower airways. Stimulation of the upper airway or disease processes in the upper airway may influence the activity of the lower airway. This proposed reflex is often termed a "nasobronchial" or "nasopulmonary" reflex. The existence and significance of this reflex are controversial, and hence the need for some discussion of this topic in the present book. In this chapter I shall describe the innervation of the upper airway, as well as the reflexes that can be initiated from the upper airway, and look at the possible nervous mechanisms that may link the upper and lower airways.

I. Sensory Nerve Supply to the Upper Airways

The term "upper airways" is not a strict anatomical designation but is used more in a functional way, to include the nasal passages, paranasal sinuses, eustachian tube and middle ear air space, pharynx (nasopharynx, oropharynx, laryngopharynx), larynx and the extra thoracic portion of the trachea (Fig. 1) (1). The pharynx can be divided into three areas: the oropharynx (from the open lips through the mouth to the posterior border of the tongue), the nasopharynx (extending from the posterior termination of the

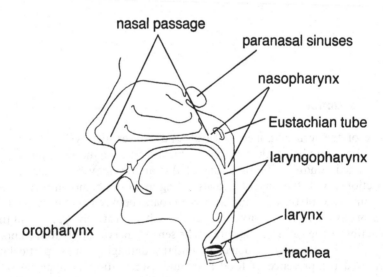

Figure 1 Nomenclature of the upper airway, which can be divided into "nasal passages" from the entrance of the nostril to the arch of the posterior end of the nasal septum, "paranasal sinuses," "eustachian tube and middle ear," "pharynx" (divided into three areas of "nasopharynx," from the arch of the septum to the tip of the soft palate, "oropharynx," from the lips back between the tongue to the tip of the palate, and "laryngopharynx," the pyriform sinuses on either side of the larynx through which food and fluids alone pass), "larynx (with its entrance at the epiglottis and arytenoids), and the "extrathoracic trachea."

nasal turbinates and the arch of the nasal septum to the inferior border of the soft palate), and the laryngopharynx (the pyriform sinuses on either side of the larynx through which food and fluids pass).

The sensory nerve supply to the upper airways is provided by the first, fifth, seventh, ninth, and tenth cranial nerves (I, olfactory; V, trigeminal; VII, facial; IX glossopharyngeal; X vagus) (Fig. 2) (2,3). The olfactory nerve enters the nasal cavity through the cribriform plate and forms a distinct olfactory area in the roof of the nasal cavity. The facial nerve supplies gustatory fibers to the tongue. The maxillary and ophthalmic divisions of the trigeminal nerve supply the nasal passages, paranasal sinuses, and anterior parts of the nasopharynx and oropharynx. The glossopharyngeal nerve supplies sensory fibers to the posterior areas of the nasopharynx and oropharynx, supplying the tympanic cavity, eustachian tube, fauces, tonsils, uvula, inferior surface of the soft palate, and posterior third of the tongue. The vagus nerve supplies the larynx and trachea with sensory fibers, and via

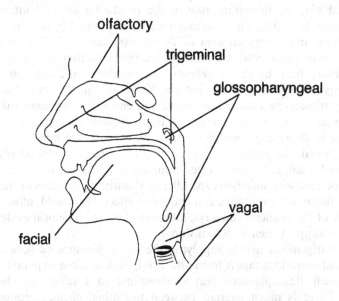

Figure 2 Distribution of the cranial nerves to the upper airway. The olfactory nerve (I) enters the nasal cavity through the cribriform plate and forms a distinct olfactory area in the roof of the nasal cavity. The maxillary and ophthalmic divisions of the trigeminal nerve (V) supply the nasal passages, the paranasal sinuses, and the anterior part of the nasopharynx and oropharynx. The facial nerve (VII) supplies gustatory fibers to the tongue. The glossopharyngeal nerve (IX) supplies the posterior area of the nasopharynx and oropharynx. The vagus nerve (X) supplies the larynx and trachea.

a small auricular branch, also supplies sensory fibers to the external acoustic meatus and tympanic membrane.

Apart from the specialized sensory receptors of the olfactory and gustatory areas, it appears that all the remaining sensory supply to the lining of the upper airway consists of bare nerve endings without any specialized form of terminal receptor. Despite this lack of specialized structure, the bare nerve endings serve as transducers for a wide range of stimuli such as physical and chemical stimulation, changes in temperature and pressure, and stimuli that cause tissue damage.

II. Sensory Receptors and Modalities of Sensation

A. Nasal Passages and Paranasal Sinuses

The nasal passages receive their sensory nerve supply from the olfactory and trigeminal nerves (2). The olfactory nerves are responsible for our sense of smell and play an important role in the regulation of food intake and reproductive behavior. The olfactory mucosa is situated in the roof of the nasal cavity and covers an area of 200 to 400 mm (2–4). The olfactory mucosa consists of specialized olfactory receptor cells that are connected to the olfactory bulb by thin myelinated nerve fibers. A discussion of the physiology of olfaction is beyond the scope of this chapter, but since olfactory stimuli can initiate autonomic and endocrine responses that may influence the lower airways, it is important to consider this sensory pathway when one is discussing possible interactions between the upper and lower airways. Nasal and paranasal sinus disease often has a profound effect on the sense of smell, and patients often complain of a loss of sense of smell and taste associated with infectious and allergic rhinitis (5). The loss of the sense of smell may cause autonomic and endocrine effects that could influence the reactivity of the bronchial airways, although there is no clinical evidence at present to support such a relationship.

The trigeminal nerves supplying the nasal passages mediate all the other nasal sensations (apart from olfaction), such as those to pain, temperature, touch, itch, pressure, and also respond to a variety of chemical stimuli. There is much overlap between trigeminal chemoreception and olfaction, and many chemicals stimulate both the sense of smell and trigeminal sensations of irritation (6). The classical view of the nonolfactory sensory innervation of the nasal passages is that trigeminal sensory nerve fibers terminate peripherally as free nerve endings within the nasal epithelium (7). The nasal trigeminal unmyelinated nerve fibers are widely distributed between the nasal epithelial cells, with branches penetrating right to the surface of the nasal respiratory epithelium.

One of the major functions of the trigeminal sensory nerve supply to the nose is to sense the characteristics of the inspired air and protect the airway from inspiration of noxious substances by initiating respiratory reflexes such as sneezing and apnea (3,8) The nasal trigeminal sensory nerves are also responsible for the major sensation of breathing, which is related to a cool sensation in the nose on inspiration (9–11). The stimulation of nasal cold receptors during inspiratory nasal airflow has an inhibitory action on respiratory drive and may influence the rhythm of breathing, especially during sleep (12,13).

B. Oropharynx, Nasopharynx, Laryngopharynx

Compared with the nasal passages and larynx, there is relatively little information available about the sensory nerve supply to the pharyngeal areas. As already discussed, the three areas of the pharynx are innervated by the trigeminal, glossopharyngeal, and vagus nerves, with some overlap of sensory fields. This, together with the complex overlap of nerves supplying the various sensory nuclei in the brain stem, makes it very difficult to define sensations in the pharynx. In general the sensations from the pharynx, except for gustation, are mediated by undifferentiated bare nerve endings that act as nociceptors and also mediate the sensations of touch and temperature.

The oropharynx is the entrance to the digestive tract, and the sensory nerve supply to this area is mainly related to gustation and sensing the physical and chemical properties of ingested material. Physical and chemical stimuli in the mouth cause reflex salivation and may also initiate vagal reflexes associated with the activity of the digestive tract (e.g., stimulation of gastric acid secretion in response to food in the mouth) (14). In this respect there is a clear reflex link between the upper and lower regions of the digestive tract.

The oropharynx acts as an airway when one is breathing through the mouth, and the cool sensation from the oral cavity on inspiration is mediated via cold receptors similar to those found in the nasal passages (10,15,16). Since the oropharynx conducts food and fluid as well as air, the temperature receptors may also be involved in the regulation of food and water intake (11).

The human nasopharynx is mainly derived from the primitive pharynx. It is divided into an anterior "nasal" and a posterior "pharyngeal" component by a junctional zone at the level of the oropharyngeal tubal orifices, where the first and third pharyngeal arches meet (17). The portion of the nasopharynx proximal to the tubal orifice is innervated by the maxillary division of the trigeminal nerve, and that posterior to the tubal orifice by the glossopharyngeal nerve. The glossopharyngeal nerve supplies motor fibers to the levator veli palatini muscles and may also supply sensory fibers to the soft palate, which forms the floor of the nasopharynx. Sensory information, from the trigeminal, glossopharyngeal, and vagus nerves is processed in the various nuclei situated in the brain stem region. There is much overlap between the nuclei situated in the reticular network of cells, and this overlap of sensory fields for the trigeminal and glosso-pharyngeal nerves, together with central processing of sensory information in the same nucleus, may explain why nasopharyngeal inflammation associated with acute upper respiratory tract infection is interpreted as a "sore throat" (18). The sensations apparent from the nasopharynx are mainly related to the presence of viscous mucus or particulate matter that triggers the sniff-like aspiration reflex.

C. Larynx

The motor and sensory innervation of the larynx and the extrathoracic portion of the trachea is provided by branches of the vagus nerve. The sensory fibers reach the larynx and trachea via the superior laryngeal nerve, which supplies mainly the cranial portion of the larynx, while the recurrent laryngeal nerve supplies the subglottal portion of the larynx and trachea (19). Most of the cell bodies of laryngeal afferents are located in the nodose ganglion (20). The central projections of these afferents synapse with cells of the nucleus of the solitary tract. The activity recorded from the whole internal branch of the superior laryngeal nerve in animals of different species shows a prominent respiratory modulation that is mainly related to the negative transmural pressure and cooling of the laryngeal epithelium during inspiration (19).

Receptors with an inspiratory discharge uniquely related to the cooling effect of inspired air have been located on the rim of the vocal folds, and application of local anesthetics blocks this activity, whereas application of 1-menthol activates the receptors in the absence of airflow and enhances the response to airflow (21). Cooling of the larynx causes a depression of ventilation, mostly owing to an increase in expiratory time that is especially pronounced in the newborn (22–24).

Sensory receptors that respond to mechanical and chemical irritant stimuli (e.g., cigarette smoke, distilled water, CO_2) have been found in the laryngeal mucosa (25). Mechanical or chemical irritation of the larynx initiates a range of protective reflexes such as cough, apnea, expiration, swallowing, bronchoconstriction, and mucus secretion (26).

The activity of most laryngeal receptors is modified by changes in osmolarity and/or ionic composition of the mucosal surface liquid. The response of laryngeal receptors to water has been studied extensively in the newborn and adult of several species (19,20). Application of water and aqueous solutions to the larynx elicits strong cardiorespiratory reflex responses (26), and inhalation of nebulized distilled water is a useful stimulus to initiate cough in human volunteers (27).

The larynx, like the rest of the upper airway, is subjected to fluctuations in airway pressure during inspiration and expiration. Large negative transmural pressures are developed during inspiratory efforts against an occluded upper airway, and this stimulus may initiate several reflexes that help to maintain the patency of the upper airway. Pressure-responsive laryngeal receptors have been described that are particularly sensitive to upper airway occlusion and initiate reflex activation of upper airway muscles (26,28).

III. Upper Airway Reflexes

The upper airway is the gateway to the respiratory system, and most of the upper airway reflexes are involved in preventing inhalation of noxious particulate matter and gases, or in preventing inhalation of food and fluid. As well as the protective reflexes initiated by noxious or potentially noxious stimuli, there are also reflexes that can be initiated by the airflow through the upper airways in relation to the cooling action of airflow or pressure changes associated with airflow.

The physiology of upper airways reflexes was extensively reviewed by Korpas and Tomori in 1979 (29) and was later reviewed by Widdicombe (3,25,30) and other authors (2,31). Much of the research on upper airway reflexes involves work on anesthetized animals. To simplify the interpretation of the results, the experiments often involve quite specific stimuli to localized areas of the upper airway. The results of these experiments help us to break down the reflexes into their various components, but the models are far removed from the situation in conscious man, where, for example, inhalation of a noxious gas or substance may provide a stimulus that varies in intensity simultaneously along the whole of the upper airway. To help simplify the understanding of the various reflexes, I have divided them into protective reflexes (sneeze, aspiration, apnea, expiration, cough) and reflexes associated with airflow (involving airway cooling or pressure changes).

A. Protective Reflexes

As noted earlier, the upper airway is the entrance to the respiratory tract, and the sensory innervation of the upper airway senses the physical and chemical properties of the inspired air. The sensory receptors have the capability of detecting any noxious or potentially noxious properties of the inspired air and, depending on the intensity of the stimulus, the airway reflexes may vary from a sneeze or cough up to apnea.

The oropharynx acts both as an airway and as a passage for food and fluid, and the presence of food and fluids in the oral cavity can trigger the swallowing reflex, which ensures that food and fluids are moved toward the esophagus rather than the larynx. The regions of the upper airway from which the various reflexes may be initiated are clearly defined (Fig. 3). The various sensations and reflexes from the upper airway may be mediated by separate and distinct pathways. One or more pathways may trigger several different reflexes according to the intensity of the stimulus. For example, mild mechanical stimulation of the nasal epithelium may be detected as a simple sensation of touch or tickle that may eventually cause sneezing and nasal secretions, but an increase in the intensity of the stimulus could cause pain associated with apnea, laryngospasm, and pronounced cardiovascular reflexes.

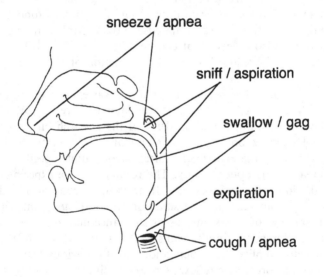

Figure 3 Reflexes arising form the upper airway. Stimulation of the nasal epithelium results in a sneeze or apnea, depending on the intensity of the stimulus. The presence of mucus in the nasaopharynx causes the sniff or aspiration reflex. Food and fluids in the oropharynx trigger swallowing, and mechanical stimulation causes the gag reflex. Mechanical stimulation of the vocal cords causes a reflex expiration. Mechanical or chemical stimulation of the laryngeal mucosa causes cough or apnea, depending on the intensity of the stimulus.

Sneeze

The sneeze is one of the most common respiratory reflexes and is associated with inhalation of dust and with the nasal inflammatory response associated with upper airway infection and allergy. Sneezing is part of a generalized response to chemical or physical stimulation of the nasal epithelium, and the response includes twitching of the nose and face, blinking, tearing, and a watery nasal secretion, often accompanied by a transient engorgement of the nasal blood vessels (32–34). Sneezing may be initiated by a number of factors such as mechanical stimulation of the nasal epithelium, cooling of the skin, bright light in the eyes, irritation of the scalp near the frontal hairline, and challenge with allergen extract, as well as by psychological causes (2). In experiments on the anesthetized cat, puffs of air have been used as a stimulus to initiate sneezing (35). The act of sneezing usually involves several brief inspirations via the mouth followed by an explosive exhalation with most of the airflow escaping via the mouth. The expiratory airflow via the mouth and nose, together with the watery nasal secretions, clears the airway of any source of irritation such as inhaled particulate matter. The sneeze reflex appears to be mediated solely by the trigeminal nerve supply to the upper airway and is mainly related to stimulation of the nasal epithelium, and possibly the anterior region of the nasopharynx.

Apnea

Apnea can be induced by physical or chemical stimulation of all parts of the upper airway, and this reflex appears to be a protective response to prevent inhalation of noxious gases, fluid, or particulate matter. The "diving response" is the reaction to water or cold stimuli applied to the face or into the nose. It was first described by Kratschmer in 1870 (36) and was reviewed in the late twentieth century by Elsner and Gooden (37).

The distinction between the diving reflex and apnea initiated by stimuli other than water or cold is not very clear, and the reflexes may share a common pathway (25). Apnea is usually accompanied by complete laryngeal closure, bradycardia, and pronounced vasoconstriction in the vascular beds of the skin, alimentary canal, kidney, and skeletal muscle, with a subsequent rise in arterial blood pressure. By moving blood flow from the peripheral circulation toward the heart and brain, the reflex prevents inhalation of water or noxious material, and protects the heart and brain from hypoxia.

Sniff, Aspiration Reflex

Unmyelinated nerve endings derived from the trigeminal and glossopharyngeal nerves, and found under the epithelium of the nasopharynx, are thought to be the sensory nerves that mediate the sniff-like aspiration reflex. Sniffing and aspiration may be elicited by mechanical deformation of the nasopharyngeal mucosa, and also occasionally by irritant gases (29). The rapidly adapting response of these nerve endings to a maintained mechanical deformation fits very well with the abrupt onset and short duration of the aspiration reflex (19). The aspiration reflex helps to clear the nasopharynx and prevents obstruction of the airway with mucus or foreign matter.

Swallow and Gag Reflexes

Swallowing and breathing are closely coordinated to prevent the accidental aspiration of food and fluid into the lungs. Swallowing is initiated voluntarily on presentation of food or fluid to the posterior area of the oropharynx, an event that triggers the reflex phase of swallowing, accompanied by inhibition of breathing and closure of the larynx. The reflex is associated with a complex pattern of muscular activity that propels food and fluid toward the esophagus and closes off the nasopharynx and larynx. Mechanical stimulation of the soft palate and fauces, via the mouth, causes the gag reflex, with palatal elevation, pharyngeal wall contraction, withdrawal of the head, coughing, retching, and eye watering (38). Surprisingly, the gag reflex is poorly described or absent in most reviews on the upper airway reflexes (25). The reflex may be exaggerated during periods of upper respiratory tract infection, especially with epiglottitis, when manipulation of the upper airway to inspect the inflamed epiglottis may be sufficient to trigger a fatal airway obstruction (39). In normal circumstances, the reflex may act to protect the airway from accidental inhalation of large food items in the mouth.

Cough

Cough is a purely vagal reflex and can be triggered by chemical irritation of the larynx and trachea or by the presence of mucus in the bronchi. The physiology of cough has been extensively reviewed by Widdicombe (30,40,41). Cough related to the upper airways is most commonly associated with acute upper respiratory tract infection or aspiration of ingested materials. The cough reflex is triggered by mechanical or chemical stimulation of laryngeal and tracheal sensory receptors (26). Cough can be initiated by inhalation of nebulized distilled water (27), and this appears to be a protective reflex similar to the nasal response to inhalation of water, since both responses prevent the entry of water into the lungs.

Cough prevents the entry of foods and fluid into the lungs, and the larynx acts as a sensitive valve at the entry to the lower respiratory tract. The laryngeal epithelium is extremely sensitive to mechanical and chemical stimuli. Inflammation of the laryngeal epithelium associated with upper respiratory tract infection, by creating a condition of hyper-reactivity, may be responsible for the dry irritating cough often associated with common cold.

Expiration Reflex

Mechanical stimulation of the vocal cords does not cause cough but initiates a transient expiratory effort called the expiration reflex. The function of this reflex may be to prevent the entry of foreign bodies into the lower respiratory tract (3,29).

B. Reflexes Associated with Airflow

Tidal airflow through the upper airway causes cooling of the airway and exposes the airway to oscillations in air pressure. The changes in temperature and pressure associated with breathing are detected by sensory nerves distributed along the upper airway.

The nasal passages are exposed to the greatest cooling action of the inspired air, for by the time the air reaches the larynx, it has been warmed and humidified by the nose. The sensation of airflow is mainly related to the cool sensation perceived from the nose, rather than from pressure sensations or sensations from chest muscles and proprioceptors. The cool sensation of nasal airflow is mediated by trigeminal nerve endings, which act as cold receptors in the skin lining the nasal vestibule and the epithelium of the nasal passages (9,42).

As well as providing a cool sensation of airflow, the cold stimulus inhibits breathing and the activity of upper airway accessory muscles (12,22). Administration of menthol causes the same cold sensation and inhibition of breathing without any change in airway temperature, and menthol is believed to stimulate and sensitize airway cold receptors by influencing calcium conductance in the sensory nerve endings (10,23,24).

The cooling of the upper airway associated with normal tidal airflow can be separated from cold air challenge, where cold air is circulated through the nasal passages or the inspired air is very cold and dry. Cold air challenge may result in nasal irritation, which leads to nasal congestion (43) and bronchoconstriction (44). The nasal irritation may be related to neurogenic inflammation caused by the release of tachykinins from trigeminal sensory nerve endings (45). The bronchoconstrictor response to nasal cold air challenge appears to be well established in the literature, but whether it is cooling of the facial skin or nasal epithelium that triggers the response is a matter of some dispute (46).

Receptors sensitive to pressure change have been described in the laryngeal epithelium, and they constitute the main element of respiratory-modulated activity of the sensory nerves to the larynx (19). Since the most compliant region of the upper airways, and the region most susceptible to inspiratory collapse, lies above the larynx, the larynx is well situated to act as pressure sensor to initiate reflex activation of upper airway muscles that stabilize and splint the airway. Stimulation of the laryngeal pressure receptors by occlusion of the upper airway has been shown to cause a reflex activation of upper airway dilating muscles, and inhibition of breathing, and both these responses limit the upper airway collapsing action of inspiratory efforts (19).

The upper airway reflexes associated with the cooling and pressure changes brought about by airflow are important in respiratory control because they influence the pattern of breathing and protect the airway from inspiratory collapse. These reflexes may be particularly important during sleep (47–49).

IV. Interactions Between the Upper and Lower Airways

Stimulation of the upper airways has been shown to induce changes in the bronchial airway in animal experiments (3,25). The animal experiments have involved applying various mechanical and chemical stimuli to the nose and larynx and monitoring changes in the lower airways. Both bronchodilator and bronchoconstrictor responses can be initiated, and the type of response depends on the intensity of the stimulus and the part of the airway to which the stimulus is applied. In healthy animals, the majority of studies indicate that nasal irritation causes bronchodilation mediated by the vagus nerve (3,25). Figure 4 illustrates two nervous mechanisms that may link the upper and lower airways. The smooth muscle of the lower airway is innervated by parasympathetic nerves derived from the vagus nerve. Stimulation of this pathway causes release of acetylcholine and bronchoconstriction. There is a continuous level of activity in the vagus nerves (vagal tone), and a reduction in vagal tone causes bronchodilation. A reduction in vagal tone leading to bronchocodilation is proposed as the mechanism for the bronchodilation often produced on stimulation of the upper airway (3,25). The smooth muscle of the lower airway is also innervated by sympathetic nerve fibers from the thoracolumbar region of the spinal cord, and stimulation of this pathway causes both release of norepinephrine and bronchodilation. The sympathetic response may also involve release of epinephrine from the adrenal medulla, and this will cause bronchodilation by relaxation of bronchial smooth muscle.

Stimuli applied to the upper airway invariably have some effects on respiration and usually slow respiratory rate or induce apnea. Inhibition of

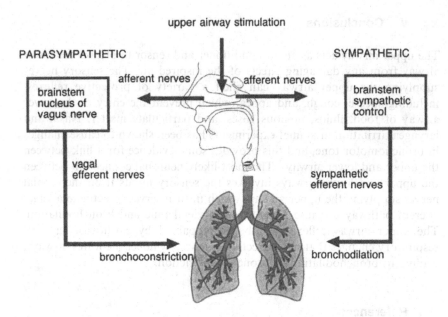

Figure 4 Nervous pathways between the upper and lower airways. Upper airway stimulation of cranial afferent nerves causes activation of parasympathetic and sympathetic reflexes. Parasympathetic vagal efferent nerves cause bronchoconstriction (a reduction in vagal tone may cause bronchodilation). Sympathetic efferent nerves cause bronchodilation.

respiration and apnea will cause hypoxia and hypercapnia, which will have direct and indirect effects on bronchial smooth muscle tone via changes in blood gases (50) and by reflex activation of sympathetic pathways (25). Activation of a generalized sympathetic cardiorespiratory response is likely to be a response to noxious stimuli applied to the upper airway, and if this is superimposed on top of a vagally mediated bronchoconstrictor response, together with apnea, which itself could alter blood gases and influence the bronchial tone, the complexity of the situation is increased appreciably. The simultaneous activation of several reflex pathways could explain why it is possible to elicit either bronchoconstriction or bronchodilation in response to nasal irritation and why both these responses are reported in the literature on animal experiments (3,51).

Unlike the nose, where chemical and mechanical irritation causes either reflex bronchoconstriction or bronchodilation, the bronchomotor response from laryngeal irritation is bronchoconstriction, and there are indications that this may be a reflex pathway separate from that initiating cough (3).

V. Conclusions

The upper airway acts as an air conditioner and sensor to protect the lower airway from any damaging effects of the inspired air. The sensory nerves supplying the upper airway can elicit a variety of protective reflexes, including sneeze, cough, and apnea, which prevent the entry to the lower airway of food, fluids, noxious gases, and particulate matter. Nasal and laryngeal irritation in animal experiments has been shown to cause changes in bronchomotor tone, and this provides some evidence for a link between the upper and lower airways. The most likely neuronal connection between the upper and lower airways involves the sensory inputs from the cranial nerves supplying the upper airway, which in turn serves to activate a vagal efferent pathway to cause a reduction in vagal tone and bronchodilation. The upper airway reflexes can be accompanied by cardiovascular and respiratory changes that may directly or indirectly affect the lower airways, leading to bronchodilation or bronchoconstriction.

References

1. Proctor DF. The upper airway. In: Proctor DF, Andersen I, eds. The Nose. Upper Airway Physiology and the Atmospheric Environment. Amsterdam: Elsevier Biomedical Press, 1982:23–43.
2. Eccles R, Neurological and pharmacological considerations. In: Proctor DF, Andersen I, eds. The Nose. Upper Airway Physiology and the Atmospheric Environment. Amsterdam: Elsevier Biomedical Press, 1982:191–214.
3. Widdicombe J. Reflexes from the upper respiratory tract. In: Cherniack N and Widdicombe J, eds. Hand Book of Physiology, The Respiratory System. Bethesda, MD: American Physiological Society, 1986, Chapter 11, p. 363–394.
4. Berglund B, Lindvall T, Olfaction. In: Proctor DF, Andersen I, eds. The Nose. Upper Airway Physiology and the Atmospheric Environment. Amsterdam: Elsevier Biomedical Press, 1982:279–305.
5. Cowart BJ, Flynn-Rodden K, McGeady SJ, Lowry LD. Hyposmia in allergic rhinitis. J Allergy Clin Immunol 1993; 91: 747–751.
6. Silver WL. Neural and pharmacological basis for nasal irritation. Ann N Y Acad Sci 1992; 641: 152–163.
7. Finger TE, Getchell ML, Getchell TV, Kinnamon JC, Affector and effector functions of peptidergic innervation of the nasal cavity. In: Green BG, Mason JR, Kare MR, eds. Irritation, Chemical Senses. New York: Marcel Dekker, 1990:1–17.
8. Angell-James JE, De Burgh-Daly M. Section of laryngology. Nasal reflexes. Proc R Soc Med 1969; 62: 1287–1293.

9. Eccles R, Effects of menthol on nasal sensation of airflow. In: Green BG, Mason JR, Kare MR, eds. Irritation, Chemical Senses. New York: Marcel Dekker, 1990:275–295.

10. Eccles R. Menthol—a spectrum of efficacy. Int Pharm J 1994; 8: 17–21.

11. Eccles R. Role of cold receptors and menthol in thirst, the drive to breathe and arousal. Appetite 2000; 34: 29–35.

12. McBride B, Whitelaw WA. Physiological stimulus to upper airway receptors in humans. J Appl Physiol 1981; 1189–1197.

13. Lavie P. Rediscovering the importance of nasal breathing in sleep or, shut your mouth and save your sleep. J Laryngol Otology 1987; 101: 558–563.

14. Johnson L. Gastric secretion. In: Johnson L, ed. Gastrointestinal Physiology. St Louis, MD: Mosby,1985:71.

15. Hensel H, Zotterman Y. The effect of menthol on the thermoreceptors. Acta , Physiol Scand. 1951; 24: 27–34.

16. Green BG. Menthol modulates oral sensations of warmth and cold. Physiol Behav 1984; 35: 427–434.

17. Chew C, Nasopharynx (postnasal space). In: Mackay I, Bull T, eds. Scott-Brown's Otolaryngology. London: Butterworths, 1987:312–340.

18. Rees GL, Eccles R. Sore throat following nasal and oropharyngeal bradykinin challenge. Acta Otolaryngol (Stockh) 1994;114: 311–314.

19. Santambrogio G, Tsubone H, Santambrogio FB. Sensory information from the upper airway—role in the control of breathing. Respir Physiol 1995; 102: 1–16.

20. Widdicombe JG, Vagal reflexes in the airway. In: Kaliner MA, Barnes PJ, eds. The Airways. Neural Control in Health and Disease. New York: Marcel Dekker, 1988:187–202.

21. Sant'Ambrogio FB, Anderson JW, Sant'Ambrogio G. Effect of l-menthol on laryngeal receptors. J Appl Physiol 1991; 70: 788–793.

22. Mathew OP, Anderson JW, Orani GP, Sant'Ambrogio FB, Sant'Ambrogio G. Cooling mediates the ventilatory depression associated with airflow through the larynx. Respir Physiol 1990; 82: 359–368.

23. Orani GP, Anderson JW, Sant'Ambrogio FB. Upper airway cooling and l-menthol reduce ventilation in the guinea pig. J Appl Physiol 1991; 70: 2080–2086.

24. Sant'Ambrogio FB, Anderson JW, Sant'Ambrogio G. Menthol in the upper airway depresses ventilation in newborn dogs. Respir Physiol 1992; 89: 299–307.

25. Widdicombe JG, Nasal and pharyngeal reflexes: protective and respiratory functions. In: Mathew OP, Sant'Ambrogio G, eds. Respiratory Function of the Upper Airway. Lung Biology in Health and Disease, Lenfant C, series ed. vol 35. New York: Marcel Dekker, 1988: 233–258.

26. Mathew O, Sant'Ambrogio, Laryngeal reflexes. In: Mathew OP, Sant' Ambrogio G, eds. Respiratory Function of the Upper Airway. Lung Biology in Health and Disease, Lenfant C, series ed. vol 35. New York: Marcel Dekker, 1988:259–302.

27. Morice AH, Higgins KS, Yeo WW. Adaption of cough reflex with different types of stimulation. Eur Respir J 1992; 5: 841–847.

28. Mathew OP. Upper airway negative-pressure effects on respiratory activity of upper airway muscles. J Appl Physiol 1984;56: 500–505.

29. Korpas J, Tomori Z. Cough and other respiratory reflexes. In: Herzog H ed. Progress in Respiration Research, Vol 12. Basel: S Karger 1979:356.

30. Widdicombe JG. Cough and related phenomena. Respir Med 1991; 85 suppl A.

31. Mathew OP, Sant'Ambogio G, eds. Respiratory Function of the Upper Airway. Lung Biology in Health and Disease. Lenfant C, series ed. Vol. 35. 1988, Marcel Dekker: New York.

32. Proetz AW. Essays on the Applied Physiology of the Nose. 2d ed. St Louis, MD: Annals Publishing, 1953.

33. Whitman BW, Packer RJ. The photic sneeze: literature review and discussion. Neurology 1993; 43: 868–871.

34. Leung AKC, Robson WLM. Sneezing. J Otolaryngol 1994; 23: 125–129.

35. Wallois F, Macron JM. Nasal air puff stimulations and laryngeal, thoracic and abdominal muscle activities. Respir Physiol 1994; 97: 47–62.

36. Kratschmer F. Über reflexe von der Nasenschleimhaut auf Athmung und Kreislauf. Sitzungsker. Akad. Wiss. Wien Math. Naturwiss. Kl. Abt. 1870; 3: 147–167.

37. Elsner R, Gooden B, Diving and asphyxia. Monographs of the Physiological Society. Vol. 40. Cambridge, UK: Cambridge University Press, 1983.

38. Hughes TAT, Wiles CM. Palatal and pharyngeal reflexes in health and in motor neuron disease. J Neurol Psychiatry 1996; 61: 96–98.

39. Hall CB, McBride JT, Upper respiratory tract infections: the common cold, pharyngitis, croup, bacterial tracheitis and epiglottitis. In: Pennington JE ed. Respiratory Infections: Diagnosis and Management. Raven Press: New York, 1988: 97–118.

40. Widdicombe JG. Neurophysiology of the cough reflex. Eur Respir J 1995; 8: 1103–1202.

41. Widdicombe JG. Afferent receptors in the airways and cough. Respir Physiol 1998; 114: 5–15.

42. Eccles R. Menthol and related cooling compounds. J Pharm Pharmacol 1994; 46: 618–630.

43. Iliopoulos O, Proud D, Norman PS, Lichtenstein LM, Kagey-Sobotka A, Naclerio RM. Nasal challenge with cold, dry, air induces a late phase reaction. Am Rev Respir Dis 1988; 138: 400–405.

44. Fontanari P, Burnet H, Zattara Hartmann M, Jammes Y. Changes in nasal resistance induced by nasal inhalation of cold dry, dry, or moist air in normal individuals. J Appl Physiol 1996; 81: 1739–1743.

45. Yoshihara S, Chan B, Yamawaki I, Geppetti P, Ricciardolo FLM, Massion PP, Nadel JA. Plasma extravasation in the rat trachea induced by cold air is mediated by tachykinin release from sensory nerves. Am J Respir Crit Care Med 1995; 151: 1011–1017.

46. Koskela H, Tukiainen H. Facial cooling but not nasal breathing of cold air, induces bronchoconstriction; a study in asthmatic and healthy subjects. Eur Respir J 1995; 8: 2088–2093.

47. Douglas NJ. Control of breathing during sleep. Clin Sci 1984; 67: 465–471.
48. White DP, Cadieux RJ, Lombard RM, Bixler EO, Kales E, Zwillich CW. The effects of nasal anesthesia on breathing during sleep. Am Rev Respir Dis 1985; 132: 972–975.
49. Berry RB, Kouchi KG, Bower JL, Light RW. Effect of upper airway anesthesia on obstructive sleep-apnea. Am J Respir Crit Care Med 1995; 151:1857–1861.
50. Whicker JH, Kern EB, Hyatt RE. Nasopulmonary reflex: evaluation in the neoparalyzed and paralyzed anesthetized dog. Ann Otol. 1978; 87: 91–98.
51. McFadden E, Physiological and pathological interactions between the upper and lower airways and bronchial asthma. In: Mygind N, Pipkorn U, Dahl R, Eds. Rhinitis and Asthma: Similarities and Differences. Copenhagen: Munksgaard, 1990:139–149.

4

Epidemiological Evidence for the Relationship Between Upper and Lower Airway Diseases

ISABELLA ANNESI-MAESANO

Institut National de la Sante et de la Recherche Medicale
Villejuif, France

Introduction

Although neither the actual size of the relationship nor the nature of the underlying mechanisms is fully known, there is convincing evidence that upper and lower airway diseases are related. In particular, few data on causation are presently available. This is partly due to the lack of sufficient appropriate investigations. Although connected, upper and lower airways are noticeably different because of differences in the target organs. There are no smooth muscles in the upper airways such as those around the bronchi and, similarly, there are no sinuslike cavities in the lower airways. Mechanisms involved in the occurrence of diseases are also dissimilar, as in the case of vasodilatation, which largely accounts for nasal blockage in rhinitis but is of little significance in pathophysiological processes of the lower airways (1).

A substantial amount of the available information on the relationship between upper and lower airway diseases has been provided by epidemiological studies in which measurements were taken from subjects and inferences made about relevant characteristics of wider populations. Overall, the epidemiological research into upper airways has been behind schedule in comparison to that into lower airways. Furthermore, supporting evidence from such studies has not been unequivocal. Carefully conducted longitudinal studies in which both upper and lower airway diseases have been accurately monitored have been rare and have concerned only certain aspects of the association (e.g., the association between hay fever and asthma). This is all the more detrimental inasmuch as correctly designed longitudinal studies are the only methods available for assessing true relationships and demonstrating causation. Nevertheless, cross–sectional studies, which have been the most frequent, can be useful because they have provided good evidence for some relationships and at the same time yield hypotheses to be addressed in further studies. Advances in the understanding of the relationship between upper and lower airway disease have also been hampered by the lack, up to now, of accurate measurements of upper airway disease. Most studies measuring whether relationships exist between upper and lower airway disease have been based on self–reports and recall of past experiences without using standardized questionnaires and, moreover, nasal patency has rarely been assessed objectively through nasal function testing (e.g., rhinomanometry or peak nasal inspiratory flow).

Evidence for the relationship between upper and lower airway disease produced by epidemiological studies is either direct or indirect. Direct evidence comprises available facts and circumstances connecting "straightforward" upper and lower airway diseases and consists of reporting numbers of individuals suffering from both. Indirect evidence provides information on relationships in which both upper and lower airway diseases are related either to another health condition or to a common factor.

This chapter summarizes the present state of knowledge on direct and indirect relationships between upper and lower airways diseases and examines the problems encountered in the investigation of such relationships. Population–based data were used.

I. Direct Evidence

Upper airway diseases constitute a heterogeneous entity for which unanimous classifications and definitions do not exist. For clinical purposes, symptoms of rhinitis—namely, sneezing, nasal obstruction, and rhinorrhea—have been classified as infectious, allergic, and vasomotor, respectively (2). Allergic rhinitis, clinically defined as a symptomatic disorder of the nose induced by an IgE–mediated inflammation after allergen exposure of the membranes lining the nose (3), has been classified as seasonal or perennial. Nonallergic rhinitis with eosinophilia is a heteregeneous syndrome consisting of at least two groups: nonallergic rhinitis with eosinophilia (NARES) and aspirin intolerance. Nasal polyps may have either an infectious (neutrophil subgroup) or allergic (eosinophil subgroup) etiology. Sinusitis is a broad term covering a condition that affects the paranasal sinuses and results from inadequate drainage usually secondary to physical obstruction, infection, or allergy. Sinusitis is discussed here in so far as it is connected with nasal disorders. These definitions and classifications have been accepted in epidemiology, which has focused its attention mainly on hay fever so far.

A. Relationships Between Self-Reported Diseases

Epidemiologic Definitions and Distribution

Standardized questionnaires in the field of respiratory medicine designed to ascertain the prevalence and severity of chronic obstructive pulmonary disease (COPD) (4–6) were the first instruments used to assess diseases of the upper airways. They entailed symptoms as well as diagnostic labels of allergic rhinitis (hay fever overall) and sometimes triggers factors for it (Table 1). Only recently, following the evaluation of the sensitivity and specificity of particular questions on nasal allergies with high clinical relevance, have more specific instruments to assess allergic rhinitis been developed (7–10). The best evaluated question for detecting noninfectious rhinitis among members of the general population is this: Have subjects had "a problem with sneezing or a runny or blocked nose" when they "did not have a cold or the flu". The positive predictive value of this question is high in detecting subjects found to have rhinitis on in-depth interviewing incorporating skin prick test assessment (7). It has been suggested that to detect allergy among those with rhinitis, questions on concomitant eye symptoms and allergen exposure, as a trigger factor, should be included. (11). The reliability of a label or reported doctor's diagnosis of allergic rhinitis is also satisfactory (12), but underestimation is common in the case of mild disease and atypical presentation. These questions were employed in isolation in various population–based studies and more recently together to implement the Score for Allergic Rhinitis (10). It has been shown, indeed, that quantitative scores are more informative than dichotomous variables in the characterization of a disease.

Large population–based studies having the potential of dealing with the comorbidity between rhinitis and asthma are as follows:

The European Community Respiratory Healthy Study (ECRHS) in young adults (20–44 years)

The International Study of Asthma and Allergies in Childhood (ISAAC) in children (6–7 years) and adolescents (13–14 years)

Table 1 Standardized Questionnaires for the Assessment of Upper and Lower Airway Diseases in Epidemiological Studies

Questionnaire[a]	Outcome investigated	
	Upper airways	Lower airways
BMRC 1960	Usual stuffy nose or catarrh in the summer	COPD
ESCC-MRC 1962 (4)	Runny nose in spring	COPD
ESCC-MRC 1967	Hay fever	COPD
ATS (1978) (5)	Hay fever confirmed by a doctor	COPD
South London Community Survey (7)	Rhinitis in the absence of cold or flu	Asthma
ECRHS (6)	Nasal allergies including hay fever in adults	Asthma in adults
ISAAC (59)	Allergic as well nonallergic rhinitis in the absence of cold or flu in children	Asthma in children
Jessen (14)	Nonallergic rhinitis	-
Annesi (9)	Allergic as well nonallergic rhinitis	COPD (as in the BMRC-ESCC) and asthma
Score for Allergic Rhinitis (10)	Allergic as well as nonallergic rhinitis	Asthma and familial resemblance of asthma

[a] BMRC, British Medical Research Council; COPD, chronic obstructive pulmonary disease; ESCC-MRC, European Steel and Coal Community–Medical Research Council; ECRHS, European Community Respiratory Health Study; ISAAC, International Study of Asthma and Allergies in Childhood; ATS, American Thoracic Society.

The National Health and Nutritional Examination (NHANES) in the United States

The Swiss Study on Air Pollution and Lung Disease in Adults (SAPALDIA)

The Swiss Study on Childhood Allergy and Respiratory Symptoms with Respect to Air Pollution, Climate, and Pollen (SCARPOL)

Presently, the WHO initiative on Allergic Rhinitis and Its Impact on Asthma (ARIA) (3) is investigating this comorbidity; owing to the multi-disciplinarity of the chosen approach, these studies are exhaustive.

Very few questionnaires have addressed upper airway symptoms and diseases other than allergies (9,13,14). The questionnaire persists as the unique method of assessing sinusitis in epidemiological studies because other instruments such as x–ray views, ultrasound, and sinus puncture cannot be used in these studies, nor can bacteriology and endoscopy. Similarly, a reported diagnosis has mostly been used in epidemiological surveys in the case of nasal polyposis for which the diagnosis is obtained either by rhinoscopy or by more invasive procedures (x–ray, endoscopy). Reliance of questions used to assess sinusitis or nasal polyps has scarcely been evaluated. In 835 children enrolled at birth in the Tucson Children's Respiratory Study, who were studied at a mean age of 8.6 years, the report of physician–diagnosed sinusitis was considered as satisfactory (15). In a study of 335 nonselected outpatients undergoing endoscopy in six hospitals in France, polyposis was confirmed in 87% of the 101 individuals having reported it on the questionnaire, which corresponded to a sensitivity of 0.88, specificity of 0.94, positive predictive value of 0.87, negative predictive value of 0.94 (Bruno Deslandes, Stéphanie Garcia–Acosta, and Isabella Annesi–Maesano, unpublished data).

Little is known about the distribution of upper airway diseases other than allergic rhinitis. According to the epidemiological literature, allergic rhinitis is a frequent disease, with cumulative prevalence ranging from 5 to 40% in the case of seasonal rhinitis and 10% or less in the case of perennial rhinitis. The incidence per year is under 1% for both. Up to 21% of people in the general population might suffer more or less regularly from nonallergic rhinitis (14). The frequency of nasal polyps was found to be about 4%. The true incidence of polyps is difficult to determine but can be inferred from the incidence of intrinsic asthma because the two conditions are related. Sinusitis prevalence has been evaluated at 10 to 30% but such figures need to be confirmed. The prevalence of active asthma is at its highest during childhood. It varies between 5 and 30% in childhood and from 2 to 11% in adulthood (16). The incidence of asthma varies with age, being highest in children, when it is about 1% per annum. Globally, it ranges between 0.3 to 0.4% per year. Overall, large geographical variations have been observed in the prevalence of all upper and lower conditions.

Allergic Rhinitis and Extrinsic Asthma

Classically, allergic rhinitis has been compared to extrinsic asthma and nonallergic rhinitis to intrinsic asthma beginning in adulthood and for which there is no provable atopy (17). The relationship between extrinsic asthma and allergic rhinitis is well established (18–21). Hay fever and asthma occur together more often than expected by chance alone (22,23). It has been observed that the probability that an asthmatic will have allergic rhinitis is higher than the probability that an individual with allergic rhinitis will have asthma, and the possibility that this is due to the natural history of the two conditions cannot be excluded (24–28). According to the literature, the prevalence figures for hay fever fluctuate between 28 and 50% among asthmatics, compared with a prevalence of 10 to 20% among nonasthmatics. Conversely, the prevalence of asthma among hay fever subjects is 13 to 38%, compared with a prevalence of 5 to 10% among non–hay fever subjects (29). A strong association between hay fever and asthma was confirmed among 12,391 adolescents aged between 11 and 18 years who answered a standardized questionnaire as a part of a nationwide health survey conducted in France in 1994 (30). Among them, the prevalences observed for asthma and hay fever were 11 and 41% respectively, whereas 5% of subjects reported asthma alone, 34% reported hay fever alone, and 7% reported both. Furthermore, 57% of those with asthma reported hay fever and 16% of those with hay fever reported asthma. Various studies reported that asthma prevalence was higher in subjects with allergic rhinitic confirmed by skin prick testing to common aeroallergens than in those with nonallergic rhinitis. In the southwest London study, 21% of 208 subjects with allergic rhinitis were found to have asthma, compared with only 7% of 119 with nonallergic rhinitis (12). Similarly, a study conducted in the United States among 142 individuals showed the prevalence of asthma to be 58% in individuals with seasonal allergic rhinitis, 10% in those with perennial allergic rhinitis, and 13% in those with vasomotor rhinitis (31). Data from 34 centers participating in the ECRHS showed that individuals with perennial rhinitis ($n = 1412$) were more likely than control subjects ($n = 5198$) to have current asthma, after adjustment for sex, age, smoking habit, family history of asthma, geographical area, and season at the time of examination [odds ratio (OR) = 8.1; 95% confidence interval (CI): 5.4–12.1 in those whose atopic status had been confirmed with skin prick test positivity] (32).

It has been hypothesized that the relationship between allergic rhinitis and extrinsic asthma depends on age, being stronger in childhood than later (12,33). In the 12,391 adolescents of the nationwide health survey conducted in France in 1994 (30), odds ratios of the associations between hay fever and asthma did not vary significantly according to age but were higher in individuals with parental asthma (Table 2). Type of onset may play a role, as assessed by data from NHANES II in which late–onset asthmatic subjects reported more allergic rhinitis than early–onset asthma: OR = 3.79 (CI: 1.53,9.41), 3.06 (1.33, 7.07) and 2.71 (1.18, 6.22) respectively. in the three groups defined) (34). It has also been suggested that the relationship between allergic rhinitis and extrinsic asthma might depend on the severity of asthma. Subjects with long–term (continuing) asthma attacks might be more likely to suffer from hay fever than subjects who suffered of asthma for only a short period of time. In our population–based sample of 12,391 adolescents, we found that the association was significantly stronger in the case of long–term asthma (OR of long–term asthma was 2.70, vs 1.89 in the other type of asthma).

Table 2 Sex-Adjusted Odds Ratio and 95% Confidence Intervals [in brackets] Between Asthma and Hay Fever According to Age and Family History of Asthma in 12,349 Adolescents Living in France

Subjects	All	No family history of asthma	Family history of asthma
<13 years	1.88	1.98	2.08
(n = 2369)	[1.46,2.41]	[1.47,2.66]	[1.25,3.48]
13–14 years	1.79	1.92	1.54
(n = 3395)	[1.45,2.19]	[1.54,2?40]	[0.99,2.39]
15–16 years	2.55	2.52	2.87
(n = 3169)	[2.04,3.18]	[1.95,3.25]	[1.91,4.32]
≥16 years	2.40	2.16	2.80
(n = 3431)	[1.93,2.97]	[1.71,2.74]	[1.86,4.22]

Source: Ref. (30).

Findings from a large British national cohort of 7225 children who were studied from birth to 16 years of age provide evidence in support of the foregoing hypothesis, since individuals with short–duration asthma reported significantly less hay fever than did those with long–standing asthma (35). Alternatively, allergic rhinitis might exacerbate asthma, as was recently suggested by data from the Asthma Outcomes Registry (36). Among 607 asthmatic subjects, 79% of whom reported seasonal or perennial rhinitis, asthma symptoms were more severe in individuals with asthma and allergic rhinitis than in those with asthma alone. The reason why some individuals with allergic rhinitis are much more prone to asthma than others has yet to be elucidated (37). Likely, genetic studies will contribute to the understanding of underlying mechanisms. With regard to the order of onset of the two diseases, various patterns have been proposed. Cross–sectional studies conducted among adult patients have showed that asthma and allergic rhinitis occur almost simultaneously (23,26,38).

Population data, however, have suggested that different timings can be expected for the two conditions. Among 3941 teenagers drawn from the general population who were interviewed with the ISAAC questionnaire in West Marne (France), 242 reported both asthma and hay fever. Supplementary questions on asthma and allergic rhinitis showed that 15% reported to have had asthma prior to hay fever, 12% hay fever prior to asthma, and 17% could not establish any temporal order. This could be due to recall bias in the case of mild conditions. The types of response did not depend on age. Childhood hay fever has also been considered to be a risk factor for asthma (39–42). This has been confirmed by longitudinal studies (Table 3). In the 1958 British cohort study followed up longitudinally, prior

Table 3   Rhinitis as a Predictor of Asthma in Follow-Up Population-Based Studies

Population	Outcomes	Measure of the association[a]	Ref
7225 (U.K.)	Allergic rhinitis, asthma at 7 years	OR = 7.1 [5.1,9.9]	43
770 (U.S.A.)	Allergic rhinitis, asthma at 5–9 years	OR = 2.9 [0.9,9.4]	39
8585 (Australia)	Allergic rhinitis, asthma at 7	OR = 3.9 [3.1,4.8]	40
1021 (U.S.A.)	Allergic rhinitis, asthma in life	RR = 3.0	41
173 cases, 2177 controls (U.S.A.)	Both allergic and nonallergic rhinitis; incident physician-confirmed asthma	Rhinitis increased the risk of development of asthma about threefold, among both atopic and nonatopic individuals and more than fivefold among patients in the highest IgE tertile	45

[a] OR, odds ratio; 95% confidence intervals in brackets; RR, relative risk.

hay fever was associated with an increased risk of subsequent asthma or wheezing illness in childhood or adolescence, and current hay fever was even more associated with asthma (43). Similarly, the risk of a history of asthma was higher if the child had a previous history of hay fever among 770 U. S. children ages 5 to 9 years (44) or 8585 Tasmanian children born in 1961 (99% of the eligible population) who were followed up prospectively (40). This was confirmed by a 23-year follow-up, which included skin prick testing, of 1021 U.S. college freshmen. In the 738 subjects who had been skin tested when they entered the study, allergic rhinitis and positive allergy skin tests were significant risk factors for developing new asthma (41). Concomitant occurrence of asthma and allergic rhinitis favors a common etiology. The onset of the two diseases in the same individual might indicate that both are manifestations of the same, simultaneously elicited reaction of the airways. The two conditions might share an underlying predisposing factor (probably atopy) which, when active, enhances the likelihood that both will be expressed. But other factors might also contribute to the concomitance of asthma and allergic rhinitis: age, genetic and immunological factors, nutrition, infections, seasonal variations, and air pollution, as well as active and passive smoking.

Nasal Symptoms and Intrinsic Asthma

The relationship between nasal symptoms and intrinsic asthma is less well documented. Recent data showed a strong association between rhinitis and asthma in nonatopic subjects with normal IgE levels, which is consistent with the epidemiological hypothesis that the association between rhinitis and asthma can not be exclusively attributed to a common allergic background. In the ECRHS data elicited from young adults, the relationship of perennial rhinitis to asthma remained very strong when the analysis was restricted to nonatopic subjects [OR = 11.6 (CI: 6.2–21.9)] as well as to those with IgE levels of 80 kIU/L or less [OR = 13.3 (6.7–26.5)] (32). Similarly, in the longitudinal cohort of the Tucson Epidemiologic Study of Obstructive Lung Diseases (n = 173 incident patients with physician–confirmed asthma and 2177 nonasthmatic controls), rhinitis was a significant risk factor for asthma [adjusted OR = 3.21 (CI: 2.2–4.7)] after adjustment for atopic status and the presence of chronic obstructive pulmonary disease (45) (Table 3). Thus, the nature of the association between rhinitis and asthma is open to interpretation.

Unexpectedly, asthma is uncommon in individuals with NARES, but there are no population–based data. Nasal polyps, whose formation is often preceded by vasomotor rhinitis, often develop in subjects with a history of asthma, particularly of the intrinsic type. Between 3 and 72% of subjects with polyps report coexisting asthma (46). The link between asthma and nasal polyps is confirmed by the fact that men have nasal polyps twice as often as women, but women have asthma with nasal polyps as often as men. In 345 unselected middle–aged policemen followed up three times between 1980 and 1990 in Paris, the presence of nasal polyps at rhinoscopy (4%) was significantly associated with asthma (20% of asthmatics among those with nasal polyps vs 6% of asthmatics among those without; p = 0.04). Furthermore, the diagnosis of asthma was a good predictor of nasal polyps seen at the endoscopy among the 335 outpatients who underwent endoscopy in six French hospitals. The probability of suffering from nasal polyposis increased significantly among asthmatics with aspirin intolerance and was modulated by trouble in smelling and by nasal treatments (Table 4) (Bruno Deslandes, Stéphanie Garcia-Acosta, and Isabella Annesi-Maesano, unpublished data). No epidemiological investigations have been conducted on the role played by nasal polyps in lower airway disease in children. In childhood, nasal polyps are associated with cystic fibrosis or primary ciliary dyskinesia. Nasal polyps occur in 8% of cases with cystic fibrosis, and they are associated with the respiratory rather than the gastrointestinal manifestations of the disease. It has been suggested that chronic hypertrophic sinus and nasal membrane disease with polyp formation are the nasal equivalent

Table 4 Probability (%) of Suffering from Nasal Polyposis According to Asthmatic Status, Problems in Smelling, Nasal Treatment, and Aspirin Intolerance for 335 Outpatients Who Underwent Nasal Endoscopy in 6 French Hospitals

	Outpatients without problems in smelling			Outpatients with problems in smelling		
	Without nasal treatment	With irregular nasal treatment	With regular nasal treatment	Without nasal treatment	With irregular nasal treatment	With regular nasal treatment
No asthma	5	12	26	20	38	63
Asthma without aspirin intolerance	14	29	53	44	66	84
Asthma with aspirin intolerance	35	57	79	72	86	95

of asthma. The kind of inflammation seen in nasal polyp tissue is similar to the response in other allergic respiratory disease and to bronchial inflammation of intrinsic asthma. This is why nasal polyposis has been proposed as a model for chronic inflammation of airways (47).

A more detailed description of the links between rhinitis and asthma is provided in the frame of the WHO initiative on Allergic Rhinitis and Its Impact on Asthma (ARIA) (3).

Relationships Among Other Disorders

It is redundant to show in detail that upper respiratory infections (URIs) of the ears, nose, and throat are related to asthma, for this relationship has been known for a long time. URIs are more frequent in asthmatics (48,49). Asthmatic children also have been reported to have an increased number of URIs compared with their nonasthmatic siblings (50). Furthermore, evidence has been presented suggesting that URIs, frequently precipitate asthma attacks in children (51), for they constitute the single most common precipitating factors in this age group (52). In adults, the association between asthma and URIs has been reported to be less striking (53,54). However, URIs have been implicated in the acute exacerbation of infections in patients with chronic bronchitis. Recently the relationships of colds to lower airway diseases such as chronic cough, chronic phlegm, persistent wheezing, and asthma were studied in a random population of 718 children in East Boston, aged 4 to 11 years (55). After adjustment for maternal smoking, age, and sex, frequent colds were significant predictors of lower respiratory tract symptoms [OR = 2.88 CI: 1.88,4.42)]. Results persisted in being significant after allowance for active smoking, a known risk factor for airway infections. It is possible that an immunological or mucosal defect common to the whole respiratory tract may explain the association between nasal disease and lower respiratory symptoms such as asthma (54).

Several studies have investigated the association between sinusitis and asthma (56,57). Studies that have considered x–ray assessment have found sinusitis in 30 to 70% of asthmatics, depending on criteria chosen for the evaluation of the radiological changes (58). But these investigations were uncontrolled, and only selected patients were studied. In epidemiological studies, after adjusting for potential confounders, sinusitis was not found to be related to asthma. Adjustment for bronchitis, hay fever, and parental asthma dispelled the idea that there might be a relationship between sinusitis and asthma in the population of 770 U.S. children aged 5 to 9 years (44). Similarly, the relationships of sinus troubles to lower airway diseases in the children of East Boston obtained after adjustment for maternal smoking, age, and sex [OR = 4.95 (CI: 1.83,13.39)] disappeared after allowance for active smoking [OR = 2.30 (CI: 0.69, 7.94)] (55). More recently in the Tucson children, although a diagnosis of sinusitis was strongly associated with a diagnosis of asthma, this association was not independent of that between sinusitis and allergic rhinitis (15), so that a common mechanism, like postnasal drip or mouth breathing, may be present in both sinusitis and allergic rhinitis.

Problems Encountered

Information gaps in reports of asthma and rhinitis consist of lack of standardization, shortage of general population studies, and biases such as recall bias and misclassification. Lack of standardized definitions of upper airway disorders as well as of intrinsic asthma in large population–based samples constitutes a major problem in the study of relationships between upper and lower airway diseases because it prevents comparison and generalization of the results obtained. However, recent studies (ISAAC, ECRHS, NHANES) have the potential to deal with this matter. The longitudinal approach has major advantages in examining the relationship between hay fever and extrinsic asthma because it avoids the recall bias inherent in any cross-sectional approach. The ECRHS should provide useful information in this respect at the end of the follow-up period. However, it cannot be excluded that knowledge of prior atopic status might bias the way in which upper and lower airway diseases are interpreted, labeled, and reported. In any event, longitudinal approaches do not eliminate self–reporting bias except in the case of standardized tools. Adjustment for potential confounders is also needed to interpret findings reliably. Problems encountered in the study of the relationship of sinusitis to asthma include definition of sinusitis and lack of adjustment for potential confounders. There is no gold standard in making a diagnosis of sinusitis. An attempt has been made to define sinusitis by means of clinical criteria (59), but these are difficult to apply in an epidemiological context and are relatively nonspecific. The studies conducted in large population samples did not assess the validity of the diagnosis. Since the other conditions, such as vasomotor rhinitis and nasal polyps, have been minimally examined, findings are not easily interpretable.

In conclusion, there is undoubtedly a clinical relationship between various upper and lower airway diseases, using epidemiological data from questionnaires. However, the geographical distribution and epidemiological associations either differ in an important respect, as in ISAAC (60), or have not yet been assessed, as in the case of nonallergic diseases.

B. Relationships Between Objective Measurements of Nasal and Lung Function

Nasal function testing is a useful investigative modality, which can provide information unavailable by other means. Two methods have been used in epidemiology to obtain objective measurements of nasal patency: anterior rhinomanometry and peak nasal inspiratory flow (PNIF). The former is well established as a useful clinical method of assessing nasal patency, but several expressions of nasal obstruction have been reported, and universal standardization has not yet been achieved (61). Posterior rhinomanometry is not used in epidemiology because pharyngeal pressure, needed to estimate nasal airway resistance, is sensed directly by a tube in the pharynx, which is badly tolerated by subjects (51). As a consequence, satisfactory recordings are not obtained in 40 to 50% of subjects. PNIF is a cheap, easily performed, and quick method suitable for the static assessment of nasal airway patency in population studies (62), but its reproducibility has not yet been sufficiently documented (63,64). However, comparisons between the two methods have shown a significant correlation (65–67). Spirometry is a standardized method of testing that is simple, inexpensive, and extremely sensitive to the physiological abnormalities that develop in upper and lower airway diseases. In comparison with many other tests of lung function, spirometric measurements have less variability, particularly the relation of forced expiratory volume in one second (FEV_1) to forced vital capacity (FVC). So far, very few comparisons have used objective assessments in population studies.

Upper Airway Disease and Lung Function

Reduction of lung function in patients with the common cold or allergic rhinitis has been extensively documented (68,69). Among the 345 policemen we surveyed, lowered FEV_1 was related also to usual and chronic rhinitis, independent of smoking, a major potential confounding factor (9). Similalry, 5-year FEV_1 decline between 1985 and 1990 was significantly related among ever smokers to allergic rhinitis and rhinitis induced by cold air independent of asthma and baseline FEV_1 level (70). Such findings are isolated and need to be renewed.

Lower Airway Disease and Nasal Function

As part of the ECRHS, 226 subjects aged 20 to 44 years, selected randomly among the inhabitants of the 18th district of Paris, performed anterior rhinomanometry tests with a pressure of 150 Pa. Nasal airway resistance (NAR), expressing the relationship between airflow and the associated pressure drop across the nasal airway, was available for 119 individuals, 4% of whom were asthmatics. The remaining 107 individuals had various problems at the test: technical failure ($n = 4$), only right nostril measurable ($n = 41$), only left nostril measurable ($n = 21$), small nostrils ($n = 7$), and nasal obstruction or cold ($n = 32$), or refusal ($n = 4$). A posteriori, it cannot be excluded that problems were partly due to the high level of pressure chosen. Data showed that average NAR was significantly higher in individual with current asthma than in others (2.94 $cmH_2O/L/s$ vs 2.03 $cmH_2O/L/s$, respectively: $p < 0.001$) (71) and personal communication). Only borderline significance was observed in the case of wheezing in the past year.

The relationships among lower airway symptoms, lung function, and PNIF level also were investigated among the policemen: 345 of them performed three maneuvers with a Youlten PNIF Meter, sniffing forcibly after a full expiration, and the best value was taken for the analysis. PNIF level was normally distributed [mean ($\pm$ SD) value = 155($\pm$ 54) L/min]. Around 40 (12%) of the men had a PNIF level as low as 100 L/min, which has been defined as a threshold value in clinical trials. Unexpectedly, PNIF was unrelated to age ($r = -0.02$) and to morphological characteristics such as height ($r = -0.01$), weight ($r = -0.06$), body mass index = weight/(height)^2 ($r = -0.07$). PNIF level was significantly diminished in men complaining of usual morning cough, day cough, and phlegm as well as shortness of breath at rest (Table 5). PNIF was also slightly diminished in men reporting asthma. Findings persisted after adjustment for smoking habit, a potential confounder (see later).

Nasal and Lung Functions

In clinical studies, rhinomanometry and lung functions have been used to evaluate the effects of exposure or treatment rather than to compare nasal and lung functions in order to raise new hypotheses on underlying mech-

Table 5 Relationships Between Peak Nasal Inspiratory Flow (PNIF) Level and Lower Respiratory symptoms for 345 middle-aged Parisian Policemen

	PNIF level (L/min)	
Symptom	NON	YES
Cough		
Morning (n = 31)	155.9 ± 54.0	135.8 ± 47.0*
Day (n = 15)	154.4 ± 53.5	129.3 ± 44.8 (p = 0.07)
Chronic (n = 10)	154.4 ± 54.0	143.0 ± 41.4
Phlegm		
Morning (n = 25)	154.8 ± 54.4	137.6 ± 42.9
Day (n = 11)	154.6 ± 53.3	122.7 ± 44.7*
Chronic (n = 5)	154.4 ± 53.6	128.0 ± 48.7
First degree (n = 8)	140.3 ± 49.5	132.5 ± 39.6
Wheezing		
In the presence of cold (n = 24)	154.3 ± 52.8	144.2 ± 62.8
In the absence of cold (n = 22)	154.8 ± 53.2	143.2 ± 59.5
Frequent (n = 7)	153.8 ± 52.2	164.3 ± 105.6
Past year (n = 26)	154.2 ± 52.4	151.5 ± 67.5
Shortness of breath		
At rest (n = 10)	154.1 ± 53.1	118.0 ± 53.5*
At night (n = 5)	154.3 ± 53.5	138.0 ± 66.1
Reactor status (n = 25)	156.2 ± 53.3	161.6 ± 46.0
Asthma (n = 25)	156.1 ± 53.4	135.6 ± 57.0 (p = 0.07)

*$p > 0.05$.
Source: Ref. 9.

anisms. Two different studies have indicated that mechanisms regulating the response of the nose to exercise are different from those involved in the response of the bronchial tree (72,73). Epidemiological data relating other markers of nasal patency to lung function are rare. Among 300 children attending a public elementary school in Vienna who underwent anterior rhinomanometry and spirometry, the nasal airflow values did not show any significant correlation with lung function, namely FVC (% pred), FEV_1 (% pred) and the ratios of FEV_1 to FVC and mean maximal expiratory flow (MEF_{50}) to FVC (74). Conversely, there are no published epidemiological data relating PNIF to lung function. In our population of 345 policemen, we find a significant association between PNIF and FEV_1 values among current smokers: the higher the FEV_1 score level, the higher the PNIF level (β = 15 ± 4 L/min, p = 0.001, in current smokers vs 6 ± 6 L/min in nonsmokers and −3 ± 5 L/min in former smokers). Further analysis taking quartiles of FEV_1 score into account showed that all nonsmokers had higher PNIF level values than former and current smokers (Fig. 1). In current smokers PNIF level ranged between 129 (±9) L/min in individuals with low FEV_1 (first quartile) and 170 (±11) L/min in individuals with high FEV_1 (last quartile). The most elevated PNIF value was found in the last quartile of FEV_1, suggesting the intervention of the "healthy smoker effect," describing the condition of smokers who continue smoking and yet are particularly healthy. Former smokers were in an intermediate position except those with the highest FEV_1 value, who had a PNIF of only 130

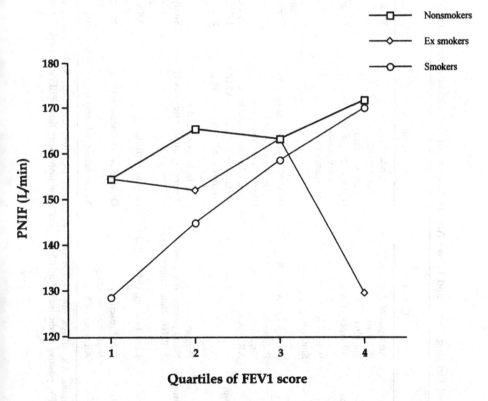

Figure 1 FEV_1 and PNIF level according to smoking habits among 345 middle-aged Parisian policemen: squares, nonsmokers; diamonds, former smokers; circles, smokers. FEV_1: Forced Expiratory Volume in 1 second; PNIF: Peak Nasal Inspiratory Flow. FEV_1 was standardized for age and height, by using a linear regression on age and height in the whole sample. FEV_1 values were then normalized (FEV_1 score) as the observed $FEV_1 - (a + b + c)/\sqrt{s^2}$, where a and b are the age and height regression coefficients, c the intercept, and s^2 the residual variance.

Table 6 Methods of Defining Upper and Lower Airway Diseases in Epidemiological Studies[a]

Method	Outcome	Comment	Epidemiological studies having used it
Clinical evaluation	All types of A and R, Polyposis, Sinusitis	Not standardized but presently gold standard	Study in France (9)
Self-report of diagnosis or diagnostic label by questionnaire	All types of A and R, Polyposis, Sinusitis	Depends on the severity of the diseases, Low specificity	Largely used in epidemiological studies: ISAAC, ECRHS, NHANES, study in France (9), SAPALDIA (116), SCARPOL (117), EGEA (118), but few data for polyposis and sinusitis
Self-report of the condition by questionnaires	All types of A and R, Polyposis, Sinusitis	High PPV (rhinoconjunctivitis, wheezing last year), High PPV in one study	Largely used in epidemiological studies (all conditions)
Allergy markers (IgE, SPT, Phadiatop, eosinophilia...)	AR, EA *vs* IA	Eosinophil count useful to diagnose NARES *vs* VMR; rarely used in epidemiology so far	ISAAC: only SPT, ECRHS, NHANES, study in France (9), SAPALDIA, SCARPOL, EGEA
	Polyposis	Role to be examined	
Function (nasal and lung)	Nasal patency (rhinometry, PNIF, rhinomanometry)	Depending on disease activity	Study in France: PNIF vs lung function ECRHS (rhinomanometry in 1 center vs lower airway disease)
	Lung function (FEV$_1$, PEF)	Easy to perform	All studies allow relating upper airway diseases to lung function
Challenge	Nasal reactivity, Bronchial reactivity	Depending on disease activity	No epidemiological data on nasal challenge
Rhinoscopy	All types of R	Not standardized, easy to perform	Study in Michigan (19), France (9)

[a]Abbreviations: A, asthma; AR, allergic rhinitis; EA, extrinsic asthma; IA, intrinsic asthma; NARES, nonallergic rhinitis with eosinophilia; VMR, vasomotor rhinitis; PPV, positive predictive value; PNIF, peak nasal inspiratory flow; PEF, oral peak expiratory flow.

($\pm$ 10) L/min. Whether PNIF level, which can be easily ascertained in epidemiological studies, allows the reliable study of the relationship between upper and lower airway diseases remains to be confirmed.

Problems Encountered

Joint data on nasal function and lower airway disease or lung function are scanty, and other investigations are urged to advance our comprehension of the relationships. Prior to that, the assessment of nasal patency in epidemiological settings should be implemented. Major problems identified in this respect concern nasal function choice and lack of standardized assessments. The choice of nasal function depends on the selected population and the circumstances encountered in the study.

Anterior rhinometry is reproducible but cannot be performed in individuals presenting nasal obstruction, thus biasing final results. PNIF seems to be more appropriate in epidemiological studies because easier to determine. However, PNIF could be problematic in some subjects because of an individual's participation in the maneuver. Reproducibility of both PNIF and rhinomanometry must be further assessed in children and elderly individuals. Measurements must be standardized in terms of either techniques or expression of the results. In the absence of common criteria, results from different studies are not comparable.

In conclusion, very few epidemiological data relate objective assessments of upper and lower airway diseases (Table 6).

II. Indirect Evidence

A. Associations with Other Conditions

The following conditions have been associated with both upper and lower airway diseases: airway hyperreactivity, immediate hypersensitivity, and allergy.

Airway Hyperresponsiveness

Human bronchial responsiveness has been analyzed as a dichotomous or a continuous variable: "reactor status" and "dose–response slope," respectively. The former considers whether the individual exhibits a postchallenge decline (PD) in lung function, (usually FEV_1 decline of 20%, expressed as $PD_{20}FEV_1$), and the latter uses an estimate of the overall slope of the dose–response relationship to better describe the phenomenon.

URIs (especially croup and bronchiolitis) in early childhood may play a role in the development of airways hyperreactivity the major characteristic of asthma (75). In adults, there is substantial evidence of an increase in bronchial hyperreactivity lasting for several weeks following URIs even in normal subjects (76). However, this has not been confirmed in epidemiological studies (9,77). The most commonly postulated explanations (78) include inflammation caused by respiratory infections in the larger airway, metabolites produced by infected cells, which interfere with the β–adrenergic tone in the airways of asthmatics, and release of mediators that sensitize lower airways.

Nonspecific bronchial hyperresponsiveness, a constant feature of asthma, is a common feature in individuals with allergic rhinitis (9,79–80, 81) and is also found in those without prior asthmatic symptoms (82,83). In the ECRHS data, bronchial hyperresponsiveness was more frequent in subjects with rhinitis without asthma than in those without rhinitis and asthma (OR = 1.7; CI: 1.2–2.6 in nonatopic subjects with IgE levels of 80 kIU/L or less) (32). Furthermore, it has been suggested that nonspecific bronchial hyperresponsiveness might be a predictor of asthma among individuals with allergic rhinitis (84–86) but data showing this were not all prospective (78,87).

To find whether airway hyperresponsiveness was associated with a greater risk of asthma in subjects with allergic rhinitis, 66 nonasthmatic patients with allergic rhinitis who had undergone inhalation challenge with methacholine were followed up for almost 2 years. Among them, the risk of developing asthma during the follow—up period was not related to bronchial hyperresponsiveness (88).

Few studies have considered factors able to modify the relationship between bronchial hyperresponsiveness and allergic rhinitis exemplified by smoking (9,89,90), immunotherapy (91,92), and allergenic exposure (93–95). In comparison to individuals with seasonal rhinitis, those with perennial rhinitis might have a higher risk of developing bronchial hyperresponsiveness (86,93). These data are isolated and entail small samples. Among the 300 Austrian children described earlier, the nasal airflow values showed a significant correlation with bronchial hyperresponsiveness (74). The consecutive decongestion test showed a marked increase in flow rates at each level, which was found to be significantly higher in children with bronchial hyperresponsiveness (p < 0.01). There was no sex–dependent difference in nasal dysfunction. Similarly, in the Parisian ECRHS sample, the mean dose–response slope was more elevated in the high NAR group than in the low NAR group (12.1%/μmol vs 2.4%/μmol; p = 0.08) (69). Subjects with nasal obstruction who could not perform rhinomanometry were not included in the analysis. However, PNIF level was not related to bronchial hyperresponsiveness in our sample of 345 policemen (Table 5). Bronchial hyperresponsiveness response was found to be significantly heightened also in nonallergic chronic rhinitis (9), but further confirmation is needed in this resepct. No epidemiological data exist on bronchial hyperresponsiveness in NARES syndrome. However, NARES patients have higher nonspecific bronchial hyperresponsiveness than others. The $PD_{20}FEV_1$ was related to chronic (lasting 3 months per year) rhinitis that was not associated with skin prick test positivity in our sample of policemen (9). The association between FEV_1 and bronchial hyperresponsiveness and nonallergic usual and chronic rhinitis supports the interplay between lung impairment and nonallergic upper airways disorders.

Other nasal conditions have been less well investigated. It has been shown that patients with nasal polyps often have increased airway responsiveness to methacholine (46,96). This was confirmed in the policemen, in whom the dose–response slope to methacholine was higher in those with polyps than in others (20.1 vs 95.5%/μmol decline in FEV_1; $p = 0.07$).

To sum up, studies suggest that bronchial hyperresponsiveness might be associated with nasal disorders independently of allergy. No epidemiological data using objective nasal hyperresponsiveness exist.

Immediate Hypersensitivity and Allergy

A relationship that is undisputed is that between immediate hypersensitivity and both asthma and allergic rhinitis, at least in childhood. Asthmatic children exhibit both raised total IgE level and increased skin prick test positivity (98). The relationship is less evident among adults. After adjustment for potential confounders, various population data have shown that total IgE level was heightened in individuals drawn from the general population with asthma, whereas skin prick test positivity was strongly associated with hay fever (99–101). These data support the concept that asthma and hay fever are related to different immunological host factors as reflected by expression of atopy phenotypes. Epidemiological differences between mechanisms may be useful pointers to the separate influences of genetic and environmental factors. A major influence on the prevalence of asthma and rhinitis may be the amount and nature of allergens in different environments. Among 5427 French subjects aged 18 to 65 years living in two areas with contrasted pollen exposure, high exposure to pollen was a risk factor for developing hay fever but not asthma after adjustment for age, sex, smoking, region, and reactivity to other allergens (102). There is information for at least two main genetic mechanisms involved in the atopic status: the specific immune response associated with the histocompatibility complex located within a chromosomal region on the short arm of chromosome 6 and the genetic control concerning the regulation of the IgE serum levels (high and low "responders"). Such mechanisms might explain the different responses observed in asthma and allergic rhinitis, respectively. Atopic dermatitis (eczema) is another condition clearly associated with asthma and allergic rhinitis in epidemiological studies. Furthermore, there is a tendency of IgE to reach higher levels in eczema with more severe respiratory allergy (103). Finally, blood eosinophil count and serum eosinophil cationic protein (S–ECP) levels, markers of both active asthma and bronchial hyperresponsiveness, were found to be closely related also to allergic rhinitis, including hay fever among subjects participating in the ECRHS in Sweden (104).

In conclusion, various allergic markers are involved in the development of extrinsic asthma and allergic rhinitis. Connections of such markers to other upper and lower airway diseases have not been examined.

B. Associations with Common Risk Factors

Various factors are potentially common to upper and lower diseases (Table 7). They can be classified as etiological agents, environmental factors, and host susceptibility. However, only a few have been considered in epidemiological studies. Most data were provided on heredity and smoking.

Heredity

Allergic disorders like asthma and allergic rhinitis are reported to be clustered in families. In a general population of rural Iowans, among the 195 asthmatics, 24% had close relatives with nasal symptoms only. Of 208 subjects with hay fever, only 28% had close relatives with allergic rhinitis only (20,29). Well–conducted analyses in 3808 pairs of Australian twins showed that genetic factors are implicated in both hay fever and asthma (correlation in genetic liability to the traits of 0.52 for men and 0.65 for women) and that some of these genetic factors are common (at least among a subgroup of individuals) to both traits (105,106). The aggregation of comorbidity between allergic rhinitis and asthma was significantly more frequent among siblings than between parents and offspring in an Italian population–based sample (107). Furthermore, the prevalence of asthma and hay fever was significantly higher among relatives of extrinsic (atopic) than among relatives of intrinsic asthmatics in a sample of the Brompton Hospital and the Doncaster Royal Infirmary (108). And the prevalence of these traits tended to be higher among siblings of extrinsic probands with one or both parents affected than among siblings of probands with neither parent affected. No data exist on family resemblance between upper and lower diseases other than allergic.

Smoking

The role of active and passive tobacco smoking has been well established in lower airway disease, including asthma (109), but very little data are

Table 7 Potential Factors Contributing to Both Upper and Lower Airway Diseases[a]

Category	Factors	Type of comorbidity	Epidemiological evidence
Etiologic agents	Allergens (pollens, molds, animals, dust mites, etc.)	AR–EA	Yes
Environmental factors	Infections	(?)	None
	Air pollution	(?)	Ecological studies for AR and EA
	Active smoking	All diseases	Few for AR and EA
	Cold air	Nonallergic (?)	None
	Passive smoking	All diseases	Few for AR and EA
	Humidity	(?)	Few
	Irritants (ammonia, chlorine, soap powder, smoke from wood stoves, etc.)	(?)	None
	Seasonal variations	AR–EA, probably also nonallergic diseases	None
	Temperature	NAR-IA, polyposis—IA	None
	Aspirin	All diseases in a different manner	Few
Variations in host susceptibility	Age		
	Airway hyperreactivity		R, polyposis and A (but few data)
	Atopy		R, polyposis and A (but few data)
	Genetic factors		All the other factors need to be studied
	Immunological factors		
	Nutrition		
	Birth order		
	Migration		

[a] A, asthma; AR, allergic rhinitis; EA, extrinsic asthma; IA, intrinsic asthma; NAR, nonallergic rhinitis; R, rhinitis.

available on the effects of tobacco smoking on upper airway disease. "Nasal catarrh" as assessed in the original British Medical Research Council questionnaire, was significantly more common in active smokers than in nonsmokers (110). Similarly, there was a close relationship between chronic nasal symptomatology and smoking habits among 27,604 French conscripts (111): 33% had a regular nasal obstruction, 14% repeated sneezing fits, and only 5% nasal manifestations related to an allergy to Graminaceae pollens. Smokers reported all upper and lower respiratory conditions more often than nonsmokers, except for allergic rhinitis only (without asthma), which was reported less often by smokers, in the NHANES II population of 11,260 white and 1482 black individuals aged 12 to 74 years (112). In the sample of policemen, we also observed that active smoking was positively related to usual and chronic rhinitis but not to allergic rhinitis (79). Individuals with allergic rhinitis were more often former smokers than were individuals without. This might be due to self–selection process by so–called healthy smokers (113). However, it cannot be excluded that individuals quit smoking because of their asthma or allergic rhinitis. However, the role of active cigarette smoking as a potential risk factor, a selection factor ("healthy smoker" effect), or a modifier (with respect to severity) of asthma and allied diseases is still discussed (109). Various studies but not all those having examined the relationship have suggested that active cigarette smoking could be a risk factor for asthma overall among adolescents. In the West

Table 8 Adjusted[a] Odds Ratios and 95% Confidence Intervals [in brackets] for Asthma and Hay Fever in Relation to Active and Passive Smoking for 3941 Teenagers of the West Marne ISAAC

	Disease		
Condition	Asthma $n = 419$	Hay fever $n = 669$	Both $n = 242$
Active smoking			
No[b]	1.00	1.00	1.00
Yes	1.39 [1.02,1.87]	1.46 [1.14,1.88]	1.61 [1.02,2.55]
	$p = 0.03$	$p = 0.003$	$p = 0.04$
Passive smoking			
No	1.00	1.00	1.00
Yes	1.06 [0.83,1.34]	1.26 [1.03,1.53]	1.12 [0.77,1.64]
	NS	$p = 0.02$	NS

[a] Adjustment made for age and sex with the logistic regression model.
[b] Referent category.

Marne ISAAC conducted among 3941 teenagers, smoking was significantly more common in individuals with asthma, hay fever, or both (Table 8). That tobacco smoking may affect also the upper airways was supported by the fact that among the policemen we observed an inverse relationship between smoking habit and PNIF level (Fig. 2). Current smokers exhibited significantly lower PNIF level values than nonsmokers. Whether tobacco smoking is responsible for upper airway impairment assessed by PNIF needs to be confirmed.

Some subjects report rhinitis symptoms after exposure to environmental tobacco smoke (ETS), but objective assessments of this response in population–based samples have been lacking. Strong evidence comes from experimental data. Exposure to sidestream tobacco smoke increased significantly chest discomfort or tightness and cough as well as nasal congestion and rhinorrhea symptoms in 10 ETS–sensitive subjects compared

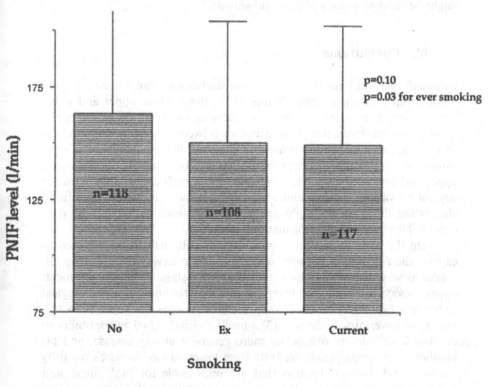

Figure 2 Peak nasal inspiratory flow level and smoking habits among 345 middle-aged Parisian policemen.

with 11 ETS–nonsensitive subjects (114). Results from population data are controversial. In the West Marne ISAAC, passive smoking was slightly related to hay fever [OR = 1.20 (CI: 1.01,1.52)] but not to asthma after allowance for age and sex (Table 8). Night cough and nasal symptoms assessed through the ISAAC questionnaire were more common in 2752 children ages 13 to 14 years exposed to smoking in New Zealand than in others (115). Inversely, among 9651 adults of the SAPALDIA study, passive smoking exposure was associated with several lower airway disorders but not with any increased risk of allergic rhinitis including hayfever, after adjustment for age, sex, body mass index, study area, atopy, and parental and sibling history (116).

In conclusion, although various factors seem to be involved in comorbidities between upper and lower airway diseases, only few have been examined so far in epidemiological settings. Preliminary data suggest that among other factors, smoking may have an influence in upper airways similar to that observed in lower airways. In any event, the associations might be masked among allergic individuals.

III. Conclusions

Although relevant data from population studies are available only for the relationship between allergic rhinitis and asthma, other upper and lower airway diseases also seem to have connections, as shown by sparse epidemiological data. In particular, associations between nasal and lung function and bronchial hyperresponsiveness might exist independently of allergic status, so supporting the hypothesis that similar processes might affect upper and lower airways. The epidemiology of such connections seems to depend on various factors, and comprehension of them might be useful in elucidating the main pathophysiological mechanisms underlying the conditions. However, other confirmations are needed.

On the basis of existing results, various patterns can be proposed to explain the association between upper and lower airway diseases (Fig. 3). Upper airway disease may be regarded as (1) a stage of lung impairment, upper airways abnormalities being the first manifestation of a pathological status that becomes prominent in larger airways over the years; (2) a risk factor for lower airway disease; (3) a marker of individual susceptibility to develop lower airway disease or more generally airway disease; and (4) another disease, completely separate from lower airway disease, caused by the same risk factors. Factors that are responsible for both upper and lower airway diseases are individual susceptibility, infections, environmental exposure (to, e.g., active and passive smoking, allergens, and

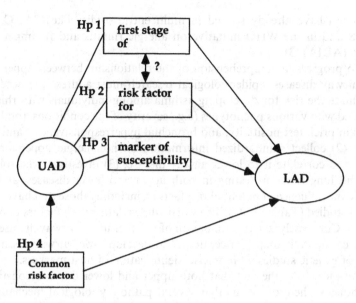

Figure 3 Patterns (Hp1–Hp4) proposed for the relationship between upper and lower airway diseases (UAD and LAD).

pollution), and some occupational factors. The present state of knowledge does not allow us to explain the nature of the connections observed between upper and lower airway diseases. In this respect, it is unfortunate that many respiratory epidemiological studies have been conducted without a precise underlying hypothesis with regard to the relationship between upper and lower airway diseases (23). The results have been that many conditions have been discarded, associations of interest have been poorly described, and furthermore confounders have rarely been considered. Future respiratory epidemiological research must reflect awareness of the relevance of designing ad hoc studies to investigate simultaneously upper and lower airway disease.

Investigating associations between upper and lower disease outcomes and their putative risk factors must involve measuring longitudinally the relevant variables with standardized methodology in representative populations and taking into account all the factors able to modify their clinical presentation. To this extent, standardization projects on upper airway disease assessment including both questionnaires and objective measurements must be advocated. Research into the epidemiology of upper airway disease would benefit from comparisons of data from different surveys obtained by using the same standardized instruments for identifying the various conditions. Such comparison have already started in multicentric studies like ISAAC and ECRHS and in the WHO initiative on allergic rhinitis and Its impact on Asthma (ARIA) (3).

To progress in comprehension of the relationship between upper and lower airway diseases, epidemiological research must address the needs to (1) estimate the risk for developing asthma among individuals with rhinitis associated with various phenotypes (e.g., severity of the conditions, total IgE level, skin prick test positivity, and bronchial hyperresponsiveness) and risk factors; (2) collect standardized information on nonallergic upper airway disease and correlate it to lower airway disease; (3) investigate the role of nasal and lung function testing in both upper and lower diseases; and (4) evaluate the influence of potential risk factors, including those that have been less well studied (Table 7). It will be worthwhile relating such factors to nasal function. Conversely, the determination of whether upper airway disease is a marker of the individual's susceptibility to develop lower airway disease is matter of genetic studies with precise identification of host markers.

Paradoxically, the fact that both upper and lower diseases constitute two wholes so heterogeneous that several pathophysiological mechanisms are involved is advantageous to the progress of the research. Maintaining the separation among the various diseases and defining new entities will contribute new evidence on the relationship between upper and lower airways disease through case–control studies and the contribution of multidisciplinary research.

Acknowledgments

I am grateful to David Moreau for assistance in analyzing data drawn from adolescents and adults living in France.

References

1. Mygind N and Bisgaard H. Applied anatomy of airways. In: Mygind N, ed. Rhinitis and Asthma: similarities and differences. Copenhagen Munksgaard, 1990: 21–37.
2. Mygind N, Weeke B. Allergic and non-allergic rhinitis. In: Middleton Jr E, Reed CE, Ellis EF, Adkinson NF, Yunginger JW, eds. Allergy: Principles and Practice. 2nd ed. St Louis, MO: Mosby, 1983:1101–1117.
3. Allergic rhinitis and its impact on asthma. ARIA Workshop Report. J Allergy Clin Immunol. 2001; 108(5): S1–S47.

4. Minette A, Brille D, Casula D et al. European Coal and Steel Community (ECSC): High Authority Questionnaire on the Study of Chronic Bronchitis and Emphysema. Luxembourg ECSC, 1967.
5. Ferris BG. Recommended respiratory disease questionnaires for use with adults and children in epidemiological research: epidemiology standardization project. Am Rev Respir Dis 1978;118:1–53.
6. Burney PGJ, Latinen LA, Perdrizet S et al. Validity and repeatability of the IUATLD (1984) bronchial symptoms questionnaire: an International comparison. Eur J Respir Dis 1989; 2:940–945.
7. Sibbald B and Rink E. Epidemiology of seasonal and perennial rhinitis: clinical presentation and medical history. Thorax 1991;46:895–901.
8. Asher MI, Keil U, Anderson HR, Beasly R, Crane J, Martinez F, Mitchell EA, Pearce N, Sibbald B, Stewrt AW, Strachan D, Weiland SK, Williams HC. International Study of Asthma and Allergies in Childhood (ISAAC): rationale and methods. Eur Respir J 1995; 8: 483–491.
9. Annesi I, Oryszczyn MP, Neukirch F, Orvoen-Frija E, Korobaeff M, Kauffmann F. Relationship of upper airways disorders to FEV_1 and bronchial hyperresponsiveness in an epidemiological study. Eur Respir J 1992; 5: 1104–1110.
10. Annesi-Maesano I, Didier A, Klossek M, Chanal I, Moreau D, Bousquet J. The score for allergic rhinitis (SFAR): a simple and valid assessment method in population studies. Allergy. 2002;57:107–14.
11. Sibbald B, Charpin D. Epidemiological identification of allergic rhinitis. Allergy 1996; 51: 293–8.
12. Sibbald B and Rink E. Labelling of rhinitis and hay fever by doctors. Thorax 1991; 46: 378–381.
13. Kern E. Use of a questionnaire for patients with nasal symptoms. Rhynology 1972; 10 : 133–377.
14. Jessen M, Janzon L. Prevalence of non-allergic nasal complaints in an urban and a rural population in Sweden. Allergy 1989; 44: 582–587.
15. Lombardi E, Stein RT. Wright AL, Morgan WJ, Martinez FD. The relation between physician-diagnosed sinusitis, asthma, and skin test reactivity to allergens in 8-year-old children. Pediatr Pulmonol 1996; 22:41–146.
16. Burr ML. Epidemiology of asthma. In: Burr ML, ed. Epidemiology of Clinical Allergy, Basel: Karger, 1993:80–102.
17. Franklin W. Perennial rhinitis. In: McKay I, ed. Rhinitis : Mechanisms and Management, Suffolk: William Clowes, 1989:117–140.
18. Rackeman F, Edwards MC, Asthma in children. N Engl J Med 1952; 246: 815–823.
19. Broder I, Higgins MW, Matthews KP, Keller JP. Epidemiology of asthma, and allergic rhinitis in a total community. Tecumseh, Michigan Ill. Second survey of the community. J Allergy Clin Immunol. 1974; 53: 127–138.
20. Smith J. Montgomery and Knowler L.A. Epidemiology of asthma and allergic rhinitis I. In a rural area. II. In a university-centered community. Am Rev Respir Dis 1965; 92: 16–31.

21. Pedersen PA, Weeke ER. Asthma and allergic rhinitis in the same patients. Allergy 1983; 38: 25–29.
22. Sibbald B, Strachan DP. Epidemiology of rhinitis. In: Busse WW, Holgate ST eds. Asthma and Rhinitis, Boston: Blackwell Scientific Publications, 1995: 32–43.
23. Annesi-Maesano I. Rhinitis and asthma. Epidemiological evidence. ACl Int 2001; 13: 147153.
24. Weeke ER, Backman A, Pedersen PA. Epidemiology, In: Mygind N, ed. Allergic and vasomotor rhinitis. Clinical Aspects, 1st ed. Copenhagen: Munksgaard, 1985: 771–809.
25. Blair H. The incidence of asthma, hay fever and infantile eczema in an East London group practice of 9145 patients. Clin Allergy 1974: 4: 389–399.
26. Edfors-Lubs ML. Allergy in 7000 twin pairs. Acta Allergol 1971; 26: 249–285.
27. Sibbald B. Epidemiology of allergic rhinitis. In: Burr ML, ed. Epidemiology of Clinical Allergy. Basel : Karger, 1993: 61–69.
28. Peckham C, Butler N. A national study of asthma in childhood. J Epidemiol Community Health 1978; 32: 79–85.
29. Smith MJ. Epidemiology and natural history of asthma, allergic rhinitis, and atopic dermatitis (eczema). In: Middleton Jr E, Reed CE, Ellis EF, Adklnson NF, Yunginger JW, eds. Allergy : Principles and Practice. 2nd ed. St Louis, MO : Mosby, 1983: 771–803.
30. Choquet M, Ledoux S. Adolescents. Enquete nationale. Paris: Les Editions INSERM,1994: 5–18.
31. Mullarkey MF, Hill JS, Webb DR. Allergic and non-allergic rhinitis: their characterization with the meaning of nasal eosinophilia. J Allergy Clin Immunol 1980; 65: 122–126.
32. Leynaert B, Bousquet J, Neukirch C, Liard R, Neukirch F. Perennial rhinitis: an independent risk factor for asthma in nonatopic subjects: results from the European Community Respiratory Health Survey. J Allergy Clin Immunol 1999;104:301–4.
33. Lundback B. Epidemiology of rhinitis and asthma. Clin Exp Allergy 1998;28 Suppl 2:3–10.
34. Gergen PJ, Turkeltaub PC, Kramer RA. Age of onset in childhood asthma: data from a national cohort. Ann Allergy 1992; 68: 507–14.
35. Kaplan BA, Mascie-Taylor CG. Predicting the duration of childhood asthma. J Asthma 1992; 29: 39–48.
36. Huse DM, Hartz SC, Klaus DH, Piercy GE, Richner R, Weiss ST. Does allergic rhinitis exacerbate asthma symptoms In adults? The Asthma Outcomes Registry. Eur Respir J.1996; 9 (suppl 23): 351s.
37. Smith JM. Epidemiology and natural history of asthma, allergic rhinitis and atopic dermatitis (eczema). In: Middleton E, Reed CE, Ellis EF eds. Allergy: Principles and Practice. 2nd ed. St Louis, MO: CV Mosby, 1983: 772–803.
38. Arsdel PP, Motulsky AG. Frequency and hereditability of asthma and allergic rhinitis in college students. Acta Genet 1959; 9: 101–114.

39. Hagy GW, Settipane GA, Risk factors for developing asthma and allergic rhinitis: a seven-year follow-up study of college students. J Allergy Clin Immunol 1976; 58: 330–336.
40. Jenkins MA, Hopper JL, Flander LB, Carlin JB, Giles GG. The associations between childhood asthma and atopy, and parental asthma, hay fever and smoking. Paediatr Perinat Epidemiol 1993; 7: 67–76.
41. Settipane RJ, Hagy GW, Settipane GA. Allergy Proc 1994; 15: 21–25.
42. Anderson HR, Bland JM, Patel S, Peckham C. The natural history of asthma in childhood. J Epidemiol Community Health 1986; 40: 121–9.
43. Anderson HR, Pottier AC, Strachan DP. Asthma from birth to age 23: Incidence and relationship to prior and concurrent atopic disease. Thorax 1992; 47: 537–542.
44. Sherman, Barr MB, Weiss ST, Segal MR, Tager IB, Speizer FE. The relationship of nasal disorders to lower respiratory tract symptoms and illness in a random sample of children. Paediatr Pulmonol 1992; 14: 91–94.
45. Guerra S, Sherrill DL, Martinez FD, Barbee RA. Rhinitis as an independent risk factor for adult-onset asthma. J Allergy Clin Immunol 2002; 109: 419–25.
46. Moloney JR. Collins J. Nasal polyps and bronchial asthma. Br J Dis Chest 1977: 71: 1–6.
47. Jordana M, Dolovich J, Ohno I. Finotto s. Denburg J. Nasal polyposis: a model for chronic inflammation. In : Asthma and rhinitis. Busse WW, Holgate ST eds. Boston: Blackwell Scientific Publications 1995: 156–166.
48. Siegel SC, Goldstein JD, Sawyer A, Glaser J. The incidence of allergy in persons who have many colds. Ann Allergy. 1952: 10: 24–30.
49. Porro E, Calamita P, Rana I, Montini L, Criscione S. Atopy and environment factors in upper respiratory infections: an epidemiological survey on 2304 school children. Int J Pediatr Otorhinolaryngol 1992; 24: 111–20.
50. Minor TE, Baker JW, Dick EC, DeMeo AN, Ouellette JJ, Cohen M, Reed CE. Greater frequency of viral infection in asthmatic children as compared with their nonasthmatic siblings. J Pediatr 1974; 85: 472–480.
51. McIntosh K, Ellis EF Hoffman LS, Lybass TG, Eller JJ, Fulginiti VA. The association of viral and bacterial respiratory infections with exacerbation of wheezing in young asthmatic children. J Pediatr 1973; 82: 578–581.
52. Carlsen KH, Orstavik I, Leegard J, Hoeg H. Respiratory virus infections and aeroallergens in acute bronchial asthma. Arch Dis Child 1984; 310: 59.
53. Halperin SA, Eggleston PA, Beasly P, Suratt P, Hendely O, Groschel M. Gwaltney JM Jr. Exacerbations of asthma in adults during experimental rhinovirus Am Rev Respir Dis 1985; 132: 976–982.
54. Hudgel DW, Langston L, Selner JC, McIntosh K. Viral and bacterial infections in adults with chronic asthma Am Rev Respir Dis 1979; 120: 393–397.
55. Barr MB, Weiss ST, Segal MR, Tager IB, Speizer FE. The relationship of nasal disorders to lower respiratory tract symptoms and illness in a random sample of children. Pediatr Pulmonol 1992; 14: 91–94.
56. Slavin RG. Relationship of nasal disease and sinusitis to bronchial asthma. Ann Allergy 1982; 49: 76–80.

57. Rachelefsky GS, Katz RM, Siegel SC. Chronic sinus disease with associated reactive airway disease in children. Paediatrics 1984; 73: 526–529.

58. Pfister R, Lutolf M, Schapowal A, Glatter B, Schmitz M, Menz G. Screening for sinus disease in patients with asthma: a computed tomography–controlled comparison of A-mode ultrasonography and standard radiography. J Allergy Clin Immunol 1994; 94: 804–809.

59. Shapiro GG, Rachelefsky GS. Introduction and definition of sinusitis. J Allergy Clin Immunol 1992: 90: 417–418.

60. ISAAC. The International Study of Asthma and Allergies in Childhood (ISAAC) Steering Commitee. Worldwide variation in prevalence of symptoms of asthma, allergic rhinoconjunctivitis, and atopic eczema. Lancet. 1998 Apr 25;351(9111):1225–32.

61. Schumacher MJ. Rhinomanometry. J Allergy Clin Immunol 1989; 83: 711–717.

62. Holmstroem M, Scadding GK, Lund VJ, Darby YC. Assessment of nasal obstruction. A comparison between rhinomanometry and nasal inspiratory peak flow. Rhinology 1990; 28: 191–196.

63. Clarcke RW, Jones AS. The limitations of peak nasal flow measurements. Clin Otolaryngology 1994; 19: 502–504.

64. Hooper RG. Forced inspiratory nasal flow–volume curves: a simple test of nasal airflow. Mayo Clin Proc 2001;76:990–4.

65. Wihl JA, Malm L. Rhinomanometry and nasal peak expiratory and inspiratory flow rate. Ann Allergy 1988; 61: 50–55.

66. Frolund L, Madsen F, Mygind N, Nielsen NH, Svendsen UG, Weeke B. Comparison between different techniques for measuring nasal patency In a group of unselected patients. Acta Oto-Laryngol 1987: 104: 175–179.

67. Enberg RN, Ownby DR. Pak nasal inspiratory flow and Wright peak flow: a comparison of their reproducibility. Ann Allergy 1991; 67: 371–374.

68. Grossmann J, Putnam S. Small airway obstruction in allergic rhinitis. J Allergy Clin Immunol 1975; 55: 49–55.

69. Morgan EJ, Hall DR. Abnormalities of lung function in hay fever. Thorax 1976; 31: 80–86.

70. Annesi I, Neukirch F, Orvoen-Frija E, Oryszczyn MP, Korobaeff M, D'Oré MF, Kauffmann F. The relevance of hyperresponsiveness but not of atopy to FEV_1 decline. Preliminary results In a working population. Bull Eur Physiopathol Respir 1987; 23: 397–400.

71. Korobaeff M, Neukirch C, Leynaert B, Henry C, Neukirch F. Nasal airflow resistance measured by rhinomanometry : Relationships to asthma and bronchial hyperresponssiveness. Eur Resp J 1995; 8 suppl 19: 33s.

72. Sthrol KP, Delker MJ, Olson LG, Flak TA, Hoekje PL. The nasal response to exercise and exercise induced bronchoconstriction in normal and asthmatic: subjects. Thorax 1988; 43: 890–895.

73. Serra-Battles J, Montserrat JM, Mullol J, Bellester E, Xauber A, Picado C. Response of the nose to exercise in healty subjects and in patients with rhinitis and asthma. Thorax 1994; 49: 128–32.

74. Kiss D, Popp W, Horak F, Wagner C, Zwick H. Nasal function and bronchial hyperresponsiveness to methacholine in children. Chest 1995; 107: 1582–1584.
75. Weiss ST, Tager IB, Munoz A, Speizer FE. The relationship of respiratory infections in early childhood to the occurrence of increased levels of bronchial responsiveness and atopy. Am Rev Respir Dis 1985; 131: 573–578.
76. Empey DW, Laitinen LA, Jacobs L, Gold WM, Nadel JA. Mechanisms of bronchial hyperreactivity in normal subjects after upper respiratory tract infection. Am Rev Respir Dls 1976; 113: 131–139.
77. Burney PGJ, Britton JR, Chinn S, Tattersfield AE, Papacosta AO, Kelson MC, Anderson F, Corfield DR. Descriptive epidemiology of bronchial reacivity in an adult population: results from a community study. Thorax 1987; 42: 38–44.
78. Busse WW. The precipitation of asthma by upper respiratory infections. Chest 1985; 87: 44.
79. Annesi-Mesano I, Oryszczyn MP, Neukirch F, Kauffmann F. Relationship of upper airway disease to tobacco smoking and allergic markers in a sample of adult men followed-up 5 years. Int Arch Allergy Immunol 1997; 114:193–201.
80. Braman SS, Barrows AA, DeCotis BA, Settipane GA, Corrao WM. Airways hyperresponsiveness in allergic rhinitis. A risk factor for asthma. Chest 1987; 91: 671–674.
81. Fish JE, Rosentahal RR, Summer WR, Bata G, Menkes H, Summer W, Permutt S, Norman P. Airway responses to methacholine in allergic and nonallergic subjets. Am Rev Respir Dis 1976; 113: 579–582.
82. Stevens WJ, Vermeire PA, Van Schil LA. Bronchial hyperreactivity in rhinitis. Eur J Respir Dis 1980; 61: 203–212.
83. Gerblich AA, Schwartz WJ, Chester EH. Seasonal variation of airway function in allergic rhinitis. J Allergy Clin lmmunol 1986; 77: 676–681.
84. Madonini E, Briattico-Vangosa G, Pappacoda A, Maccagni G, Cardani A, Saporiti F. Seasonal increase of bronchial reactivity in allergic rhinitis. J Allergy Clin Immunol 1987; 79: 358–363.
85. Ramsdale EH, Morris MM, Roberts RS, Tech M, Hargreave FE. Asymptomatic bronchial hyperresponsiveness in rhinitis. J Allergy Clin Immunol. 1985; 75: 573–577.
86. Svenonius E, Arborelius M, Kautto R, LiIja B. Lung function studies In children with allergic rhinitis. Allergy 1982: 37: 87–92.
87. Giazdonskl R. Chronic atopic rhinitis is a preliminary stage of asthma. Fate of patients after several years of observation. Acta Otolaryngol 1984; 38: 143–146.
88. Prieto L, Berto JM, Gutierrez V. Airway responsiveness to methacholine and risk of asthma in patients with allergic rhinitis. Ann Allergy 1994; 72 : 534–539.
89. Buczko GB, Zamel N. Combined effect of cigarette smoking and allergic rhinitis on airways responsiveness to inhaled methacholine. Am Rev Respir Dis 1984; 129: 15–16.
90. Lu-Yuan L. Acute effects of cigarette smoke on the upper airways. In: Mathew OP and Sant'Ambrogio G, eds. Respiratory Function of the Upper Airway. New York: Marcel Dekker, 1988: 561–597.

91. Grammer LC, Shaughnessy MA, Shaughnessy JJ, Patterson R. Asthma as a variable in a study of immunotherapy for allergic rhinitis. J Allergy Clin Immunol 1984; 73: 557–560.

92. Rak S, Löwhagen O, Venge P. The effect of immunotherapy on bronchial hyperresponsiveness and eosinophil cationic protein in pollen allergic patients. J Allergy Clin Immunol. 1988; 470–480.

93. Boulet LP, Morin D, Milot J, Turcotte H. Bronchial responsiveness increases after seasonal antigen exposure in non-asthmatic subjects with pollen-induced rhinitis. Ann Allergy 1989: 63: 114–119.

94. Allen Bruce C, Rosenthal RR, Lichtenstein LM, Norman PS. Quantitative inhalation bronchial challenge in ragweed hay fever patients: a comparison with ragweed allergic asthmatics. J Allergy Clin Immunol 1975; 56: 331–337.

95. Verdiani P, Di Carlo S, Baronti A. Different prevalence and degree of nonspecific bronchial hyperreactivity between seasonal and perennial rhinitis. J Allergy Clin Immunol 1990; 86: 576–582.

96. Miles-Laurence R, Kaplan M, Chang K. Methacholine sensitivity in nasal polyposis and the effet of polypectomy. J Allergy Clin Immunol 1982; 69: 102A.

97. Haahtela T, Heiskala M, Suoniemi I. Allergic disorders and immediate skin test reactivity in Finland. Allergy 1980; 35: 433–441.

98. Kjellman NI, Croner S, Falth-Magnusson K, Odelram H, Bjorksten B. Prediction of allergy in infancy. Allergy Proc 1991; 12: 245–249.

99. Burrows B, Martinez FD, Halonen M, Barbee RA, Cline MG. Association of asthma with serum IgE levels and skin-prick test reactivity to allergens. N Engl J Med 1989; 320: 271–277.

100. Tollerud DJ, O'Connor GT, Sparrow D, Weiss ST. Asthma, hay fever, and phlegm production associated with distinct patterns of allergy skin test reactivity, eosinophilia and serum IgE levels. The Normative Aging Study. Am Rev Respir Dis. 1991; 144: 776–781.

101. Vervloet D, Haddi E, Tafforeau M, Lanteaume A, Kulling G, Charpin D. Reliability of respiratory symptoms to diagnose atopy. Clin Exp Allergy 1991; 21: 733–737.

102. Charpin D, Highes B, Mallea M, Sutra JP, Balansard G, Vervloet D. Seasonal allergic symptoms and their relation to pollen exposure in soul-east France. Clin Exp Allergy 1993: 23: 435–439.

103. Johnson EE, Irons JJ, Paterson R, Roberts M. J Allergy Clin Immunol 1974; 54: 94–97.

104. Bjornsson E, Janson C, Hakansson L, Enander I, Venge P, Boman G. Serum eosinophil cationic protein in relation to bronchial asthma in a young Swedish population. Allergy 1994; 49: 730–6.

105. Duffy DL, Martin NG, Battistutta D, Hopper JL, Mathews JD. Genetics of asthma and hay fever in Australian twins. Am Rev Respir Dis 1990; 142: 1351–1358.

106. Hopper JL, Hannah MC, Macaskill GT, Mathews JD. Twin concordance for

a binary trait: Ill. A bivariate analysis of hay fever and asthma. Genet Epidemiol 1990; 7: 277–289.

107. Annesi-Maesano I, Cotichini R, Stazi MA. Early gene–environment interaction into asthma and allergic rhinitis comorbidity. Chest 2001; 120:1755.

108. Sibbald B and Turner Warwick M. Factors influencing the prevalence of asthma among first degree relatives of extrinsic and intrinsic asthmatics. Thorax 1979; 34: 332–337.

109. Viegi G, Annesi-Maesano I, Mateelli G. Epidemiology of asthma. Eur Resp Monograph 2003; 23: 1–25.

110. Huhti E, Takala J, Nuntinen J, Poukkala A. Chronic respiratory disease in rural men. An epidemiologic survey at Hankasalmi, Finland. Ann Clin Res 1978; 10: 87–94.

111. Dor P, Armaud A, Barre, Charpin J. Fréquence des rhinites chronique dans une population d'adultes jeunes. Influence de l'allergie pollinique et du tanac. Poumon Coeur 1980; 36: 179–181.

112. Turkeltaub PC, Gergen PJ. Prevalance of upper and lower respiratory conditions in the US population by social and environmental factors: data from the second National Health and Nutrition examination Survey 1976 to 1980 (NHANES II). Ann Allergy 1991; 67: 147–154.

113. Kauffmann F, Annesi I, Oryszczyn MP. The realationship between allergy and smoking. In : Van Gorcum ed. Bronchitis IV. Groningen: Assen, 1989: 57–70.

114. Bascom R, Kulle T, Kagey-Sobotka A, Proud D. Upper respiratory tract environmental tobacco smoke sensitivity. Am Rev Resp Dis 1991; 143: 1304–1311.

115. Moyes CD, Waldon J, Ramadas D, Crane J, Pearce N. NZ Med J 1995; 108: 358–361.

116. Leuenberger P, Schwartz J, Ackermann-Liebrich U, Blaser K, Bolognini G, Bongard JP, Brandi O,Braun P, Bron C, Brutsche M et al. Am J Respir Crit Care Med 1994; 150: 1222–1228.

117. Braun-Fahrlander C, Wulthrich B, Gassner M, Grize L, Sennhauser FH, Varonier HS, Vuille JC. Validation of a rhinitis symptom questionnaire (ISAAC core questions) in a population of Swiss school children visiting the school health services. SCARPOL-team. Swiss Study on Childhood Allergy and Respiratory Symptom with respect to Air Pollution and Climate. International Study of Asthma and Allergies in Childhood. Pediatr Allergy Immunol 1997; 8(2): 75–82.

118. Kauffmann F, Dizier MH, Annesi-Maesano I, Bousquet J, Charpin D, Demenais F, Ecochard D, Feingold J, Gormand F, Grimfeld A, Lathrop M, Matran R, Neukirch F, Paty E, Pin I, Pison C, Scheinmann P, Vervloet D, Lockhart A. EGEA (Epidemiological Study on the Genetics and Environment of Asthma, Bronchial Hyperresponsiveness and Atopy)—descriptive characteristics. Clin Exp Allergy. 1999; 29 suppl 4: 17–21.

5

Comparative Pathogenesis of Upper and Lower Airway Allergic Disease

K. RAJAKULASINGAM

Homerton University Hospital
London, United Kingdom

STEPHEN R. DURHAM

Imperial College of Science,
Technology and Medicine
at the National Heart and
Lung Institute
London, United Kingdom

Introduction

Rhinitis and asthma have steadily increased in prevalence in the last 50 years. Also consultations and admissions for these diseases have continued to rise. These increases are in contrast to the availability of effective medications for both asthma and rhinitis and to the number of preventive factors known today. The upper and lower airways have a common respiratory epithelium and are more likely to share a common mucosal susceptibility to disease. Thus, it is not uncommon to see the occurrence of both asthma and rhinitis in the same patient. It is estimated that around 50 to 80% of asthmatics have concurrent rhinitis (1), although this figure varies depending on the diagnostic criteria, the population studied, the sample size, and other environmental factors (2). It is therefore important to understand the comparative pathogenesis of these two conditions, and this chapter focuses on the most common forms, atopic asthma and rhinitis.

Although it is often stated that because the nose is an integral part of the airways, the findings in the nose mirror those in the bronchi, there are important differences between the two sites in terms of both anatomy and inflammatory cell responses. The anatomical and physiological differences between the two airways are discussed in detail in Chapter 2. In brief, the nose and bronchi share a common pseudostratified columnar epithelium, with submucosal glands present in abundance in the upper airways. There are similarities between the nose and lower airways in response to nonspecific irritants. Inhalation of an irritant substance induces itching, sneezing, and rhinorrhea in the nose. On the other hand, cough, bronchoconstriction, and mucus hypersecretion occur in the lower airways in response to the inhalation of an irritant. Another important difference is seen in the mucosal circulation of the upper and lower airways. The nasal submucosa is richly vascularized and has a complex vascular structure with arterioles beneath the basement membrane feeding subepithelial and glandular capillary networks, which empty via cavernous sinusoids into the draining venules. There are also arteriovenous anastomoses diverting blood directly from the arterial to the venous system. The superficial capillaries are fenestrated and can allow rapid exudation of protein-rich fluid into the nasal cavity, thereby contributing to nasal secretions. The cavernous sinuses, which comprise plexi of venous capacitance vessels, are at their densest concentration in the mucosa of the inferior and middle turbinates. Their capacitance volume is under neural regulation, with an intrinsic neural tone limiting the sinusoidal capacity. The venous drainage of the trachea drains into the systemic veins and that for the bronchi mainly into the pulmonary vasculature. There is no smooth muscle within the upper airways, since changes in the venous capacitance volume affect turbinate size and thus alter the nasal airflow and nasal airways resistance, whereas smooth muscle constriction is an important determinant of lower airway narrowing.

I. Role of Atopy, IgE, and Its Receptors

Atopy, defined as positive skin tests and radioallergosorbent tests (RAST) to common aeroallergens, is a significant risk factor for the development of asthma and rhinitis (3,4). In addition, long-term follow-up studies show that allergic rhinitis, both seasonal and nonseasonal, is a significant risk factor for developing new asthma (3,4). Further population studies link total serum IgE concentrations with the incidence of asthma symptoms and bronchial hyperresponsiveness (5,6). In contrast, the allergen-specific IgE (RAST) rather than total IgE relates best to the symptoms of allergic rhinitis. On the other hand, bronchial biopsy studies show that atopy per se is a risk factor for developing mucosal inflammation (7). Despite the presence of convincing evidence for the association of atopy, asthma, and rhinitis, a significant number of patients with asthma and rhinitis demonstrate no evidence of atopy to common aeroallergens. Although it is plausible that this group of patients may have allergy to unidentified allergens, the pathogenesis of this "nonatopic" asthma and rhinitis may still be mediated by IgE, but not driven by allergen exposure.

An important characteristic of IgE is its ability to bind to mast cells and basophils with high affinity through its Fc portion to the IgE receptor (FcεRI). In sensitized individuals, the interaction of FcεRI-bound IgE with the relevant antigen elicits an immediate reaction characterized by mast cell degranulation and release of preformed mediators and cytokines. Apart from mediating the immediate response, the allergen-induced late phase skin reaction has also been shown to be IgE dependent (8,9). In support of this, a recent study has demonstrated upregulation of FcεRI receptors in the nasal submucosa at 6 h following allergen challenge in seasonal rhinitics, although the baseline expression is not different from that of normal controls (10). On the other hand, a somewhat earlier study in stable, mild asthmatics has demonstrated elevated numbers of FcεRIα$^+$ cells in the bronchial submucosa (11). In both studies, the majority of FcεRI$^+$ cells were mast cells, followed by macrophages and a small contribution from eosinophils and dendritic cells. Evidence from studies of nasal mucosal biopsy samples suggests that IgE may be produced locally by B cells in the mucosa during late responses (12,13) and during natural exposure (14). This local IgE synthesis can be inhibited by topical steroids (14). There is also evidence that IgE may be expressed locally in the bronchial mucosa at both the message (15) and the protein (16) level. These studies add further support for IgE and its high affinity receptor FcεRI in mediating late phase responses and ongoing inflammation in atopic asthma and rhinitis.

II. Early and Late Phase Responses to Allergen

The interaction of allergen with appropriately sensitized mucosa results in the release of inflammatory mediators that interact with nerves, blood vessels, and glands to produce symptoms of mucosal allergy. Following allergen provocation, early asthmatic and nasal responses begin within 10 mins, peak between 10 and 30 mins, and resolve between 1 and 3 h. The spontaneous recurrence of a reaction without further provocation, termed late phase response (LPR), first reported by Blackley in 1873 (17), has gained increasing attention. At least three patterns of airway responses are possible following allergen provocation: isolated early response (ER), early followed by late (dual) response, and isolated late responses (18). Late nasal and asthmatic responses usually begin between 3 and 4 h of provocation, peak during the next few hours, and clear within approximately 24 h depending on the severity (18–20). Late asthmatic responses occur in about 50% of patients following allergen inhalation tests (20) and are usually detectable by monitoring the forced expiratory volume in one second (FEV_1). The existence of nasal LPR after allergen challenge has been examined in very few studies (21–23). The prevalence of nasal LPR differs between 5 and 50% among the studies. LPRs in the nose are more difficult to quantify and usually manifest by nasal obstruction and late increase in some proinflammatory mediators in nasal lavage (24,25). It is not clear why LPR occurs in some subjects but not in others, and the significance of this phenomenon in naturally occurring disease is not clearly known. The human LPR provides a suitable in vivo model for exploring the mechanisms underlying the pathogenesis of asthma and rhinitis. The immediate response of the airways to allergen conforms to a type I hypersensitivity reaction (26,27), occurring through the interaction of IgE bound to mast cells and basophils with relevant allergen. This results in release of several mediators producing local and systemic reactions (22). Although the exact pathophysiology of the LPR is still unknown, present evidence suggests that it is an IgE-dependent process associated with the cellular phase of the inflammatory reaction in the airways (18,20). In keeping with this, LPRs in the upper and lower airways are inhibited by anti-inflammatory drugs and are associated with prolonged increases in airway responsiveness to inhaled histamine or methacholine.

Factors predicting late phase responses in the nose and airways are not entirely clear. Although there are no relevant studies in the nose, studies in asthmatics support the view that LPR is dependent on allergen dose (28,29). A series of studies, conducted mostly in the bronchi, has addressed the question of quantitative and/or qualitative differences between dual and early-only reactors. Boulet et al. (30) reported that dual asthmatic responders had higher levels of antigen-specific IgE levels without α difference in the size of the cutaneous ER between the groups. Further studies related the development of an LPR after bronchial allergen provocation to the presence of specific serum IgG1 and IgG4 antibodies (31,32). The magnitude of the early response in asthmatics is largely predictable on the basis of the level of airway responsiveness to nonspecific stimuli such as histamine and skin sensitivity to allergen (33). On the other hand, no such simple relationship exists for the LPR, which may occur independently of an early response and at a lower allergen dose. A subsequent study in the nose demonstrated no significant relationship between the total amount of mediators released in nasal fluid and symptoms generated during the early phase between early-only and dual responders, suggesting equivalent degrees of mast cell activation (34). Furthermore, neither the amount of mediators generated during LPR nor the symptomatic response was predicted by skin sensitivity or serum IgE levels. On the other hand, following nasal allergen challenge, a significant correlation was observed between the amount of mediators released in nasal lavage and symptoms generated during the early response and the corresponding amount during LPR (34). This finding was in agreement with studies of late phase skin reactivity in which the intensity of the early response reflects the LPR (35). Despite this, to date, no single factor distinguishes early-only responders from dual responders to antigen provocation.

III. Bronchial and Nasal Hyperresponsiveness

Bronchial hyperresponsiveness (BHR) has been recognized as a key pathophysiological feature of bronchial asthma (36). Another clinical manifestation of this condition is the exaggerated diurnal variation in airway caliber resulting in the characteristic symptoms of nocturnal wheeze and early morning chest tightness (37). BHR was originally described in asthmatics 24 h after allergen challenge (38). This effect was later shown to occur predominantly in patients who had demonstrated LPR after allergen inhalation challenge (39). Further studies demonstrated that LPR in asthmatics was associated with an increase in BHR as early as 3 h after allergen inhalation (i.e., before the onset of LPR) (40,41). This early BHR correlated with the magnitude of the subsequent LPR (40) and the accompanying reduction in peripheral eosinophil count (42). On the other hand, it is not known whether nasal reactivity to histamine or other agonists occurs earlier following allergen challenge before the development of nasal LPR. The findings in the lower airways, however, support the view that tissue events that underlie the LPR may occur before the LPR is clinically evident.

The degree of airways responsiveness in asthma is usually measured as the provocative concentration or dose of a bronchoconstrictor substance causing a 20% fall in FEV_1 (PC_{20} or PD_{20}). Substances such as histamine and methacholine are the agents commonly used to measure bronchial reactivity with good reproducibility. The extent of histamine or methacholine reactivity correlates well with different indices of asthma severity such as treatment requirements, symptoms of bronchial irritability, and the diurnal variation in peak expiratory flow (32), and the test may be useful in monitoring the response to antiasthma therapy.

In contrast to the lower airways, attempts to discriminate between patients and healthy subjects using nasal hyperresponsiveness have led to conflicting results (43–47). Because these investigations differ from each other in the provocation technique, in the way of assessing the symptoms and in the selection of the patient population, comparisons of studies are almost impossible, and at present a standard way of assessing nasal hyperresponsiveness after provocation is not available. If all these studies are taken together, there appears to be considerable overlap between rhinitic and normal subjects.

IV. The Role of Inflammatory Cells in Asthma and Rhinitis

Historically, the mast cell has been linked to asthma and rhinitis through the capacity of this cell to be activated by an IgE-dependent mechanism to release an array of inflammatory mediators. Recently, more evidence has been found to support important roles for other cells, especially lymphocytes, eosinophils, monocytes, macrophages, platelets, epithelial cells, and dendritic cells (Fig. 1). It is probably unhelpful to argue that one particular inflammatory cell is important in the pathogenesis of allergic inflammation,

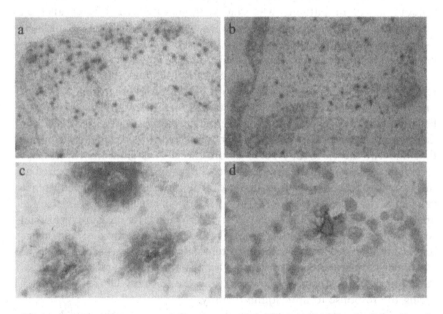

Figure 1 Immunohistology of nasal mucosa in allergic rhinitis. Sections (6 μm) have been immunostained with specific monoclonal antibodies to demonstrate (a) eosinophils (MBP×200), (b) Il-5 mRNA positive cells (predominantly T lymphocytes), (c) Tryptase-only and tryptase and chymase positive mast cells (×1000), and (d) a dendritic (Langerhans) cell (CD1a ×1000).

since mast cells, lymphocytes, and eosinophils are probably all important, although their exact place in the sequence of events remains to be established (Fig. 2).

A. Mast Cells

Mast cells have been associated with type I allergic reactions mediated via surface-bound IgE. The numbers of mast cells in the bronchial and nasal submucosa of both asthmatics and rhinitics are not different from those of nonatopic controls (7,48). In patients with seasonal allergic rhinitis, epithelial accumulation of mast cells occurs about a week after exposure to pollen (49,50). On the other hand, earlier studies in stable asthma showed no significant difference in epithelial mast cell numbers between asthmatic and healthy controls (7,48,51). In contrast, as in rhinitis, two recently published studies have demonstrated the presence of increased numbers of epithelial mast cells in asthma (52,53). Similarly, mast cell numbers in bronchoalveolar lavage (BAL) have also been shown in some but not all studies to be elevated in asthma (54,55). The varying findings seen in the limited number of studies performed so far may reflect differing states of disease activity.

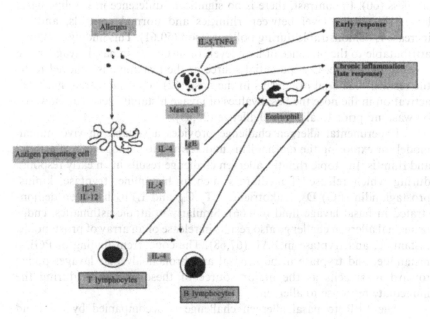

Figure 2 Schematic diagram of involvement of inflammatory cells and their products following provocation with allergen.

Also, different methods used to identify and quantitate the mast cells may partly explain disparities in the results.

On the other hand, the foregoing studies have clearly demonstrated evidence of varying degrees of mast cell degranulation indicating secretory activity by electron microscopy, and this is considered to be a characteristic feature of both asthmatic and rhinitic mast cells, distinguishing them clearly from those of normal control subjects (7,48,50,51). Almost all the mast cells in the bronchial mucosa of normal airways contain secretory granules in which tryptase is the predominant neutral protease, compatible with their classification as MC_T cells, which outnumber tryptase and chymase$^+$ mast cells (MC_{TC}) by a ratio of 8:1 (56). On the other hand, both MC_T and MC_{TC} subtypes of mast cells are present in comparable numbers within the nasal mucosa of atopic rhinitics (57). Following nasal allergen challenge, there is a trend for a decrease in mucosal MC_T mast cells in rhinitics consistent with the occurrence of degranulation (57).

In vitro and in vivo studies have provided convincing evidence that IgE-triggered mediator release from mast cells is largely responsible for immediate nasal and bronchial responses provoked by allergen (58,59). In keeping with this, raised levels of histamine can be detected in BAL of atopic asthmatics even in stable disease, and this correlates with bronchial responsiveness (60). In contrast, there is no significant difference in baseline nasal lavage histamine level between rhinitics and normal controls, and no increase is demonstrable during pollen season (50,61). This finding is mainly attributable to the presence of high levels of histamine in nasal lavage in the absence of disease. One potential source of the histamine is believed to be the resident bacterial organisms in the nose (62). To demonstrate mast cell activation in the nose the basal values of lavage histamine levels are lowered by washing prior to allergen challenge (25,63).

Experimental allergen challenge provides a suitable in vivo human model for exploring the mechanisms underlying the pathogenesis of asthma and rhinitis. In atopic rhinitis, allergen challenge results in an early response during which release of mediators such as histamine, tryptase, kinins, prostaglandin (PG) D_2, leukotriene (LT) C_4, and LTB_4 has been demonstrated in nasal lavage fluid (64–66). Similarly in atopic asthmatics, endobronchial allergen challenge also results in release of an array of prostanoids, histamine, and tryptase in BAL (67,68). The concurrent finding of PGD_2, histamine, and tryptase in both nasal and bronchoalveolar lavages points toward mast cells as the major source of these mediators during the immediate response to allergen.

The LPR to nasal allergen challenge is accompanied by a second increase in the concentrations of histamine and TAME (N-α-p-tosyl-L-arginine methyl ester hydrochloride)-esterase but differs from the early response in the lack of PGD_2 production and in the amount of kinin production (25). Since basophils do not produce PGD_2, this study suggests an important role for basophils as the late source of histamine during nasal LPR. Similarly, in the lower airways, a second increase of mediators is demonstrable after allergen challenge (67). These studies therefore support a role for mast cells in the LPR of asthma and rhinitis.

The identification of histamine in nasal lavage following allergen challenge and the known efficacy of oral antihistamines confirms a primary role for histamine in allergic rhinitis. Histamine has direct and indirect nasal effects, inducing itching, sneezing, rhinorrhea, and transient nasal blockage following nasal insufflation. Like histamine, mediators such as bradykinin, PGD_2, and LTC_4 are also known to cause symptoms and signs of rhinitis (69–71). The involvement of nonhistamine mediators is strengthened by the incomplete therapeutic effect of antihistamines on nasal blockage in naturally occurring disease (72).

In the airways, although inhalation of histamine induces bronchospasm, oral antihistamines offer little protection against bronchospasm in asthma. These findings indicate that mechanisms other than the direct action of histamine contribute to the pathogenesis of asthma. Recent evidence indicates that the activation of mast cells, induced by the cross-linking of cell-surface-bound IgE following allergen exposure in a sensitized individual not only releases the classical granule-associated preformed mediators but also results in the local release of cytokines. Consistent with this, there is direct evidence for immunological release of interleukin 4 (IL-4) from purified human mast cells in vitro (73) and indirect evidence for release of tumor necrosis factor α (TNF-α) from nasal mast cells (74). Furthermore, within both the upper and lower airways, immunohistochemical staining has identified the presence of interleukins (IL-4, IL-5, IL-6) and TNFα co localized to tissue mast cells (75,76). These studies also provide evidence, obtained by using one specific monoclonal antibody (3H4), for enhanced expression of IL-4 in atopic asthma and rhinitis. Furthermore, TNF-α expression in mast cells is found to be increased by sevenfold in asthmatics. These findings support an important role for mast cells in maintaining the chronicity of allergic inflammation seen in asthma and rhinitis.

B. Eosinophils

For over 100 years eosinophils have been associated with allergic disease. Increasing evidence demonstrates that eosinophils are pathologically associated with inflammation, and eosinophilia is considered to be a cardinal feature of both asthma and rhinitis. Asthma is associated with blood, tissue, BAL, and sputum eosinophilia, and the degree of eosinophilia correlates with bronchial hyperresponsiveness (56,77,78). Similarly, nasal tissue and lavage eosinophilia are demonstrable in both seasonal and perennial allergic rhinitis (57,79,80). Yet, tissue eosinophilia occurs to a lesser extent in perennial allergic rhinitis than in seasonal disease. Unlike what is observed in asthma, no clear association is demonstrable between tissue or nasal lavage eosinophilia and nasal hyperresponsiveness (81,82). Mild to moderate bronchial eosinophilia occurs without symptoms of asthma in rhinitic subjects who are sensitive to house dust mites (7), and these eosinophils show ultrastructural features of degranulation. On the other hand, nasal tissue eosinophilia does not occur in seasonal atopic rhinitics out of season (57). Therefore, the presence or absence of asthmatic symptoms in atopic rhinitics may be related to quantitative differences in airway responsiveness to allergens (83).

Both pulmonary segmental allergen challenge in asthmatics and nasal allergen challenge in rhinitics result not only in the recruitment of eosinophils but also in the release of eosinophil granule proteins. Tissue eosinophilia following allergen provocation occurs within hours. Eosinophils recovered from patients with asthma possess an increased propensity to degranulate as a consequence of "priming" (84,85). Degranulation of activated eosinophils results in the release of toxic cationic proteins, lipid mediators such as LTC_4, LTD_4, and platelet-activating factor (PAF), and oxygen metabolites (86–88). The eosinophil granule proteins, major basic protein (MBP), eosinophil-derived neurotoxin (EDN), eosinophil peroxidase (EPO), and eosinophil cationic protein (ECP), all damage respiratory epithelium and pneumatocytes (89). Despite prominent tissue infiltration by eosinophils and the possible toxic effects of eosinophil granule proteins, epithelial integrity remains normal in allergic rhinitis (90). In contrast, in asthma the bronchial epithelium is disrupted and damaged (51,90). There is no obvious explanation for this dichotomy seen in asthma and rhinitis. However the nose is a "dirty" organ and constantly exposed to irritants, whereas the lower airways are protected and sterile. One explanation may be a more rapid turnover of the epithelium within the nose in response to irritant exposure. This is speculation, however, since there is no evidence. The toxic effect of ECP is said to be less than other granule proteins (89). MBP is found in increased amounts in BAL and nasal lavage following allergen challenge (91,92).

Autopsy studies in fatal asthma demonstrate the presence of large number of eosinophils and striking MBP deposition in bronchial mucosa (93,94). In particular, the effects of MBP on respiratory epithelium mimic the pathology of asthma (91). Furthermore, the amount of MBP in BAL correlates with the number of desquamated epithelial cells and the degree of BHR (91). There is no clear understanding of the mechanism(s) by which eosinophil granule protein cause BHR and other changes. In primates both MBP and EPO have been shown to directly stimulate the respiratory epithelium, thereby causing smooth muscle contraction and increased sensitivity of the muscle to methacholine. A recent study suggests that BHR in asthma may be due to the ability of MBP to selectively block M2 cholinergic receptors (97) or due to the generation of bradykinin, a potent bronchoconstrictor in asthmatics (98). In addition to its toxic properties, MBP activates platelets, neutrophils, mast cells, and basophils (89).

In addition to the secretion of cationic proteins, eosinophils can synthesize a variety of cytokines, chemokines, and neuropeptides (89). These in turn amplify and regulate local immune responses. Furthermore, eosinophils may express major histocompatibility complex (MHC) class II proteins and are capable of presenting antigen to stimulate MHC-restricted T-lymphocyte responses (78,99). Yet, the interaction of eosinophils with other cells involved in the immune response is poorly understood.

C. Lymphocytes

Since T lymphocytes are the only cells that recognize antigenic material, they have a central role to play in both allergic rhinitis and asthma. Recent studies demonstrate that both asthma and rhinitis are associated with activation of a distinct subset of T cell called TH2-type cells. Both CD4 and CD8 are the most numerous cells present in the nasal and bronchial mucosa in both normal and atopic subjects. Although the total numbers of these cells do not differ between normal and disease states, activated T lymphocytes (CD25$^+$) are present in increased amounts in bronchial biopsy specimens and in the BAL of asthmatics (56,100). Changes in T-cell populations in BAL occur as early as 10 min after allergen challenge (101), suggesting that activation of T lymphocytes may be an early event in the development of airway inflammation. Consistent with T-cell populations in other mucosal tissues, most T cells in the airways bear the CD45RO surface marker associated with memory T cells (48,102). Flow cytometric analysis of BAL from asthmatics also reveals increased expression of CD25 (identifying IL-2R) by CD4$^+$ cells. Furthermore, the degree of activation of CD4$^+$ lymphocytes correlates with the number of eosinophils on BAL fluid, as well as the severity of asthma symptoms and the degree of BHR (103), implying a role for T cells in the eosinophilic infiltrate in asthma. This link is strengthened by the demonstration, by in situ hybridization, of mRNA for IL-5 in biopsy samples from asthmatics that correlated with the number of CD25$^+$, EG2$^+$ cells, and total eosinophils (104).

Relatively very few studies of biopsies of the nasal mucosa in allergic rhinitis have addressed the role of T cells and their activation status in the mucosa. Unlike results obtained with asthmatics, these studies do not show evidence of out-of-season activation of T cells in seasonal rhinitics (57,105). Nasal allergen challenge in seasonal rhinitic subjects results in a small but significant increases in $CD4^+$ and $CD25^+$ cells and unlike asthma, there is no correlation between the degree of T-cell activation and nasal symptoms (57). Increases in T-cell numbers and in macrophages and TH2-type cytokines such as IL-4 and IL-5 are observed in both atopic and aspirin-sensitive perennial rhinitis (106,107).

Activation of peripheral blood T cells occurs in mild asthmatics, and this correlates with the degree of peripheral blood eosinophilia (108). Furthermore, CD4 lymphocytes in peripheral blood from patients with severe asthma demonstrate increased expression of activation markers, and these changes resolve with improvement in lung function (109). Unlike in asthmatics, no significant changes in $CD4^+$, and CD25 cells in peripheral blood are demonstrable in allergic rhinitis (57). These studies indicate that activated lymphocytes tend to compartmentalize in the tissue in allergic rhinitis, whereas in asthma, lymphocyte activation is evident in both bronchial mucosa and peripheral blood.

Studies of T-cell clones from both rhinitics and asthmatics support the hypothesis that there is selective activation of a subgroup of helper cells. T lymphocytes in BAL and bronchial biopsy samples from atopic asthmatics demonstrate evidence of activation of gene clusters for IL-3, IL-4, and IL-5 and granulocyte–macrophage colony-stimulating factor, (GM-CSF), a pattern compatible with predominant activation of the TH_2-like T-cell population (103,110,111). Similarly in patients with atopic perennial rhinitis, in situ hybridization studies in the nasal mucosa have confirmed preferential increases in cytokine mRNA cells positive for IL-3, IL-4, IL-5, and GM-CSF (112). Furthermore, TH2-type cytokines have also been detected in nasal lavage following allergen challenge (113). These cytokines enhance allergic response by activating mast cells and eosinophils. IL-4 is responsible for B-cell isotype switching in favor of IgE production (114) and may also play a role in eosinophil recruitment (115). IL-5 promotes differentiation of eosinophils, activates mature eosinophils, and selectively enhances eosinophil degranulation and adhesion to vascular endothelium (116). Recent studies have confirmed that T cells harvested from BAL during late asthmatic responses produce 10-fold more TH2 cytokines (IL-5) than equivalent numbers of T cells in peripheral blood collected at the same time (117). Moreover these T cells remain susceptible to the effects of inhibitory cytokines such as IL-12 and interferon-γ (118), which may have indications for local (topical) anticytokine therapy, although preliminary results have been disappointing (119,120).

Taken together, these observations are consistent with the view that T-lymphocyte activation and expression of TH2 cytokines may contribute to tissue eosinophilia and local IgE-dependent events in asthma and rhinitis.

D. Other Cells

Alveolar macrophages are the most numerous cells in BAL in normal lungs and in those of asthmatics. These macrophages are phenotypically and functionally distinct from those of normal subjects. These cells are known to release increased amounts of reactive oxygen species and IL-1 (121). Following allergen challenge, human alveolar macrophages obtained from asthmatics vigorously release superoxide anion (122). Furthermore, increases in tissue macrophages have commonly been reported (53,102) in asthmatics. Expression of HLA-DR (marker of cell activation) is also increased in asthmatics (102). These data suggest that alveolar macrophages from asthmatics are activated and that, following antigen challenge, there are changes in the macrophage cell population that facilitate the development of airway inflammation. Macrophages are also found in the human nasal mucosa (105,123). Furthermore, increases in the number of macrophages has been reported in the nasal mucosa in a nasal allergen challenge model and in seasonal allergic rhinitis (124).

The role of neutrophils in promoting allergic inflammation is less clear. Although most studies report no significant increase in the proportion or number of neutrophils in BAL fluids from asthmatics (67,124), another study reported increases in BAL neutrophils in symptomatic asthmatics (125). Moreover, BAL neutrophilia is commonly seen within a few hours of antigen challenge in asthmatics subjects (62) and is known to present as late as 48 h following segmental allergen challenge (126).

Neutrophils are also found in nasal mucosa. The number of neutrophils on the mucosal surface increases some hours after allergen challenge (92,105). As a marker of neutrophil activation, the level of myeloperoxidase (MPO) increases in nasal lavage fluid during seasonal exposure to allergen (127). Although in primate models there is a close association between airway neutrophilia and inflammation, which results in the physiological changes of airway hyperresponsiveness and airflow limitation, there are no data that directly address this issue in human airways disease. On the contrary, topical corticosteroid therapy in rhinitics, which inhibits allergen-induced late responses, results in a corresponding increase in nasal mucosal neutrophils, in contrast to the observed decrease in eosinophils (128). This result might call into question earlier thinking about the role of neutrophils in the development of LPR.

E. Nasobronchial Interactions

In a recent series of elegant studies from Rotterdam, the influence of allergen provocation to the nose on cellular infiltration, adhesion molecule expression, and cytokine provocation was investigated in biopsy samples of both the nasal and bronchial mucosa at 24 h after challenge (129). Nasal challenge resulted in significant increases in tissue IL-5 and eosinophils in both the upper and lower airway. Similarly, nasal challenge resulted in increases in expression of the vascular cell and intercellular adhesion molecules VCAM-1 and ICAM-1 in both nose and lung. Conversely, segmental provocation of the lower airways via the fiberoptic bronchoscope resulted in inflammatory changes in both lower and upper airways (130). Taken together, these data provide evidence for the "united airways" hypothesis and suggest a causal link between allergen-induced inflammation in rhinitis and asthma, the implication being that treatment of allergic rhinitis may have a beneficial effect in allergic asthma (131).

V. Role of Epithelium in Asthma and Rhinitis

Recent evidence suggests that the airway epithelium, which has traditionally been regarded as a physical barrier preventing the entry of inhaled foreign particles into the submucosa, may play a much more important role as a physicochemical barrier that influences both the pathogenesis and the etiology of allergic rhinitis and asthma. In comparison to controls, subjects suffering from both atopic asthma and perennial rhinitis demonstrate greater reticular basement membrane thickness in both nasal and bronchial epithelium (132). This feature was still maintained for those patients treated with topical corticosteroids. Moreover, this change is more pronounced in bronchial than in nasal biopsies (132). The nasal epithelium in patients with perennial rhinitis is significantly thickened, in comparison to that in the tissue of either normal subjects or seasonal allergic rhinitics during or out of pollen season (133). It is possible that the difference in the thickness between the epithelium of seasonal allergic and perennial rhinitic subjects may be a result of the difference in the duration of exposure to allergen. On the other hand, extensive damage to the epithelium may be present even in the mildest asthmatic subjects (134–136). Although these findings suggest that upper and lower airway inflammation is associated with an increased thickness of the reticular membrane, factors like mesenchymal cells (e.g., fibroblasts, myofibroblasts) and protease–antiprotease balance may operate in the lower airways, accounting for the enhanced basement membrane thickness seen in the bronchi. Patients with both asthma and rhinitis also show enhanced bronchial epithelial shedding when compared with control subjects. Epithelial shedding is a prominent histopathological feature of airway inflammation in asthma, and it correlates to the severity of the disease (136,137). Treatment with inhaled corticosteroids improves bronchial epithelial shedding in asthmatics, and repair of the damaged airway epithelium is seen to occur as an exacerbation of asthma resolves (138). On the other hand, nasal epithelial shedding is not seen in allergic rhinitis (132). Although the reason for this dichotomy is not known, nasal and bronchial mucosa clearly seem to behave differently in terms of epithelial shedding and thickness of reticular membrane.

Development of the inflammatory response in the nasal and bronchial mucosa may be due to the ability of the epithelial cells to generate and release specific inflammatory mediators like leukotrienes, prostaglandins (139,140), and cytokines, as well as to express specific "inflammatory" cell adhesion molecules and MHC class II antigens (141–143). In addition to interactions with antigens and secretion of arachidonate mediators, the epithelium produces cytokine mediators, which may both upregulate and perpetuate the inflammatory state in asthma (144–146). Other evidence suggests that airway epithelial cells and cell lines are capable of synthesizing GM-CSF, IL-1, and TNF-α (147,148). Studies suggest that human airway epithelial cells are capable of expressing messenger ribonucleic acid (mRNA) for IL-1, IL-3, IL-5, TNF-α, and GM-CSF in vitro (148–150). Imunocytochemical evaluation demonstrated that these cytokines were mostly produced by nonciliated epithelial cells in the lavage (151). Furthermore, ICAM-1 has been shown to be expressed on several human airway epithelial cell types (141,152).

Nitric oxide (NO) has been recognized as an important signaling molecule and may play a key role in host defense and in the pathophysiology of airway diseases. There is a close analogy between the nose and the lungs in terms of NO levels in asthma and rhinitis. Levels of nasal and exhaled NO are elevated in patients with allergic rhinitis and asthma, respectively (153–157). The functional significance of increased production of NO in both asthma and allergic rhinitis is not clearly understood. However, treatment with topical nasal and inhaled corticosteroids results in reduction of NO levels in both groups of patients (153,158,159). The source of increased NO in both nose and lungs in these patients may be derived from the high level of inducible NO synthase (iNOS) expressed in nasal and airway epithelial cells (160,161). Proinflammatory cytokines are known to induce iNOS expression in cultured human airway epithelial cell in vitro as a result of increased transcription of the iNOS gene (162,163). The mechanism of increased iNOS expression in asthma and rhinitis may be similar, in as much as similar proinflammatory cytokine profiles are detected in both nasal and bronchial lavages, in patients with both rhinitis and asthma (73–81).

Although both nasal and bronchial epithelial cells have been cultured in vitro by several groups, a major difficulty experienced by many workers in the field has been to consistently grow these cells to confluency, such that large numbers can be harvested for further study. Epithelial cells harvested from asthmatic subjects secrete more GM-CSF than epithelial cells harvested from nonasthmatic volunteers (164).

Taken together, these studies suggest that the damage to the epithelium, as seen in asthma, may be the direct result of the mediators secreted by several inflammatory cells. It is also probable that the epithelial cells play an important role in the growth, differentiation, maintenance, migration, and activation of cell types in nasal and bronchial mucosa.

VI. Mechanisms of Cellular Infiltration

The development of inflammation involves a highly complex series of events, at both the tissue and the cellular level, in response to a diverse variety of stimuli. It is now recognized that adhesion between leukocytes, vascular endothelium, and target cells is critical to the inflammatory response process. Initially, the circulating inflammatory cells bind to the endothelium of mucosal vessels by interaction between complementary adhesion molecules on the inflammatory cell and endothelial cell surfaces. This is followed by cell migration through the endothelial gaps involving interaction between the cell and matrix proteins and additional complex interaction with chemokines. Unlike in animal models, distribution and intensity of expression of ICAM-1 and endothelial leukocyte adhesion molecule 1 (ELAM-1) in bronchial biopsy specimens are comparable between asthmatics and healthy volunteers (165), while increased baseline expression of ICAM-1 and VCAM-1 in nasal biopsy specimens is demonstrable in perennial allergic rhinitis (166). This observed difference between rhinitic and asthmatic airways may be explained in terms of the severity of the inflammation and allergen exposure. On the other hand, segmental allergen challenge in asthmatics results in increased expression of ICAM-1 and E-selectin at 6 h (167). Furthermore, there is also an upregulation for leukocyte-function-associated antigen 1 (LFA-1), the ligand for ICAM-1. These studies point to adhesion mechanisms as being important to the pathogenesis of asthma and rhinitis. In support of this, pretreatment with anti-ICAM antibodies attenuates allergen-induced LPR and eosinophilia in primates (168). Further assessment of the role of adhesion mechanisms in allergic airway diseases, however, must await studies in which anti-ICAM antibodies are used in humans.

Cellular recruitment and persistence at allergic sites also depends on chemotaxis in response to a distinct group of agents referred to as chemokines. These chemokines are basic, heparin-binding polypeptides, which are subdivided into two subfamilies, CXC and CC, depending on the position of two cysteine residues near the N-terminus. The CC branch includes RANTES, I-309, monocyte chemotactic proteins 1, 2, and 3 (MCP-1, -2, -3), macrophage inflammatory proteins 1α and 1β (MIP-1α) and (MIP-1β), and eotaxin (101,169,170). Most of these cytokines are not normally expressed in unstimulated cells and have attracted considerable interest for a putative role in allergic inflammation. RANTES, MCP-1, the recently described MCP-4, and eotaxin all induce potent chemotactic responses for eosinophils both in vivo and in vitro. Eotaxin, in particular, is considered to be eosinophil specific (105,170–172). The presence of a specific receptor for these chemokines on eosinophils (e.g., CCR3) (169) represents a specific therapeutic target, since antagonism is likely to inhibit many eosinophil–chemokine interactions, which require this receptor. Recently, the CC chemokine receptors CCR4 and CCR8, as well as CCR3, have been demonstrated on human peripheral blood (173), nasal (174), and bronchial (175–177) T lymphocytes. At present, it is not clear whether these receptors are specific for TH2 (as opposed to TH1) T cells (173) and/or whether they may represent tissue-specific homing receptors for T cells during allergic inflammation.

VII. Microvascular Leakage and Plasma Protein Exudation

Plasma exudation has long been known to be a cardinal factor in inflammation. A role for exuded plasma proteins and peptides in rhinitis is supported by a substantial accumulation of data, and plasma exudation may be a better correlate of the disease state than the presence of several mediators (178). Inflammatory mucosal provocations in the nose and airways produce exudative responses without disrupting the epithelial lining and without increasing the airway tissue penetration of luminal material whereby a largely nonsieved plasma enters the lumen (179–181). Therefore such provocations are being proposed as a primary mucosal defense mechanism. This process allows immunoglobulins, kinins, coagulation peptides, complement, and other peptides to operate on the mucosal surface of the airway. If exaggerated, plasma exudation may become pathogenic in atopic diseases of the airways.

The permeability of venules in the nasal mucosa can be increased by irritants acting via sensory neurones (182). This effect may be produced either through a central neural reflex, associated with efferent parasympathetic cholinergic neurotransmission, or via antidromic release of neuropeptides from sensory neurones. This axonal pathway has not been clearly demonstrated in humans. The role of sensory nerves in causing plasma exudation has been clearly documented in several animal studies. In rats, nasal challenge with capsaicin, an extract of red hot pepper, induces plasma exudation mediated via nonmyelinated "C" nerve fibers (183). This effect is believed to be due to the release of sensory neuropeptides such as substance P, neurokinins, and calcitonin gene-related peptide (CGRP). In an animal model, nasal challenge with substance P induced plasma leakage, which was inhibited by pretreatment with capsaicin or substance P antagonist (184). Consistent with this, studies undertaken in humans have demonstrated the presence of receptors for substance P, neurokinin A, and CGRP in the nasal mucosa (185). Furthermore, substance P has been found in increased amounts in nasal lavage fluid following nasal allergen challenge (186). Despite this, nasal challenge with capsaicin in humans does not induce plasma exudation (187). Therefore the role of neural pathways in causing plasma leakage in allergic rhinitis remains unclear.

Like histamine, other inflammatory mediators such as bradykinin, platelet-activating factor (PAF), and leukotrienes can also increase the microvascular permeability to macromolecules in the nose. In animals, mediator antagonists have been shown to inhibit antigen-induced airway microvascular leakage. The specific 5-lipoxygenase inhibitor A-63162 has been shown to inhibit airway microvascular leakage to a greater extent than airflow obstruction following inhalation of ovalbumin in sensitized guinea pigs (188). However, mediator antagonists other than antihistamines have not been shown to be effective in inhibiting plasma leakage in allergic rhinitis.

Microvascular leakage is also thought to play an important role in asthma. The underlying mechanisms of this phenomenon are similar to that of rhinitis. The observed wall thickness of the airways in asthma is probably due to a combination of mucosal thickening and liquid filling of intraluminal spaces (189). Furthermore, mathematical models suggest that smooth muscle constriction alone produces only relatively modest increases in small-airway resistance, whereas when the same degree of constriction is coupled with airway wall thickening dramatic increases in resistance may take place (190). BHR is known to occur in congestive cardiac failure, and the underlying mechanism is thought to be due to mucosal thickening, since this is improved by prior treatment with α-adrenergic agonists (191). This study supports a role for mucosal edema in the pathogenesis of BHR. However, adrenaline, a known effective agent against microvascular leakage, has not been shown to more effective than inhaled salbutamol in acute asthma (192). Therefore the role of microvascular leakage in human asthma is still under investigation.

VIII. Comparative Effects of Therapeutic Agents

The understanding of the mechanisms of both asthma and rhinitis has enabled us to rationalize treatment for these conditions. However, the implications of the comparative pathology of asthma and rhinitis to the response to treatment are unclear. Patients with infrequent symptoms of asthma may require only bronchodilator therapy. Similarly, patients with occasional symptoms of rhinitis may require only symptomatic use of oral antihistamines. Use of both antihistamines and bronchodilator represents the "drug for relief" approach. In patients with persistent symptoms, topical corticosteroids are the mainstay of treatment, and their use represents the "drug for prevention" approach. Antihistamines are effective in relieving many of the symptoms of rhinitis, including rhinorrhea and itching. Similarly, drugs with mast-cell-stabilizing properties such as cromoglycate are also effective in mild allergic rhinitis. These finding would suggest that mild upper airways allergic disease is a process driven predominantly by mast cells. However, antihistamines offer only limited relief in nasal blockage, indicating the contribution of other important mechanisms in allergic rhinitis. Antihistamines have very mild bronchodilating properties and are not very effective in asthma. In contrast, β_2-adrenergic agonists have a strong bronchodilator property in asthma but no effect in rhinitis, since the upper airways lack smooth muscle. In both asthma and rhinitis, mucosal inflammation responds well to treatment with topical steroids, and this correlates with improvement in symptoms. Treatment with topical steroids inhibits T-lymphocyte activation and eosinophil recruitment and activation. Furthermore, topical steroids also inhibit allergen-induced increases in TH2-type cytokines, particularly IL-4 (193), and seasonal increases in expression of TH2-type cytokines during pollen season (194,195).

Although T-cell activation is demonstrated in both rhinitis and asthma, as discussed earlier, it is not a predominant finding in allergic rhinitis, at least in terms of IL-2R expression (57). On the other hand, activation of T lymphocytes in the bronchial mucosa is a feature of increasingly severe disease and probably accounts for the need to treat this condition with corticosteroids. In contrast, cytokine production (IL-4, IL-5) is comparable in both rhinitis and asthma, the principal cell source in both sites being the T cells (at mRNA level), with lesser contributions from mast cells and eosinophils (196). However, persistent T-cell activation can be demonstrated in severe asthma despite the use of high doses of steroids (197). A recent study indicates that there is selective dysregulation of gene expression of TH2-type cytokines in steroid-resistant asthma (198). Whether similar patterns account for severe forms of rhinitis remains to be determined.

Immunotherapy is highly effective in the treatment of selected patients with seasonal allergic rhinitis and may confer benefit for at least 1 to 3 years following discontinuation (199). Two position papers, one by the European Academy of Allergology and Clinical Immunology (200) and the other by the World Health Oranization (201), add valuable evidence for the role of immunotheraphy in the treatment of atopic rhinitis. Recent studies suggest that immunotherapy may act by promoting TH1 response with production of interferon-γ (202–204). On the other hand, the benefit of immunotherapy in the treatment of atopic asthma is variable, with two recent studies demonstrating either modest (205) or no significant benefit (206) in comparison to placebo treatment. However, a well-conducted meta-analysis of randomized controlled trials (207) demonstrated a role for immunotherapy in asthma. Earlier studies supported a role for leukotriene antagonists in the treatment of both asthma and rhinitis (208,209). Since then, an abundance of studies have become available supporting a definite role for leukotriene receptor antagonists (LTRAs) in the treatment of asthma (210,211). On the other hand, only a handful of studies have investigated these substances in the treatment of allergic rhinitis. The evidence favoring the use of LTRAs in allergic rhinitis amounts to a few studies showing only a modest benefit (212). Long-term studies are, therefore, needed to investigate the role of LTRAs in the treatment of allergic rhinitis.

IX. Conclusions

Studies of the pathology of asthma and rhinitis demonstrate some important similarities but also differences between the two clinical conditions. Although it is recognized that asthma and rhinitis occur commonly in the same patient, the relationship between them is not clearly understood.

Many of the inflammatory mechanisms, including IgE-dependent mast cell activation, tissue eosinophilia, and recruitment of CD4$^+$ T cells that express TH2-type cytokines, are virtually identical, although they may differ in intensity, presumably owing to differences in disease intensity or methodology. The striking difference between the two is the different anatomy and differing effector organ responses to these inflammatory mechanisms, especially the predominance of the vasculature and submucosal glands in the nose and, in contrast, the presence of bronchial smooth muscle as a principal effector tissue in the large airways. Both asthma and rhinitis respond well to topical corticosteroid treatment. The factor or factors determining whether atopic disease is expressed in the upper or lower airways or indeed, as often the case, in both parts of the airways, are not known and further research should focus on the differences between these two conditions, especially differences in cellular activity, end organ responses, and the influence of treatments.

References

1. The World Health Organisation Initiative. Allergic Rhinitis and Its Impact on Rhinitis and Asthma (ARIA). Eds: Bousquet J, van Cauwenberge P, Khaltaev N. J Allergy Clin Immunol 2001; 108:S147–S334.
2. Kapsali T, Horowitz E, Diemer F, Togias A. Rhinitis is ubiquitious in allergic asthma. J Allergy Clin Immunol 1997; 99 (pt 2); S138 (abstr).
3. Hagy GW, Settipane GA, Risk factors for developing asthma and allergic rhinitis; a 7 year follow up study of college students. J Allergy Clin Immunol 1976; 58: 330–336.
4. Haggy GW, Settipane GA. Bronchial asthma, allergic rhinitis and allergy skin test among college students. J Allergy 1969; 44: 323–332.
5. Burrows KM, Martinez FD, Halonen M, Barbee RA, Cline MG. Association of asthma with serum IgE levels and skin test reactivity to allergens. N Engl J Med 1989; 320: 271–277.
6. Sears MR, Burrows B, Flannery EM, Herbison GP, Hewitt CJ, Holdaway MD. Relation between airway responsiveness and serum IgE in children with asthma and in apparently normal children. N Engl J Med 1991; 325: 11067–11071.
7. Djukanovic R, Lai CKW, Wilson JW, Britten KM, Wilson SJ, Roche WR, Howarth PH, Holgate ST. Bronchial mucosal manifestations of atopy: a comparison of markers of inflammation between atopic asthmatics, atopic non-asthmatics and healthy controls. Eur Respir J 1992; 5: 538–544.
8. Dolovich J, Hargreave FE, Chalmers R, Shier KJ, Gouldie J, Bienenstock J. Late cutaneous responses in isolated IgE-dependent reactions. 1973; 52: 38.
9. Solley GO, Gleich GJ, Jordan RE and Schroeter AL. The late phase of the immediate wheal and flare skin reaction: its dependence upon IgE antibodies. J Clin Invest 1976; 58: 408.
10. Rajakulasingam K, Durham SR, Humbert M, O'Brien F, Taborda-Barata L, Kay AB and Grant JA. High affinity IgE receptors (FcɛRI) in human allergen-induced rhinitis: upregulation of mRNA and protein and co-localisation to mast cells, macrophages, eosinophils and dendritic cells. J Allergy Clin Immunol 1997; 100(1): 78–86.
11. Humbert M, Grant JA, Taborda-Barata L, Durham SR, Pfister R, Menz G, Barkans J, Ying S and Kay AB. High affinity immunoglobulin E (FcɛRI) receptor bearing cells in bronchial biopsies from atopic and non-atopic asthma. Am J Respir Crit Care Med 1996; 153: 1931–1937.
12. Durham SR. Gould HJ, Thienes CP, Jacobson MR, Masuyama K, Rak S, Lowhagen O, Schotman E, Cameron L, Hamid QA. Expression of ɛ germ-line transcripts and mRNA for the ɛ heavy chain of IgE in nasal B cells and the effects of topical corticosteroid. Eur J Immunol 1997; 27: 2899–2906.
13. Smurthwaite L, Walker SN, Wilson DR, Birch DS, Merrett TG, Durham SR,

Gould HJ Persistent IgE synthesis in the nasal mucosa of hayfever patients. Eur J Immunol 2001; 31: 3422–3431.

14. Cameron L, Durham SR, Jacobson Mr, Masuyama K, Juliusson S, Gould HJ, Lowhagen O, Minshall EM, Hamid QA. Expression of IL-4, Cε RNA and Iε RNA in the nasal mucosa of patients with seasonal rhinitis: effect of topical corticosteroids. J Allergy Clin Immunol 1998; 101: 330–336.

15. Ying S, Humbert M, Meng Q, Menz G, Pfister R, Gould HJ, Kay AB, Durham SR. Local expression of ε germ-line gene transcripts (Iε) and RNA for the ε heavy chain of IgE (Cε) in the bronchial mucosa in atopic and non-atopic asthma. J Allergy Clin Immunol 2001; 107: 686–692.

16. Wilson DR, Merrett TG, Varga EM, Smurthwaite L, Gould HJ, Kemp M, Hooper J, Till SJ, Durham SR. Increases in allergen-specific IgE in BAL after segmental allergen challenge in atopic asthmatics. Am J Respir Crit Care Med 2002; 165: 22–26.

17. Blackley CH. Experimental Researches on the Causes and Nature of Catarrhus Aestivus. London: Bailliere, Tindal, Cox 1873.

18. O'Byrne PM, Dolovich J and Hargreave FE. Late asthmatic responses. Am Rev Respir Dis 1987; 136: 740–751.

19. Booij-Noord H, Orie NGM, de Vries K. Immediate and late bronchial obstructive reactions to inhalation of house dust and protective effects of disodium cromoglycate and prednisolone. J Allergy Clin Immunol 1971; 48: 344–354.

20. Hargreave FE. Late-phase asthmatic responses and airway inflammation. J Allergy Clin Immunol 1989; 83: 525–527.

21. Pelikan Z. Late and delayed responses of the nasal mucosa to allergen challenge. Ann Allergy 1978; 41: 37–47.

22. Dvoracek JE, Yunginger JW, Kern EB, Hyatt RE and Gleich GJ. Induction of nasal late-phase reactions by insufflation of ragweed-pollen extract. J Allergy Clin Immunol 1984; 73: 363–368.

23. Richerson HB, Rajtora DW, Penick JD, Dick FR, Yoo TJ, Kammermeyer JK and Anuras JS. Cutaneous and nasal allergic responses in ragweed hay fever: lack of clinical and histological correlations with late-phase reactions. J Allergy Clin Immunol 1979; 64: 67–77.

24. Gronborg H, Bisgaard H, Romeling F and Mygind N. Early and late nasal symptom response to allergen challenge. The effect of pre-treatment with a glucocorticoid spray. Allergy 1993; 48: 87–93.

25. Naclerio RM, Proud D, Togias AG, Adkinson NF.Jr, Meyers DA, Sobotka AK, Plant M, Norman PS and Lichtenstein LM. Inflammatory mediators in late antigen-induced rhinitis. N Engl J Med 1985; 313: 65–70.

26. Coombs RRA, Gell PGH. Classification of allergic reactions responsible for clinical hypersensitivity and disease. In: Gell PGH, Coombs RRA and Lackman PJ, eds. Clinical Aspects of Immunology. Blackwell Ltd. Oxford, UK: 1975; 761–782.

27. Lichtenstein LM, Osler AG. Studies on the mechanism of hypersensitivity phenomena. IX. Histamine release from leukocytes by ragweed antigen. J Exp Med 1964; 120: 507–530.

28. Lai CK, Beasley R, Holgate ST. The effect of an increase in inhaled allergen dose after terfenadine on the occurrence and magnitude of the late asthmatic response. Clin Exp Allergy 1989; 19: 209–216.

29. Lai CK, Twentyman OP, Holgate ST. The effect of an increase in inhaled allergen dose after rimiterol hydrobromide on the occurrence and magnitude of the late asthmatic response and the associated change in non-specific bronchial responsiveness. Am Rev Respir Dis 1989; 140: 917–923.

30. Boulet LP, Roberts RS, Dolovich J, Hargreave FE. Prediction of late asthmatic responses to inhaled allergen. Clin Allergy 1984; 14: 379–385.

31. Gwynn CM, Ingram J, Almousawi T, Stanworth DR. Bronchial provocation tests in atopic patients with allergen-specific IgG4 antibodies. Lancet 1982; 1: 254–256.

32. Ito K, Kudo K, Okudaira S, Yoshinoya S, Morita Y, Nakagawa T, Akiyama K, Urata C, Hayakawa T, Ohta et al. IgG1 antibodies to house dust mite (*Dermatophagoides farinae*) and late asthmatic responses. Int Arch Allergy Appl Immunol 1986; 81: 69–74.

33. Cockcroft DW, Murdock KY, Kirby J, Hargreave FE. Prediction of airway responsiveness to allergen from skin sensitivity to allergen and airway responsiveness to histamine. Am Rev Respir Dis 1987; 135: 264–267.

34. Iliopoulos O, Proud D, Adkinson Jr NF, Norman PS, Kagey-Sobotka A, Lichtenstein LM, Naclerio RM. Relationship between the early, late, and rechallenge reaction to nasal challenge with antigen: observations on the role of inflammatory mediators and cells. J Allergy Clin Immunol 1990; 86; 851–861.

35. Umemoto L, Poothullil J, Dolovich J, Hargreave FE. Factors which influence late skin-allergic responses. J Allergy Clin Immunol 1978; 58: 60–65.

36. Boushey MA, Holtzman J, Sheller JR, Nadel JA. Bronchial hyperreactivity, state of the art. Am Rev Respir Dis 1980; 121: 389–413.

37. Ryan G, Latimer KM, Dolovich J, Hargreave FE. Bronchial responsiveness to histamine: relationship to diurnal variation of peak flow rate, improvement after bronchodilator, and airway calibre. Thorax, 1982; 37: 423–429.

38. Cockcroft DW, Ruffin RE, Dolovich J, Hargreave FE. Allergen-induced increase in non-allergic bronchial reactivity. Clin Allergy 1977; 7: 503–513.

39. Cartier A, Thomson NC, Frith PA, Roberts R, Hargreave FE. Allergen-induced increase in bronchial responsiveness to histamine: relationship to the late asthmatic response and change in airway calibre. J Allergy Clin Immunol 1982; 70: 170–177.

40. Durham SR, Craddock CF, Cookson WF, Benson M. Increases in airway responsiveness to histamine precede allergen-induced late asthmatic responses. J Allergy Clin Immunol 1988; 82: 764–770.

41. Bernstein DI, Ploysongsang Y, Mittman RJ. The relationship between airway responsiveness measured before and after the allergen-induced late asthmatic response. Chest 1992; 101: 437–441.

42. Cookson WO, Craddock CF, Benson MK, Durham SR. Falls in peripheral eosinophil counts parallel the late asthmatic response. Am Rev Respir Dis 1989; 139: 458–462.

43. Asakura K, Enomoto K, Ara H, Azuma E, Kataura A. Nasal responsiveness to methacholine stimulation in allergic rhinitis patients. Arch Otolaryngol 1984; 239: 273–278.

44. Borum P. Nasal methacholine challenge: a test for the measurement of nasal reactivity. J Allergy Clin Immunol 1979; 63: 253–257.

45. Clement PAR, Stoop AP, Kaufman L. Histamine threshold and nasal hyperreactivity in non-specific allergic rhinopathy. Rhinology 1985; 23: 35–42.

46. Corrada OJ, Gould CAL, Kassab JY, Davies RJ. Nasal responses of rhinitic and non-rhinitic subjects to histamine and methacholine; a comparative study. Thorax 1986; 41: 863–868.

47. Mullens RJ, Olson LG, Sutherland DC. Nasal histamine challenges in symptomatic allergic rhinitis. J Allergy Clin Immunol 1989; 83: 955–959.

48. Djukanovic R, Wilson JW, Britten KM, Wilson SJ, Walls AF, Roche WR, Howarth PH, Holgate ST. Quantitation of mast cells and eosinophils in the bronchial mucosa of symptomatic atopic asthmatics and healthy control subjects using immunohistochemistry. Am Rev Respir Dis 1990; 142: 863–871.

49. Enerback L, Pipkorn U, Granerus G. Intraepithelial migration of nasal mucosal mast cells in hay fever. Int Arch Allergy Appl Immunol 1986; 80: 44–51.

50. Pipkorn U, Karlsson G, Enerback L. The cellular response of the human allergic mucosa to natural allergen exposure. J Allergy Clin Immunol 1988; 82: 1046–1054.

51. Beasley R, Roche WR, Roberts JA, Holgate ST. Cellular events in the bronchi in mild asthma and after bronchial provocation. Am Rev Respir Dis 1989; 139: 806–817.

52. Yang JP, Wong BJO, Dolovich J, Denburg JA, Ramsdale EH, Hargreave FE. Intraepithelial mast cells in allergic and non-allergic asthma: assessment using bronchial brushings. Am Rev Respir Dis 1993; 148: 80–86.

53. Ollerenshaw SL, Woolcock AJ. Characteristics of the inflammation in biopsies from large airways of subjects with asthma and subjects with chronic airflow limitation. Am Rev Respir Dis 1992; 145: 922–927.

54. Wardlaw AJ, Dunnette S, Gleich GJ, Collins JV, Kay AB. Eosinophils and mast cells in bronchoalveolar lavage in subjects with mild asthma. Relationship to bronchial hyperreactivity. Am Rev Respir Dis 1988; 137: 62–69.

55. Kirby JG, Hargreave FE, Gleich GJ, O'Byrne PM. Bronchoalveolar cell profiles of asthmatic and non-asthmatic subjects. Am Rev Respir Dis 1987; 136: 379–383.

56. Bradley BL, Azzawi M, Jacobson MR, Assoufi B, Collins JV, Irani AM, Schwartz LB, Durham SR, Jeffery PK, Kay AB. Eosinophils, T-lymphocytes, mast cells, neutrophils, and macrophages in bronchial biopsy specimens from atopic subjects with asthma: comparison with biopsy specimens from subjects without asthma and normal control subjects and relationship to bronchial hyperresponsiveness. J Allergy Clin Immunol 1991; 88: 661–674.

57. Varney VA, Jacobson MR, Sudderick RM, Robinson DS, Irani A-M R,

Schwartz LB, Mackay IS, Kay AB, Durham SR. Immunohistology of the nasal mucosa following allergen-induced rhinitis. Identification of activated T lymphocytes, eosinophils and neutrophils. Am Rev Respir Dis 1992; 170–176.

58. Lai CKW, Holgate ST. The mast cell in asthma. In: Kay AB, ed. Clinical Immunology and Allergy: the Allergic Basis of Asthma. London: Bailliere Tindall, 1988; 37–65.

59. Gomez E, Corrado OH, Baldwin DL, Swanton AR, Davies RJ. Direct in vivo evidence for mast cell degranulation during allergen-induced reactions in man. J Allergy Clin Immunol 1986; 78: 637–645.

60. Casale TB, Wood D, Richerson HB, Trapp S, Metzger WJ, Zavala D, Hunninghake GW. Elevated bronchoalveolar lavage fluid histamine levels in allergic asthmatics are associated with methacholine bronchial responsiveness. J Clin Invest 1987; 79: 1197–1203.

61. Linder A, Strandberg K, Deuschel H. Variations in histamine concentrations in nasal secretion in patients with allergic rhinitis. Allergy 1988; 43: 119–126.

62. Sheinman BD, Devalia JL, Crook SJ, Davies RJ. De novo generation of histamine in sputum and the effects of antibiotics. Agents Actions 1986; 17: 449–453.

63. Andersson M, Nolte H, Olsson M, Stahiskov P, Pipkorn U. Measurement of histamine in nasal lavage fluid; comparison of a glass fibre based fluoromertic method with two radio-immunoassays. J Allergy Clin Immunol 1990; 86: 815–820.

64. Creticos PS, Adkinson NF, Sobotka AK, Proud D, Meier HL, Naclerio RM, Lichtenstein LM, Norman PS. Nasal challenge with ragweed pollen in hay fever patients. J Clin Invest 1985; 76: 2247–2253.

65. Naclerio RM, Meier HL, Sobotka AK, Adkinson NF, Meyers DA, Norman PS, Lichtenstein LM. Mediator release after nasal airway challenge with allergen. Am Rev Respir Dis 1983; 128: 597–602.

66. Julisson S, Holmberg K, Baumgarten CR, Olsson M, Enauder I, Pipkorn U. Tryptase in nasal lavage fluid after local allergen challenge. Relationship to histamine levels and TAME-esterase activity. Allergy 1991; 46: 459–465.

67. Liu MC, Hubbard WC, Proud D, Stealey BA, Galli SJ, Sobotka AK, Bleecker ER, Lichtenstein LM. Immediate and late inflammatory responses to ragweed antigen challenge of the peripheral airways in allergic asthmatics. Cellular, mediator and permeability changes. Am Rev Respir Dis 1991; 144: 51–58.

68. Wenzel SE, Westcott JY, Smith HR, Larsen GL. Spectrum of prostanoid release after bronchoalveolar allergen challenge in atopic asthmatics and in control groups: an alteration in the ratio of bronchoconstrictive to bronchoprotective mediators. Am Rev Respir Dis 1989; 139: 450–457.

69. Harrison K, Robinson C, Brewster H, Howarth PH. Comparative effects of prostaglandin D_2, 9a 11B PGF_2 and histamine on nasal airflow. In: Prostaglandins and related compounds. 7th International conference proceedings. 1990: 323.

70. Miadonna A, Tedeschi A, Leggiere E, Lorini M, Folco G, Sala A, Qualizza R, Froldi M, Zanussi C. Behaviour and clinical relevance of histamine and

leucotrienes C_4 and B_4 in grass pollen–induced rhinitis. Am Rev Respir Dis 1987; 136: 357–362.

71. Doyle WJ, Boehm BS, Skoner DP. Physiologic responses to intranasal dose–response challenges with histamine, methacholine, bradykinin and prostaglandin in adult volunteers with and without nasal allergy. J Allergy Clin Immunol 1990; 86: 924–935.

72. Howarth PH. Allergic rhinitis: a rational choice of treatment. Respir Med 1989; 83: 179–188.

73. Bradding P, Feather IH, Howarth PH, Mueller R, Roberts JA, Britten K, Bews JPA, Hunt TC, Okayama Y, Heusser CH, Bullock GR, Church MK, Holgate ST. Interleukin-4 is localised to and released by human mast cells. J Exp Med 1992; 176: 1381–1386.

74. Bradding P, Mediwake R, Feather IH, Madden J, Church MK, Holgate ST, Howarth PH. TNFα is localised to nasal mucosal mast cells and is released in acute allergic rhinitis. Clin Exp Allergy 1995; 25(5): 406–415.

75. Bradding P, Feather IH, Wilson S, Bardin PG, Heusser CH, Holgate ST and Howarth PH. Immunolocalisation of cytokines in the nasal mucosa of normal and perennial rhinitic subjects. The mast cells as a source of IL-4, IL-5 and IL-6 in human allergic inflammation. J Immunol 1993; 151: 3852–3865.

76. Bradding P, Roberts JA, Britten KM, Montefort S, Djukanovic R, Mueller R, Heusser CH, Howarth PH, Holgate ST. Interleukin-4, -5, and -6 and tumor necrosis factor-α in normal and asthmatic airways: evidence for the human mast cell as a source of these cytokines. Am J Respir Cell Mol Biol 1994; 10: 471–480.

77. Spry CFJ, Kay AB, Gleich GJ. Eosinophils. Immunol Today 1992; 13: 384–387.

78. Weller PF. Eosinophils: structure and functions. Curr Opin Immunol 1994; 6: 85–90.

79. Lim MC, Taylor RM, Naclerio RM. The histology of allergic rhinitis and its comparison to nasal lavage. Am J Respir Crit Care Med 1995; 151: 136–144.

80. Naclerio RM, Baroody FM, Kagey-Sabotka A, Lichtenstein LM. Basophils and eosinophils in allergic rhinitis. J Allergy Clin Immunol 1994; 94: 1303–1309.

81. Klementsson H, Andersson M, Venge P and Pipkorn U. Allergen-induced changes in nasal secretory responsiveness and eosinophil granulocytes. Acta Otolaryngol 1991; 111: 776–784.

82. Klementsson H, Andersson M, Baumgarten C, Venge P, Pipkorn U. Changes in non-specific nasal reactivity and eosinophil influx and activation after allergen challenge. Clin Exp Allergy 1990; 20: 539–547.

83. Bonavia M, Crimi E, Quaglia A, Brusasco V. Comparison of early and late asthmatic responses between patients with allergic rhinitis and mild asthma. Eur Respir J 1996; 9: 905–909.

84. Carlson M, Hakansson L, Peterson C, Stalenheim G, Venge P. Secretion of granule proteins from eosinophils and neutrophils is increased in asthma. J Allergy Clin Immunol 1991; 87: 306–312.

85. Carlson M, Hakansson L, Kampe M, Stalenheim G, Peterson C, Venge P. Degranulation of eosinophils from pollen-atopic patients with asthma is increased during pollen season. J Allergy Clin Immunol 1992; 89: 131–139.
86. Ayars GH, Altman LC, McManus MM, Agosti JM, Baker C, Luchtel DL, Loegering DA, Gleich GJ. Injurious effect of the eosinophil peroxide–halide system and major basic protein on human nasal epithelium in vitro. Am Rev Respir Dis 1989; 140: 125–131.
87. Lee TH, Austen KF. Arachidonic acid metabolism by the 5-lipoxygenase pathway and the effects of alternative dietary fatty acids. Adv Immunol 1986; 39: 145–175.
88. Shaw RJ, Walsh GM, Cromwell O, Moqbel R, Spry CJF and Kay AB. Activated human eosinophils generate SRS-A leukotrienes following physiological (IgG-dependent) stimulation. Nature 1985; 316: 150–152.
89. Martin LM, Kita H, Leiferman KM, Gleich GJ. Eosinophils in allergy: role in disease, degranulation, and cytokines. Int. Arch. Allergy Immunol 1996; 109: 207–215.
90. Laitinen LA, Heino M, Laitinen A, Kava T, Haahtela T. Damage of the airway epithelium and bronchial reactivity in patients with asthma. Am Rev Respir Dis 1985; 131: 599–606.
91. Wardlaw AJ, Dunnette S, Gleich GJ, Collins JV, Kay AB. Eosinophils and mast cells in bronchoalveolar lavage in mild asthma: relationship to bronchial hyperreactivity. Am Rev Respir Dis 1988; 137: 62–69.
92. Bascom R, Pipkorn U, Proud D, Dunnette S, Gleich GJ, Lichtenstein LM, Naclerio RM. Major basic protein and eosinophil-derived neurotoxin concentrations in nasal lavage fluid after antigen challenge: effect of systemic corticosteroids and relationship to eosinophil influx. J Allergy Clin Immunol 1989; 84: 338–346.
93. Azzawi M, Johnston PW, Majumdar S, Kay AB, Jeffery PK. T lymphocytes and activated eosinophils in airway mucosa in fatal asthma and cystic fibrosis. Am Rev Respir Dis 1992; 145: 1477–1482.
94. Filley WV, Holley KE, Kephart GM, Gleich GJ. Identification of immunofluorescence of eosinophil granule major basic protein in lung tissues of patients with bronchial asthma. Lancet 1982; ii: 11–12.
95. Frigas E, Loegering DA, Gleich GJ. Cytotoxic effects of the guinea pig eosinophil major basic protein on tracheal epithelium. Lab Invest 1980; 42: 35–43.
96. Gundel RH, Letts LG, Gleich GJ. Human eosinophil major basic protein induces airway constriction and airway hyperresponsiveness in primates. J Clin Invest 1991; 87: 1470–1473.
97. Jacoby DB, Gleich GJ, Fryer AD. Human eosinophil MBP is an endogenous allosteric antagonist at the inhibitory muscarinic M2 receptor. J Clin Invest 1993; 91: 1314–1318.
98. Coyle AJ, Ackerman SJ, Burch R, Proud D, Irvin CG. Human eosinophil granule major basic protein and synthetic polycations induce airway hyperresponsiveness in vivo dependent on bradykinin generation. J Clin Invest 1995; 95: 1735–1740.

99. Weller PF, Rand TH, Barret T, Elovic A, Wong DT, Finberg RW. Accessory cell function of human eosinophils, HLA-DR dependent MHC-restricted antigen presentation and interleukin 1α expression. J Immunol 1993; 150: 2554–2562.

100. Wilson JW, Djukanovic R, Howarth PH, Holgate ST. Lymphocyte activation in bronchoalveolar lavage and peripheral blood in atopic asthma. Am Rev Respir Dis 1992; 145: 958–960.

101. Gratziou C, Carroll M, Walls A, Howarth PH, Holgate ST. Early changes in T lymphocytes recovered by bronchoalveolar lavage after local allergen challenge of asthmatic airways. Am Rev Respir Dis 1992; 145: 1259–1264.

102. Poston RN, Chanez P, Lacoste JY, Lichfield T, Lee TH, Bousquet J. Immunohistochemical characterisation of the cellular infiltration in asthmatic bronchi. Am Rev Respir Dis 1992; 145: 918–921.

103. Robinson DS, Bentley AM, Hartnell A, Kay AB, Durham SR. Activated memory T helper cells in bronchoalveolar lavage fluid from patients with atopic asthma: relation to asthma symptoms, lung functions, and bronchial responsiveness. Thorax. 1993; 48: 26–32.

104. Hamid Q, Azzawi M, Ying S, Moqbel R, Wardlaw AJ, Corrigan CJ, Bradley B, Durham SR, Collins JV, Jeffery PK, Kay AB. Expression of mRNA for interleukin-5 in mucosal biopsies from asthma. J Clin Invest 1991; 87: 1541–1546.

105. Rajakulasingam K, Hamid Q, O'Brien F, Shotman E, Jose PJ, Williams TJ, Jacobson M, Barkans J, Durham SR. RANTES in human allergic rhinitis: evidence for synthesis and release after allergen challenge and relationship to tissue eosinophilia. Am J Respir Crit Care Med 1997; 155(2): 696–703.

106. Varga EM, Jacobson MR, Till SJ, Masuyama K, O'Brien F, Rak S, Lowhagen O, Scadding GK, Hamid QA, Durham SR. Cellular infiltration and cytokine mRNA expression in perennial allergic rhinitis. Allergy 1999; 54: 338–345.

107. Varga EM, Jacobson Mr, Masuyama K, Kay AB, Rak S, Till SJ, Darby Y, Hamid Q, Lund V, Scadding GK, Durham SR. Inflammatory cell populations and cytokine mRNA expression in the nasal mucosa of aspirin sensitive rhinitics. Eur Respir J 1999; 3: 610–615.

108. Walker C, Virchow JC Jr, Bruijnzeel PLB, Blaser K. T-cell subsets and their soluble products regulate eosinophilia in allergic and non-allergic asthma. J Immunol 1991; 146: 1829–1835.

109. Corrigan CJ, Hartnell A, Kay AB. T lymphocyte activation in acute severe asthma. Lancet 1988; 1: 1129–32.

110. Sun Ying, Durham SR, Corrigan CJ, Hamid Q, Kay AB. Phenotype of cells expressing mRNA for TH2-type (interleukin 4 and interleukin 5) and TH1-type (interleukin-2 and interferon γ) cytokines in bronchoalveolar lavage and bronchial biopsies from atopic asthmatic and normal control subjects. Am J Respir Cell Mol Biol 1995; 12: 477–487.

111. Robinson DS, Hamid Q, Ying S, Tsicopoulos A, Barkans J, Bentley AM, Corrigan C, Durham SR, Kay AB. Predominant Th-2 like bronchoalveolar

T-lymphocyte population in atopic asthma. N Engl J Med 1992; 326: 298–304.

112. Durham SR, Sun Ying, Varney VA, Jacobson MR, Sudderick RM, Mackay IS, Kay AB, Hamid QA. Cytokine mRNA expression for IL-3, IL-4, IL-5 and GM-CSF in the nasal mucosa after local allergen provocation: relationship to tissue eosinophilia. J Immunol 1992; 148: 2390–2394.

113. Sim TC, Reece LM, Kimberly A, Hilsmeier J, Grant AJ, Alam R. Secretion of chemokines and other cytokines in allergen-induced nasal responses: inhibition by topical steroid treatment. Am J Respir Crit Care Med 1995; 152: 927–933.

114. Del Prete GF, Maggi E, Parronchi P, Chretien A, Tiri D, Macchia M, Ricci J, Bachereau J, de Vries, Romagnani S. IL-4 is an essential factor for the IgE synthesis induced in vitro by human T cell clones and their supernatants. J Immunol 1988; 140: 4193–4198.

115. Schleimer RP, Sterbinsky SA, Kaiser J, Bickel CA, Klunk DA, Tomioka D, Newman W, Luscinskas FW, Gimbrone MA Jr, McIntyre BW, Bochner BS. IL-4 induces adherence of human eosinophils and basophils but not neutrophils to endothelium. Association with expression of VCAM-1. J Immunol 1992; 148: 1086–1092.

116. Wardlaw AJ, Moqbel R, Kay AB. Eosinophils: biology and role in disease. Adv Immunol 1995; 60: 151–266.

117. Till SJ, Durham SR, Rajakulasingam K, Humbert M, Huston D, Dickason R, Kay AB, Corrigan C. Allergen-induced proliferation and interleukin-5 production by bronchoalveolar lavage and blood T cells after segmental allergen challenge. Am Rev Respir Crit Care Med 1998; 158(2): 404–411.

118. Varga EM, Wachholz P, Nouri-Aria KT, Verhoef A, Corrigan CJ, Till SJ, Durham SR. T cells from human allergen-induced late asthmatic responses express IL-12 receptor beta2 subunit mRNA and respond to IL-12 In vitro. J Immunol 2000; 165: 2877–2885.

119. Bryan SA, O'Connor BJ, Matti S, Leckie MJ, Kanabar V, Khan J, Warrington SJ, Renzetti L, Rames A, Bock JA, Boyce MJ, Hansel TT, Holgate ST, Barnes PJ. Effects of recombinant human interleukin-12 on eosinophils, airway hyperresponsiveness and the late asthmatic response. Lancet 2000; 356: 2149–2153.

120. Leckie MJ, ten Brinke A, Khan J, Diamant Z, O'Connor BJ, Walls CN, Mathur AK, Cowley HC, Chung KF, Djukanovic R, Hansel TT, Holgate ST, Sterk PJ, Barnes PJ. Effects of an interleukin-5 blocking monoclonal antibody on eosinophil airway hyperresponsiveness and the late asthmatic response. Lancet 2000; 356: 2144–2148.

121. Pujol J-L, Cosso B, Daures J-P, Clot J, Michel FB, Godard P. Interleukin-1 release by alveolar macrophages in asthmatic patients and healthy subjects. Int Arch Allergy Appl Immunol 1990; 91: 207–210.

122. Calhoun WJ, Bush RK. Enhanced reactive oxygen species metabolism of airspace cells and airway inflammation following antigen challenge in human asthma. J Allergy Clin Immunol 1990; 86: 306–313.

123. Juliusson S, Bachert C, Klementsson H, Karlsson G, Pipkorn U. Macrophages on the nasal mucosal surface in provoked and naturally occurring allergic rhinitis. Acta Otolaryngol (Stockh) 1991; 11: 946–953.

124. Walker C, Kaegi MK, Braun P, Blaser K. Activated T-cells and eosinophilia in bronchoalveolar lavages from subjects with asthma correlated with disease severity. J Allergy Clin Immunol 1991; 88: 935–942.

125. Broide DH, Gleich GJ, Cuomo AJ, Coburn DA, Fedeman EC, Schwartz LB, Wasserman SI. Evidence of ongoing mast cell and eosinophil degranulation in symptomatic asthma airway. J Allergy Clin Immunol 1991; 88: 637–648.

126. Sedgwick JB, Calhoun WJ, Gleich GJ, Kita H, Abrams JS, Schwartz LB, Volovitz B, Ben-Yaakov M, Busse WW. Immediate and late airway response of allergic rhinitis patients to segmental allergen challenge: characterisation of eosinophils and mast cells mediators. Am Rev Respir Dis 1991; 144; 1274–1281.

127. Linder A, Venge P, Deuschl H. Eosinophil cationic protein and myeloperoxidase on the nasal mucosa surface in patients with hay fever during natural allergen exposure. Allergy 1987; 42: 583–590.

128. Rak S, Jacobson MR, Sudderick RM, Masuyama K, Juliusson S, Kay AB, Hamid Q, Lowhagen O, Durham SR. Influence of prolonged treatment with topical corticosteroid (fluticasone propionate) on early and late phase nasal responses and cellular infiltration in the nasal mucosa after allergen challenge. Clin Exp Allergy 1994; 94; 24(10): 930–939.

129. Braunstahl GJ, Overbeek SE, Kleinjan A, Prins J-B, Hoogsteden HC, Fokkens WJ. Nasal allergen provocation induces adhesion molecule expression and tissue eosinophilia in upper and lower airways. J Allergy Clin Immunol 2001; 107: 469–476.

130. Braunstahl GJ, Overbeek SE, Fokkens WJ, Kleinjan A, McEwen AR, Walls AF, Hoogsteden HC, Prins J-B. Segmental bronchoprovocation in allergic rhinitis patients affects mast cell and basophil numbers in nasal and bronchial mucosa. Am J Respir Crit Care Med 2001; 164: 858–865.

131. Welsh PW, Stricker WR, Chu-Pin C et al. Efficacy of beclomethasone nasal solution, flunisolide and cromolyn in relieving symptoms of ragweed allergy. May Clin Proc 1987; 62: 125–134.

132. Chanez P, Vignola AM, Vic P, Guddo F, Bonsignore G, Godard P, Bousquet J. Comparison between nasal and bronchial inflammation in asthmatic and control subjects. Am J Respir Crit Care Med 1999; 159: 588–595.

133. Calderon M, Lozewicz S, Chalstrey S, Davies RJ. Infiltration by lymphocytes in the nasal mucous membrane in allergic rhinitis. Thorax. 1992; 47: 232p.

134. Latinen LA, Heino M, Laitinen A, Kava T, Haahtela T. Damage of the airway epithelium and bronchial reactivity in patients with asthma. Am Rev Respir Dis 1985; 131: 599–606.

135. Beasley R, Roche WR, Roberts JA, Holgate ST. Cellular events in the bronchi in mild asthma and after bronchial provocation. Am Rev Respir Dis 1989; 139: 806–817.

136. Montefort S, Roche WR, Holgate ST. Bronchial epithelial shedding in asthmatics and non-asthmatics. Respir Med 1993; 87: 9–11.

137. Jeffrey PK, Wardlaw AJ, Nelson FC, Collins JV, Kay AB. Bronchial biopsies in asthma: an ultrastructural, quantitative study and correlation with hyprereactivity. Am Rev Respir Dis 1989; 140: 1745–1753.

138. Zahm JM, Chevillard M, Puchelle E. Wound repair of human surface respiratory epithelium. Am J Respir Cell Mol Biol 1991; 5: 242–248.

139. Holtzman MJ, Aizwa H, Nadel JA, Goetzl EJ. Selective generation of leukotriene B_4 by tracheal epithelial cells from dogs. Biochem Biophys Res Commun 1983; 114: 1071–1076.

140. Eling TE, Danilowicz RM, Hence DC, Sivarajah K, Yankaskas JR, Boucher RC. Arachidonic acid metabolism by canine tracheal epithelial cells: product formation and relationship to chloride secretion. J Biol Chem 1986; 261: 12841–12849.

141. Altman LC, Dumler K, Baker C. Expression of intercellular adhesion molecule-1 (ICAM-1) on human nasal epithelial cell cells (HNE). (abstract). J Allergy Clin Immunol 1991; 87: 304.

142. Manolitsas N, Devalia JL, d'Ardenne AJ, McAulay AE, Davies RJ. Expression of adhesion receptors in asthmatic and normal bronchial epithelium. (abstract). Clin Exp Allergy 1991; 22: 120.

143. Stoop AE, Hameleers DMH, van Run PEM, Biewenga J, van der Baan S. Lymphocytes and nonlymphoid cells in the nasal mucosa of patients with nasal polyps and of healthy subjects. J Allergy Clin Immunol 1989; 84: 734–741.

144. Ohnishi M, Ruhno J, Bienenstock J, Dolovich J, Denburg JA. Haemopoetic growth factor production by cultured cells of human nasal polyp epithelial scrapings: kinetics, cell source, and relationship to clinical status. J Allergy Clin Immunol 1989; 83: 1091–1100.

145. Cox G, Ohtoshi T, Vancheri et al. Promotion of eosinophil survival by human bronchial epithelial cells and its modulation by steroids. Am J Respir Cell Mol Biol 1991; 4: 525–531.

146. Soloperto M, Mattoso VL, Fasoli A, Mattoli S. A bronchial epithelial cell–derived factor in asthma that promotes eosinophil activation and survival as GM-CSF. Am J Physiol Lung Cell Mol Physiol 1991; 260: L530–L538.

147. Churchill L, Friedman B, Schleimer RP and Proud D. Granulocyte macro-phage–colony stimulating factor (GM-CSF) production cultured human tracheal epithelial cells. (abstract). J Allergy Clin Immunol 1990; 85: 233.

148. Devalia JL, Campbell AM, Sapsford RJ et al. Effect of nitrogen dioxide on synthesis of inflammatory cytokines expressed by human bronchial epithelial cells, in vitro. Am J Respir Cell Mol Biol 1993; 9: 271–278.

149. Devalia JL, Pan XQ, Sapsford RJ, Davies RJ. Expression of interleukin-5, granulocyte–macrophage colony stimulating factor and granulocyte–colony stimulating factor by cultured human bronchial epithelial cells. (abstract). Thorax 1991; 46: 53P.

150. Hamid Q, Azzawi M, Ying S et al. expression of mRNA for interleukin-5

in mucosal bronchial biopsies from asthma. J Clin Invest 1991; 87: 1541–1546.

151. Mattoli S, Mattoso VL, Soloperto M, Allegra L, Fasoli A. Cellular and biochemical characteristics of bronchial lavage fluid in symptomatic non-allergic asthma. (abstract). J Allergy Clin Immunol 1991; 87: 794.

152. Sapsford RJ, Devalia JL, McAulay AE, d'Ardenne AJ, Davies RJ. Expression of alpha 1–6 integrin cell-surface receptors on normal human bronchial biopsies and cultured bronchial epithelial cells. (abstract). J Allergy Clin Immunol 1991; 87: 303.

153. Kharitonov SA, Rajakulasingam K, O'Connor BJ, Durham SR, Barnes PJ. Nasal nitric oxide is increased in patients with asthma and allergic rhinitis and may be modulated by nasal glucocorticoids. J Allergy Clin Immunol 1997; 99(pt 1): 58–64.

154. Lundberg J, Farkas-Szallasi T, Weitzberg E et al. High nitric oxide production in human paranasal sinuses. Nat Med 1995; 1: 370–373.

155. Martin U, Bryden K, Devoy M, Howarth PH. Exhaled nitric oxide levels are increased in association with symptoms of seasonal and perennial rhinitis. Am J Respir Crit Care Med 1995; 151: A128.

156. Kharitonov SA, Yates D, Robbins RA, Logan-Sinclair R, Shinebourne E, Barnes PJ. Increased nitric oxide in exhaled air of asthmatic patients. Lancet 1994; 343: 133–135.

157. Alving K, Weitzberg E, Lundberg JM. Increased amount of nitric oxide in exhaled air of asthmatics. Eur Respir J 1993; 6: 1268–1270.

158. Yates DH, Kharitonov SA, Robbins RA, Thomas PS, Barnes PJ. Effect of a nitric oxide synthase inhibitor and a glucocorticosteroid on exhaled nitric oxide. Am J Respir Crit Care Med 1995; 152: 892–896.

159. Kharitonov SA, Yates D, Barnes PJ. Regular inhaled budesonide decreases nitric oxide concentration in the exhaled air of asthmatic patients. Am J Respir Crit Care Med 1996; 153(1): 454–457.

160. Furukawa K, Saleh D, Giaid A. Expression of nitric oxide synthase in human nasal mucosa. Am J Respir Crit Care Med 1995; 1: 370–373.

161. Hamid Q, Springall DR, Riveros-Moreno V et al. Induction of nitric oxide synthase in asthma. Lancet 1993; 342: 1510–1513.

162. Robbins RA, Barnes PJ, Springall DR et al. Expression of inducible nitric oxide synthase in human bronchial epithelial cells. Biochem Biophys Res Commun 1994; 203: 209–218.

163. Asano K, Chee CBE, Gaston B et al. Constitutive and inducible nitric oxide synthase gene expression, regulation and activity in human lung epithelial cells. Proc Natl Acad Sci U S A 1994; 91: 10089–10093.

164. Solperto M, Mattoso VL, Fasoli A and Mattoli S. A bronchial epithelial cell–derived factor in asthma that promotes eosinophil activation and survival as GM-CSF. Am J Physiol Lung Cell Mol Physiol 1991; 260: L530–L538.

165. Montefort S, Roche WR, Howarth PH, Djukanovic R, Gratziou C, Carroll M, Smith L, Britten KM, Haskard DO, Lee TH, Holgate ST. Intercellular adhesion molecule-1 (ICAM-1) and endothelial leucocyte adhesion molecule-

1(ELAM-1) expression in the bronchial mucosa of normal and asthmatic subjects. Eur Respir J 1992; 5: 815–823.

166. Montefort S, Feather IH, Wilson SJ, Haskard DO, Lee TH, Holgate ST, Howarth PH. The expression of leucocyte–endothelial adhesion molecules is increased in perennial allergic rhinitis. Am J Respir Cell Mol 1992; 7: 393–398.

167. Montefort S, Gratziou C, Goulding D, Polosa R, Haskard DO, Howarth PH, Holgate ST, Caroll M. Bronchial biopsy evidence for leucocyte infiltration and upregulation of leucocyte endothelial cell adhesion molecules 6 hours after local allergen challenge of sensitised asthmatic airways. J Clin Invest 1994; 93: 1411–1421.

168. Wegner CD, Gundel RH, Reily P, Haynes N, Letts LG, Rothlein R. Intercellular adhesion molecule (ICAM-1) in the pathogenesis of asthma. Science 1990; 247: 456–459.

169. Zhang L, Redington AE, Hogate ST. RANTES: a novel mediator of allergic inflammation? Clin Exp Allergy 1994; 24(10): 899–904.

170. Jose PJ, Griffiths-Johnson DA, Collins PD, Walsh DT, Moqbel R, Totty N.F, Truong O, Hsuan JJ, Williams TJ. Eotaxin: A potent chemoattractant cytokine detected in a guinea pig model of allergic airways inflammation. J Exp Med 1994; 179: 881–887.

171. Lamkhioued B, Renzi PM, Rothenberg M, Luster AD, Hamid Q. Eotaxin is increased in the airways and bronchoalveolar lavage fluid of asthmatic patients. Am J Respir Crit Care Med 1997; 155(4): A816 (abstract).

172. Humbert M, Ying S, Corrigan CJ, Menz G, Barkans J, Pfister R, Meng Q, Van Damme J, Opdenakker G, Durham SR, Kay AB. Bronchial mucosal expression of the genes encoding chemokines RANTES and MCP-3 in symptomatic atopic and non-atopic asthmatics: relationship to the eosinophil-active cytokines interleukin (IL)-5, granulocyte macrophage-colony-stimulating factor, and IL-3. Am J Respir Crit Care Med 1997; 16(1): 1–8.

173. Kim CH, Rott L, Kunkel EJ, Genovese MC, Andrew DP, Wu L, Butcher EC. Rules of chemokine receptor association with T cell polarisation in vivo. J Clin Invest 2001; 108: 1331–1339.

174. Till SJ, Jopling LA, Wachholz P, Robson RL, Qin S, Andrew DP, Wu L, van Neerven J, Williams TJ, Durham SR, Sabroe I. T cell phenotypes of the normal nasal mucosa: induction of TH2 cytokines and CCR3 expression by IL-4. J Immunol 2001; 166: 2303–2310.

175. Nouri-Aria KT, Wilson DW, Francis JN, Jopling LA, Jacobson MR, Hodge M, Andrew DP, Till SJ Varga EM, Williams TJ, Pease JE, Lloyd C, Sabroe I, Durham SR. CCR4 in human allergen-induced late responses in the skin and lung. Eur J Immunol 2002; 32(7): 1933–1938.

176. Campbell JJ, Brightling CE, Symon FA, Qin S, Murphy KE, Hodge M, Andrew DP, Wu L, Butcher EC, Wardlaw AJ. Expression of chemokine receptors by lung T cells from normal and asthmatic subjects. J Immunol 2001; 166: 2842–2848.

177. Panina-Bordignon P, Papi A, Mariani M, Di Lucia P, Casoni G, Bellettato C, Buonsanti C, Miotto D, Mapp C, Villa A, Arigoni G, Fabbri LM, Sinigaglia

F. The C–C chemokine receptors CCR4 and CCR8 identify airway T cells of allergen-challenged atopic asthmatics. J Clin Invest 2001; 107: 1357–1364.

178. Persson CGA. Plasma exudation and asthma. Lung 1988; 166: 1–23.

179. Erjefalt I, Persson CGA. Allergen, bradykinin and capsaicin increase outward but not inward macromolecular permeability of guinea pig tracheobronchial mucosa. Clin Exp Allergy 1991; 21: 217–224.

180. Greiff L, Wollmer P, Pipkorn U, Persson CGA. Absorption of ^{51}Cr-EDTA across the human nasal airway barriers in the presence of topical histamine. Thorax 1991; 46: 630–632.

181. Luts A, Sundler F, Erjefalt I, Persson CGA. The airway epithelial lining in guinea pigs is intact promptly after the mucosal crossing of a large amount of plasma exudate. Int Arch Allergy Appl Immunol 1990; 91: 385–388.

182. Lundberg JM, Saria A. Capsaicin induced desensitization of the airway mucosa to cigarette smoke, mechanical and chemical irritants. Nature 1983; 302: 251–253.

183. Lundblad L, Anggard A, Lundberg JM. Effects of antidromic trigeminal nerve stimulation in relation to parasympathetic vasodilation in cat nasal mucosa. Acta Physiol Scand 1983; 119: 7–13.

184. Lundblad L, Saria A, Lundberg JM, Anggard A. Increased vascular permeability in rat nasal mucosa induced by substance P and stimulation of capsaicin-sensitive trigeminal neurons. Acta Otolaryngol 1983; 96: 479–484.

185. Baraniuk JN. Neural control of human nasal secretion. Pulm Pharmacol 1991; 4: 20–31.

186. Nieber K, Rathsack R, Henning R, Mullier ST, Slapke J, Oehme P, Schilling W, Baumgarten C, Kunkel G. Substance P in bronchoalveolar lavage and nasal lavage fluids after allergen provocation in patients with asthma. Allergologie 1990; 12: 60.

187. Rajakulasingam K, Polosa R, Lau LCK, Church MK, Holgate ST, Howarth PH. The nasal effects of bradykinin and capsaicin: influence on microvascular leakage and role of sensory nerve fibres. J Appl Physiol 1992; 72(4): 1418–1424.

188. Hui KP, Lotvall J, Chung KF, Barnes PJ. Attenuation of inhaled allergen-induced microvascular leakage and airflow obstruction in guinea pigs by a 5-lipoxygenase inhibitor. Am Rev Respir Dis 1991; 143: 1015–1019.

189. Pare PD, Wiggs BR, James A, Hogg JC and Bosken C. The comparative mechanics and morphology of airways in asthma and in chronic pulmonary disease. Am Rev Respir Dis 1991; 143: 1189–1193.

190. Wiggs BR, Bosken C, Pare PD, James A, Hogg JC. A model of airway narrowing in asthma and in chronic obstructive pulmonary disease. Am Rev Respir Dis 1992; 145: 1251–1258.

191. Cabanes L, Weber S, Matran R, Regnard J, Richard MO, Degeorges M, Lockhart A. Bronchial hyperresponsiveness to methacholine in patients with impaired left ventricular function. N Engl J Med 1990; 323: 940–945.

192. Coupe MO, Guly U, Brown F, Barnes PJ. Nebulised adrenaline in acute severe asthma: comparison with salbutamol. Eur J Respir Dis 1987; 71: 227–232.

193. Masuyama K, Jacobson MR, Rak S, Meng Q, Sudderick RM, Kay AB, Lowhagen O, Hamid Q, Durham SR. Topical glucocorticosteroid (fluticasone propionate) inhibits cytokine mRNA expression for interleukin-4 (IL-4) in the nasal mucosa in allergic rhinitis. Immunology 1994; 82: 192–199.

194. Jacobson MR, Juliusson S, Balder B, Lowhagen O, Durham SR. Topical corticosteroid (fluticasone propionate) inhibits seasonal symptoms and tissue eosinophilia in patients with summer hay fever. Clin Exp Allergy 1994; 24: 978.

195. Jacobson MR, Hamid Q, Rak S, Sudderick RM, Lowhagen O, Durham SR. Topical corticosteroid (fluticasone propionate) inhibits cytokine messenger RNA expression for GM-CSF in the nasal mucosa in allergen-induced rhinitis. Clin Exp Allergy 1994; 24: 989.

196. Ying S, Durham SR, Barkans J, Masuyama J, Jacobson MR, Rak S, Lowhagen O, Moqbel R, Kay AB, Hamid Q. T cells are the principal source of interleukin-5 mRNA in allergen-induced rhinitis. Am J Respir Crit Care Med 1993; 9(4): 356–360.

197. Vrugt B, Wilson S, Underwood JM et al. Increased expression of interleukin-2 receptor in peripheral blood and bronchial biopsies from severe asthmatics. Eur Respir J 1994; 7: 239 A.

198. Leung DYM, Martin RJ, Szefler SJ, Sher ER, Ying S, Kay AB, Hamid Q. Dysregulation of interleukin 4, interleukin 5 and interferon γ gene expression on steroid resistant asthma. J Exp Med 1995; 181: 33–40.

199. Durham SR, Walker SM, Varga EM, Jacobson MR, O'Brien F, Noble W, Till SJ, Hamid Q, Nouri-Aria K. Long-term clinical efficacy of grass pollen immunotherapy. N Engl J Med 1999; 341: 468–475.

200. Malling H-J, Weeke B. European Academy of Allergology and Clinical Immunology (EAACI) position paper: Immunotherapy. 1993, 48, suppl. 14, 9–35.

201. Bousquet J, Lockey RF, Malling H-J, ed. Allergen immunotherapy: therapeutic vaccines for allergic diseases. A WHO position paper. Allergy, 1998; 53: suppl. 44, 1–42.

202. Durham SR, Ying S, Varney VA, Jacobson MR, Sudderick RM, Mackay IS, Kay AB and Hamid Q. Grass pollen immunotherpy inhibits allergen-induced infiltration of CD4$^+$ T lymphocytes and eosinophils in the nasal mucosa and increases the number of cells expressing messenger RNA for interferon-gamma. J Allergy Clin Immunol 1996; 97(6): 1356–1365.

203. Wilson DR, Nouri-Aria KT, Walker SM, O'Brien F, Jacobson MR, Durham SR. Grass pollen immunotherapy: symptomatic improvement correlates with reductions in eosinophils and IL-5 mRNA expression in the nasal mucosa during the pollen season. J Allergy Clin Immunol 2001; 107: 971–976.

204. Wachholz P, Nouri-Aria KT, Wilson DR, Verhoef A, Till SJ, Durham SR. Grass pollen immunotherapy for hayfever is associated with increases in local nasal but not peripheral Th1/Th2 cytokine ratios. Immunology 2002; 105: 56–62.

205. Creticos PS, Reed CE, Norman PS, Khoury J, Adkinson NF, Buncher CR, Busse WW, Bush RK, Gadde J. Ragweed immunotherapy in adult asthma. N Engl J Med 1996; 334: 501–506.

206. Adkinson NF, Eggleston PA, Eney D, Goldstein EO, Schuberth KC, Bacon JR, Hamilton RG, Weiss ME, Arshad H, Meinert CL, Tonascia J, Wheeler B. A controlled trial of immunotherapy for asthma in allergic rhinitis. N Engl J Med 1997; 336: 324–331.

207. Abramson MJ, Puy RM, Weiner JM. Is allergen immunotherapy effective in asthma? A meta-analysis of randomised controlled trial. Am J Respir Crit Care Med 1995; 15194: 969–74.

208. Tomaoki J, Kondo M, Sakai N, Nakata J, Takemura H, Nagai A, Takizawa T, Konno K. Leukotriene antagonist prevents exacerbation of asthma during reduction of high-dose inhaled corticosteroid. The Tokyo Joshi-Idai Asthma Research Group. Am J Resp Crit Care Med 1997; 155(4): 1235–1240.

209. Donnelly AL, Glass M, Minkwitz MC, Casale TB. The leukotriene D4-receptor antagonist ICI 204, 219, relieves symptoms of acute allergic rhinitis. Am J Respir Crit Care Med 1995; 151(6): 1734–1739.

210. Drazen JM, Elliot I, O'Byrne PM. Treatment of asthma with drugs modifying the leukotriene pathway. N Engl J Med 1999; 340:197–206.

211. Lipworth BJ. Leukotriene-receptor antagonists. Lancet 1999; 353: 57–62.

212. Sander C, Rajakulasingam K. Leukotriene receptor antagonists for the treatment of allergic rhinitis. Clin Exp Allergy 2002; 32(1): 4–7.

6

Pathogenetic Links Between Rhinitis and Asthma

JEAN BOUSQUET
and PASCAL DEMOLY

Hopital Arnaud de Villeneuve
Montpellier, France

A. MAURIZIO VIGNOLA

Instituto di Fisiopatologia Respiratoria
Palermo, Italy

Introduction

Asthma and allergies including rhinoconjunctivitis and atopic dermatitis are common throughout the world, with resultant morbidity and cost. The nasal and bronchial mucosa present similarities, and most patients with asthma also have rhinitis (1–3), suggesting the concept of "one airway, one disease." On the other hand, not all patients with rhinitis present asthma, and there are some differences between rhinitis and asthma.

I. Rhinitis and Nonspecific Bronchial Hyperreactivity

Many patients with allergic rhinitis have unique physiological behavior separating them from patients with asthma and from normal subjects: they have increased bronchial sensitivity to methacholine or histamine (5,6), especially during and slightly after the pollen season (7,8). There are large differences in the magnitude of airway reactivity between asthmatics and rhinitics, however, which are not explained by the allergen type or degree of reactivity (9,10).

II. Common Causative Agents in Rhinitis and Asthma

Among the causative agents inducing asthma and rhinitis, some [e.g., allergens and aspirin (11)] are well known to affect both the nose and the bronchi. Most inhaled allergens are associated with nasal (4) and bronchial symptoms, but in epidemiological studies differences have been observed. Although there are some recent concerns (12), the prevalence of IgE sensitization to indoor allergens (house dust mites and cat allergens) is positively correlated with both the frequency of asthma and its severity (13,14). *Alternaria* (15,16) and insect dusts (17) have also been found to be linked with asthma, but pollen sensitivity has not been found to be associated with asthma in epidemiological studies (18,19). On the other hand, pollen sensitivity is always associated with rhinitis (4).

Occupational diseases represent an interesting model to study the relationships between rhinitis and asthma. Subjects with occupational asthma may often report symptoms of rhinoconjunctivitis. Rhinitis is less pronounced than asthma with low molecular weight agents. On the other hand, rhinitis more often appears before asthma in the case of high molecular weight agents such as small mammals (20–22), raw green beans (23), flour (24,25) and latex (26,27). In many patients nasal symptoms occur before bronchial ones, making it possible to prevent the development of asthma. In addition, rhinitis caused by some low molecular weight agents is associated with or develops into occupational asthma (28–31), highlighting the importance of cessation of allergen exposure in occupational allergic rhinitis to prevent asthma.

III. Nasal Inflammation in Patients with Asthma

In normal subjects, the structure of the airways mucosa presents similarities between the nose and the bronchi. Both nasal and bronchial mucosa are characterized by a pseudostratified epithelium with columnar, ciliated cells resting on a basement membrane. Underneath the epithelium, in the sub-mucosa, vessels and mucous glands are present with structural cells (fibroblasts), some inflammatory cells (essentially monocytic cells, lymphocytes, and mast cells) (32,33) and nerves.

There are also differences between the nose and the bronchi. In the nose, there is a large supply of subepithelial capillary and arterial system and venous cavernous sinusoids. The high degree of vascularization is a key feature of the nasal mucosa, and changes in the vasculature may lead to severe nasal obstruction (34). On the other hand, smooth muscle is present from the trachea to the bronchioles, explaining bronchoconstriction in asthma (35).

Recent progress achieved in the cellular and molecular biology of airways diseases has yielded clear documentation of the critical role of inflammation in the pathogenesis of asthma and rhinitis. The same inflammatory cells appear to be present in the nasal and bronchial mucosa (36). A growing number of studies show that the inflammation of nasal and bronchial mucosa is sustained by a similar inflammatory infiltrate, which is represented by eosinophils, mast cells, T lymphocytes, and cells of the monocytic lineage (36–39). The same proinflammatory mediators (histamine, CysLT), TH2 cytokines (interleukins 4, 5, and 13; granulocyte–macrophage colony-stimulating factor) (36,40–42), chemokines (RANTES and eotaxin) (43) and adhesion molecules (44–46) appear to be involved in nasal and bronchial inflammation of patients with rhinitis and asthma.

However there are major differences between the sites. Although the nasal and bronchial mucosa are exposed to the same noxious environment (and the nose even more so), epithelial shedding is more pronounced in the bronchi than in the nose of the same patients suffering from asthma and rhinitis (47). The magnitude of inflammation may not be identical. In patients with moderate to severe asthma, eosinophilic inflammation is more pronounced in the bronchi than in the nose (47), whereas in patients with mild asthma, inflammation appears to be similar in both sites. Moreover, eosinophilic inflammation of the nose exists in asthmatics with or without nasal symptoms (48). On the other hand, features of airways remodeling appear to be less extensive in the nasal mucosa than in the bronchial mucosa.

To determine whether nasal inflammation in asthma was related to asthma or was found commonly in other bronchial diseases, nasal inflammation and sinus involvement were studied in patients with chronic obstructive pulmonary disease (COPD). Less than 10% of patients with COPD have nasal symptoms. Nasal inflammation assessed by means of mucosal biopsy samples is usually not detectable in these patients (50). CT images show few abnormalities in COPD. Thus, nasal and sinusal inflammation seen in asthmatics is related to asthma and is not a feature of all bronchial diseases (49).

IV. Bronchial Inflammation and Asthma in Patients with Rhinitis

A. Bronchial Biopsies in Patients with Rhinitis

Some studies have examined the bronchial mucosa in atopic nonasthmatic patients or in patients with allergic rhinitis. They all combined to indicate that there was a slight increase of the basement membrane size (51) and a moderate eosinophilic inflammation (52).

Natural exposure to pollen during season provokes an increase in airway responsiveness in nonasthmatic subjects with seasonal allergic rhinitis and also induces inflammatory cell recruitment and expression of interleukin 5 (IL-5), leading to bronchial inflammation (53).

B. Bronchial Allergen Challenge in Patients with Rhinitis

Endobronchial allergen challenge was carried out in patients with seasonal rhinitis who had never presented asthma before. These patients developed a bronchoconstriction, and lavage carried out serially after challenge demonstrated the occurrence of proinflammatory mediators and cytokines as well as the recruitment of inflammatory cells (54,55).

Pulmonary inflammation after segmental ragweed challenge was examined in allergic asthmatic and nonasthmatic subjects (56). A total of 46 ragweed-allergic subjects took part in these studies. Subjects had normal or nearly normal pulmonary function, were on no chronic medication, and were characterized with respect to their skin sensitivity to intradermal ragweed injection, their nonspecific responsiveness to methacholine, and the presence (or absence) of a late asthmatic response after whole-lung antigen challenge. In both groups, a marked inflammatory response measured in fluid from bronchoalveolar lavage (BAL) (total cells, macrophages, lymphocytes, eosinophils, and neutrophils per milliliter, total protein, albumin, urea, or eosinophil cationic protein) 24 h after challenge was seen only in the subgroup of subjects who demonstrated a late airway reaction after whole-lung antigen challenge, regardless of disease classification.

C. "Thunderstorm-Induced Asthma"

The foregoing studies combine to indicate that although patients with nasal symptoms can only react if the allergen is properly administered into the airways, it may be argued, however, that the doses of allergen inducing these bronchial reactions are far greater than those naturally occurring during allergen exposure. This situation seems to exist in thunderstorm-induced asthma (57–60), which has been associated with grass pollen allergy (57,61, 62). The aerodynamic size of pollen grains is from 10 to 100 μm, and since only a fraction can be deposited into the bronchi, most patients present only rhinitis, without asthma. However, when exposed to water, pollen allergens are released in submicrometer-sized particles, the starch granules, which can reach the lower airways and induce asthma (63).

V. "Bidirectional" Relationship Between Nasal and Bronchial Inflammation

Subjects with occupational asthma often report nasal symptoms. Fifteen subjects with occupational asthma (8 due to high -molecular -weight agents such as flour and guar gum, and 7 due to isocyanates) underwent inhalation challenges by means of closed-circuit devices on two occasions, 2 to 4 weeks apart, in random fashion. On one occasion, they inhaled through the nose and, on another, through the mouth (64). Inhalation of occupational agents through the mouth or nose resulted in similar asthmatic responses, caused a significant nasal response in terms of symptoms, and produced an increase in nasal resistance as well inducing significant changes in nasal inflammatory cells and mediators.

To analyze further the aspects of nasobronchial cross-talk, inflammation and the expression of adhesion molecules were studied in nasal and bronchial mucosa after allergen provocation. In a first study, endobronchial allergen challenge induced nasal and bronchial symptoms as well as reductions in pulmonary and nasal function (65). In this study, the number of eosinophils increased in the challenged bronchial mucosa, in the blood, and in the nasal mucosa 24 h after bronchial challenge. Moreover, eotaxin-positive cells in the nasal lamina propria and enhanced expression of IL-5 in the nasal epithelium were found 24 h after bronchial challenge.

In a second study, bronchial and nasal biopsy specimens were taken before and 24 h after nasal provocation (66). At 24 h, an influx of eosinophils was detected in nasal epithelium and lamina propria, as well as in bronchial epithelium and lamina propria. Increased expression of intercellular adhesion molecule (ICAM-1) and increased percentages of ICAM-1$^+$, VCAM-1$^+$, and E-selectin$^+$ vessels were seen in nasal and bronchial tissue of patients with allergic rhinitis (AR). The number of mucosal eosinophils correlated with the local expression of ICAM-1, E-selectin, and VCAM-1 in patients with AR.

These studies show that nasal or bronchial allergen provocation results in generalized airway inflammation (66).

VI. Systematic Nature of Allergic Inflammation

Two major mechanisms contribute to the increased number of eosinophils in the inflamed airways of allergic subjects: recruitment and persistence of inflammatory cells into the airways and the presence of bone marrow progenitors in the inflamed airway tissues.

A. Bone Marrow Involvement

In patients with allergic diseases, allergen provocation can activate a systemic response that provokes inflammatory cell production by the bone marrow (67). There is considerable evidence in animal models and humans that the bone marrow plays an integral role in allergic inflammation (68). In response to allergen exposure in the airway, bone marrow (white blood cell) progenitors proliferate and differentiate, which leads to persistent increases in eosinophil numbers. Signaling between the lung and bone marrow after allergen exposure provides further support for the proposition that allergy is a systemic disease. Although the nature of the signal-mediating activation of bone marrow after airway allergen exposure is unknown, several pathways have been implicated, including allergen-induced hemopoietic growth factors, cell trafficking, and stimulation of resident bone marrow cells. A common thread in all these pathways is the importance of IL-5.

After release and differentiation of progenitor cells, eosinophils, basophils, and mast cells are typically recruited to tissues in atopic individuals. An understanding at the molecular level of the signaling process that leads to these systemic responses between the target organ, especially the airways, and the bone marrow may open up new avenues of therapy for allergic inflammatory disease (69,70).

Studies that support the critical involvement of the bone marrow in the development of eosinophilic inflammation of the airways point out the systemic nature of these conditions.

B. In Situ Hemopoiesis

The second important mechanism, termed "in situ hemopoiesis" (71), depends on the production of hemopoietic cytokines by inflamed tissues from patients with allergic rhinitis (72–74) and nasal polyposis (75), which, generating a particular local "microenvironment," promote the differentiation and maturation of eosinophil progenitors that populate the nasal or the bronchial mucosa (76,77). It is therefore likely that a truly "systemic" response to the application of inflammatory stimuli to the nasal mucosa should be associated with an activation of the aforementioned mechanisms.

VII. Rhinitis and Asthma: A Continuum of Disease?

There are similarities and differences between the nasal and bronchial mucosa in rhinitis and asthma. It appears that most asthmatics present rhinitis, whereas only a fraction of rhinitis patients present clinically demonstrable asthma even though a greater number of patients have nonspecific bronchial hyperreactivity. It seems that the epithelial–mesenchymal trophic unit exists from the nose to the bronchiolar–alveolar junction and that the same inflammatory cells are present throughout the airways, suggesting a continuum of disease.

However, there are differences in terms of exposure to allergens and noxious agents, the nose being more exposed than the lower airways. There are also major structural differences between the nasal and the bronchial mucosa, since in the former there is a large vascular supply whereas in the latter there is smooth muscle. Airway smooth muscle is of paramount importance in asthma owing to its contractile properties; in addition, however, it may contribute to the pathogenesis of the disease by increased proliferation (78), as well as by the expression and secretion of proinflammatory mediators and cytokines (79).

It is therefore possible that the difference between rhinitis and asthma is that in the former there is an epithelial–mesenchymal trophic unit (80), whereas in the latter there is an epithelial–mesenchymal–muscular trophic unit.

References

1. Vignola AM, Chanez P, Godard P, Bousquet J. Relationships between rhinitis and asthma. Allergy 1998;53(9):833–9.
2. Simons FE. Allergic rhinobronchitis: the asthma–allergic rhinitis link. J Allergy Clin Immunol 1999;104(3 Pt 1):534–40.
3. American Thoracic Society Workshop. Immunobiology of Asthma and Rhinitis. Pathogenic factors and therapeutic options. Am J Respir Crit Care Med 1999; 160(5):1778–87.
4. Sibbald B, Rink E. Epidemiology of seasonal and perennial rhinitis: clinical presentation and medical history. Thorax 1991;46(12):895–901.
5. Townley R, Ryo U, Kolotin B, Kang B. Bronchial sensitivity to methacholine in current and former asthmatic and allergic rhinitis patients and control subjects. J Allergy Clin Immunol 1975;56:429-37.
6. Leynaert B, Bousquet J, Henry C, Liard R, Neukirch F. Is bronchial hyperresponsiveness more frequent in women than in men? A population-based study. Am J Respir Crit Care Med 1997;156(5):1413–20.
7. Sotomayor H, Badier M, Vervloet D, Orehek J. Seasonal increase of carbachol airway responsiveness in patients allergic to grass pollen. Reversal by corticosteroids. Am Rev Respir Dis 1984;130(1):56–8.
8. Boulet LP, Morin D, Milot J, Turcotte H. Bronchial responsiveness increases after seasonal antigen exposure in non-asthmatic subjects with pollen-induced rhinitis. Ann Allergy 1989;63(2):114–9.
9. Witteman AM, Sjamsoedin DH, Jansen HM, van-der-Zee JS. Differences in nonspecific bronchial responsiveness between patients with asthma and patients with rhinitis are not explained by type and degree of inhalant allergy. Int Arch Allergy Immunol 1997;112(1):65–72.
10. Dahl R, Mygind N. Mechanisms of airflow limitation in the nose and lungs. Clin Exp Allergy 1998;2:17–25.
11. Szczeklik A, Stevenson DD. Aspirin-induced asthma: advances in pathogenesis and management. J Allergy Clin Immunol 1999;104(1):5–13.
12. Pearce N, Douwes J, Beasley R. Is allergen exposure the major primary cause of asthma? Thorax 2000;55(5):424–31.

13. Sporik R, Holgate ST, Platts-Mills TA, Cogswell JJ. Exposure to house-dust mite allergen (Der p I) and the development of asthma in childhood. A prospective study. N Engl J Med 1990;323(8):502–7.

14. Peat JK, Tovey E, Toelle BG, Haby MM, Gray EJ, Mahmic A, et al. House dust mite allergens. A major risk factor for childhood asthma in Australia. Am J Respir Crit Care Med 1996;153(1):141–6.

15. Peat J, Tovey E, Mellis C, Leeder S, Woolcock A. Importance of house dust mite and *Alternaria* allergens in childhood asthma: an epidemiological study in two climatic regions of Australia. Clin Exp Allergy 1973;23:812–20.

16. Neukirch C, Henry C, Leynaert B, Liard R, Bousquet J, Neukirch F. Is sensitization to *Alternaria alternata* a risk factor for severe asthma? A population-based study. J Allergy Clin Immunol 1999;103(4):709–11.

17. Rosenstreich DL, Eggleston P, Kattan M, Baker D, Slavin RG, Gergen P, et al. The role of cockroach allergy and exposure to cockroach allergen in causing morbidity among inner-city children with asthma [see comments]. N Engl J Med 1997;336(19):1356–63.

18. Gergen PJ, Turkeltaub PC. The association of individual allergen reactivity with respiratory disease in a national sample: data from the second National Health and Nutrition Examination Survey, 1976–80 (NHANES II). J Allergy Clin Immunol 1992;90(4 Pt 1):579–88.

19. Charpin D, Hughes B, Mallea M, Sutra JP, Balansard G, Vervloet D. Seasonal allergic symptoms and their relation to pollen exposure in south-east France. Clin Exp Allergy 1993;23(5):435–9.

20. Chan-Yeung M, Malo JL. Occupational asthma. N Engl J Med 1995;333(2):107–12.

21. Malo JL, Lemiere C, Desjardins A, Cartier A. Prevalence and intensity of rhinoconjunctivitis in subjects with occupational asthma. Eur Respir J 1997;10(7):1513–5.

22. Seward JP. Medical surveillance of allergy in laboratory animal handlers. Ilar J 2001;42(1):47–54.

23. Daroca P, Crespo JF, Reano M, James JM, Lopez-Rubio A, Rodriguez J. Asthma and rhinitis induced by exposure to raw green beans and chards. Ann Allergy Asthma Immunol 2000;85(3):215–8.

24. Gorski P, Krakowiak A, Ruta U. Nasal and bronchial responses to flour-inhalation in subjects with occupationally induced allergy affecting the airway. Int Arch Occup Environ Health 2000;73(7):488–97.

25. Heederik D, Houba R. An exploratory quantitative risk assessment for high molecular weight sensitizers: wheat flour. Ann Occup Hyg 2001;45(3):175–85.

26. Kujala V. A review of current literature on epidemiology of immediate glove irritation and latex allergy. Occup Med (Lond) 1999;49(1):3–9.

27. Larese Filon F, Bosco A, Fiorito A, Negro C, Barbina P. Latex symptoms and sensitisation in health care workers. Int Arch Occup Environ Health 2001;74(3):219–23.

28. Piirila P, Estlander T, Hytonen M, Keskinen H, Tupasela O, Tuppurainen M. Rhinitis caused by ninhydrin develops into occupational asthma. Eur Respir J 1997;10(8):1918–21.

29. Piirila P, Estlander T, Keskinen H, Jolanki R, Laakkonen A, Pfaffli P, et al. Occupational asthma caused by triglycidyl isocyanurate (TGIC). Clin Exp Allergy 1997;27(5):510–4.
30. Moscato G, Galdi E, Scibilia J, Dellabianca A, Omodeo P, Vittadini G, et al. Occupational asthma, rhinitis and urticaria due to piperacillin sodium in a pharmaceutical worker. Eur Respir J 1995;8(3):467–9.
31. Quirce S, Baeza ML, Tornero P, Blasco A, Barranco R, Sastre J. Occupational asthma caused by exposure to cyanoacrylate. Allergy 2001;56(5):446–9.
32. Igarashi Y, Goldrich MS, Kaliner MA, Irani AM, Schwartz LB, White MV. Quantitation of inflammatory cells in the nasal mucosa of patients with allergic rhinitis and normal subjects. J Allergy Clin Immunol 1995;95(3):716–25.
33. Jeffery P. Bronchial biopsies and airway inflammation. Eur Respir J 1996;9:1583–7.
34. Holmberg K, Bake B, Pipkorn U. Nasal mucosal blood flow after intranasal allergen challenge. J Allergy Clin Immunol 1988;81(3):541–7.
35. King GG, Pare PD, Seow CY. The mechanics of exaggerated airway narrowing in asthma: the role of smooth muscle. Respir Physiol 1999;118(1):1–13.
36. Bousquet J, Jeffery PK, Busse WW, Johnson M, Vignola AM. Asthma. From bronchoconstriction to airways inflammation and remodeling. Am J Respir Crit Care Med 2000;161(5):1720–45.
37. Bentley AM, Menz G, Storz C, Robinson DS, Bradley B, Jeffery PK, et al. Identification of T lymphocytes, macrophages, and activated eosinophils in the bronchial mucosa in intrinsic asthma. Relationship to symptoms and bronchial responsiveness. Am Rev Respir Dis 1992;146(2):500–6.
38. Bentley AM, Jacobson MR, Cumberworth V, Barkans JR, Moqbel R, Schwartz LB, et al. Immunohistology of the nasal mucosa in seasonal allergic rhinitis: increases in activated eosinophils and epithelial mast cells. J Allergy Clin Immunol 1992;89(4):877–83.
39. Durham SR, Ying S, Varney VA, Jacobson MR, Sudderick RM, Mackay IS, et al. Cytokine messenger RNA expression for IL-3, IL-4, IL-5, and granulocyte/macrophage-colony-stimulating factor in the nasal mucosa after local allergen provocation: relationship to tissue eosinophilia. J Immunol 1992; 148(8):2390–4.
40. Bradding P, Roberts JA, Britten KM, Montefort S, Djukanovic R, Mueller R, et al. Interleukin-4, -5, and -6 and tumor necrosis factor-alpha in normal and asthmatic airways: evidence for the human mast cell as a source of these cytokines. Am J Respir Cell Mol Biol 1994;10(5):471–80.
41. Bradding P, Feather IH, Wilson S, Bardin PG, Heusser CH, Holgate ST, et al. Immunolocalization of cytokines in the nasal mucosa of normal and perennial rhinitic subjects. The mast cell as a source of IL-4, IL-5, and IL-6 in human allergic mucosal inflammation. J Immunol 1993;151(7):3853–65.
42. Baraniuk JN. Pathogenesis of allergic rhinitis. J Allergy Clin Immunol 1997;99(2):S763–72.
43. Minshall EM, Cameron L, Lavigne F, Leung DY, Hamilos D, Garcia-Zepada EA, et al. Eotaxin mRNA and protein expression in chronic sinusitis and allergen-induced nasal responses in seasonal allergic rhinitis. Am J Respir Cell Mol Biol 1997;17(6):683–90.

44. Vignola AM, Campbell AM, Chanez P, Bousquet J, Paul-Lacoste P, Michel FB, et al. HLA-DR and ICAM-1 expression on bronchial epithelial cells in asthma and chronic bronchitis. Am Rev Respir Dis 1993;148(3):689–94.
45. Montefort S, Holgate ST, Howarth PH. Leucocyte–endothelial adhesion molecules and their role in bronchial asthma and allergic rhinitis. Eur Respir J 1993;6(7):1044–54.
46. Canonica GW, Ciprandi G, Pesce GP, Buscaglia S, Paolieri F, Bagnasco M. ICAM-1 on epithelial cells in allergic subjects: a hallmark of allergic inflammation. Int Arch Allergy Immunol 1995;107(1–3):99–102.
47. Chanez P, Vignola AM, Vic P, Guddo F, Bonsignore G, Godard P, et al. Comparison between nasal and bronchial inflammation in asthmatic and control subjects. Am J Respir Crit Care Med 1999;159(2):588–95.
48. Gaga M, Lambrou P, Papageorgiou N, Koulouris NG, Kosmas E, Fragakis S, et al. Eosinophils are a feature of upper and lower airway pathology in non-atopic asthma, irrespective of the presence of rhinitis [in process citation]. Clin Exp Allergy 2000;30(5):663–9.
49. Bresciani M, Paradis L, Des Roches A, Vernhet H, Vachier I, Godard P, et al. Rhinosinusitis in severe asthma. J Allergy Clin Immunol 2001;107(1):73-80.
50. Vachier I, Chiappara G, Mezziane H, Vignola A, Grid F, Grid P, et al. Bronchial and nasal inflammation in asthma and COPD. Am J Respir Crit Care Med 2000;333 (A161):A50.
51. Chakir J, Laviolette M, Boutet M, Laliberte R, Dube J, Boulet LP. Lower airways remodeling in nonasthmatic subjects with allergic rhinitis. Lab Invest 1996;75(5):735–44.
52. Djukanovic R, Lai CK, Wilson JW, Britten KM, Wilson SJ, Roche WR, et al. Bronchial mucosal manifestations of atopy: a comparison of markers of inflammation between atopic asthmatics, atopic nonasthmatics and healthy controls. Eur Respir J 1992;5(5):538–44.
53. Chakir J, Laviolette M, Turcotte H, Boutet M, Boulet LP. Cytokine expression in the lower airways of nonasthmatic subjects with allergic rhinitis: influence of natural allergen exposure. J Allergy Clin Immunol 2000;106(5 Pt 1): 904–10.
54. Calhoun WJ, Jarjour NN, Gleich GJ, Stevens CA, Busse WW. Increased airway inflammation with segmental versus aerosol antigen challenge. Am Rev Respir Dis 1993;147(6 Pt 1):1465–71.
55. Calhoun WJ, Reed HE, Moest DR, Stevens CA. Enhanced superoxide production by alveolar macrophages and air-space cells, airway inflammation, and alveolar macrophage density changes after segmental antigen broncho-provocation in allergic subjects. Am Rev Respir Dis 1992;145(2 Pt 1): 317–25.
56. Shaver JR, O'Connor JJ, Pollice M, Cho SK, Kane GC, Fish JE, et al. Pulmonary inflammation after segmental ragweed challenge in allergic asthmatic and nonasthmatic subjects. Am J Respir Crit Care Med 1995;152(4 pt 1):1189–97.
57. Packe GE, Ayres JG. Asthma outbreak during a thunderstorm. Lancet 1985;2(8448):199–204.

58. Venables KM, Allitt U, Collier CG, Emberlin J, Greig JB, Hardaker PJ, et al. Thunderstorm-related asthma—the epidemic of 24/25 June 1994. Clin Exp Allergy 1997;27(7):725–36.
59. Anto JM, Sunyer J. Thunderstorms: a risk factor for asthma attacks [editorial; comment]. Thorax 1997;52(8):669–70.
60. Bauman A. Asthma associated with thunderstorms [editorial; comment]. Br Med J 1996;312(7031):590–1.
61. Celenza A, Fothergill J, Kupek E, Shaw RJ. Thunderstorm associated asthma: a detailed analysis of environmental factors [see comments]. Br Med J 1996;312 (7031):604–7.
62. Knox RB. Grass pollen, thunderstorms and asthma. Clin Exp Allergy 1993;23(5):354–9.
63. Suphioglu C, Singh MB, Taylor P, Bellomo R, Holmes P, Puy R, et al. Mechanism of grass-pollen-induced asthma. Lancet 1992;339(8793):569–72.
64. Desrosiers M, Nguyen B, Ghezzo H, Leblanc C, Malo JL. Nasal response in subjects undergoing challenges by inhaling occupational agents causing asthma through the nose and mouth. Allergy 1998;53(9):840–8.
65. Braunstahl GJ, Kleinjan A, Overbeek SE, Prins JB, Hoogsteden HC, Fokkens WJ. Segmental bronchial provocation induces nasal inflammation in allergic rhinitis patients. Am J Respir Crit Care Med 2000;161(6):2051–7.
66. Braunstahl GJ, Overbeek SE, Kleinjan A, Prins JB, Hoogsteden HC, Fokkens WJ. Nasal allergen provocation induces adhesion molecule expression and tissue eosinophilia in upper and lower airways. J Allergy Clin Immunol 2001; 107(3):469–76.
67. Denburg JA, Sehmi R, Saito H, Pil-Seob J, Inman MD, O'Byrne PM. Systemic aspects of allergic disease: bone marrow responses. J Allergy Clin Immunol 2000;106(5 Suppl):S242–6.
68. Inman MD. Bone marrow events in animal models of allergic inflammation and hyperresponsiveness. J Allergy Clin Immunol 2000;106(5 suppl):S235–41.
69. Gaspar Elsas MI, Joseph D, Elsas PX, Vargaftig BB. Rapid increase in bone-marrow eosinophil production and responses to eosinopoietic interleukins triggered by intranasal allergen challenge. Am J Respir Cell Mol Biol 1997;17 (4):404–13.
70. Inman MD, Ellis R, Wattie J, Denburg JA, O'Byrne PM. Allergen-induced increase in airway responsiveness, airway eosinophilia, and bone-marrow eosinophil progenitors in mice [see comments]. Am J Respir Cell Mol Biol 1999;21(4):473–9.
71. Denburg JA, Otsuka H, Ohnisi M, Ruhno J, Bienenstock J, Dolovich J. Contribution of basophil/mast cell and eosinophil growth and differentiation to the allergic tissue inflammatory response. Int Arch Allergy Appl Immunol 1987;82(3–4):321–6.
72. KleinJan A, Dijkstra MD, Boks SS, Severijnen LA, Mulder PG, Fokkens WJ. Increase in IL-8, IL-10, IL-13, and RANTES mRNA levels (in situ hybridization) in the nasal mucosa after nasal allergen provocation. J Allergy Clin Immunol 1999;103(3 Pt 1):441–50.

73. Varga EM, Jacobson MR, Till SJ, Masuyama K, O'Brien F, Rak S, et al. Cellular infiltration and cytokine mRNA expression in perennial allergic rhinitis. Allergy 1999;54(4):338–45.

74. Lee CH, Lee KS, Rhee CS, Lee SO, Min YG. Distribution of RANTES and interleukin-5 in allergic nasal mucosa and nasal polyps. Ann Otol Rhinol Laryngol 1999;108(6):594–8.

75. Bachert C, Wagenmann M, Hauser U, Rudack C. IL-5 synthesis is upregulated in human nasal polyp tissue. J Allergy Clin Immunol 1997;99(6 Pt 1):837–42.

76. Robinson DS, Damia R, Zeibecoglou K, Molet S, North J, Yamada T, et al. CD34($^+$)/interleukin-5Rα messenger RNA$^+$ cells in the bronchial mucosa in asthma: potential airway eosinophil progenitors. Am J Respir Cell Mol Biol 1999;20(1):9–13.

77. Cameron L, Christodoulopoulos P, Lavigne F, Nakamura Y, Eidelman D, McEuen A, et al. Evidence for local eosinophil differentiation within allergic nasal mucosa: inhibition with soluble IL-5 receptor. J Immunol 2000;164(3): 1538–45.

78. Panettieri R, Jr., Murray RK, Eszterhas AJ, Bilgen G, Martin JG. Repeated allergen inhalations induce DNA synthesis in airway smooth muscle and epithelial cells in vivo. Am J Physiol 1998;274(3 Pt 1):L417–24.

79. Chung KF. Airway smooth muscle cells: contributing to and regulating airway mucosal inflammation? [in process citation]. Eur Respir J 2000;15(5):961–8.

80. Holgate ST, Davies DE, Lackie PM, Wilson SJ, Puddicombe SM, Lordan JL. Epithelial–mesenchymal interactions in the pathogenesis of asthma. J Allergy Clin Immunol 2000;105(2 pt 1):193–204.

7

Viral Infections
Effects on Nasal and Lower Airway Functions

IMRAN R. HUSSAIN and SEBASTIAN L. JOHNSTON

National Heart and Lung Institute, Imperial College of Science,
    Technology and Medicine
London, United Kingdom

Introduction

The common respiratory viruses are a diverse group of viruses that encompass RNA, DNA, enveloped, and nonenveloped viruses. These viruses cause symptoms associated with the "common cold": cough, nasal stuffiness, sneezing, coryza, pharyngitis, throat irritation, and mild fever.

Rhinovirus and coronavirus, the main etiological agents of the common cold, initially were thought to be relatively benign infectious agents. More recent studies have shown that respiratory viral infections, the majority of which are rhinovirus (RV) and coronavirus, are the commonest cause of asthma exacerbations in both children (1) and adults (2). The better known respiratory viruses, influenza virus, parainfluenza virus (PIV), respiratory syncytial virus (RSV), and adenovirus, are all well known to cause diseases with a significant lower respiratory tract (LRT) component, such as bronchiolitis (3), croup, and pneumonia (3–5). Each of these latter viruses has been shown to infect the lower airway mucosa, but regarding the most common respiratory viruses, this has been controversial for rhinoviruses, and there is no evidence available for coronaviruses.

Each of the common respiratory viruses is associated with upper respiratory tract infections (URTI) throughout life, with frequency and severity depending on many factors such as virus type or subtype, season, age, and both individual and community levels of immunity. Each of the common respiratory viruses may also be able to cause significant infection of the lower airways in any individual, but whether the predominant infection/illness affects the URT or the LRT may be determined by a balance of several factors, including the following:

Virus dose
Levels of host immunity (both innate and specific) in upper and lower
   airway
Cellular tropism of the virus in question
Route of inoculation
Particle size of droplets (i.e., > 5 µm leads to URTI, < 5 µm leads
   to LRTI)

Virus infection of the URT may result in pathological or physiological change in the LRT either as a result of direct infection of the LRT with virus or as a result of LRT consequences of URTI that are not related to infection of the LRT with virus but are consequent upon neural reflexes or circulatory responses to the URTI. This chapter reviews the similarities and differences between viral infections of the URT and LRT, addresses the question of whether LRT responses during URTI (such as asthma exacerbations) are consequent upon LRTI, and considers differences and similarities in relation to these questions among the different respiratory viruses.

One of the major difficulties in considering these questions in relation to rhinovirus infection has been diagnosing infection in the first place. The limitations in methodology also lead to difficulties in demonstrating infection in lower respiratory tract samples, while permitting confidence that the sample was not contaminated with virus from the URT during sampling.

I. Identification of Respiratory Viruses in Samples

To answer the question of whether infection of the lower respiratory tract is necessary to alter lower respiratory tract function, methodology is required that can accurately identify respiratory viruses in upper and lower airway samples.

One of the difficulties in establishing the cause of an infection of the respiratory tract is isolating the organism. Techniques such as cell culture of the virus are complex, and many of the viruses have differing cell culture requirements and can be very fastidious. For example, neither rhinoviruses nor coronaviruses, which account for approximately 60 and 10 to 15% of URTIs, respectively, will grow well in the standard cell cultures in use in most diagnostic laboratories.

In addition, the rapid transfer of samples from infected subject to cell culture is important, since delay in transfer can lead to a significant reduction in the yield of the organisms (6). Community studies, which theoretically have the benefit of prompt reporting of symptoms, can show reduced virus isolation rates if there is a delay between reporting and sampling (6). All these difficulties complicate virus diagnosis and mean that negative results are frequently false negatives due to technical limitations.

The use of serology is not straightforward for respiratory viruses either: rhinoviruses alone have over 100 different serotypes that can cause clinical symptoms, making diagnosis by rising antibody titers completely impractical. Furthermore, serology is not capable of indicating the timing of infection or whether infection is present in the URT, the LRT, or both.

New methodologies, such as the use of the polymerase chain reaction (PCR), have provided a major advance in the detection of respiratory viruses and have contributed to demonstrating their significance in the pathogenesis of exacerbations of asthma (1). But although, the use of this technique gives an indication of the presence of the viral genome in the samples, it does not indicate whether there is live virus present or whether viral replication is taking place. PCR is also very sensitive, and positive results in samples taken from the lower airway may therefore be positive because of contamination with virus from the upper airways, which may very easily have occurred during the sampling procedure (7).

II. Viral Infection and the Upper Airways

All the viruses being discussed have tropism for the respiratory mucosa. Most of the cell types that are infected have not been fully delineated, but the nasal epithelium is infected by all these organisms. Infection of the nasal mucosa causes classical coryzal symptoms, an increase in nasal discharge, congestion/blockage, and sneezing, and it may lead to otitis media or pharyngitis.

The site of subsequent spread of the virus infection may depend on the site of the original inoculum. Nasal inoculation may lead to secondary otitis media, while oral inoculation may lead to pharyngitis. RSV infection has been shown to be associated with exudative otitis media, with virus isolated in the exudate (8). Studies that have tried to establish an association between URTI and otitis media have given variable rates of viral infection, most

Table 1 Virus Serotypes for the Common Respiratory Viruses and Association with Respiratory Infections

Virus	Number of serotypes	Upper respiratory tract diseases[a]				Lower respiratory tract diseases[a]			
		Common cold	Sinusitis	Pharyngitis	Otitis media	Croup	Bronchiolitis	Bronchitis	Pneumonia
Rhinovirus	100[+]	+++++	+++	+++	+++	+	+++	++++	+
Coronavirus	229E, OC43	++++	+++	+++	++	+		++	+
Parainfluenza	1–4 (with 4A and 4B)	++	+	++	+	++++	+++	+++	++
Influenza	A,B,C (further subtyping by hemagglutinin and neuraminidase)	+++	+	++	+	+++	++	+++++	+++++
Respiratory syncytial virus	A and B	+++		+	+++	++	+++++	++	+++
Adenovirus	50[+] serotypes	+	+	+++++	++	++	+	+	++
Enterovirus	Polio 1-3 Echoviruses (31 serotypes) Coxsackie virus (A, B main serotypes)	++	+	+++	+	+	+	+	+

[a] Strength of association between virus and disease goes from the highest (++++) to weakest (+).

likely because of variability in the sampling and virus detection methods. Originally RSV was thought to be the most common etiological agent. With the availability of improved techniques, however, rhinovirus has been shown to be of increasing importance (9,10). Most recent studies find respiratory viruses associated with approximately a third of all cases of secretory otitis media, and the majority of these are concurrent with or subsequent to an episode of URTI (11,12).

In the past, poor sampling methods and inadequate virological detection methods used to study otitis media made it difficult to draw firm conclusions from the literature regarding which viruses are the most common etiological agent, of this condition. With the use of PCR and better sampling techniques, it is now apparent that most cases of culture-negative otitis media are of respiratory virus etiology (see Table 1). RSV and parainfluenza and influenza viruses have all been shown to infect the middle ear (13) during upper respiratory tract infection. Rhinovirus is the commonest etiological cause for upper respiratory tract infections, has been linked with up to 35% of the cases of acute otitis media (14), and is also associated with a higher risk of development of a middle ear effusion (15).

III. Studies Investigating Immune Responses to Respiratory Virus Infection of the Upper Airway

Studies of immune responses to respiratory virus infections can be broken down into studies that investigate infection in vitro or in vivo. The in vitro studies can be further subdivided into those that used primary epithelial cells and those that used cell lines established from the airway. The in vivo studies can be divided into studies of natural infection in a defined population or of experimental infection of a population. The studies highlighted support the notion that responses seen with in vitro infection are similar to those seen with in vivo infection (where it has been possible to study this), and therefore that in vitro studies do represent a satisfactory model for in vivo infections. Table 2 presents a summary of all studies.

A. Upper Respiratory Tract: In Vitro Infection

In vitro infection studies comparing different organisms have tended to give broadly similar results across different virus types. For studies of the nasal epithelium, cell lines or primary nasal epithelium have been used.

Recent studies have investigated the regulation of intercellular adhesion molecule 1 (ICAM-1), the major receptor for 90% of RV serotypes, and have shown that expression can be increased with respiratory virus infection (16). ICAM-1 is one of the cellular adhesion molecules that is critical in

Table 2 Experimental Rhinovirus Infection Studies

Study	Virus	Infecting dose (TCID$_{50}$)	Method of Infection[a]	Study population[b]	Change to resting lung function with infection	Other findings[c]
Blair, 1976 (77)	HRV13/15	100	A	N (21)	No change	Reduction in diffusion capacity with clinical illness
Summers, 1992 (81)	HRV2/EL	100	A	N (16) + atopic (11)	No change	Trend towards increased BHR in atopics, but not statistically significant
Doyle, 1992 (79)	HRV 39	100	A	AR (20) + N (18)	No change	No difference in viral shedding, illness scores, middle ear pressures and nasal patency
Doyle, 1994 (80)	HRV 39	100	A	AR (20) + N (18)	No change	No difference with either histamine or cold air challenge
Fraenkel, 1995 (84)	HRV 16	100	A	Asthmatic (6) + N (11)	No change	Increased BHR
Skoner, 1996 (82)	HRV 39	100	A	AR (50) + N (46)	No change	D2-3 maximal symptoms, no change in methacholine responsiveness
Lemanske, 1989 (85)	HRV 16	640-6400	A + B	AR (10)	No change	Development of LAR in 7 subjects, no increase in plasma histamine post antigen challenge
Calhoun, 1991 (86)	HRV 16	5-32	A + B	AR (8)	No change	Increase in histamine in antigen challenge, inc. in eosinophils post infection BHR to both methacholine and histamine, development of LAR post viral infection

Calhoun, 1994 (146)	HRV 16	$1\text{-}32 \times 10^3$	A + B	AR (7) + N (5)	No change	Increase in BAL histamine, TNFα and eosinophils post infection, no significant increase in tryptase
Cheung, 1995 (83)	HRV 16	3×10^4	A + B + C	Asthmatic (14)	No change	Increased BHR, peak symptoms at D2-3, lymphopenia D2 – normal by D7/15
Grunberg, 1997 (61)	HRV 16	$0.5\text{-}2.9 \times 10^4$	A + B + C	Asthmatic (27)	No change	Peak symptoms D2-3, associated with maximal asthmatic symptoms and fall in FEV$_1$, lymphopenia on D2 assoc. with asthma and change in IL-8
Grunberg, 1999 (94)	HRV16	$0.25\text{-}1.45 \times 10^4$	A + B + C	Asthmatic (27)	Fall in FEV$_1$	Fall in FEV$_1$ on D2, associated with an increase in histamine responsiveness
Bardin, 2000 (95)	HRV16	2×10^3	A	N (11) + AR (5) + asthmatic (6)	Fall in PEF in 6 subjects	Fall in PEF in 6 subjects, including N(2), AR(1) and asthmatic (3), with histamine responsiveness

[a] A, droplet instillation; B, inhalation via atomizer; C, nebulization.
[b] AR, allergic rhinitic; N, normal (nonatopic).
[c] BHR, bronchial hyperresponsiveness; LAR, late allergic response; BAL, bronchoalveolar lavage.

causing inflammatory cell adhesion to vascular endothelium and extrava-sation from the bloodstream. The nasal mucosa has low level expression of ICAM-1, though on culture primary nasal epithelium does increase its ex-pression of ICAM-1 (17). Certain eosinophil products, such as major basic protein (MBP) and eosinophil cationic protein (ECP) can also upregulate the expression of ICAM-1 on nasal epithelium (17).

B. Upper Respiratory Tract: Mediator Release

Infection of the respiratory epithelium leads to the initiation of a cascade of events that will lead to acute inflammation with vascular leakage and mucus secretion induced by kinins, histamine, prostaglandins, and leukotrienes. In addition, there is recruitment of inflammatory cells to the site of infection, and further pathological changes follow this. In recent years the role of cytokines and chemokines (chemotactic cytokines) as effectors in this system has been realized. The respiratory epithelium is a potent source of many of these peptides and as such is now thought of as an initiator of the inflammatory response, not just an inert barrier. There have been several studies investigating both in vitro and in vivo infection and cytokine responses with a variety of viral infections.

The cytokine responses of the respiratory epithelium have been most extensively studied in RSV infection. The results from these experiments can serve as an indication of the response to other viral infections.

Results from in vitro experimentation on upper airway cell lines, or from the use of primary nasal tissue, are shown in Table 3. These show that RSV infection can lead to the production of interleukin 8 (IL-8) (18), RANTES (18–20), and tumor necrosis factor α (TNF-α) (18). The first two cytokines are both important as neutrophil and eosinophil chemo-attractants, respectively. Constitutive production by nasal explant tissue of the neutrophil attractant growth-related protein α (GRO α) and the lymphocyte attractant monocyte chemotactic protein 1 (MCP-1) has also been reported, but this was effect not increased with RSV infection (21).

C. Upper Respiratory Tract: In Vivo Infection

Infection of the upper respiratory tract leads to epithelial shedding of infected cells in some viral infections. Infection by adenovirus, influenza virus, and RSV leads in each case to cytopathic effect. Infection of the nasal mucosa is often patchy (22), with different areas affected during the illness, perhaps accounting for the variable results shown by studies that have taken biopsy samples from individuals experimentally infected with rhinovirus. Some studies have shown that in the early stages of infection, there is a neutrophil infiltrate into the nasal mucosa, often occurring before symptoms

Table 3 Cytokine and Chemokine Production by Respiratory Virus Infection

Virus	In vitro				In vivo
	Upper airway epithelial cells	Lower airway epithelial cells	Mononuclear cells	Macrophages and monocytes	
Adenovirus	IL-8 (120)	IL-8 (121,122)	IFN-γ (119)	IL-1β, TNF-α (123)	IL-6, IL-8, TNF-α (101); TGF-β (102)
Coronavirus					IFN-γ (10,103)
Enterovirus			IFN-γ, TNF-α, IL-1-β, IL-2, IL-10 (127)		
Influenza	IL-6, IL-8, RANTES (32), eotaxin (45)	IL-6, IL-8, RANTES (104); IFN-α/β (129)	IL-1β, IFN-α, IFN-β, IFN-γ, TNF-α(105)	IL-1β, IL - 6, IFN-α/β, MCP-1, MIP-1α, MIP-1β, RANTES, IP-10, TNF-α (106–109); (not IL-8, GRO-α)	IL-6, IL-8, TNF-α, IFN-α (not IL-1β, TGF-β) (88,110)
Parainfluenza	IL-11 (38)				
Rhinovirus		IL-1β, (31), IL-6, IL-8 (111); IL-11 (38), GM-CSF (48,49,112), RANTES, IL-16 (41), MIP-1α, eotaxin, eotaxin-2 (50), G-CSF, ENA-78, GRO-α (47)	IL-8 (112)	IL-8(112)	IL-1β (113), IL-6, IL-8 (77); IL-11 (38), RANTES (37); TNF-α, MIP-1α (37)
RSV	IL-1β, IL-6, IL-8, RANTES, TNF-α (15–17)	IL-1α, IL-1B, IL-6, IL-8 (37); IL-11 (38), IFN-β, IFN-γ, TNF-α, RANTES (17); MIP-1α, MCP-1 (42), I309, *exodus*-1, TARC, MDC, I-TAC, fractalkine, MIP-1β, GRO-αβ/γ (44)	HRF (114), IL-1ra (115), IL-2, IL-5 (116), IFN-α, low IFN-γ (116)	IL-1ra (115), IL-6, IL-8 (117); IL-10, IL-12 (118); TNF-α (117), IFN a/b/g (119)	IL-1β, IL-6, IL-8 (26); IL-10 (53), IL-11 (38), TNF-α (27, 28), RANTES (120), MIP-1α, MCP-1 (32)

(22,23). Studies that have shown similar findings have used other techniques such as flow cytometry to identify the leukocyte subpopulations that are present during infection (24,25). In one study of asthmatic children with proven viral infection, increased levels of myeloperoxidase (MPO) and IL-8 were found in nasal aspirates and both correlated with symptom severity (26). These findings have also been reported in a study where experimental rhinovirus infection has been induced in an older nonasthmatic population (27). Other studies have not been able to demonstrate an inflammatory infiltrate associated with experimental infection (28).

The results from the in vivo studies of children infected with RSV show findings broadly similar to those of in vitro studies. There are increased nasal lavage levels of IL-1β, IL-6, and IL-8 (29), and mRNA transcripts for these cytokines were shown to be increased on biopsy samples that were taken at the same time (29). The foregoing results were replicated in a study of middle ear effusions, where increased levels of IL-1β, IL-6, and also TNF-α were observed (30). RANTES levels are increased in lavage specimens from children with RSV URTI (20), as are the levels of the proinflammatory cytokines IL-6 and TNF-α (31). Experimental infection of adults with RSV has confirmed nasal lavage fluid levels of IL-8 and RANTES but has also demonstrated an increase in levels of macrophage inflammatory protein 1α (MIP-1α) and MCP-1 in nasal lavage fluid (32).

There is firm evidence of neutrophil recruitment and activation in the upper airways associated with both rhinovirus and RSV infection; there is also a nonspecific response in the upper airways, with production of IL-6 and TNF-α. The findings are similar for both viruses and suggest that the initial response would be observed in other respiratory viruses as well. More importantly, the local production of RANTES by RSV (20) and other virus infections including rhinovirus (33), shows that the upper airway response also includes the recruitment of lymphocytes and eosinophils to the site of infection. These cells are likely to be critical to the development of airway changes and further cytokine production, as well as to the development of mucosal damage.

IV. Studies Investigating Immune Responses to Respiratory Virus Infection of the Lower Airway

The immune responses to lower respiratory tract infection have been intensively explored in vitro mainly using established cell lines. In vivo studies have not been as extensive as the in vivo upper respiratory tract studies, since more invasive procedures are required to sample the lower airways.

A. Lower Respiratory Tract: In Vitro Infection

Most studies investigating lower airway responses to viral infection have studied cell lines. The cell lines have either been the type II alveolar cell carcinoma cell line A549, or an SV40-transformed bronchial epithelial cell line, either the 16HBE cell line or the BEAS-2B cell line. Viral infection of primary cells has also been studied for the respiratory viruses RV (34,35), RSV (19), and influenza (36).

ICAM-1 is constitutively expressed on A549 cells, but respiratory virus infection further upregulates its expression. Rhinovirus infection can lead to an upregulation of both ICAM-1 and vascular cell adhesion molecule 1 (VCAM-1) (34), as can RSV (37) and adenovirus infection (38). ICAM-1 expression can also be increased on A549 cells through other pathways, such as local release of interferon gamma (IFN-γ), or TNF-α (39). Thus respiratory virus infection may cause both a direct increase in adhesion molecules, such as ICAM-1 in URT and LRT epithelial sites, and also an indirect increase via other factors that are also produced by the infection.

B. Lower Respiratory Tract: Mediator Release

In this section we use RSV infection as a representative model of cytokine production by the respiratory epithelium. The results from in vitro studies of lower respiratory cell lines that have been infected with RSV are similar to the upper airway results. Results from studies that have used the alveolar cell line A549 have shown that IL-1α, IL-1β, IL-6, IL-8 (40),and IL-11 (41), as well as TNF-α (40) and the chemokines RANTES (20) and MIP-1α and MCP-1 (42), can all be induced by RSV infection. Results for the bronchial BEAS-2B cell line show an almost identical pattern (where the same cytokines have been studied), with increases in IL-6, IL-8 (43), and RANTES (20). These results do suggest that the response to RSV infection of the lower and upper airway epithelium in terms of cytokines released are very similar. Recently, Zhang et al. used cDNA microarrays to demonstrate the broad cytokine response that occurs following RSV infection of epithelial cells, with increases seen in *exodus-1*, TARC, MDC, MIP-1β, GRO-$\alpha/\beta/\gamma$, ENA-78, I-TAC, and fractalkine (44).

As a comparison, the results for infection with influenza virus show that with infection of both nasal primary cells and primary bronchial tissue there is RANTES production (36). Infection of established bronchial epithelial cell lines with the same virus type leads to the upregulation of mRNA and subsequent protein production of IL-6, IL-8, RANTES (36), and eotaxin (45). Similar results have recently been observed with in vitro infection of primary bronchial epithelial cells with rhinovirus, with the induction of IL-6, IL-8, RANTES, and IL-16 being observed (46). Rhinovirus infection of epithelial cell lines produces the foregoing cytokines, as well as granulocyte colony-stimulating factor (G-CSF) (47), granulocyte–macrophage colony-stimulating factor (GM-CSF) (48,49), growth protein α (GRO-α), epithelial neutropil-activating protein 78 GRO-α (ENA-78), MIP-1α (47), eotaxin, and eotaxin-2 (50).

C. Lower Respiratory Tract: In Vivo Infection

There are no reported studies investigating cytokine production from experimental human RSV lower airway infection. Indeed, there have been no studies of experimental RSV infection for a number of years. A few studies have looked at the cytokine response in children with bronchiolitis. Smith et al. (51) reported a fall in mRNA levels (corrected for housekeeping gene expression) of a variety of inflammatory cytokines from tracheal epithelial cells in response to RSV infection. The cytokines that showed this response were IL-1β, IL-6, IL-8, TNF-α, IFN-γ, and GM-CSF. The main reason for this finding is likely to be that since epithelial cells collected by aspiration are shed, their mRNA is likely to be degrading, and this may have accounted for the lower mRNA levels in children with RSV bronchiolitis (51). One other study has shown that the nasopharyngeal aspirate cytokine levels are closely correlated to the levels obtained by endotracheal aspiration, though not as extensive a profile was studied (52). Sheeran et al. (53), who studied cytokine levels in children intubated with RSV bronchiolitis, compared nasal washes with tracheal aspirates and demonstrated a broad inflammatory response, with IL-6, IL-8, IL-10, MIP-1α, and RANTES all being elevated in both samples. This has been confirmed for IL-8, RANTES, and MIP-1α by Harrison et al. (54), investigating the tracheal aspirates of children with RSV bronchiolitis only. More recent studies have confirmed these results and also demonstrated an increase in IL-4 and IL-5 (55) and MCP-1 (56), as well as TNF-α (57) in the nasal aspirates of children with RSV bronchiolitis.

Experimental infection of 12 volunteers with influenza A showed that increased levels of IL-4 (nonsignificant) and IL-6 were produced (58). More recent studies have demonstrated the production of both neutrophil- and eosinophil-attracting chemokines, IL-8, MCP-1, and MIP-1α/β (59,60). Experimental rhinovirus infection has also shown an increase in IL-6 production, as well as IL-8 production, within 2 days of virus challenge (61,62). Natural virus infection has been shown to induce IL-8 production; in this study the predominant infecting virus was influenza virus (63).

D. Upper and Lower Respiratory Tract: In Vivo Infection

A study that compared infants who had had RSV infection with significant LRT involvement with those with predominantly URT involvement showed evidence of immune activation in both groups. The production of soluble ICAM-1 and CD25 (IL-2 receptor) in the serum of infected children was studied. There were no significant differences between the two groups, though the study may not have been sensitive enough and was looking at relatively broad measures, which would not have reflected the changes at the epithelial level (64). Cytokine levels were not assayed in this study.

One recent study has shown some changes between children with proven RSV upper respiratory tract symptoms without bronchiolitis and those with proven RSV bronchiolitis (taken as a marker of lower respiratory tract infection). The mononuclear cell cytokine response in the first 2 days of infection showed that significantly higher levels of IFN-γ and IL-18 were produced by the mononuclear cells of children with an upper respiratory tract infection than of children with bronchiolitis. This pattern was reversed for the mononuclear cell IL-4 levels (65).

No studies have investigated the cellular responses in URT and LRT infections simultaneously; some studies have shown similar events taking place, though samples were not temporarily related. In URTI due to rhinovirus, there is evidence of neutrophil influx and activation, with increased levels of MPO and IL-8, which correlated to disease severity and symptoms (26). Rhinovirus LRTI also shows increased levels of neutrophil attractants following rhinovirus infection (61).

Similar findings were observed when eosinophil activation and degranulation were investigated. Rhinovirus URT infection is associated with increased levels of MBP (major basic protein) in children (33). Eosinophil activation is seen in RSV URTI and also LRTI, with increased levels of RSV-specific IgE as well as eosinophil degradation products (66,67).

E. Upper and Lower Infection: Conclusion

Most viral infections cause increased production of a variety of different cytokines, as highlighted in this section. Each of the different cytokines produced plays a part in epithelial cellular immune responses to viral infection, causing neutrophil, eosinophil, and lymphocyte recruitment and activation.

These results confirm the earlier statements: first, that the use of cell lines (or primary cells) is a valid technique for investigating the respiratory mucosal responses to virus infection, and second that the responses of the upper and lower respiratory mucosa to respiratory virus infection are similar.

V. Physiological Response of the Upper Respiratory Tract to Infection

The upper airway response to virus infection is due to the release of a variety of inflammatory mediators secondary to infection of the epithelium by the virus. These mediators may also be implicated in linking the upper and lower airways.

Kinins, such as bradykinin, are known to produce several of the symptoms that are associated with viral URTI including rhinorrhea, nasal obstruction, and sore throat and are elevated in both natural (68) and experimental infections (69). The first two symptoms are due to an increase in vascular permeability and vasodilatation. Histamine has an effect on causing rhinorrhea as well, but its major effect is to cause sneezing. Increased levels of histamine have not been observed during experimental rhinovirus infection (24), except in atopic subjects (70). Symptoms such as sneezing and coughing can be reproduced by the administration of prostaglandins D_2 and $F_{2\alpha}$ (71), with partial blocking of these symptoms accomplished by the administration of nonsteroidal anti-inflammatory drugs (NSAIDs). Cholinergic reflexes cause early nasal discharge through their innervation of the submucosal glands, which can be blocked by intranasal administration of the anticholinergic agent ipratropium bromide (72). Mucus hypersecretion and nasal blockage may also be caused by increased leukotriene production (73), though the effect of leukotriene antagonists has not been investigated in connection with efforts to reduce the symptoms associated with respiratory viral infections.

Although the relative contributions of individual mediators are not clear from current data, the physiological symptom complex associated with virus infection is likely to be due to the release of several mediators that act in concert to cause nasal blockage, sneezing, cough, and rhinorrhea.

VI. Physiological Response of the Lower Respiratory Tract to Infection

Few data are available on the release of mediators in the lower airways following viral infection. One study has shown an increase in allergen-induced histamine release in bronchalveolar lavage (BAL) specimens following rhinovirus infection (74), establishing a response similar to that seen in the upper airway.

A. Natural Infection

Empey et al. (75) showed that though there was no change in resting airway resistance (R_{AW}) following rhinovirus infection, and no change in bronchial hyperresponsiveness (BHR) to saline, there was increased responsiveness to histamine. In this study 9 of 16 normal subjects developed BHR to histamine, which lasted up to 4 weeks. By the termination of the study, all the subjects' BHR had returned to baseline.

Little et al. (76) showed similar findings during an epidemic outbreak of influenza A in 44 subjects. As with the Empey study, an increase in airway reactivity was seen in subjects who developed a URTI without LRTI symptoms.

B. Experimental Infection

Early experimental rhinovirus infection studies may not have administered a large enough dose of virus (77–79), with only 30 to 50% of subjects developing clinical illness following challenge. The low infectivity rate may have accounted for the lack of significant changes between challenged and unchallenged groups. When clinically symptomatic upper airway rhinovirus infection was established, there were significantly increased responses to nasal administered histamine (80).

Studies that have investigated alterations in lower airway BHR have also been hampered by the poor induction of clinically symptomatic infection if low viral dose or inadequate virus administration method was used. Summers (81) and Skoner (82) and their colleagues were unable to show statistically significant changes in BHR following infection, though Cheung et al. (83), who used triple administration of virus, reported significant changes not only in BHR, but also in maximal airway narrowing.

The late asthmatic response (LAR) for inhaled allergen is not seen in all asthmatic subjects and is thought to be due to the recruitment of inflammatory cells (lymphocytes and eosinophils) to the small-airway submucosa (84). This response is thought to be a good model for the pathogenesis of chronic inflammation in asthma. Two studies have shown the development of LAR responses following viral URTI; both used the double administration method for the virus challenge. The study by Lemanske et al. (85) showed an increase in LAR from 1 of 10 to 8 of 10 subjects following rhinovirus infection, while Calhoun et al. (86) showed an increase from 1 of 8 to 5 of 8. A subsequent study by Calhoun's group (74) showed that the levels of BAL histamine recovered following antigen challenge rose postinfection, as did levels of TNF-α and eosinophils.

VII. Virus Infection of the Upper Airways: Lower Airway Functional Changes

The preceding section highlighted the similarities in the immune responses of the epithelia of the upper and lower airways. Studies that have investigated the functional airway changes in response to respiratory virus infection can also be divided into two broad categories: studies that have investigated normal subjects and those that have investigated asthmatic/atopic subjects. The results with normal and asthmatic individuals give both different and similar results, indicating that the changes in the lower respiratory tract are greater in asthmatics but can be observed in both populations.

A. Natural Infections

Normal Subjects

Many of the early studies that investigated the response of static lung function tests, such as forced expiratory volume in one second (FEV_1), peak expiratory flow (PEF), and airway resistance (R_{AW}), failed to demonstrate changes in respiratory function following respiratory virus infection (75,87,88). The results of these studies suggest that normal subjects do not develop changes in resting airway tone following infection. In a more recent observational study, of normal nonatopic subjects monitored closely, with twice daily peak flow recordings during naturally occurring viral infections, falls in peak expiratory flow rate of around 9.5% were observed during viral URTI (89), significantly lower than the fall observed in atopic asthmatic individuals with URTI (14.1%, $p = 0.03$).

Atopic/Asthmatic Subjects

Similarly, early studies of asthmatic populations were not able to demonstrate changes in either static or dynamic pulmonary lung function tests associated with virus infections (90,91). More recent population studies of adult and pediatric populations of asthmatic subjects have shown a fall in PEF associated with URTI in both populations. Initial information was obtained from a study by Morris (5). More recent studies by Nicholson (2), and Johnston (1) and their collegues support the first study for adult and pediatric populations, respectively. The latter study was able to show that viral URTI is implicated in the vast majority of childhood asthma exacerbations. Not unexpectedly, static lung function tests do change in asthmatic individuals: a median fall in PEF of 35% was reported (1). Other studies have confirmed the change in static pulmonary function tests associated with viral infection (92,93).

Investigators using more rigorous techniques have been able to show the extent of alterations in pulmonary function during virus infections. Earlier studies may not have been able to show significant changes because they were unable to confirm all virus infections. These data suggest that the asthmatic response seems to be quantitatively increased in comparison to the normal response.

B. Experimental Infection

Functional Changes

The experimental infection and study of volunteers allows the pathophysiology of the acute infection to be studied closely in a controlled way, with measurements being accurately timed with respect to the onset of infection. Nevertheless, there is great variability in the reported results. There are several key protocol differences between experimental infection studies, and some of these may account for some of the variation. Specifically, the study populations are variable; there are differences in the virus serotypes used (though most human rhinovirus infection studies have used RV-16 and RV-39); and there are several different methods and doses of virus inoculation.

Administration methods vary, with three main types. The simplest is droplet administration of virus directly into the nose. This can be combined with nasal inhalation via an atomizer, which may lead to pharyngitis and possibly LRTI as well. The final method is the use of the first two, with the addition of nebulized virus administered over 2 days. The last method has the highest chance of active administration of virus into the lower airways and increases the chances of the subject developing an LRTI.

The infective dose of the virus is often expressed as the $TCID_{50}$; this is defined as the dose needed to cause infection of 50% of tissue cultures. The infecting dose of the virus varies from 100 $TCID_{50}$ (77) through to 3×10^4 $TCID_{50}$ (83). The 300-fold differences in viral dose administered in these studies could be enough to account for the differences in results reported.

Study populations have varied from normal subjects to stable asthmatic subjects. Some studies have used atopic rather than asthmatic individuals, presumably to investigate subjects that are safer to infect. The reported experimental rhinovirus infection studies are summarized in Table 2.

A study that used triple inoculation has demonstrated that experimental RV infection does significantly reduce airway calibre (94), a finding that had not been shown before 1999. Other recent studies have demonstrated changes in lung function after experimental rhinovirus infection. Bardin et al. have been able to demonstrate a fall in PEF in following RV-16 inoculation: the changes were seen in 6 out of 16 subjects, who included 2 normal subjects, and atopic and 3 atopic asthmatic subjects (95). The subjects in whom a fall in PEF is seen also demonstrate an increase in airway responsiveness as measured by histamine challenge. Grunberg et al. demonstrated a fall in serial FEV_1 following RV-16 infection in atopic asthmatics; this was maximal on day 2 after challenge and was associated with an increase in airway hyperresponsiveness (94).

Experimental infection and subsequent study of asthmatic hyper-responsiveness to bradykinin showed that repeated bradykinin challenge over several days led to tachyphylaxis, but RV-16 infection abolished this tachyphylaxis (61). This suggests that there is an increased sensitivity to bradykinin following RV-16 infection, though this effect is not seen in all studies (81).

The foregoing studies show that experimental virus infection can lead to a fall in PEF and FEV_1, an increase in BHR to both histamine and methacholine, and the development of the LAR in atopic individuals. The development of these changes does seem to require that the virus be administered in large enough doses to cause clinically symptomatic infection.

Histological Changes

Rhinovirus infection is associated with an accumulation of inflammatory cells in the lower airways in both normal and asthmatic subjects (84). There were also increases in airway reactivity to histamine in the asthmatic subjects. A separate study that investigated the response of rhinovirus infection on nasal lavage contents showed increased levels of IL-6, IL-8 and ECP. This was associated with increased bronchial hyperreactivity (96), though measures of lower respiratory tract cellular recruitment were not studied. A study by Seymour et al. has demonstrated, by immunohisto-chemistry of bronchial biopsy samples taken from nonatopic subjects infected with HRV-16, that there is an increase in macrophages positive for 5-lipoxygenase (LO) and eosinophils and an increase in macrophages, positive for cyclooxygenase 2 (COX-2), eosinophils, and mast cells. There was also an increase in the BAL fluid cysteinyl leukotrienes, which may contribute to the lower airway inflammation reportedly associated with rhinovirus infection (97).

There is evidence that rhinovirus infection is associated with cellular changes in the lower airway and that this is associated with airway reactivity changes seen in the experimental infection studies. What is not clear from these studies is whether the functional, physiological, and immunological changes observed in the lower airway during rhinovirus URTI are a result of direct LRT infection or occur via indirect mechanisms. For this reason, several studies have attempted to investigate the capacity of rhinovirus to infect the lower respiratory tract.

VIII. Methodology for Eliminating URT Contamination

A variety of methods have been tried to try to obtain LRT samples without URT contamination. Originally methods such as tracheal aspiration (98) and lung puncture (99) were tried, but these techniques are associated with appreciable discomfort and morbidity. Postmortem studies have succeeded in bypassing the upper airways by obtaining samples directly from lung tissue, but these have limited application! Double-lumen catheters have been introduced via bronchoscopy, protected from the upper airway by a polyethylene glycol (PEG). However, when bacterial cultures were taken by this method, Halperin et al. showed that there was 73% oropharyngeal contamination on subsequent culture of the lavage specimens (7).

Even if LRT sampling could be performed without URT contamination, viral diagnostic procedures have been so limited with respect to the most common respiratory tract viruses, rhinoviruses, and coronaviruses that no useful data have been available until the recent development of more sensitive techniques, such as PCR.

In one study bronchoalveolar lavage was used to sample and PCR to detect respiratory viruses. After the BAL samples had been processed and cells separated from the fluid, the cells were washed to reduce the viral particle contamination of the samples that may have occurred during the passage of the bronchoscope through the upper airways (100). In this study eight allergic volunteers were experimentally challenged with rhinovirus. Reverse transcriptose-PCR and Southern blotting served to identify rhinovirus in all subjects 2 and 4 days after challenge, while all prechallenge samples were negative. However, despite the precautions taken, URT contamination could not be excluded, in as much as washing cells in in vitro studies is known not to remove virus that is already attached.

To try to eliminate the confounding influence of URT contamination in the diagnosis of LRTI, a recent rhinovirus experimental infection study obtained mucosal biopsy samples at bronchoscopy and used in situ hybridization (ISH), a technique that detects viral RNA or DNA tissues. Viral gene products demonstrated in tissue by this means would provide clear evidence of viral replication in the LRT.

Nasal mucosal studies of experimental rhinovirus infection have used of in situ hybridization (ISH) to demonstrate rhinovirus within epithelial cells (101) and rhinoviral replication (102). ISH techniques have been applied to lower airway samples to confirm rhinovirus localization and replication in the lower airways (103). Figure 1 shows lower respiratory tract biopsy specimens, taken before and during experimental RV colds, that were probed for rhinovirus by means of ISH techniques.

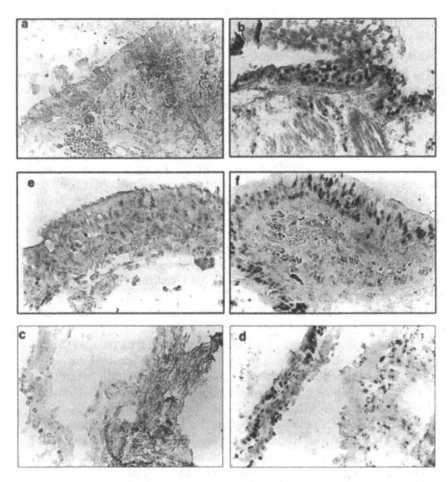

Figure 1 In situ hybridization for rhinovirus RV-16 in sections of human bronchial biopsy samples. Negative bronchial biopsy samples were taken before infection from three subjects: – (A), (C), and (E) are compared with RV-16-positive biopsy samples from the respective subjects obtained during experimental RV-16 infection (B), (D), and (F). The hybridization signal for RV-16 is visible as black color in the cells and is localized mainly on epithelium. Magnification, × 400. (From Ref. 46.)

There is now also evidence that rhinovirus can infect airway smooth muscle in vitro, via binding to ICAM-1. This leads to an increase in the constrictor response to acetylcholine and an attenuated relaxation response to isoproterenol (104). Thus rhinovirus can directly act on airway smooth muscle and alter its tone, suggesting that direct local effects at the level of the lower airway may be important.

Thus, there are methods that can be used for sampling the lower airways with minimal risk of contamination from the upper airways and confounding of the results. If these methods are used, the identification of viral genome can reliably be ascribed to lower respiratory tract infection.

IX. Linking of the Upper and Lower Airways

Although there is now good evidence of rhinovirus replication in the lower respiratory tract, the cellular and functional changes observed in the lower respiratory tract that are associated with a rhinoviral or any other viral URTI may also be linked by indirect means. Several different mechanisms may be involved in this possible linkage, such as the production of circulating factors, neurogenic links between the upper and lower airways, and factors produced in the upper airways that are transferred by inhalation to the lower airways.

A. Circulating Factors

Histamine and bradykinin are found in the circulation and may be involved in the remote linkage of the upper and lower airways. An ex vivo study of basophils from subjects infected with rhinovirus showed increased histamine release, suggesting that this may be a possible mechanism for increased hyperresponsiveness (105,106).

Busse (107) has shown in an ex vivo study that there is alteration of the sensitivity of β-adrenoreceptors present on mononuclear cells following rhinovirus infection, indicating that rhinovirus infection can lead to a down-regulation of the sensitivity of β-adrenoreceptors. There is no evidence that rhinovirus can alter the β-adrenoreceptor sensitivity in vivo, although the foregoing findings suggest that such change may occur and could lead to an alteration in the resting tone airways during viral infections and narrower airways.

B. Indirect Links: Cytokines

The principal mediators of inflammation, the cytokines, which tend to be short-lived, and often strongly bound to albumin, are elevated in bacterial pulmonary infections. They are biologically active at very low concentrations, and increased levels of plasma IL-1 and TNF-α are likely to be involved in the febrile and arthralgic responses to viral upper respiratory infections. It is therefore quite possible that increased circulating levels of cytokines resulting from URT infection may result in biological changes in the lower airway. Few studies have studied serum cytokine levels during viral URTI or LRTI. One study of experimental influenza A infection reported an increase in serum TNF-α and IL-6 levels; the maximal rise was 2 to 3 days postchallenge (108). However there is insufficient evidence to support or refute the hypothesis that circulating cytokines are present at levels sufficient to lead to remote inflammatory cell activation.

C. Neurogenic Links

The nervous innervation of the lungs has been difficult to study directly in humans, and much of the available information has been derived from animal models. If there were indirect neurogenic links, then local infection of the respiratory epithelium could lead to local changes in the upper airway that would cause alterations in lower airway reactivity and airway function via neural pathways, rather than by local infection of the LRT.

There is evidence that disruption of the local nerve innervation can cause local effects in the lungs. This would support virus infection in the lower respiratory tract, leading to local changes in the lower airways. There may be an alteration in the parasympathetic supply to the lungs, either a reduction in presynaptic M_2 receptor functioning or an alteration in M_2 innervation. This is thought to be a result of MBP (major basic protein) release by eosinophils (109). The nonadrenergic noncholinergic (NANC) nervous system may also be affected by local viral infection. Substance P and neurokinin A are the major mediators of the sensory C fibers. With the loss of epithelium, the major source of neutral endopeptidase, which degrades substance P and neurokinin A, their levels can increase, leading to an increase in the constrictor tone of the NANC system.

If neuronal links exist between the upper and lower airways, URTI may indirectly lead to alterations in lower airway functions. For many years neuronal links between the upper and lower airways have been suggested. In fact, asthma was postulated as being a nasal response (110). Several studies have shown that the lower airways do react to changes in the nasal environment (111,112) and that changes can occur in response to exercise, cold air (111), or histamine challenge (113). Yan et al. (114) showed that the nasal administration of histamine led to a fall in FEV_1. This study and one by Fontanari et al. (115) showed that this response was present in normal individuals as well as asthmatic individuals, though the response in asthmatic individuals was greater, with the largest response seen in asthmatic individuals with rhinitic symptoms. The work of Yan and Fontanari and their colleagues showed a correlation between nasal cold-air-induced bronchoconstriction and airway hyperresponsiveness. Others, however, have shown these effects without demonstrating a clear correlation (116). Nasal cold air is a vagally mediated response and is used in the in vivo studies of M2 receptor function (109). Recent studies by Braunstahl et al. (117,118) have demonstrated in nonasthmatic subjects with allergic rhinitis that segmental bronchial provocation (SBP) with allergen (117) induces nasal inflammation, with an increase in circulating eosinophils, as well as a local increase in eosinophils in nonchallenged bronchial mucosa and nasal lamina propria. The opposite is also seen: with nasal allergen challenge in subjects with nonasthmatic allergic rhinitis, there was an increase in ICAM-1 and VCAM-1 expression both in nasal and bronchial mucosa, and there was an increase in mucosal eosinophils in both nasal and bronchial epithelia (118). These changes in the lower and upper airway could not be demonstrated in control sham-challenged subjects (117,118).

There is a great deal of evidence that viral infections may be causing an alteration in the local nervous system network in the lung, and that they may be exerting an influence over a greater distance. Much work still needs to be undertaken to fully dissect the interaction between the effects of the virus locally and remotely. Most evidence points to local viral effects causing the lower airway response directly, though there is evidence that indirect effect may play a role as well.

X. Timing of Symptoms in Upper Airway Infection

Can the timing of the development of symptoms help in establishing whether upper airway infections are linked to lower airway infections? Most studies rely on symptom reporting to classify an infection as either a URTI or as a an LRTI. One of the most commonly reported symptoms that is reported, cough, often classified as a an LRT symptom, was reported in 70% of URTIs (1). Lower airway symptoms are thought to follow upper airway symptoms, though there are few data to support the anecdotal evidence of this timing. Johnston's study (1) shows that of 269 reported episodes of URT or LRT symptoms associated with viral infections, 184 were combined URTI and LRTI (70%), while only 16 of 269 (6%) were only LRTI and 69 of 269 (24%) were URTI only. This suggests that often there is infection of both upper and lower airways, though to have isolated LRTI is also possible.

Using data from Johnston's study (1), allows us to study relationships between the timing of upper airway symptoms and a fall in peak flow (seen in 141 of 269 episodes) in the asthmatic subjects, (Fig. 2a). There is a median one-day delay between the reporting of symptoms and the fall in peak flow, suggesting that in most cases URT infection precedes LRTI. However, falls in peak flow preceded URT symptoms in 14% of cases, perhaps suggesting that LRT infection preceded URT infection in these cases. LRT symptom reporting had the same temporal relationship with falls in PEF as did

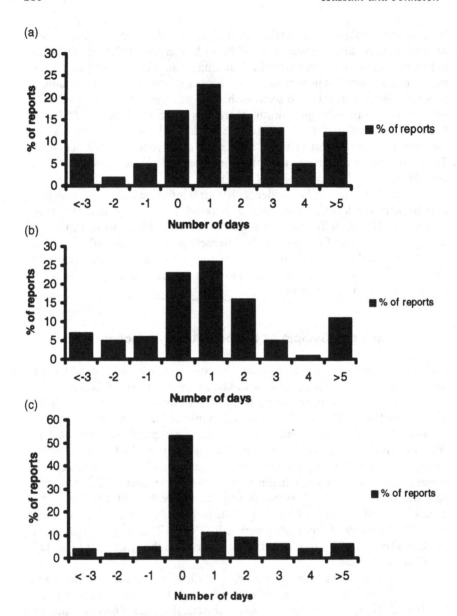

Figure 2 (a) Number of days by which upper respiratory symptoms preceded a fall in PEF. (b) Number of days by which lower respiratory symptoms preceded a fall in PEF. (c) Number of days by which upper respiratory symptoms preceded lower.

reporting of URT symptoms (Fig. 2b), and the median reporting time of lower respiratory tract symptoms and upper respiratory tract symptoms is indeed usually simultaneous (Fig. 2c). However, once again LRT symptoms preceded URT symptoms in a significant (38%) percentage. We believe that the relative timing illustrated for PEF drops and URT symptoms is more likely to reflect the true sequence of events than that illustrated for LRT symptoms and URT symptoms, since, when triggered by an overall load of symptoms, children recording diary cards may start to record symptoms irrespective of their source, rather than accurately assessing upper and lower respiratory symptoms separately on a daily basis, as instructed. It is likely that the objective PEF recordings do not suffer from this triggering effect. It is interesting to note that these data combined demonstrate that in a significant percentage of cases, LRT symptoms or a fall in PEF precede URT symptoms. Whether the mechanisms involved are direct or indirect, however, is not clear.

XI. Conclusion

There is a large body of evidence to support direct infection of the lower respiratory tract by most respiratory viruses including rhinoviruses. Infection of lower respiratory tract cells leads to inflammatory responses similar to those observed in upper respiratory tract cells both in vitro and in vivo. There are many local pathophysiological responses that can cause symptoms. There is increasing evidence that levels of inflammatory mediators released by local tissue infection correlate with the symptoms reported by individuals.

Though most investigations have focused on the direct effect of virus infections on the pathology and physiology of the lower airway, indirect effects of upper airway infection may play a significant role on the lower airway as well. Some evidence exist for indirect effects, but more research needs to be conducted to clarify their role in airway response to virus infections.

References

1. Johnston SL, Pattemore PK, Sanderson G, Smith S, Lampe F, Josephs L, Symington P, O'Toole S, Myint SH, Tyrrell DA, Holgate ST. Community study of role of viral infections in exacerbations of asthma in 9–11 year old children. Br Med J 1995; 310:1225-1228.
2. Nicholson KG, Kent J, Ireland DC. Respiratory viruses and exacerbations of asthma in adults. Br Med J 1993; 307:982–986.

3. Nicholson KG. Impact of influenza and respiratory syncytial virus on mortality in England and Wales from January 1975 to December 1990. Epidemiol Infect 1996; 116:51–63.

4. Knott AM, Long CE, Hall CB. Parainfluenza viral-infections in pediatric outpatients: seasonal patterns and clinical characteristics. Pediatr Infect Dis J 1994; 13:269–273.

5. Morris DJ, Cooper RJ, Barr T, Bailey AS. Polymerase chain-reaction for rapid diagnosis of respiratory adenovirus infection. J Infect 1996; 32:113–117.

6. Horn ME, Brain EA, Gregg I, Inglis JM, Yealland SJ, Taylor P. Respiratory viral infection and wheezy bronchitis in childhood. Thorax 1979; 34:23–28.

7. Halperin SA, Suratt PM, Gwaltney JM, Groschel DHM, Hendley JO, Eggleston PA. Bacterial cultures of the lower respiratory-tract in normal volunteers with and without experimental rhinovirus infection using a plugged double catheter system. Am Rev Respir Dis 1982; 125:678–680.

8. Heikkinen T, Waris M, Ruuskanen O, Putto-Laurila A, Mertsola J. Incidence of acute otitis media associated with group A and B respiratory syncytial virus infections. Acta Paediatr 1995; 84:419–423.

9. Arola M, Ruuskanen O, Ziegler T, Mertsola J, Nanto-Salonen K, Putto-Laurila A, Viljanen MK, Halonen P. Clinical role of respiratory virus infection in acute otitis media. Pediatrics 1990; 86:848–855.

10. Pitkaranta A, Arruda E, Malmberg H, Hayden FG. Detection of rhinovirus in sinus brushings of patients with acute community-acquired sinusitis by reverse transcription-PCR. J Clin Microbiol 1997; 35:1791–1793.

11. Harsten G, Prellner K, Lofgren B, Kalm O. Serum antibodies against respiratory tract viruses in episodes of acute otitis media. J Laryngol Otol 1991; 105:337–340.

12. Uhari M, Hietala J, Tuokko H. Risk of acute otitis media in relation to the viral etiology of infections in children. Clin Infect Dis 1995; 20:521–524.

13. Heikkinen T, Thint M, Chonmaitree T. Prevalence of various respiratory viruses in the middle ear during acute otitis media. N Engl J Med 1999; 340:260–264.

14. Pitkaranta A, Virolainen A, Jero J, Arruda E, Hayden FG. Detection of rhinovirus, respiratory syncytial virus, and coronavirus infections in acute otitis media by reverse transcriptase polymerase chain reaction. Pediatrics 1998; 102:291–295.

15. Pitkaranta A, Jero J, Arruda E, Virolainen A, Hayden FG. Polymerase chain reaction-based detection of rhinovirus, respiratory syncytial virus, and coronavirus in otitis media with effusion. J Pediatr 1998;133: 390–394.

16. Matsuzaki Z, Okamoto Y, Sarashina N, Ito E, Togawa K, Saito I. Induction of intercellular adhesion molecule-1 in human nasal epithelial cells during respiratory syncytial virus infection. Immunology 1996; 88:565–568.

17. Altman LC, Ayars GH, Baker C, Luchtel DL. Cytokines and eosinophil-derived cationic proteins up-regulate intercellular-adhesion molecule-1 on human nasal epithelial cells. J Allergy Clin Immunol 1993; 92:527–536.

18. Black HR, Yankaskas JR, Johnson LG, Noah TL. Interleukin-8 production by cystic fibrosis nasal epithelial cells after tumor necrosis factor-alpha and respiratory syncytial virus stimulation. Am J Respir Cell Mol Biol 1998; 19:210–215.

19. Becker S, Koren HS, Henke DC. Interleukin-8 expression in normal nasal epithelium and its modulation by infection with respiratory syncytial virus and cytokines tumor necrosis factor, interleukin-1, and interleukin-6. Am J Respir Cell Mol Biol 1993; 8:20–27.

20. Becker S, Reed W, Henderson FW, Noah TL. RSV infection of human airway epithelial cells causes production of the beta-chemokine RANTES. Am J Physiol 1997; 272:L512–L520.

21. Saito T, Deskin RW, Casola A, Haeberle H, Olszewska B, Ernst PB, Alam, R, Ogra PL, Garofalo R. Respiratory syncytial virus induces selective production of the chemokine RANTES by upper airway epithelial cells. J Infect Dis 1997; 175:497–504.

22. Turner RB, Winther B, Hendley JO, Mygind N, Gwaltney JM, Jr. Sites of virus recovery and antigen detection in epithelial cells during experimental rhinovirus infection. Acta Otolaryngol Suppl (Stockh) 1984; 413:9–14.

23. Winther B, Farr B, Turner RB, Hendley JO, Gwaltney JM Jr, Mygind N. Histopathologic examination and enumeration of polymorphonuclear leuko-cytes in the nasal mucosa during experimental rhinovirus colds. Acta Otolaryngol Suppl (Stockh) 1984; 413:19–24.

24. Naclerio RM, Proud D, Kagey Sobotka A, Lichtenstein LM, Hendley JO, Gwaltney JM Jr. Is histamine responsible for the symptoms of rhinovirus colds? A look at the inflammatory mediators following infection. Pediatr Infect Dis J 1988; 7:218–222.

25. Levandowski RA, Weaver CW, Jackson GG. Nasal-secretion leukocyte populations determined by flow cytometry during acute rhinovirus infection. J Med Virol 1988; 25:423–432.

26. Teran LM, Johnston SL, Schroder J-M, Church MK, Holgate ST. Role of nasal interleukin-8 in neutrophil recruitment and activation in children with virus-induced asthma. Am J Respir Crit Care Med 1997; 155:1362–1366.

27. Turner RB, Weingand KW, Yeh CH, Leedy DW. Association between interleukin-8 concentration in nasal secretions and severity of symptoms of experimental rhinovirus colds. Clin Infect Dis 1998; 26:840–846.

28. Fraenkel DJ, Bardin PG, Johnston SL, Wilson S, Sanderson G, Holgate ST. Nasal biopsies in human rhinovirus-16 infection—an immunohistochemical study. Am Rev Respir Dis 1993; 147:A460.

29. Noah TL, Henderson FW, Wortman IA, Devlin RB, Handy J, Koren HS, Becker, S. Nasal cytokine production in viral acute upper respiratory infection of childhood. J Infect Dis 1995; 171:584–592.

30. Okamoto Y, Kudo K, Ishikawa K, Ito E, Togawa K, Saito I, Moro I, Patel, JA, Ogra PL. Presence of respiratory syncytial virus genomic sequences in middle ear fluid and its relationship to expression of cytokines and cell adhesion molecules. J Infect Dis 1993; 168:1277–1281.

31. Matsuda K, Tsutsumi H, Okamoto Y, Chiba C. Development of interleukin 6 and tumor necrosis factor alpha activity in nasopharyngeal secretions of infants and children during infection with respiratory syncytial virus. Clin Diagn Lab Immunol 1995; 2:322–324.

32. Noah TL, Becker S. Chemokines in nasal secretions of normal adults experimentally infected with respiratory syncytial virus. Clin Immunol 2000; 97:43–49.

33. Teran LM, Seminario MC, Shute JK, Papi A, Compton SJ, Low JL, Gleich GJ, Johnston SL. RANTES, macrophage-inhibitory protein 1-alpha, and the eosinophil product major basic protein are released into upper respiratory secretions during virus-induced asthma exacerbations in children. J Infect Dis 1999; 179:677–681.

34. Papi A, Johnston SL. Respiratory epithelial cell expression of vascular cell adhesion molecule-1 and its up-regulation by rhinovirus infection via NF-kappa B and GATA transcription factors. J Biol Chem 1999; 274:30041–30051.

35. Terajima M, Yamaya M, Sekizawa K, Okinaga S, Suzuki T, Yamada N, Nakayama K, Ohrui T, Oshima T, Numazaki Y, Sasaki H. Rhinovirus infection of primary cultures of human tracheal epithelium: role of ICAM-1 and IL-1 beta. Am J Physiol Lung Cell Mol Physiol 1997; 17:L749–L759.

36. Matsukura S, Kokubu F, Kubo H, Tomita T, Tokunaga H, Kadokura M, Yamamoto T, Kuroiwa Y, Ohno T, Suzaki H, Adachi M. Expression of RANTES by normal airway epithelial cells after influenza virus A infection. Am J Respir Cell Mol Biol 1998; 18:255–264.

37. Chini BA, Fiedler MA, Milligan L, Hopkins T, Stark JM. Essential roles of NF-kappa B and C/EBP in the regulation of intercellular adhesion molecule-1 after respiratory syncytial virus infection of human respiratory epithelial cell cultures. J Virol 1998; 72:1623–1626.

38. Pilewski JM, Sott DJ, Wilson JM, Albelda SM. ICAM-1 expression on bronchial epithelium after recombinant adenovirus infection. Am J Respir Cell Mol Biol 1995; 12:142–148.

39. Arnold R, Konig W. ICAM-1 expression and low-molecular-weight G-protein activation of human bronchial epithelial cells (A549) infected with RSV. J Leukoc Biol 1996; 60:766–771.

40. Arnold R, Humbert B, Werchau H, Gallati H, Konig W. Interleukin-8, interleukin-6, and soluble tumour necrosis factor receptor type release from a human pulmonary epithelial cell line (A549) exposed to respiratory syncytial virus. Immunology 1994; 82:126–133.

41. Einarsson O, Geba GP, Zhu Z, Landry M, Elias JA. Interleukin-11 stimulation in-vivo and in-vitro by respiratory viruses and induction of airways hyperresponsiveness. J Clin Invest 1996; 97:915–924.

42. Olszewska-Pazdrak B, Casola A, Saito T, Alam R, Crowe SE, Mei F, Ogra, PL, Garofalo RP. Cell-specific expression of RANTES, MCP-1, and MIP-1-alpha by lower airway epithelial cells and eosinophils infected with respiratory syncytial virus. J Virol 1998; 72:4756–4764.

43. Noah TL, Wortman IA, Becker S. The effect of fluticasone propionate on respiratory syncytial virus- induced chemokine release by a human bronchial epithelial cell line. Immunopharmacology 1998; 39:193–199.

44. Zhang YH, Luxon BA, Casola A, Garofalo RP, Jamaluddin M, Brasier AR. Expression of respiratory syncytial virus-induced chemokine gene networks in lower airway epithelial cells revealed by cDNA microarrays. J Virol 2001; 75:9044–9058.

45. Kawaguchi M, Kokubu F, Kuga H, Tomita T, Matsukura S, Suzaki H, Huang SK, Adachi M. Influenza virus A stimulates expression of eotaxin by nasal epithelial cells. Clin Exp Allergy 2001; 31:873–880.

46. Papadopoulos NG, Bates PJ, Bardin PG, Papi A, Leir SH, Fraenkel DJ, Meyer J, Lackie PM, Sanderson G, Holgate ST, Johnston SL. Rhinoviruses infect the lower airways. J Infect Dis 2000; 181:1875–1884.

47. Griego SD, Weston CB, Adams JL, Tal-Singer R, Dillon SB. Role of p38 mitogen-activated protein kinase in rhinovirus-induced cytokine production by bronchial epithelial cells. J Immunol 2000; 165:5211–5220.

48. Kim J, Connolly KR, Porter JD, Siekierski ES, Proud D. Nitric oxide inhibits rhinovirus-induced granulocyte macrophage colony-stimulating factor production in bronchial epithelial cells. Am J Respir Cell Mol Biol 2001;24: 317–325.

49. Sanders SP, Siekierski ES, Casolaro V, Proud D. Role of NF-kappa B in cytokine production induced from human airway epithelial cells by rhinovirus infection. J Immunol 2000;165:3382–3394.

50. Papadopoulos NG, Papi A, Meyer J, Stanciu LA, Salvi S, Holgate ST, Johnston SL. Rhinovirus infection up-regulates eotaxin and eotaxin-2 expression in bronchial epithelial cells. Clin Exp Allergy 2001;31: 1060–1066.

51. Smith PK, Hussain IR, Lovejoy M, Forsyth K, Johnston SL. Presence of pro-allergic cytokine mRNA from mononuclear lymphocytes from respiratory syncytial virus bronchiolitis. Am J Respir Crit Care Med 1998; 157:A287.

52. Joshi P, Kakakios A, Jayasekera J, Isaacs D. A comparison of IL-2 levels in nasopharyngeal and endotracheal aspirates of babies with respiratory syncytial viral bronchiolitis. J Allergy Clin Immunol 1998; 102:618–620.

53. Sheeran P, Jafri H, Carubelli C, Saavedra J, Johnson C, Krisher K, Sanchez PJ, Ramilo O. Elevated cytokine concentrations in the nasopharyngeal and tracheal secretions of children with respiratory syncytial virus disease. Pediatr Infect Dis J 1999; 18:115–122.

54. Harrison AM, Bonville CA, Rosenberg HF, Domachowske JB. Respiratory syncytical virus–induced chemokine expression in the lower airways: eosinophil recruitment and degranulation. Am J Respir Crit Care Med 1999; 159: 1918–1924.

55. Sung RYT, Hui SHL, Wong CK, Lam CWK, Yin J. A comparison of cytokine responses in respiratory syncytial virus and influenza A infections in infants. Eur J Pediatr 2001;160:117–122.

56. Garofalo RP, Patti J, Hintz KA, Hill V, Ogra PL, Welliver RC. Macrophage inflammatory protein-1 alpha (not T helper type 2 cytokines) is associated

with severe forms of respiratory syncytial virus bronchiolitis. J Infect Dis 2001; 184:393–399.

57. Hornsleth A, Loland L, Larsen LB. Cytokines and chemokines in respiratory secretion and severity of disease in infants with respiratory syncytial virus (RSV) infection. J Clin Virol 2001; 21:163–170.

58. Gentile D, Doyle W, Whiteside T, Fireman P, Hayden FG, Skoner D. Increased interleukin-6 levels in nasal lavage samples following experimental influenza A virus infection. Clin Diagn Lab Immunol 1998; 5:604–608.

59. Fritz RS, Hayden FG, Calfee DP, Cass LM, Peng AW, Alvord WG, Strober W, Straus SE. Nasal cytokine and chemokine responses in experimental influenza A virus infection: results of a placebo-controlled trial of intravenous zanamivir treatment. J Infect Dis 1999; 180:586–93.

60. Skoner DP, Gentile DA, Patel A, Doyle WJ. Evidence for cytokine mediation of disease expression in adults experimentally infected with influenza A virus. J Infect Dis 1999; 180:10–4.

61. Grunberg K, Smits HH, Timmers MC, de Klerk EP, Dolhain RJ, Dick EC, Hiemstra PS, Sterk PJ. Experimental rhinovirus 16 infection. Effects on cell differentials and soluble markers in sputum in asthmatic subjects. Am J Respir Crit Care Med 1997; 156:609–616.

62. Avila PC, Abisheganaden JA, Wong H, Liu J, Yagi S, Schnurr D, Kishiyama JL, Boushey HA. Effects of allergic inflammation of the nasal mucosa on the severity of rhinovirus 16 cold. J Allergy Clin Immunol 2000; 105:923–932.

63. Pizzichini MMM, Pizzichini E, Efthimiadis A, Chauhan AJ, Johnston SL, Hussak P, Mahoney J, Dolovich J, Hargreave FE. Asthma and natural colds—inflammatory indices in induced sputum: a feasibility study. Am J Respir Crit Care Med 1998; 158:1178–1184.

64. Smyth RL, Fletcher JN, Thomas HM, Hart CA. Immunological responses to respiratory syncytial virus infection in infancy. Arch Dis Child 1997; 76:210–214.

65. Legg J, Hussain IR, Johnston SL, Warner JO. Deficient production of interferon-gamma, IL-12 and IL-18 in RSV bronchiolitis. Am J Respir Crit Care Med 2002:in press.

66. Counil FP, Lebel B, Segondy M, Peterson C, Voisin M, Bousquet J, Arnoux B. Cells and mediators from pharyngeal secretions in infants with acute wheezing episodes. Eur Respir J 1997; 10:2591–2595.

67. Sigurs N, Bjarnason R, Sigurbergsson F. Eosinophil cationic protein in nasal secretion and in serum and myeloperoxidase in serum in respiratory syncytial virus bronchiolitis: relation to asthma and atopy. Acta Paediatr 1994; 83:1151–1155.

68. Proud D, Naclerio RM, Gwaltney JM Jr, Hendley JO. Kinins are generated in nasal secretions during natural rhinovirus colds. J Infect Dis 1990; 161:120–123.

69. Naclerio RM, Proud D, Lichtenstein LM, Kagey Sobotka A, Hendley JO, Sorrentino J, Gwaltney JM Jr. Kinins are generated during experimental colds. J Infect Dis 1988; 157:133–142.

70. Igarashi Y, Skoner DP, Fireman P, Kaliner MA. Analysis of nasal secretions during experimental rhinovirus upper respiratory infections. J Allergy Clin Immunol 1993; 92:722–731.

71. Doyle WJ, Boehm S, Skoner DP. Physiologic response to intranasal dose–response challenge with histamine, methacholine, bradykinin, and prostaglandin in adult volunteers with and without nasal allergy. J Allergy Clin Immunol 1990; 86:924–935.

72. Borum P, Olsen L, Winther B, Mygind N. Ipratropium nasal spray: a new treatment for rhinorrhea in the common cold. Am Rev Respir Dis 1981; 123:418–420.

73. Bisgaard H, Olsson P, Bende M. Effect of leukotriene D4 on nasal mucosal blood flow, nasal airway resistance and nasal secretion in humans. Clin Allergy 1986; 16:289–298.

74. Calhoun WJ, Dick EC, Schwartz LB, Busse WW. A common cold virus, rhinovirus-16, potentiates airway inflammation after segmental antigen bronchoprovocation in allergic subjects. J Clin Invest 1994; 94:2200–2208.

75. Empey DW, Laitinen LA, Jacobs L, Gold WM, Nadel JA. Mechanisms of bronchial hyperreactivity in normal subjects after upper respiratory tract infection. Am Rev Respir Dis 1976; 113:131–139.

76. Little JW, Hall WJ, Douglas RGJ, Mudholkar GS, Speers, DM, Patel K. Airway hyperreactivity and peripheral airway dysfunction in influenza A infection. Am Rev Respir Dis 1978; 118:295–303.

77. Blair HT, Greenberg SB, Stevens PM, Bilunos PA, Couch, RB. Effects of rhinovirus infection of pulmonary function of healthy human volunteers. Am Rev Respir Dis 1976; 114:95–102.

78. Bush RK, Busse W, Flaherty D, Warshauer D, Dick EC, Reed CE. Effects of experimental rhinovirus 16 infection on airways and leukocyte function in normal subjects. J Allergy Clin Immunol 1978; 61:80–87.

79. Doyle WJ, Skoner DP, Fireman P, Seroky JT, Green I, Ruben F, Kardatzke DR, Gwaltney JM. Rhinovirus-39 infection in allergic and nonallergic subjects. J Allergy Clin Immunol 1992; 89:968–978.

80. Doyle WJ, Skoner DP, Seroky JT, Fireman P, Gwaltney JM. Effect of experimental rhinovirus-39 infection on the nasal response to histamine and cold-air challenges in allergic and nonallergic subjects. J Allergy Clin Immunol 1994; 93:534–542.

81. Summers QA, Higgins PG, Barrow IG, Tyrrell DAJ, Holgate ST. Bronchial reactivity to histamine and bradykinin is unchanged after rhinovirus infection in normal subjects. Eur Respir J 1992; 5:313–317.

82. Skoner DP, Doyle WJ, Seroky J, Fireman P. Lower airway responses to influenza-A virus in healthy allergic and nonallergic subjects. Am J Respir Crit Care Med 1996; 154:661–664.

83. Cheung D, Dick EC, Timmers MC, Deklerk EPA, Spaan WJM, Sterk PJ. Rhinovirus inhalation causes long-lasting excessive airway narrowing in response to methacholine in asthmatic subjects in-vivo. Am J Respir Crit Care Med 1995; 152:1490–1496.

84. Fraenkel DJ, Bardin PG, Sanderson G, Lampe F, Johnston SL, Holgate ST. Lower airways inflammation during rhinovirus colds in normal and in asthmatic subjects. Am J Respir Crit Care Med 1995; 151:879–886.
85. Lemanske RF Jr, Dick EC, Swenson CA, Vrtis RF, Busse WW. Rhinovirus upper respiratory infection increases airway hyperreactivity and late asthmatic reactions. J Clin Invest 1989; 83:1–10.
86. Calhoun WJ, Swenson CA, Dick EC, Schwartz LB, Lemanske JR, Busse WW. Experimental rhinovirus 16 infection potentiates histamine release after antigen bronchoprovocation in allergic subjects. Am Rev Respir Dis 1991; 144:1267–1273.
87. Picken JJ, Niewoehner DE, Chester EH. Prolonged effects of viral infections of the upper respiratory tract upon small airways. Am J Med 1972; 52:738–746.
88. Fridy WW Jr, Ingram RH Jr, Hierholzer JC, Coleman MT. Airways function during mild viral respiratory illnesses. The effect of rhinovirus infection in cigarette smokers. Ann Intern Med 1974; 80:150–155.
89. Corne JM, Marshall C, Smith S, Schreiber J, Sanderson G, Holgate ST, Johnston SL. Frequency, severity, and duration of rhinovirus infections in asthmatic and nonasthmatic individuals: a longitudinal cohort study Lancet 2002; 359:831–834.
90. Julius MH. T-dependent B-cell activation—molecules involved in mediating interaction and introduction signals. Ann Immunol 1984; 135:85–88.
91. Jenkins CR, Breslin AB. Upper respiratory tract infections and airway reactivity in normal and asthmatic subjects. Am Rev Respir Dis 1984; 130:879–883.
92. Haby MM, Peat JK, Woolcock AJ, Sokhandan M, McFadden ERJ, Huang YT, Mazanec MB. Effect of passive smoking, asthma, and respiratory infection on lung function in Australian children. The contribution of respiratory viruses to severe exacerbations of asthma in adults. Pediatr Pulmonol 1994; 18:323–329.
93. Kondo S, Ito M, Saito M, Sugimori M, Watanabe H. Progressive bronchial obstruction during the acute stage of respiratory tract infection in asthmatic children. Chest 1994; 106:100–104.
94. Grunberg K, Timmers MC, de Klerk EP, Dick EC, Sterk PJ. Experimental rhinovirus 16 infection causes variable airway obstruction in atopic asthmatic subjects. Am J Respir Crit Care Med 1999; 160:1375–1380.
95. Bardin PG, Fraenkel DJ, Sanderson G, van Schalkwyk EM, Holgate ST, Johnston SL. Peak expiratory flow changes during experimental rhinovirus infection. Eur Respir J 2000; 16: 980–985.
96. Grunberg K, Timmers MC, Smits HH, de Klerk EP, Dick EC, Spaan WJ, Hiemstra PS, Sterk PJ. Effect of experimental rhinovirus 16 colds on airway hyperresponsiveness to histamine and interleukin-8 in nasal lavage in asthmatic subjects in vivo. Clin Exp Allergy 1997; 27:36–45.
97. Seymour ML, Gilby N, Bardin PG, Fraenkel DJ, Sanderson G, Penrose GF, Holgate ST, Johnston SL, Sampson AP. Rhinovirus infection increases

5-lipoxygenase and cyclooxygenase-2 in bronchial biopsy specimens from nonatopic subjects. J Infect Dis 2002; 185:540–544.

98. Spencer CD, Beaty HN. Complications of transtracheal aspiration. N Engl J Med 1972; 286:304–306.

99. Klein JO. Diagnostic lung puncture in the pneumonias of infants and children. Pediatrics 1969; 44:486–492.

100. Gern JE, Galagan DM, Jarjour NN, Dick EC, Busse WW. Detection of rhinovirus RNA in lower airway cells during experimentally induced infection. Am J Respir Crit Care Med 1997; 155:1159–1161.

101. Arruda E, Boyle TR, Winther B, Pevear DC, Gwaltney JM, Hayden FG. Localization of human rhinovirus replication in the upper respiratory tract by in-situ hybridization. J Infect Dis 1995; 171:1329–1333.

102. Bardin PG, Johnston SL, Sanderson G, Robinson BS, Pickett MA, Fraenkel DJ, Holgate ST. Detection of rhinovirus infection of the nasal-mucosa by oligonucleotide in-situ hybridization. Am J Respir Cell Mol Biol 1994; 10:207–213.

103. Bates PJ, Bardin PG, Fraenkel DJ, Sanderson G, Holgate ST, Johnston SL. Localization of rhinovirus in the bronchial epithelium of experimentally-infected human volunteers. Am J Respir Crit Care Med 1998; A25.

104. Hakonarson H, Maskeri N, Carter C, Hodinka RL, Campbell D, Grunstein MM. Mechanism of rhinovirus-induced changes in airway smooth muscle responsiveness. J Clin Invest 1998; 102:1732–1741.

105. Thomas LH, Lareus SE, Bardin PG, Fraenkel DJ, Holgate ST, Warner JA. The effect of viral infection on histamine-release from human basophils. Am Rev Respir Dis 1993; 147:A554.

106. Skoner DP, Fireman P, Doyle WJ. Urine histamine metabolite elevations during experimental colds. J Allergy Clin Immunol 1997; 99:1703.

107. Busse WW. Decreased granulocyte response to isoproterenol in asthma during upper respiratory infections. Am Rev Respir Dis 1977; 115:783–791.

108. Hayden FG, Fritz RS, Lobo MC, Alvord WG, Strober W, Straus SE. Local and systemic cytokine responses during experimental human influenza A virus infection—relation to symptom formation and host defense. J Clin Invest 1998; 101:643-649.

109. Jacoby DB, Gleich GJ, Fryer AD. Human eosinophilic major basic protein is an endogenous allosteric antagonist at the inhibitory muscarinic M2 receptor. J Clin Invest 1993; 91:1314–1318.

110. Sluder G. Asthma as a nasal reflex. J Am Med Assoc 1919; 73:589–593.

111. Deal EC Jr, McFadden ERJ, Ingram RHJ, Breslin FJ, Jaeger JJ. Nasopulmonary mechanics—experimental evidence of the influence of the upper airway upon the lower. Am Rev Respir Dis 1980; 1980:621–628.

112. Ogura JH, Harvey JE. Nasopulmonary mechanics—experimental evidence of the influence of the upper airway upon the lower. Acta Otolaryngol (Stockh) 1971; 71:123–132.

113. Welliver R, Wong DT, Choi TS, Ogra PL. Natural history of para-influenza virus—infection in childhood. J Pediatr 1982; 101:180–187.

114. Yan K, Salome C. The response of the airways to nasal stimulation in asthmatics with rhinitis. Aust N Z J Med 1982; 12:682.

115. Fontanari P, Zattara-Hartmann MC, Burnet H, Jammes Y. Nasal eupnoeic inhalation of cold, dry air increases airway resistance in asthmatic patients. Eur Respir J 1997; 10:2250–2254.

116. McFadden ER. Nasal–sinus–pulmonary reflexes and bronchial asthma. J Allergy Clin Immunol 1986; 78:1–3.

117. Braunstahl GJ, Kleinjan A, Overbeek SE, Prins JB, Hoogsteden HC, Fokkens WJ. Segmental bronchial provocation induces nasal inflammation in allergic rhinitis patients. Am J Respir Crit Care Med 2000; 161:2051–2057.

118. Braunstahl GJ, Overbeek SE, KleinJan A, Prins JB, Hoogsteden HC, Fokkens WJ. Nasal allergen provocation induces adhesion molecule expression and tissue eosinophilia in upper and lower airways. J Allergy Clin Immunol 2001; 107:469–476.

119. Diaz PV, Calhoun WJ, Hinton KL, Avendano LF, Gaggero A, Simon V, Arredondo SM, Pinto R, Diaz A. Differential effects of respiratory syncytial virus and adenovirus on mononuclear cell cytokine responses. Am J Respir Crit Care Med. 1999; 160:1157–64.

120. Amin R, Wilmott R, Schwarz Y, Trapnell B, Stark J. Replication-deficient adenovirus induces expression of interleukin-8 by airway epithelial cells in-vitro. Hum Gene Ther 1995; 6:145–153.

121. Keicho N, Elliott WM, Hogg JC, Hayashi S. Adenovirus E1A upregulates interleukin-8 expression induced by endotoxin in pulmonary epithelial cells. Am J Physiol Lung Cell Mol Physiol 1997; 16:L1046–L1052.

122. Noah TL, Wortman IA, Hu PC, Leigh MW, Boucher RC. Cytokine production by cultured human bronchial epithelial cells infected with a replication-deficient adenoviral gene transfer vector or wild-type adenovirus type 5. Am J Respir Cell Mol Biol 1996; 14:417–424.

123. Kristoffersen AK, Sindre H, Mandi Y, Rollag H, Degre M. Effect of adenovirus 2 on cellular gene activation in blood-derived monocytes and macrophages. Apmis 1997; 105:402–409.

124. Mistchenko AS, Diez RA, Mariani AL, Robaldo J, Maffey AF, Bayley Bustamante G, Grinstein S. Cytokines in adenoviral disease in children—association of interleukin-6, interleukin-8, and tumor-necrosis-factor-alpha levels with clinical outcome. J Pediatr 1994; 124:714–720.

125. Mistchenko AS, Koch ERR, Kajon AE, Tibaldi F, Maffey AF, Diez RA. Lymphocyte subsets and cytokines in adenoviral infection in children. Acta Paediatr 1998; 87:933–939.

126. Linden M, Greiff L, Andersson M, Svensson C, Akerlund A, Bende M, Andersson E, Persson CGA. Nasal cytokines in common cold and allergic rhinitis. Clin Exp Allergy 1995; 25:166–172.

127. Vreugdenhil GR, Wijnands PG, Netea MG, van der Meer JW, Melchers WJ, Galama JM. Enterovirus-induced production of pro-inflammatory and T-helper cytokines by human leukocytes. Cytokine 2000; 12:1793–1796.

128. Adachi M, Matsukura S, Tokunaga H, Kokubu F. Expression of cytokines on

human bronchial cells induced by influenza virus. Int Arch Allergy Immunol 1997; 113:307–311.

129. Julkunen I, Melen K, Nyqvist M, Pirhonen J, Sareneva T, Matikainen S. Inflammatory responses in influenza A virus infection. Vaccine 2000;19:S32–S37.

130. Lundemose JB, Smith H, Sweet C. Cytokine release from human peripheral-blood leukocytes incubated with endotoxin with and without prior infection with influenzavirus—relevance to the sudden-infant-death syndrome. Int J Exp Pathol 1993; 74:291–297.

131. Lehmann C, Sprenger H, Nain M, Bacher M, Gemsa D. Infection of macrophages by influenza A virus: characteristics of tumour necrosis factor-alpha (TNF alpha) gene expression. Res Virol 1996; 123–130.

132. Sprenger H, Meyer RG, Kaufmann A, Bussfeld D, Rischkowsky E, Gemsa D. Selective induction of monocyte and not neutrophil-attracting chemokines after influenza A virus infection. J Exp Med 1996; 184:1191–1196.

133. Hofmann P, Sprenger H, Kaufmann A, Bender A, Hasse C, Nain M, Gemsa D. Susceptibility of mononuclear phagocytes to influenza A virus infection and possible role in the antiviral response. J Leukoc Biol 1997; 61:408–414.

134. Bussfeld D, Kaufmann A, Meyer RG, Gemsa D, Sprenger H. Differential mononuclear leukocyte attracting chemokine production after stimulation with active and inactivated influenza A virus. Cell Immunol 1998; 186:1–7.

135. Kragsbjerg P, Jones I, Vikerfors T, Holmberg H. Diagnostic-value of blood cytokine concentrations in acute pneumonia. Thorax 1995; 50:1253–1257.

136. Subauste MC, Jacoby DB, Richards SM, Proud D. Infection of a human respiratory epithelial cell line with rhinovirus. Induction of cytokine release and modulation of susceptibility to infection by cytokine exposure. J Clin Invest 1995; 96:549–557.

137. Johnston SL, Papi A, Monick MM, Hunninghake GW. Rhinoviruses induce interleukin-8 mRNA and protein production in human monocytes. J Infect Dis 1997; 175:323–329.

138. Proud D, Gwaltney JM Jr, Hendley JO, Dinarello CA, Gillis S, Schleimer RP. Increased levels of interleukin-1 are detected in nasal secretions of volunteers during experimental rhinovirus colds. J Infect Dis 1994; 169:1007–1013.

139. Chonmaitree T, Lettbrown MA, Weigent DA, Richardson L. Effect of respiratory syncytial virus (rsv) on leukocyte histamine release—role of interferon (IFN). Pediatr Res 1986; 20:A306.

140. Roberts NJ, Prill AH, Mann TN. Interleukin-1 and interleukin-1 inhibitor production by human macrophages exposed to influenza-virus or respiratory syncytial virus—respiratory syncytial virus is a potent inducer of inhibitor activity. J Exp Med 1986; 163:511–519.

141. Anderson LJ, Tsou C, Potter C, Keyserling HL, Smith TF, Ananaba G, Bangham CR. Cytokine response to respiratory syncytial virus stimulation of human peripheral blood mononuclear cells. J Infect Dis 1994; 170:1201–1208.

142. Arnold R, Werner F, Humbert B, Werchau H, Konig W. Effect of respiratory

syncytial virus-antibody complexes on cytokine (IL- 8, IL-6, TNF-alpha) release and respiratory burst in human granulocytes. Immunology 1994; 82:84–191.

143. Konig B, Streckert HJ, Krusat T, Konig W. Respiratory syncytial virus G-protein modulates cytokine release from human peripheral blood mononuclear cells. J Leukoc Biol 1996; 59:403–406.

144. Krilov L, Godfrey E, Mcintosh K. Interferon (IFN) Production by monocyte macrophages in response to respiratory syncytial virus (RSV) and parainfluenza type 3 (PI3). Pediatr Res 1985; 19:A298.

145. Tristram DA, Hicks W, Hard R. Respiratory syncytial virus and human bronchial epithelium. Arch Otolaryngol Head Neck Surg 1998; 124:777–783.

146. Calhoun WJ, Dick EC, Schwartz LB, Busse WW. A common cold virus, rhinovirus-16, potentiates airway inflammation after segmental antigen bronchoprovocation in allergic subjects. J Clin Invest 1994; 94:2200–2208.

8

Experimental Animal Models of Upper–Lower Airways Interactions

CHARLES G. IRVIN

University of Vermont
Burlington, Vermont, U.S.A.

Introduction

Sinusitis and rhinitis are significant health care issues. Yet so little is known about the mechanisms that cause these inflammatory disorders or even how to best treat these entities. To increase our understanding of this important disease, in vivo animal models or systems are often pivotal advancement of knowledge and developing new approaches to therapy.

Animal experiments can be the crucial "proof of concept" needed to prove or disprove mechanistic hypotheses (1–3). In this regard, animal systems have been invaluable in establishing cause-and-effect relationships, inasmuch as clinical studies rarely go beyond descriptive or correlative findings. In fact, the exponential increase in medical knowledge is, in part, credited to the use of animals in research (4). For instance, of the 82 Nobel Prizes in medicine or physiology awarded between 1901 and 1982, animal experiments contributed to 71% of the research. As a final, but very pertinent example, it was largely through the use of animal systems that inflammation and inflammatory mediators took center stage to explain asthma pathogenesis (2,3) and led directly to similar experiments in humans that showed the importance of inflammation in asthma.

Animal models serve many key purposes. First, they allow for a further refinement of hypotheses on mechanisms that are responsible for biological or pathological phenomena. Second, animal studies allow us to address questions or issues that are impossible or, at the least, extremely difficult to obtain from clinical studies or trials. Third, animal models allow us to obtain data critical to the development of new and unproven therapeutic interventions. So while an animal model has certain real limitations, the insight gained often leads to important advances in mechanistic knowledge. Such was clearly the case for the role of inflammation in asthma pathogenesis, and such will likely be the case in unraveling the mechanisms important in causing or maintaining rhinitis and sinusitis.

Asthma is a reasonably well described disease entity that exhibits certain pathological or pathophysiological features. To be useful, a relevant animal model needs only to exhibit some of the features of the disease (1). It is probably totally unreasonable to expect that an animal model will be exactly identical to the human condition; hence, referring to an animal as "having" asthma or sinusitis except in the broadest of terms is incorrect. For sinusitis and rhinitis, unlike asthma, there is absent a clear consensus about the features that would specifically characterize these disorders. Yet, using the same notions that have been used for animal models of asthma, a relevant process to study rhinitis/sinusitis in the nose and sinus of an experimental animal needs cause only

1. Acute inflammation, consisting of swelling and diapedisis of inflammmatory cells (type unspecified)
2. Chronic, persistent inflammation
3. Airflow obstruction associated to either acute or chronic inflammation

At first glance these requirements seem rudimentary, but because so little is known, this is all that is currently needed. With these caveats in mind, we will turn to the purpose of this chapter, which is to use findings derived from experiments in laboratory animals to explore the relationship and mechanisms of sinus–lower airways interaction.

I. Creating a Relevant Model: The Problems

It must be clearly understood from the onset that animals do not have the well-developed sinuses of humans (5); however, it is thought that the nasal passages of animals serve similar functions. In addition, the nasal passages in animals perform important temperature-regulating functions. The anatomy of the nasal/upper respiratory passages of animals shows marked interspecies differences (5). There are also significant age-dependent changes in structure. Since the majority of the current and future work will most likely be in smaller laboratory animals, the discussion is confined to rabbits, rats, and mice. The majority of the information detailing the structure of the nose and sinuses has been derived from dissection and measurements of the gross structures. Precise anatomical descriptions for various animal species can be found in standard texts and references (6–11); beyond this little more is known, however, since the anatomy of the nose and sinuses has not been as extensively explored.

A. Epithelium: Structure and Function

Rabbit

The nasal epithelium of the rabbit, like the mouse, has a predominance of Clara cells, which make up significant parts of the epithelium of the nose. Like the rat and mouse, rabbits have few submucosal glands.

Rat

Rats have been widely used for inhalation toxicology investigations, and as a result there is considerable information for this species (12). The rat nasal passages, like those of rabbits, exhibit somewhat more structural complexity than those of the mouse. Unlike the rabbit, the rat has predominance of serous cells, but like the mouse and rabbit, has few submucosal glands (13).

Mouse

Because of the reagents, antibodies, and transgenic techniques available, mice have been and will become increasingly used for studies (13). Anatomy and cellular structure of the murine nasal passages are less well described, however, than those of other laboratory animal species. Based on body size, the nasal cavity of the mouse is proportionately larger (7:1) than that of the rat (5:1). The functional reason for this difference is unknown, but the mouse breathes very rapidly (5–6 Hz), and a large nasal passage would provide more efficient gas humidification. It has been reported that about 40% of the nasal passage of mouse is olfactory epithelium (14). While 3.5% of the nasal cavity of the rat is squamous epithelium, the mouse has about 20%; therefore, the mouse has more respiratory epithelium available for air filtration. The epithelium of the nasal passages of the mouse also has a predominance of Clara cells and few submucosal glands.

It has been speculated that the significant amount of nonciliated cuboidal epithelium in rodents provides protection against xenobiotics owing to high amounts of cytochrome P450-dependent monooxygenase (13) present in these cells. This is in sharp contrast to primate species. There are also considerable differences in the cell types, cellular composition, and gross and subgross morphology of the nasal passages between mice and rats and mice and primates.

B. Nerves

Neural innervation of the sensory type originates from the trigeminal nerves via both the ophthalmic and maxillary branches. Nonmylineated nerve fibers are frequently found within the epithelium and are responsible for a myriad of reflexes. Autonomic neural innervation can include parasympathetic, sympathetic, nonadrenergic inhibition, and noncholinergic excitation. In general, very little is known about the function of these nerves beyond some of the stimuli that activate autonomic reflexes. The sole exception is the rabbit, where investigations by J. H. Widdicombe beginning in the 1960s provided some information (15–17). Of interest in mice, the presence of neural peptides appears to be especially complicated (18,19), but the function of such a complicated network of peptides in this species is again unknown.

II. Asthma and Sinusitis

Elsewhere we have outlined the factors indicating that upper respiratory tract disease processes in humans are linked largely through circumstantial evidence (20) that provides indisputable evidence that sinusitis and rhinitis and other disorders of the upper respiratory tract are strongly associated with asthma. Yet, there is little definitive information linking upper respiratory tract inflammation directly to asthma. Even if sinusitis does play a causal role in asthma, the exact mechanisms remain uncertain (20,21).

Numerous anecdotal and epidemiological studies have reported a high coincidence of asthma with either rhinitis or sinusitis. Bullen (22), Gottlieb (23), and Weille (24) reported that 26 to 70% of asthmatic adults had coexistent sinusitis, and more recent studies corroborate these findings (25–27). Despite this clear association between sinusitis or rhinitis and asthma, there continues to be a poor appreciation and, indeed many doubt, that upper airways disease is a *cause* of asthma (20,21). The strongest evidence in favor of such a relationship comes from an array of clinical investigations indicating that specific treatment of the nasal/sinus passages helps patients with asthma (28–34). In refractory cases, surgical intervention can often effect a remission of asthma (28,34,35). These studies provide more convincing evidence for a causal link between sinusitis and asthma but still lack the definitive proof one would like.

Another point of view is that significant upper respiratory tract disease is merely another manifestation of global airways disease (21,36). Lower airways hyperresponsiveness can be demonstrated in about 15 to 56% of individuals who have only allergic rhinitis (37–39). On the other hand, several investigators have shown no alteration in lower airways function in patients with allergic rhinitis and asthma (40–42). Thus, the actual causal role of the upper respiratory tract in precipitating or enhancing disease in the lungs still remains controversial.

III. Rabbit Model of Asthma and Sinusitis

A. Asthma

A model of the late asthmatic response was initially developed in the rabbit to investigate the immunopathogenesis of the response to the airways to antigen (43–45). Animals can be rendered immune by injections of adjuvant and antigen (*Alternaria* or ragweed) and then subjected to an inhalation challenge of the same antigen. The physiological and pathological findings following antigen challenge were qualitatively similar to the responses that occur in atopic asthmatics after bronchial challenge with antigen. As in man, the rabbit develops a delayed airflow limitation or late asthmatic response (LAR) that usually is greater than the airflow limitation observed during the initial time points or immediate asthmatic response (IAR) (45). That the mechanisms involved might be similar to those involved in man is suggested by the reaction of this model to common antiasthma drugs. Cromolyn sodium blocked the IAR and LAR, while corticosteroids inhibit only the LAR, and β-adrenergic agents are ineffective in reversing the airflow limitation once the LAR has occurred (43,45).

Histopathologically, this model also parallels the physiological events in man, since granulocytes have been be recovered from bronchoalveolar lavage (BAL) or observed within the large and small airways (46,47), where within the bronchioles, 80% of the granulocytes were eosinophils. Thus, in this animal model, the LAR has been associated with significant increases in granulocytes within both bronchi and bronchioles, as well as a heightened airways responsiveness to an inhaled agonist. Rabbits, when made neutropenic with the administration of nitrogen mustard, exhibited an IAR but no LAR or increase in responsiveness (48). Moreover, neutrophil-rich populations of white cells appearing at the time of ragweed exposure were transferred into control (non-ragweed-immune) rabbits, which had neither asthmatic responses nor changes in airways responsiveness after exposure, or into ragweed-immune rabbits, which now had early and late decreases in lung function, as well as a marked increase in airways responsiveness. It would appear that in this rabbit model, both the late response and the subsequent increase in airways responsiveness is absolutely dependent on the presence of inflammatory granulocytes.

Immunization and antigen challenge represents a realistic approach to the study of asthma pathogenesis (1–3,49), but the approach is not without problems. The most important of these are the time, costs, and energy required to manipulate such models. Accordingly, researchers have employed any number of other inflammatory stimuli. Ozone exposures cause both inflammation and hyperresponsiveness in dogs (49–51), guinea pigs (52), and rats (53). Toluene diisocyanate (TDI) will cause inflammation and airways hyperresponsiveness in quinea pigs (49,54), but whether these effects are granulocyte dependent is unclear (55). Endotoxin produces airways hyperresponsiveness in sheep (56,57) and in certain inbred strains of rats (58), a result that has been associated with increased airways responses to inhaled agonists.

We have also investigated the ability of a modified complement fragment, C5a des Arg, to induce inflammation and subsequent airways dysfunction (59) in the rabbit. C5a des Arg is the fifth component of complement, which has had the terminal arginine removed. C5a des Arg is also a potent phlogistic factor but, unlike C5a does not have a direct spasmogenic effect on smooth muscle. When administered to rabbit airways, this molecule caused an inflammatory lesion of the airways, bronchospasm, and an increased responsiveness to inhaled histamine (59). Granulocyte depletion abrogated the effects of C5a des Arg. Yet, the presence of inflammatory cells airways does not always automatically translate to physiological dysfunction, as we showed in the sham-treated animals, which also developed airways inflammation but without an increase in airways responsiveness.

Our current operational scheme (Fig. 1) shows a much more involved process. Aside from the importance of cellular activation, some of the additional features include the following:

1. Granulocyte activation probably involves both a process of "priming" and then "triggering."
2. The exact spectrum of mediators involved is dependent on activation and probably is critical to the specificity of the reponse.
3. These mediators probably target structures other than the smooth muscle.
4. In all likelihood, the mechanisms that control the occurence of airway narrowing are quite different from the mechanisms that determine heightened airways responsiveness, two events that can be dissociated.

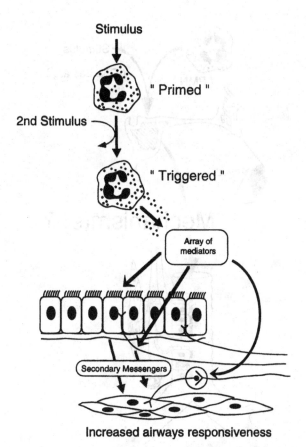

Figure 1 A current working hypothesis of the relationship between inflammatory cells and mediator release in affecting increased airways responsiveness. Cells likely pass through a two-step process where first "priming" occurs by exposure to the primary stimulus. The secondary then "triggers" the release (or greater amounts) of a spectrum of mediators. This spectrum of mediators targets a variety of tissues, which may include the generation of secondary messengers.

B. Sinusitis

Our purpose in developing an animal model of sinusitis (60,61) was twofold: first, to develop a model in which sinusitis and airways hyperresponsiveness could be associated and, second, to investigate some of the postulated mechanisms that might explain this association (Fig. 2).

Rabbits underwent pulmonary function testing (46,48,59), and a histamine dose–response relationship was determined to establish a baseline. Animals were then assigned randomly to the various treatment groups.

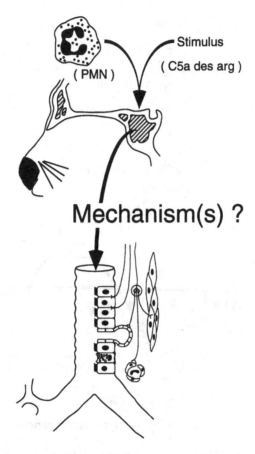

Figure 2 Unanswered questions concerning the mechanistic link between upper airways inflammation and lower airways responsivesness are (1) What is released from the inflammatory process within the nose and sinuses that increases responsiveness? and (2) How do those products increase responsiveness?

As a control, the maxillary sinus on each side was injected with a sterile saline (Fig. 3) and then the animal was positioned prone and the head elevated. Sixteen hours post treatment, animals were reanesthetized and retested. Rabbits that received sinus injections of the saline–protein diluent demonstrated no change in airway responsiveness (Fig. 4A). The baseline EC_{50} (mean $\pm$ SEM) for specific pulmonary conductance (SGL) was 2.39 $\pm$ 0.5 compared with postsaline, 2.39 $\pm$ 0.6 mg/mL (NS).

In another group of rabbits, the maxillary sinus was injected with human recombinant C5a des Arg. Rabbits that received C5a Arg, posi-

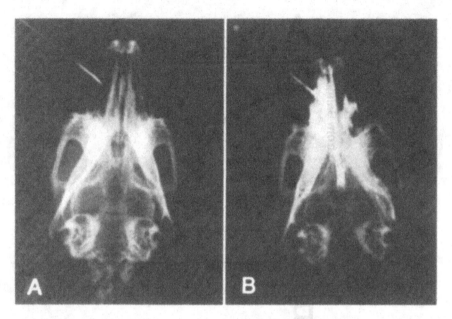

Figure 3 Radiographs of a rabbit head. (A) Needle is passed into the paranasal sinus. (B) Radiocontrast has been injected; Note passage of material to the contralateral side.

tioned head up, showed a marked increase in airways responsiveness [EC_{50} SGL pretreatment was 5.35 ± 1.0 vs posttreatment 1.44 ± 0.5 mg/mL ($p = 0.005$)] (Fig. 4B). The sinus lavage fluid showed a predominance of polymorphonuclear cells. However, sinus lavage following saline injection was similar to that of normal, unmanipulated rabbits: that is, no evidence of granulocyte inflammation.

C. Mechanisms Linking Sinusitis to Lower Airways Dysfunction

Several mechanisms might account for our observation that an inflammatory process in the upper airways was associated with hyperresponsiveness of the lower airways. Astutely, many of these mechanisms were first proposed by Gottlieb in 1925 (23). Based on his simple clinical observations as a physician in private practice, he had postulated several mechanisms that might link upper airways processes to lower airways symptoms (Table 1). Of the mechanisms postulated by Gottlieb, we thought the most likely were reabsorption of inflammatory products and subsequent delivery via the circulation to the lower airways, elicitation of a nasobronchial

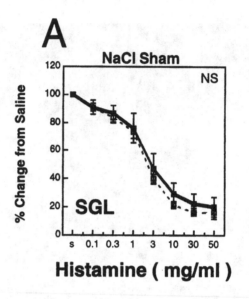

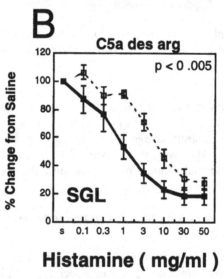

Figure 4 Following the injection of saline (NaCl sham) or 30 μg of human C5a des Arg into each paranasal sinus, the animals have airways responsiveness to inhaled histamine determined prior to treatment (dashed lines). (A) Following injection of saline, there is no shift in the dose response curves. (B) Following C5a des Arg, the dose–responsive curve shifts left and the change is significant. Open symbols and bars are prechallenge and closed symbols and bars are postchallenge. Data points are mean ± SEM. In both experiments the animals were positioned head-up for induction SGL. (Adapted from Ref. 60.)

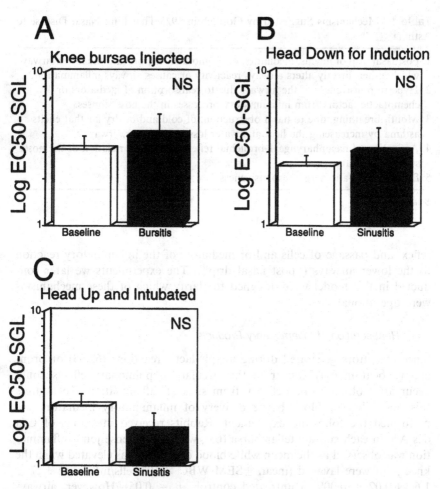

Figure 5 C5a des Arg (30 μg each sinus) was injected into both knee bursae (A) or sinuses (B, C), and determinations of the histamine dose–response characteristics were made 16 h later. Airway responsiveness (Log EC_{50}-SGL) was not increased following induction of bursitis, suggesting that the responsible factors are not absorbed and conveyed to the lung by the circulations. Further, responsiveness was not increased if the animal was positioned head down (B) or positioned head up and intubated prior to C5a des Arg injection (C). Prevention with either method (B or C) of passage of materials from the nose and sinuses appears to prevent airways hyperresponsiveness. (Adapted from Ref. 60.)

Table 1 Mechanisms Suggested by Gottlieb in 1925 That Link Nasal Disease to Asthma

1. Postnasal drip of mucus, mediators, or chemotactic factors into the lower airways which either directly alters airways reactivity or causes airways inflammation.
2. Hyperresponsiveness of the airways due to reabsorption of mediators or chemotactic factors from inflammatory processes in the nose sinuses.
3. Mouth breathing, due to nasal obstruction, of cold and/or dry air that elicits asthma by increaseing the heat and water loss in the lower airways.
4. Activation of nasopharyngeal–bronchial reflexes due to stimulation of the nose, sinuses, or pharynx.
5. Diminished β-adrenergic responsiveness.

Source: Ref. 23.

reflex, and passage of cells and/or mediators of the inflammatory reaction to the lower airways ("post nasal drip"). The experiments we later conducted in this model were designed to clarify which of these mechanisms were operational.

Reabsorption of Inflammatory Products

Since mediators generated during anaphylactic reactions (62,63) or bronchoprovocation (64) appear in the circulation, pulmonary effects could occur after blood-borne delivery from sites of inflammation. To address this possibility of blood-borne delivery of inflammatory mediators, we performed the following experiment. Rabbits received injections of C5a des Arg in each suprapatellar bursa (65), where an intense joint inflammation was observed as the mean white blood cell count was elevated when the knee joint were lavaged (mean $\pm$SEM WBC $\times$ 10^6 cells/mL/joint: 3.27 $\pm$ 1.6 vs 0.02 $\pm$ 0.009 in untreated controls, p = 0.05). However, airways responsiveness to histamine was unchanged (EC_{50} pre 3.70 $\pm$ 0.9 vs post 3.95 $\pm$ 1.0 mg/mL p = NS) (Fig. 5A).

A failure to show an increase in airways responsiveness provides circumstantial evidence that reabsorption of inflammatory mediators may not be an important mechanism in this model. However, this negative finding could have been due either to the small quantities of inflammatory mediators present, or alternatively, to inadequate amount of mediators, which might have been reabsorbed and rapidly metabolized in the vascular space. Of interest, we did observe in the occasional animal a marked increase in responsiveness (49). Thus, although this mechanism may be operative in some forms of lower airways obstruction, data to support its contribution in the setting of upper respiratory tract inflammation in the current model could not be demonstrated.

Nasobronchial Reflexes

Activation of a nasobronchial reflex is suggested as the second mechanism that might potentially explain how an inflammatory process in the upper airways would lead to a change in lower airways function. Sluder in 1919 (66) first proposed such a reflex arc, comprising a sensory limb consisting of receptors in the nose, sinuses, and pharynx that project afferent signals through the trigeminal, facial, and glossopharyngeal nerves to the medulla. From there, connections are made to the vagal nucleus, from which efferent impulses project to the lower airways via the vagus nerve, resulting in bronchoconstriction (67). Following nasal provocation with irritant agents, such reflexes have been clearly demonstrated in both animals (68–70) and humans (71–73). Further, a nasobronchial reflex has been shown to be operative in an animal model of viral upper respiratory tract infection (74) or antigen challenge (75). In man, such reflexes could not be demonstrated under conditions of allergen-induced nasal inflammation (40–42). We performed the following experiment in the rabbit system, to indirectly address the postulate that neural reflexes originating in the upper airways caused the observed increase in lower airways responsiveness.

Rabbits underwent injections of C5a des Arg in each maxillary sinus while positioned head down for 40 mins. When positioned in this way for the induction period, these animals failed to show airways hyperresponsiveness even though there was similar sinusitis present.

We must conclude that in this model of experimental sinusitis, there was no evidence for either bronchoconstriction or nonspecific airways hyperresponsiveness due to the sinus inflammation alone, which argues against either a reflex or an absorption of mediators from the sinuses, even though nasobronchial reflexes are known to exist in this species (16,17).

"Postnasal Drip"

Passage ("postnasal drip") of the chemotactic factors, inflammatory cells, or their products into the lower airways was the third mechanism investigated to explain the association between sinusitis and airways hyperresponsiveness observed in this model.

An endotracheal tube was placed prior to sinus injections of C5a des Arg to physically block the passage of cells or mediators from the nose to the lower airways. These intubated animals demonstrated a degree of sinusitis nearly identical to that of a group of animals that were positioned head up, but unintubated. Yet these animals were not hyperresponsive (Fig. 5C). Animals which were placed head down also failed to increase airways responsiveness (Fig. 5B), which makes it unlikely that either the reabsorption of mediators from the sinuses or activation of a nasobronchial reflex is a significant operational mechanism.

Multiple secretagogues, including potent bronchoconstrictors, are generated within the nose following nasal allergen challenge (76,77). Despite this, several studies showed no change in pulmonary function after nasal allergen or histamine provocation in patients with hay fever or asthma (40,42). Several explanations for the negative results of these clinical studies are suggested by the findings of the rabbit model. One is the possibility that insufficient time was allowed for the development of lower airways dysfunction. In the rabbit, alterations in lung function were observed at 16 h, but not earlier, at 4 h (data not presented). Second, as we have shown in human studies (78), a significant result would have been detected in these studies if the correct outcome variable used in these clinical studies had been measures of airways responsiveness.

What Is Conveyed from the Nose to the Lungs?

Passage of some signal from the inflammatory process into the lower airways best explained the results of these animal studies. Silent pulmonary aspiration of nasopharyngeal secretions occurs frequently in normal humans during sleep (79) or depressed consciousness (80). Postnasal drip is often implicated as a principal cause of chronic cough (81).

Since we had previously demonstrated that increased lower airways responsiveness can be induced in rabbits following direct pulmonary inhalation of aerosolized complement fragments (59), the results of our study may be due merely to passage of the chemotactic factor to the lower airways. We addressed this concern with two different approaches. The first evidence that chemotactic factors were not involved was that recovery of significant numbers of inflammatory cells from the lower airways, with lavage, could not be demonstrated in any of the groups. Enumeration of BAL cellularity shows no significant differences in total numbers of white blood cells (polymorphonuclear cells PMN), mononuclear cells, or eosinophils compared with controls (i.e., unmanipulated, untreated rabbits). Second, examination of the lungs immediately after sacrifice showed no gross evidence of inflammation.

We conclude that first, the increase in lower airways responsiveness is not due to the mere dripping of the chemotactic signal into the lower airways. If that had been the case, we should have found a significant pathological lesion in the airways and recovered significant numbers of granulocytes with lavage, but we did not. Second, a failure to show inflammation in the lower airways when coupled with the known adhesiveness of stimulated inflammatory cells (57,62) suggests that the increase in lower airways responsiveness is also not due to the passage of inflammatory cells from the sinuses to the lung. There is also the clear indication that airways dysfunction can be caused by a mechanism that is associated with a distal site of inflammation. In the conditions of these experiments, sinus/nasal inflammation, a signal that is not chemotactic, is physically transported to the lower airways, where a significant effect is observed. These findings are important because they show a situation of lungs that are dysfunctional but not inflamed. If this occurs in humans, then lavage or biopsy results of the lower airways may be less definitive than they appear.

IV. Rat Model of Asthma and Sinusitis

In a series of studies (75,82–85) the laboratory of J. G. Martin has developed a well-characterized animal model of both lower airways dysfunction (asthma) and upper airways dysfunction (sinusitis). The major impetus for the development of such a model was to investigate the contribution of the upper airways to the total respiratory system response to various bronchomotor agonist and antigens. Moreover, it is known that laryngeal narrowing and responses within the nose and sinuses are important to the asthmatic response in humans (86–88), and so these studies on rats may be relevant.

Selective challenge of the upper and lower airways was accomplished by an ingenious exposure system in which the rat's muzzle was inserted into an exposure box. The pressure drop between the box and trachea defined the upper airways response, whereas the pressure drop from the tracheal cannula to an esophageal catheter detects changes in the lower airways. By rearranging the exposure from the nose to the tracheal cannula, a differential exposure to the nose or lungs could be accomplished (75,82).

Several interesting observations were made prior to any specific challenges. The upper airways resistance of the rat accounts for about 80% of the total respiratory system resistance, in comparison to 45% in guinea pigs, 50% in cats, and 70% in humans (82). Upper airways resistance was also dependent on the phase of respiration; for upper airways resistance, expiratory was much greater than inspiratory resistance, and the former exhibited a linear pressure–flow relationship. These findings have not been completely explained. As in humans, a component of upper airways resistance was shown to be glottic closure (82,83).

The response of upper airways resistance to challenge was demonstrated to be large for all models of challenge, but there were marked differences between types of challenge agent. Following challenge with methacholine (82), the upper airways resistance was much larger than the lower airways resistance (Fig. 6). While the expiratory resistance response was larger, this was not uniformly observed in all animals. Unlike methacholine, antigen challenge (75) in sensitized animals was due to changes in the inspiratory phase of respiratory and highly correlated to the response in the lower airways ($r = 0.94$; $p < 0.001$). The antigen response is also characterized by a late phase reaction that was consistently observed but highly variable in time of onset, magnitude, and duration (83). The response in the lower airways was delayed by half an hour, was shorter, and did not correlate in magnitude to the upper airways response. This latter finding suggests that different mechanisms are operational in the nose and in the lower airways.

The mechanism of this upper airways response in the rat is unclear. While the response to methacholine might be nasal secretions, which were

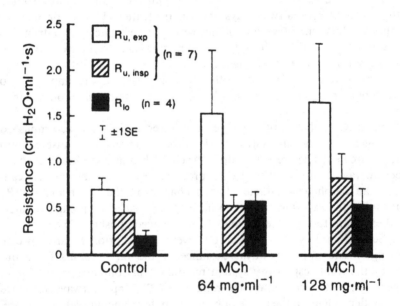

Figure 6 Comparison of the response of positioned resistance in the rat to methacholine (MCH) challenge. Upper airways partitioned into resistance (R_u) and lower airway resistance (R_{lo}) was measured following methacholine challenge selectively administered to the nose and upper airways. Note the increase in lower airways resistance even though these airways were not directly challenged. (Data from Ref. 82.)

indeed observed following methacholine challenge (75), the major site of airway narrowing was felt to be the larynx. Treatment with atropine prior to antigen exposure (75) diminished the lower airways response and the expiratory upper airway response, but not the upper airway inspiratory response (Fig. 7). These results clearly show that each aspect of the upper airway response is differentially regulated. It is clear that reflexes are operational in the nose of the rat as expiratory upper airways resistance increased following methacholine challenge to the lower airway, (Fig. 8). Most intriguing was the loss of correlation between upper and lower airways responses upon treatment with atropine ($r = 0.94$ vs 0.07), suggesting that reflexes arise from the nose and project to the lung and coordinate the upper and lower airways responses. Again, the exact purpose of such an integrated response is unclear.

The data clearly illustrate several points. First, that the response in the nose is very significant in this species. Second, that even in this species of rodent, the mechanical resistance of the nose is very complex and is controlled by several mechanisms that are at best unclear. A third point these studies make is that the response of the upper airways shows both strain and

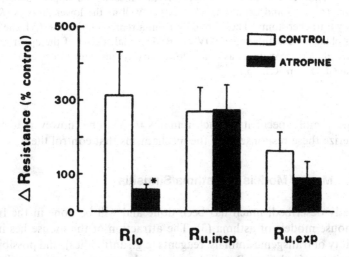

Figure 7 The change in resistance of the lower airways (R_{lo}) or upper airways, both inspiratory ($R_{u, insp}$) and expiratory ($R_{u, exp}$), in rats challenged with antigen (OVA) as a control (open bars). If the rats were premedicated with atropine (solid bars), the response in the nose was not blocked by altering the response in the lower airways even though the response in the lower airways was decreased. Asterisk is $p < 0.05$. (Data from Ref. 75.)

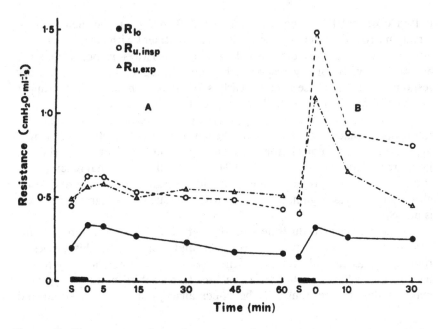

Figure 8 Time course of the changes in resistance of the upper airway, both inspiratory ($R_{u, insp}$) and expiratory ($R_{u, exp}$), as well as the lower airways (R_{lo}) as divided by a tracheostomy. These are data from a representative rat. (A) The lower airway is challenged with antigen (OVA). (B) The challenge is of the upper airway. Note marked increase in upper as well as lower airways resistance when either airway is challenged. (From Ref. 75.)

challenge stimuli specificity. Much remains to be done, however, to better characterize these responses and the mechanisms that control them.

V. Mouse Models of Asthma/Sinusitis

As already described, much has been done and will be done in the future using mouse models of asthma (3). The attraction of the mouse lies in the availability of transgenic animals, reagents (e.g., antibodies), and possibilities for genetic manipulation. By using various schemes of antigen sensitization and aerosol exposure, a constant and significant response to antigen can be observed (89–92). Others have shown the antigen response in mouse airways conforms to the TH_1/TH_2 parenchyma (3,93). Much has been learned and much will be learned with mouse systems concerning lower airways response (3,93).

Very little is known about the response of the nose and sinus to antigen or challenges in the mouse. It is common practice in some laboratories to instill antigen into the nose rather than into the lung (94,95). In addition, several recent publications show the feasibility of using bacterial inoculations in the mouse sinuses to develop a rhinosinusitis model (96,97). Renz and colleagues (89) have shown that following 20 days of antigen exposure, while the airways are relatively free of inflammation or structural changes (Fig. 9), the nose shows marked alterations of structure and, in particular, a thickening of the epithelium (Fig. 10). Clearly, this demonstrates the impact of antigen exposure on nasal structure. Since the data are reminiscent of those from the rabbit model in that there is lower airway dysfunction without local inflammation, it is tempting to speculate that the changes in lower airway function in this system may also be due to a similar "postnasal drip" mechanism.

In a recent study (91), we evaluated the use of a noninvasive approach to assess lung function in the mouse. Since the antigen exposures were whole-body exposures, we presume that a major site of deposition would be the nasal passages (98). We showed that there is a very significant response

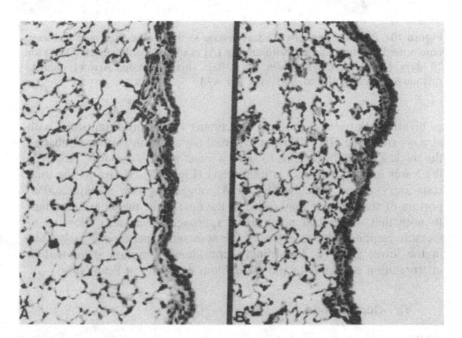

Figure 9 Photomicrographs of longitudinal sections of lobar airways taken from mice challenged 20 days with antigen (OVA) (B), or unsensitized (A), sections stained with hematoxylin and eosin. Magnification 400×. (From Ref. 89.)

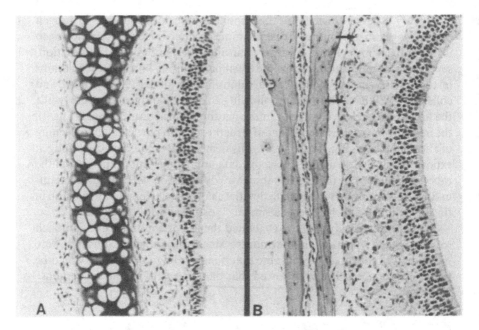

Figure 10 Photomicrographs of nasal passage sections taken from mice that were unsensitized and unchallenged with antigen (A) challenged with antigen (OVA) for 20 days (B). Hematoxylin–eosin stain 400× magnification. Arrows indicate submucosal gland proliferation. (From Ref. 89.)

in breathing pattern as the flow and timing of the breathing slows with airways challenge (91). When we bypassed the upper airways by intubating the trachea, we still were able to show a lower airways response. However, the lower airways response is diminished (Fig. 11B) relative to the total respiratory system response (Fig. 11A), suggesting that a major (50%) portion of the response may reside in the nose. It is, therefore, important to note that using such noninvasive approaches may also allow us to measure responses due to events in the nose and upper airways only—not in the lower airways. Accordingly, considerable caution is advised in interpretation of such data and the dubious end point of Penh (99).

VI. Conclusions

While sinusitis and other inflammatory diseases of the upper respiratory tract have long been associated with asthma, there is little direct evidence that links these processes mechanistically (21,20).

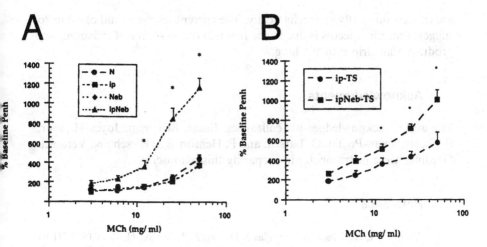

Figure 11 The response of a breathing parameter, the enhanced pause (Penh) to inhaled methacholine. Mice were sensitized and challenged with antigen (OVA). (A) Mice were not tracheotomized when challenged with antigen: N, control untreated; IP (intraperitoneal antigen) sensitized to antigen only; Neb, aerosol challenge of antigen only; IP Neb, sensitized and challenged with antigen. (B) IP-TS (TS, tracheostomy) indicates mice that were sensitized but not challenged, whereas IP Neb-TS mice were challenged with antigen. These mice were tracheotomized for the measurements of responsiveness to methacholine. Note that when IP Neb-TS is compared with IP Neb, bypassing the upper airways diminishes the response. This suggests that a significant proportion of the response in the intact animal is due to an upper airway response. (Data from Ref. 91.)

Clear, valid reasons for employing animal models to study human disease processes exist. Yet, limitations exist for any animal model of a human disease, and the models described here are not exceptions. Furthermore, it must be recalled that important species differences exist which limit strict application of results to the human condition. In reality, there is not one best model; each model has merit, since relevant questions can be addressed and important conclusions can be derived. Indeed, it should be remembered that the current recognition that asthma is largely an inflammatory process came from animal experiments. Studies in animal systems show evidence for a plausible mechanism involved in the response the association of sinusitis and asthma. Whether these findings explain the common clinical association in humans of upper airways disease to lower airways dysfunction in sinusitis and asthma remains to be determined.

It is perhaps appropriate to speculate at this point about the anecdotal, but dramatic, improvement in the asthma of patients with sinusitis who are treated surgically or mechanically. The current results would cause us to suggest that this success is due to the removal of the source of inflammatory products that drip into the lung.

Acknowledgments

The author acknowledges his colleagues, Susan Brugman, Joyce Honour, P. Giclas, Yuan-Po Tu, G. Larsen, and P. Henson. Sue Hirsch and Veronica Gardiner were instrumental in preparing this manuscript.

References

1. Wanner A, Abraham W, Douglas J, Drazen J, Richerson H, Ram JS. NHLBI Workshop summary: models of airways hyperresponsiveness. Am Rev Respir Dis 1990; 141: 253–257.
2. Larsen GL. Experimental models of reversible airway obstruction. In: Crystal RG, West JB, eds. The Lung: Scientific Foundations. New York: Raven Press, 1991; 953–965.
3. Tu Y-P, Larsen GL, Irvin CG. Utility of mice in investigating asthma pathogenesis. Eur Respir Rev 1995; 5(29): 224–230.
4. Nicoll CS, Russell SM. Mozart Alexander the Great, and the animal rights/liberation philosophy. FASEB J 1991; 5: 2888–2892.
5. Gross EA, Morgan KT. Architecture of nasal passages and larynx. In: Parent RA, ed. Comparative Biology of the Normal Lung. Boca Raton, FL: CRC Press, 1992.
6. Negus VE. The Comparative Anatomy of the Nose and Paranasal Sinuses. Livingston Press, Edinburgh, UK, 1958.
7. Miller MB. Miller's Anatomy of the Dog. Philadelphia: WB Saunders, 1979.
8. Hebel R, Stromberg MW. Anatomy of the Laboratory Rat. Baltimore: William & Wilkins, 1976.
9. Cooper G, Schiller. Anatomy of the Guinea Pig. Cambridge, MA: President and Fellows of Harvard College, 1975.
10. Popesko P, Rajtova V, Horak J. A Color Atlas of Anatomy of Small Laboratory Animals. Volume One: Rabbit and Guinea Pig. London: Wolfe Publishing, 1990.
11. Popesko P, Rajtova V, Horak J. A Color Atlas of Anatomy of Small Laboratory Animals. Volume Two: Rat, Mouse and Hamster. London: Wolfe Publishing, 1990.
12. Toxicology of the Nasal Passages. Barrow CS, ed. New York: Hemisphere, 1986.
13. Harkema JR. Epithelial cells of the nasal passages. In: Parent RA, ed., Comparative Biology of the Normal Lung. Boca Raton, FL: CRC Press, 1992.

14. Gross EA, Swenberg JA, Field S, Popp JA. Comparative morphometry of the nasal cavity in rats and mice. J Anat 1982; 135: 83.
15. Widdecombe JG. Regulation of tracheobronchial smooth muscle. Physiol Rev 1963; 43: 1–120
16. Widdicombe JG. The physiology of the nose. Clin Chest Med 1986; 7(2):159–170.
17. Karczewski W, Widdicombe JG. The role of the vagus nerve in the respiratory and circulatory responses to intravenous histamine an phenyl diguanide in rabbits. J. Physiol 1969; 201: 271–291.
18. Uddman RE, Sundher F. Neuropeptides in the airways: a review. Am Rev Respir Dis 1987; 136: 53.
19. Uddman RE, Malm L, Sundher F. Substance-P containing nerves, nerve fibers in the nasal mucosa. Arch Otorhinolaryngol 1983; 238: 9.
20. Adinoff AD, Irvin CG. Upper respiratory tract disease and asthma. Sem Respir Med 1987; 8(4): 308–314.
21. McFadden ER. Nasal–sinus–pulmonary reflexes and bronchial asthma. J Allergy Clin Immunol 1986; 78(1): 1–3.
22. Bullen SS. Incidence of asthma in 400 cases of chronic sinusitis. J Allergy 1932; 4: 402–407.
23. Gottlieb MJ. Relation of intranasal disease in the production of bronchial asthma. JAMA 1925; 85(2): 105–107.
24. Weille FL. Studies in asthma: nose and throat in 500 cases of asthma. N Engl J Med 1936; 215: 235–239.
25. Rachelefsky GS, Goldberg M, Katz RM, Boris G, Gyepes MT, Shapiro M, Mickey MR, Finegold SM, Siegel SC. Sinus disease in children with respiratory allergy. J Allergy Clin Immunol 1978; 61: 310–314.
26. Adinoff AD, Wood RW, Buschman D, Cummings NP. Chronic sinusitis in childhood asthma: correlation of symptoms, x-ray, cultures and response to treatment. Pediatr Res 1983; 17: 373.
27. Schwartz HJ. Thompson JS, Sher TH, Ross RJ. Occult sinus abnormalities in the asthmatic patient. Arch Intern Med 1987; 147: 2194–2196.
28. Slavin RG, Cannon RE, Friedman WH, Palitang E, Sundaram M. Sinusitis and bronchial asthma. J Allergy Clin Immunol 1980; 60: 250–257.
29. Friedman R, Ackerman M, Wald E, Cassellmant M, Friday G, Fireman P. Asthma and bacterial sinusitis in children. J Allergy Clin Immunol 1984; 74: 185–189.
30. Phipatanakul CS, Slavin RG. Bronchial asthma produced by paranasal sinusitis. Arch Otolaryngol 1974; 100: 109–112.
31. Businco L, Fiore L, Frediani T, Artuso A, diFazio A, Bellioni P. Clinical and therapeutic aspects of sinusitis in children with bronchial asthma. Int J Pediatr Otorhinolaryngol 1981; 3: 287–294.
32. Cummings NP, Lere JL, Wood R, Adinoff A. Effect of treatment of sinusitis on asthma and bronchial reactivity: results of a double-blind study. J Allergy Clin Immunol 1983; 73(suppl): 143 (abstr).
33. Rachelefsky GS, Katz RM, Siegel SC. Chronic sinus disease with associated reactive airways disease in children. Pediatrics 1984; 73: 526–529.

34. Werth G. The role of sinusitis in severe asthma. Immun Allergy Pract 1984; 7(3): 45–49.

35. Juntunen K, Tarkkanen J, Makinon J. Caldwell Luc operation in the treatment of childhood bronchial asthma. Laryngoscope 1984; 94: 249–251.

36. Friday GA, Fireman P. Sinusitis and asthma: clinical and pathogenetic relationships. Clin Chest Med 1988; 9(4): 557–565.

37. Fish JE, Rosenthal R, Menkes H. Airway responses to methacholine in allergic and nonallergic subjects. Am Rev Respir Dis 1976; 113: 579–586.

38. Townley RG, Ryo VY, Kolotbin BM, Kangi B. Bronchial sensitivity to methacholine in current and former asthmatic and allergic rhinitic patients and control subjects. J Allergy Clin Immunol 1975; 56: 429–442.

39. Cockcroft DW, Killian DN, Mellon JJA, Hargreave PE. Bronchial reactivity to inhaled histamine: a method and clinical survey. Clin Allergy 1977; 7: 235–243.

40. Schumacher MJ, Cota KA, Taussig LM. Pulmonary response to nasal challenge testing of atopic subjects with stable asthma. J Allergy Clin Immunol 1986; 78: 30–35.

41. Hoehne JH, Reed CE. Where is the allergic reaction in ragweed asthma? J Allergy Clin Immunol 1971; 48(1): 36–39.

42. Rosenberg GL, Rosenthal RR, Norman PS. Inhalation challenge with ragweed pollen in ragweed-sensitive asthmatics. J Allergy Clin Immunol 1983; 71(3): 302–310.

43. Larsen GL. The rabbit model of the late asthmatic response. Chest 1985; 87: 184S–188S.

44. Larsen GL, Shampain MP, Marsh WR, Behrens BL. An animal model of the late asthmatic response to antigen challenge. In: Kay AB, Austen KF, Lichtenstein LM, eds. Asthma: physilogy, Immunopharmacology, and Treatment, 3rd International Symposium. London: Academic Press, 1984; 245–262.

45. Shampain MP, Behrens BL, Larsen GL, Henson PM. An animal model of late pulmonary responses to Alternaria challenge. Am Rev Respir Dis 126: 493–498.

46. Marsh WR, Irvin CG, Murphy KR, Behrens BL, Larsen GL. Increases in airway reactivity and pulmonary inflammation following the late asthmatic response in an animal model. Am Rev Respir Dis 1985; 131(6): 875–879.

47. Behrens BL, Clark RAF, Presley DM, Graves JP, Feldsien DC, Larsen GL. Comparison of the evolving histopathology of early and late cutaneous and asthmatic responses in rabbits following a single antigen challenge. Lab Invest 1987; 56: 101–113.

48. Murphy KR, Wilson MC, Irvin CG, Glezen LS, Marsh WR, Haslett C, Henson PM, Larsen GL. The requirement for polymorphonuclear leukocytes in the late asthmatic response and heightened airway reactivity in an animal model. Am Rev Respir Dis 1986; 134: 62–68.

49a. Kay AB, Nadel JA, Henson PM, Irvin CG, Hunninghake GW, Lichtenstein

LM. The role of inflammatory cells and their mediators in bronchial hyper-responsiveness. In: Holgate ST, ed. The Role of Inflammatory Processes in Airway Hyperresponsiveness. London: Blackwell Publications, 1989; 151–178.

49b. Holtzman MN, Fabbri LM, O'Byrne PM. Importance of airway inflammation for hyperresponsiveness induced by ozone. Am Rev Respir Dis 1983; 127: 686–690.

50. Fabbri LM, Aizawa H, Alpert SE et al. Airway hyperresponsiveness and changes in cell counts in bronchoalveolar lavage after ozone exposure in dogs. Am Rev Respir Dis 1984; 129: 288–291.

51. O'Byrne PM, Walters EH, Gold BD, Aizawa HA, Fabbri LM, Alpert SE, Nadel JA, Holtzman MJ. Neutrophil depletion inhibits airway hyper-responsiveness induced by ozone exposure. Am Rev Respir Dis 1984; 130: 214–219.

52. Murlas C, Roum JH. Sequence of pathologic changes in the airway mucosa of guinea pigs during ozone-induced bronchial hyperreactivity. Am Rev Respir Dis 1985; 131: 314–320.

53. Evans TW, Brokaw JJ, Chung KF, Nadel JA, McDonald DM. Ozone-induced bronchial hyperresponsiveness in the rat is not accompanied by neutrophil influx or increased vascular permeability in the trachea. Am Rev Respir Dis 1988; 138: 140–144.

54. Cibulas W Jr, Murlas CG, Miller ML et al. Toluene-diisocyanate-induced airway hyperreactivity and pathology in the guinea pig. J Allergy Clin Immunol 1986; 77: 828–834.

55. Thompson JE, Scypinski LA, Gordon T, Sheppard D. Hydroxyurea inhibits airway hyperresponsiveness in guinea pigs by granulocyte-independent mechanism. Am Rev Respir Dis 1986; 134: 1213–1216.

56. Hutchinson AA, Hinson JM Jr, Brigham KL, Snapper JR. Effect of endotoxin on airway responsiveness to aerosol histamine in sheep. J Appl Physiol 1983; 54: 1463–1468.

57. Hinson JM Jr, Hutchinson AA, Brigham KL, Meyrick BO, Snapper JR. Effect of granulocyte depletion on pulmonary responsiveness to aerosol histamine. J Appl Physiol 1984; 56: 411–417.

58. Pauwels R, Van Der Straeten M, Weyne J, Bazin H. Genetic factors in non-specific bronchial reactivity in rats. Eur J Respir Dis 1985; 66: 98–104.

59. Irvin CG, Berend N, Henson PM. Airways hyperreactivity and inflammation produced by aerosolization of human C5a des Arg. Am Rev Respir Dis 1986; 134: 777–783.

60. Brugman SM, Larsen GL, Henson PM, Irvin CG. Increased lower airways responsiveness associated with sinusitis in a rabbit model. Submitted for publication.

61. Corren J, Honour J, Irvin CG. Activated neutrophils are crucial for development of airways hyperresponsiveness in sinusitis. Am Rev Respir Dis 1990; 141(4): A177.

62. Webster RO, Hong SR, Johnston RB, Henson PM. Biological effects of the

human complement fragments C5a and C5a des Arg on neutorphil function. Immunopharmacology 1980; 2: 201–219.

63. Valentine MD, Lichtenstein LM. Anaphylaxis and stinging insect hypersensitivity. JAMA 1987; 258(20): 2881–2885.

64. Lee TH, Hagadura T, Papageorgiu N, Iikura Y, Kay AB. Exercise-induced late asthmatic reaction with neutrophil chemotactic activity. N Engl J Med 1983; 308(25): 1502–1505.

65. Haslett C, Jose PJ, Giclas PC, William TJ, Henson PM. Cessation of neutrophil infux in C5a induced experimental arthritis is associated with loss of chemoattractant activity from the joint space. J Immunol 1989; 142: 3510–3517.

66. Sluder G. Asthma as a nasal reflex. JAMA 1919; 73: 589–591.

67. Settipane GA. Rhino-sino-bronchial reflex. Immunol Allergy Pract 1985; VII(12): 29–32.

68. Whicker TH, Kern EB. The nasopharyngeal reflex is the awake animal. Ann Otol 1973; 82: 255–358.

69. Rall JE, Gilbert NC, Trup R. Certain aspects of the bronchial reflexes octained by stimulation of the nasopharynx. J Lab Clin Med 1945; 30: 953–956.

70. Nadel JA, Widdicombe JG. Reflex effects of upper airway initiation for total lung resistance and pressure. J Appl Physiol 1962; 17: 861–865.

71. Kaufman J, Wright GW. The effect of nasal and nasopharyngeal irritation on airway resistance in man. Am Rev Respir Dis 1969; 100: 626–630.

72. Nolte P, Berger D. On vagal bronchoconstriction in asthmatic patients by nasal irritation. Eur J Respir Dis 1983; 64(suppl); 128: 110–114.

73. Ogura SH, Nelson JR, Dammkoehler R, Kawasaki M, Togawa K. Experimental observations of the relationships between upper airway obstruction and pulmonary function. Trans Am Laryngol Assoc 1964; 85: 40–64.

74. Buckner CK, Songsiridej V, Dick EC, Busse WW. In vitro and in vivo studies on the use of the guinea pig as a model for virus-provoked airway hyperreactivity. Am Rev Respir Dis 1985; 132: 305–310.

75. Bellofiore S, Di Maria GU, Martin JG. Changes in upper and lower airway resistance after inhalation of antigen in sensitized rats. Am Rev Respir Dis 1987; 136: 363–368.

76. Peters SP, Naclerio RM, Togias A, Schleimer RP, MacGlashan DW, Kagey-Sobotka Adkinson NF, Normer PS, Lichtenstein LM. In Vitro and in vivo model systems for the study of allergic and inflammatory disorders in man. Chest 1985; 87(5)(suppl): 162s–171s.

77. Naclerio RM, Proud D, Togias AG, Adkinson NF, Meyers DA, Kagey-Sobotka A, Plaut M, Norman PS, Lichtenstein LM. Inflammatory mediators in late antigen-induced rhinitis. N Engl J Med 1985; 313: 65–70.

78. Corren J, Adinoff A, Irvin CG. Changes in bronchial responsiveness to methacholine following nasal provocation with allergen. J Allergy Clin Immunol Accepted for publication.

79. Huxley EJ, Viroslar J, Gray WR, Pierce AK. Pharyngeal aspiration in normal adults and patients with depressed conciousness. Am J Med 1978; 64: 654–658.

80. Bardin PG, VanNeerhan BB, Joubert. Absence of pulmonary aspiration of sinus contents in patients with asthma and sinusitis. J Allergy Clin Immunol 1990; 85:82–88.

81. Irwin RS, Corrao WM, Pratter MR. Chronic persistent cough in the adult: the spectrum and frequency of causes and successfull outcome specific therapy. Am Rev Respir Dis 1991; 123: 413–417.

82. Di Maria GU, Wang CG, Bates JHT, Guttman R, Martin JG. Partitioning of airway responses to inhaled methacholine in the rat. J Appl Physiol 1987; 62: 1317–1323.

83. Xu LJ, Eidelman DH, JHT, Martin JG. Late response of the upper airway of the rat to inhaled antigen. J Appl Physiol 1990; 69: 1360–1365.

84. Xu LJ Sapienza S, Du T, Wasserman S, Martin JG. Comparison of upper and lower airway responses of two sensitized rat strains to inhaled antigen. J Appl Physiol 1992; 73: 1608–1613.

85. Eidelman DH, Bellofiore S, Martin JG. Late airways response to antigen challenge in sensitized inbred rats. Am Rev Respir Dis 1988; 137: 1033–1037.

86. Campbell AH, Imberger H, Jones B. Increased upper airway resistance in patients with airway narrowing. Br J Dis Chest 1976; 70: 58–65.

87. Higgenbottam T, Payne J. Glottis narrowing in lung disease. Am Rev Respir Dis 1982; 125: 746–750.

88. Lisboa C, Jardim J, Angus E, Macklem PT. Is extrathoracic airway obstruction important in asthma? Am Rev Respir Dis 122:115–121, 1980.

89. Renz H, Smith HR, Henson JE, Ray BS, Irvin CG, Gelfand EW. Aerosolized antigen exposure without adjuvant causes increased IgE production and airways hyperresponsiveness in the mouse. J Allergy Clin Immunol 1992; 89(6): 1127–1138.

90. Irvin CG, Tu Y-P, Sheller JR, Funk CD. 5-Lipoxygenase products are necessary for ovalbumin-induced airways responsiveness in mice. Am J Physiol 1997; 272: 1053–1058.

91. Hamelmann E, Schwarze J, Takeda K, Oshiba A, Larsen GL, Irvin CG, Gelfand EW. Noninvasive measurement of airway responsiveness in allergic mice using barometric plethysmography: Am J Respir Crit Care Med 1997; 156: 766–775.

92. Takeda K, Hamelmann E, Joetham A, Shultz LD, Larsen GL, Irvin CG, Gelfand EW. Development of eosinophilic airway inflammation and airway hyperresponsiveness in mast cell–deficient mice. J Exp Med 1997; 186: 449–454.

93. Gelfand EW, Irvin CG. News & Views Editorial: T Lymphocytes: setting the tone of the airways. Nat Med 1997; 3: 382–383.

94. Iwasaki T, Tanaka A, Itakura A, Yamashita N, Ohta K, Matsuda H, Uma M. Atopic NC/nga mice as a model for allergic asthma: severe allergic responses by single intranasal challenge with protein antigen. J Vet Med Sci 2001; 63: 413–419.

95. Henderson WR, Tange L, Chu S, Tsao S, Chiang GKS, Jones F, Jorva M, Pae C, Wang H, Chi EY. A role for cysteinyl leukotrienes in airway remodeling in a mouse asthma model. J Respir Crit Care Med 2002; 165: 108–116.
96. Jacob A, Faddis BT, Chole RA. Chronic bacterial rhino-sinusitis: description of a mouse model. Arch Ortolaryngol Head Neck Surgery 2001; 127:657–664.
97. Bomer K, Brichta A, Baroody F, Boonlayangoor S, Xi L, Nacierio RM. A mouse model of acute bacterial rhino-sinusitis. Arch Otolaryngol Head Neck Surg 124: 1227–1232, 1998.
98. Schlesinger RB. Comparative deposition of inhaled aerosols in experimental animals and humans: a review. J Toxicol Environ Health 1985; 15: 197–214.
99. Bates JHT, Irvin CG. Measuring Lung Function in Mice: The Phenotyping Uncertainty Principle. J Appl Physiol, 2003 (in press).

9

Diagnostic Evaluation of Sinusitis in Patients with Asthma

SHELDON SPECTOR
and MICHAEL DIAMENT

DALE RICE

University of California
Los Angeles, California, U.S.A.

University of Southern California
Los Angeles, California, U.S.A.

I. Symptoms and Signs of Sinusitis

The symptoms of sinusitis will vary somewhat, depending on age of the patient and chronicity of the disease. Cough is a common symptom, as well as nasal congestion, headache, pain in the facial area that is made worse with bending over, and tooth pain. Fatigue and malaise can be prominent, especially when the symptoms are persistent. In this respect, a common presentation is a "cold that won't go away." Upper respiratory infections should last, typically, about 5 days. So, if symptoms persist past this period of time, suspect sinusitis.

Common signs of sinusitis include a purulent nasal discharge, and/or purulent pharyngeal discharge. Indeed, drainage can occur mainly toward the posterior pharynx, rather than anteriorly. Occasionally an unhappy spouse suggests the diagnosis is due to "fetorosis" (foul breath) apparent with close contact.

Williams et al. described five independent predictors of sinusitis: maxillary toothache (odds ratio 2:9), transillumination (odds ratio 2:7), poor response to nasal decongestants or antihistamines (odds ratio 2:4), colored nasal discharge reported by the patient (odds ratio 2:2), and mucopurulence seen during examination (odds ratio 2:9). The overall clinical impression was more accurate than any single finding (1).

Shapiro and Rachelefsky used major criteria in proposing a definition of sinusitis based on various symptoms and signs (2). The presence of two major criteria or one major and two or more minor criteria constitute the diagnosis. The major criteria include purulent nasal discharge, purulent pharyngeal drainage, and cough. The minor criteria include periorbital edema, headache, facial pain, toothache, earache, soreness of the throat, foul breath, increased wheeze, and fever. Some of the minor criteria point out the effect of sinusitis on associated organs such as the ear and the lung. There is an important relationship between asthma and sinusitis in which treatment of the latter improves the former (3).

II. Nasal Cytology

Nasal cytology reflects both nasal and sinus pathology and, thereby has limited ability to characterize sinus disease per se. It is most often employed to differentiate an allergic process from an infectious one and serves as a simple screening tool in comparison to more sensitive and costly diagnostic procedures such as sinus radiographs and computed tomography (CT).

There are several methods of collecting nasal secretions. The patient can blow into wax paper or Saran Wrap, the sample can be collected by swab or brush, or the sample can be collected by nasal lavage or with a Rhinoprobe (Synbiotics Corporation, San Diego, CA). Less cellular material is collected from blowing (4).

Once the sample has been collected, it must be stained. Following cytofixation or heat fixation, a Hansel stain is used to identify eosinophils. Other commonly used stains, such as hematoxylin–eosin, acidified toluidine blue, or Nay–Grunwald–Giemsa stain, can be used to identify other elements, including mast cells, basophils, neutrophils, goblet cells, epithelial cells, and Charcot–Leyden crystals. Certain medications such as topical corticosteroids may affect the findings, a factor that should be considered when one is interpreting the results or nasal cytology.

Nasal cytology helps to define the presence and type of sinusitis (5). These include allergic rhinitis and/or sinusitis, nonallergic rhinitis with eosinophilia (NARES syndrome), and bacterial sinusitis. There are semiquantitative and subjective methods for quantitating the nasal cytology (6–8).

Studies defining the sensitivity and specificity of nasal cytology for various diseases are limited. Establishing a gold standard in allergic rhinitis requires a global assessment of clinical history and evaluation of allergen-specific IgE. Once this has been done, the sensitivity of finding eosinophils in the nasal secretions is high, but the sensitivity may be low, depending on recent exposure to allergens. In one study, nasal eosinophilia (> 20% of all cells recovered) was found in 43% of patients with allergic rhinitis, but 0% of controls with nonallergic rhinitis (8). In a similar cytological study, numerous eosinophils, both isolated and in clusters, were found in the allergic rhinitis patients. In poorly defined diseases with negative specific IgE studies, the presence of eosinophils leads to the diagnosis of the NARES syndrome by default. Although the successful use of topical corticosteroids for this disease helps in its confirmation, failure to respond to this therapy does not rule out the diagnosis. Correlation of nasal cytology with mucociliary clearance has been examined in one study in which the presence of eosinophilia was significantly associated with decreased saccharin clearance (9). It was once thought that the eosinophilia found in nasal smears of infants would confuse the interpretation of their nasal smears. A recent study (10) suggests that eosinophilia is not a common occurrence in infants, so when sinusitis is being investigated in younger children, nasal cytology is useful.

Comparison studies of nasal cytology with global and radiographic assessments of sinusitis are also limited. Wilson and coworkers (11) used a Rhinoprobe curette in evaluating 55 adult and pediatric asthma and allergy patients. They reported a specificity of 90% when positive cytology [> 6 polymorphonucleophils per high power field (PMN/HPF) and bacteria] was compared with a positive x-ray (asymmetry, mucoperiosteal thickening, opacification, or air–fluid levels). However, 33% of patients with under 6PMN/HPF had a positive x-ray (sensitivity of 67%). Gill and Neilburger (12) examined 300 allergy patients (2–69 years old) and found that 5 or more PMN per high power field was associated with a higher incidence of positive radiographs with a sensitivity of 86%, but specificity was only 40%. Cytology was done by collecting nasal secretions on wax paper or by cotton swab. Jong and coworkers, in their search for a screening test in children with chronic sinusitis, used a wax paper blow with a Rhinoprobe to compare quantitative nasal cytology. They found that more than 5 PMN/HPF on Rhinoprobe cytology significantly correlated with radiographic sinusitis (13). While it is generally possible to discriminate among upper respiratory infections for allergy on clinical grounds, these data must be balanced against the observation that acute viral infections can lead to neutrophilic nasal secretions and transiently abnormal imaging studies (14). Further, it is certainly possible for patients to have concurrent allergy and bacterial si-nusitis. If the clinical picture persuasively favors the diagnosis of bacterial sinusitis, a predominance of eosinophils present on the nasal smear should not deter the physician from treating with antimicrobial therapy. In some cases fungi on the smear may be informative about the rare cases of allergic fungal disease being the etiology of sinusitis.

One of the greatest applications of nasal cytology is in the clinical studies of therapeutic agents. In such studies there have been variable changes noted in comparison to other subjective and objective criteria (see e.g., Refs. 6 and 15). Such studies are most useful when a patient is pretreated with a drug and then challenged with an allergen (16). The acuteness of this process leads to a better interpretation of changes in nasal cytology and their implications for nasal obstruction.

Limitations of the procedures include lack of data regarding reproducibility of the sample and variability on the two sides of the nose. Future studies should assess comparisons between nasal cytology and CT scans, endoscopy, or bilateral cultures.

In summary, nasal cytology is most useful in the evaluation of sinusitis, especially when it contains predominantly eosinophils or neutrophils. If the clinical data support the histological findings, the presence of eosinophils suggests a diagnosis of allergic rhinosinusitis or NARES, while the presence of neutrophils supports the diagnosis of bacterial rhinosinusitis. Quantitation of cells requires good sample collection and an experienced observer. While further studies are desirable to establish the optimal collection methods and more standardized quantitation methods with concurrent radiographic studies of the sinuses, it is likely that the complex interrelationship of allergy, anatomy, immunity, and infectious disease will limit nasal cytology to a supportive role in clinical diagnosis.

III. Sinus Ultrasound

A-mode ultrasonography is based on the principle that reflection of ultrasound waves occurs at the boundary of two media with differing acoustic impedances. Acoustic impedance depends on the velocity of the sound in the medium, and on the density of the medium. Air acts as a total reflector; thus, all structures behind an air-filled cavity are not accessible to ultrasound examination. A fluid-filled sinus cavity transmits most of the ultrasound waves through to the back wall of the sinus, where they are reflected by the bone. There is a correlation between the interval separating the initial echo and the reflected echo, and the distance of the reflecting boundary from the skin surface. In this way, A-mode ultrasound elicits a one-dimensional scan, allowing the axis of the transducer that is displayed on an oscilloscope. A-mode ultrasound has been compared in various studies to the gold standard of the time. Thus, Rohr and co-workers correlated A-mode ultrasound with radiography in the diagnosis of maxillary sinusitis and concluded that the ultrasound was primarily useful in the detection of secretions within the sinus, and not mucosal thickening (17). Depending on the device employed, the specificities were over 90%, but the overall sensitivities varied from 30 to 60%. The maxillary sinus was usually assessed in these authors' study, since the number of patients with frontal sinusitis was minimal.

In a more recent study, Pfister and coworkers compared A-mode ultrasound and standard radiography with the present gold standard, computed tomography (18). In their study of 19 patients, CT showed at least some minimal mucosal thickening in the paranasal sinuses in 74% and, of the maxillary sinuses in 61% of the patients. Compared with the results of computed tomography, plain view radiography gave a specificity of 86.7% for the maxillary sinuses. Although all cases of severe mucosal thickening were detected, sensitivity for minimal mucosal hyperplasia was low (52.2%). By contrast, A-mode ultrasonography demonstrated a sensitivity of 70%, but a specificity of only 22%. The authors suggest that the primary usefulness of A-mode ultrasonography is as a follow-up in selected patients who have known anatomical characteristics, rather than as an initial scan for patients whom there would be insufficient evaluation of mucosal hyperplasia.

Thus, in both of the studies (17,18), it is suggested that A-mode ultrasound is most useful as a follow-up procedure or alternative when x-ray or ST

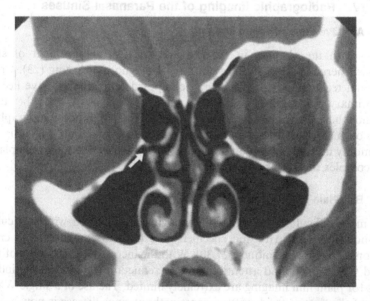

Figure 1 A normal coronal section from a CT scan in a 37-year-old female demonstrating a patent air passage (arrow) through the right osteomeatal unit. Note mild deviation of the mid septum to the left in this patient, who has no evidence of sinus disease.

scan is undesirable, such as with a pregnant patient. Other investigators believe that A-mode ultrasound has value as a screening procedure (19) but do not consider it to be an adequate substitute for radiography (20,21).

Most of the generalizations concerning ultrasound have involved the maxillary sinuses, since the incidence of involvement in these sinuses is greater than in the others. In one study preoperative ultrasonography of the frontal sinus was compared with the surgical findings in 27 frontal sinuses. These Dutch investigators found ultrasonography to be a reliable method for the demonstration or exclusion of mucosal swelling and accumulated fluid (sensitivity 92%, specificity 93) (22).

In summary, ultrasound of the paranasal sinuses can provide useful information such as the presence of an air–fluid level (Fig. 1). Examples of its applicability include determination of the presence of sinus disease in a pregnant patient for whom a radiograph would be contraindicated and suspected persistence of sinus disease in a patient for whom other diagnostic procedures might be undesirable. Sinusitis in such a patient could safely be followed sequentially.

IV. Radiographic Imaging of the Paranasal Sinuses

A. Overview of Sinus Imaging

Along with the changes in medical and surgical management of sinus disease, there has been a major shift in its diagnostic imaging (23). Cross-sectional techniques, primarily x-ray computed tomography, have become the primary modalities (24–26). Plain film x-ray diagnosis, once the standard, now has very limited indications (27–30). Plain film polytomography is only of historical interest. Magnetic resonance imaging (MRI) is less commonly utilized but has an important role in the evaluation of neoplasms and complex infections (26,31–35).

B. Plain Film Imaging

The main difficulty with plain film imaging is that even with meticulous technique, its sensitivity and specificity are poor in comparison to cross-sectional imaging techniques (27,30). With the increasing availability of high speed CT scanners and attention to dose reduction techniques, the indications for plain film imaging are extremely limited. The use of a single Waters view of the sinuses to identify patients without sinus disease is now a questionable practice (Fig. 2). The technique has limited sensitivity and specificity and is unable to identify isolated disease in the ethmoid and sphenoid sinuses (Fig. 3)—which is increasingly recognized with cross-sectional techniques (36). Selection of patients for imaging should be based on the

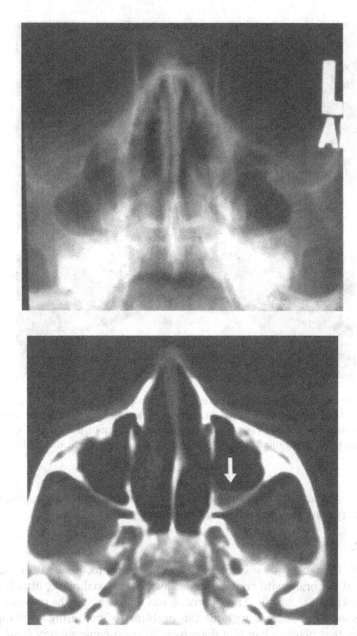

Figure 2 A 25-year-old male with fever and facial pain. A Waters view (a) was interpreted as normal although the inferior maxillary recesses are obscured by the overlying temporal bones. An axial CT section (b) clearly demonstrates an air–fluid level (arrow) in the left maxillary antrum.

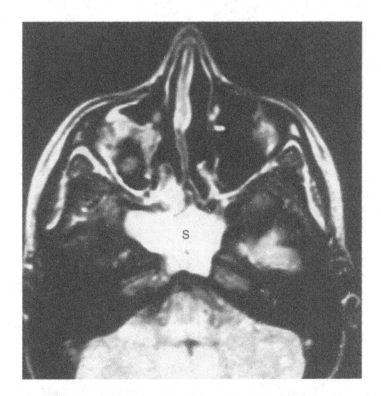

Figure 3 A 40-year-old female referred for nonspecific headache. An axial T2-weighted MRI section shows opacification of the sphenoid sinus (S) and irregular mucosal thickening in the right maxillary antrum. Culture of the surgical specimen was positive for aspergillus. The patient had no underlying medical condition.

presence and severity of symptoms and signs, supplemented by appropriate laboratory tests and possibly nasal endoscopy (37).

C. Sinus CT Imaging

Initially, CT technique was an extension of the protocols used for examination of the brain with contiguous sections in the axial plane, usually of 5 mm thickness (24,38–40). This approach was able to assess the presence and severity of sinus disease without the problems of confusing overlapping densities that plague plain film diagnosis. As endoscopic surgery came into wider use, direct coronal sections (Figs. 1 and 4) were utilized to provide anatomical details for presurgical planning which are much better appreciated in this plane (25,41–43).

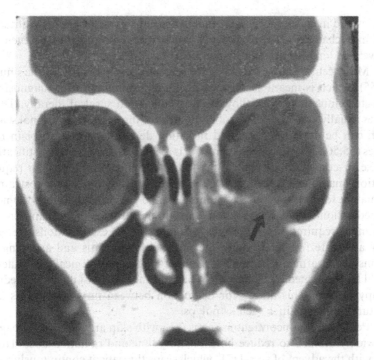

Figure 4 A coronal CT section showing opacification of the left maxillary antrum in a 6-year-old male who presented with low grade fever and left lid swelling. There is destruction of the medial and superior (arrow) bony margins of the sinus, with extension of the disease process into the orbit. A neoplasm was suspected, but the surgical specimens demonstrated pyogenic sinusitis with osteomyelitis.

Many patients are referred for evaluation of sinus disease because of incidental opacification noted on CT or MRI studies of the brain. In many cases, the clinical significance of these abnormalities, especially if there is only minor mucosal thickening, is doubtful (44–50). Some degree of sinus opacification is a common finding, especially in children (44,46). Sinus opacification can also accompany uncomplicated upper respiratory tract infections, including the common cold (51,52).

The significance of CT as a presurgical planning technique is not limited to the diagnosis of sinus opacification and fluid. Its primary importance is to determine the presence of structural abnormalities that may impede sinus drainage and the presence of anatomical variants, which are relatively common, that might influence surgical planning and technique. Presurgical or "complete" sinus CT examination should be performed only after maximal medical therapy. This allows for the resolution of inflammatory changes and makes it more likely that persistent soft tissue abnormalities are structural changes, such as polyps, which would be resistant to even intensive and long-term medical treatment.

Many centers now offer so-called screening or limited CT of the sinuses (53–55), which is meant to serve as an initial examination for diagnosis of suspected sinusitis or for follow-up of medical and surgical therapy. These studies usually consisted of a limited number of direct axial or coronal scans, which can be done at a cost and radiation dose comparable to plain film studies (55,56). If low cost screening CT is available, there is little justification for use of conventional plain film studies. Younger children who require sedation may be a special case, but even they can usually restrained adequately so that high speed scanning can be performed without the need for medication. While such limited scans do not provide the full anatomical assessment required for presurgical planning, these examinations are generally adequate for determining the presence of sinusitis and assessing its response to treatment. In nonemergent situations, presurgical CT imaging should be performed after the patient has had the benefit of maximal medical therapy (42,57). This allows for distinction between fluid and mucus and structural abnormalities such as polyps.

Performing noncontiguous scans (i.e., with skip areas between images) was widely utilized to reduce both imaging time and radiation dose. However, with the advent of spiral CT, which scans the patient continuously as he or she moves through the scanner, this practice has been largely abandoned. Since modern spiral CT scanners can usually image the sinuses in 5 to 30 s, there is little advantage to performing noncontiguous imaging—except to reduce radiation dose. Radiation, which is a serious concern in patients who require repeated studies, can be minimized by selection of proper x-ray technique (41,58–64). In general, sinus imaging can be done with much lower dose settings than are used for CT of the brain.

Modern "multislice" spiral CT scanners can also perform so-called isotropic scans, which utilize sections less than one millimeter thick to allow reconstruction of scans in arbitrary planes without significant loss of spatial resolution (65). However, this technique should not be used routinely, since it does require a higher radiation dose (66). Most scanning for infectious disease can be done without intravenous contrast enhancement (41). Contrast is only used when extension beyond the sinuses, as commonly occurs with fungal infections or neoplasm, is suspected.

D. MRI Imaging

MRI is capable of providing images in any plane without the need to flex or extend the patient's neck, which may be uncomfortable or impossible for patients who are combative or have cervical abnormalities. However, until recently the spatial resolution possible with this technique was inadequate for evaluation of small bony structures (26,31,32,35,67,68), a critical factor in presurgical planning. Newer work (69) suggests that MRI may be able to have a primary role in screening and presurgical evaluation of patients with sinusitis, but issues of cost, access, and longer imaging times are still likely to limit its use to selected cases. In comparison to CT, MRI does provide superior assessment of soft tissue disease when inflammation or neoplasm extends beyond the sinuses (Fig. 5)—especially into the intracranial space (31,32,68,70–73). MRI may also be able to characterize sinus secretion, differentiating between fluid, soft tissue, and mucus, and between desiccated chronic collections (33,74,75).

E. Radiologic Classification of Severity

Classification schemes have been developed to give a semiquantitative assessment of the severity of sinus involvement (44,76,77). These generally are based on the percentage of the volume of the pneumatized sinuses that are filled with soft tissue and fluid or on the depth of mucosal thickening within the maxillary antra. Such schemes are primarily used in research studies. In clinical practice, the radiologist should describe the extent and character of opacification of the individual sinuses and any anatomical abnormalities and variants that may predispose to persistent or recurrent disease. The nasopharyngeal airway should be evaluated for polyps, severe septal deviation, or other abnormalities that may obstruct sinus drainage—especially in the area of the ostiomeatal units, which form the common drainage pathway for the antra and anterior ethmoids (41,78–80). However, many anatomical variants of the sinuses and nasal airway may not be clinically significant: there are conflicting reports about their prevalence in control populations who have chronic sinusitis (45,81–83).

F. Stereotactic CT Imaging

Stereotactic CT of the sinuses, a specialized surgical planning technique, is a recent development. Patients who are scheduled for endoscopic surgery undergo a spiral CT scan in the axial plane with a custom frame placed on their head (84–86). The same frame is placed on the patient's head during surgery and the CT data are transferred to a computer in the operating room to provide a "virtual" image of the endoscope's position. This allows the surgeon to know the position of the tip of the endoscope even when it is not in view and, more importantly, the relative location of the scope and adjacent vital structures such as the orbits and skull base.

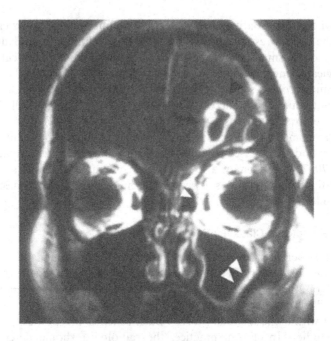

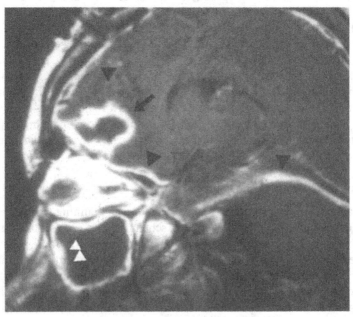

G. Summary

The evolution of imaging techniques for sinus disease is similar to that for intracranial abnormalities. Conventional plain film studies have almost been completely replaced by cross-sectional imaging techniques. For almost all uncomplicated infectious and allergic sinus disease, the study of choice is CT without contrast enhancement. The details of section thickness and imaging plane largely depend on clinical presentation, available technology, and patient characteristics. Contrast-enhanced CT studies and MRI play a valuable role when extension beyond the confines of the paranasal sinuses is known or suspected.

V. Endoscopy of the Nose and Sinuses

A. Background

Historically, physical examination of the nasal airway and the paranasal sinuses has proven challenging. The use of a handheld speculum and head lamp allows for examination of the anterior nasal passage but does not generally provide good visualization of the upper recesses of the nose or the sinus ostia. In the early 1980s, the Hopkins rod endoscope, previously used to examine the larynx, was modified into a size and variety of angles that made the instrument suitable for examining the nasal passages. This new development represented a major breakthrough in the diagnosis and treatment of nasal and sinus disorders. Table 1 lists the equipment used in nasal endoscopy today.

B. Purpose of Endoscopy

While endoscopy of the nose and sinuses is an invaluable aid for inspecting potential inflammatory or neoplastic disorders, a second function of the endoscope is as an operative tool. With the advent of the rigid endoscope, many procedures can be done through a transnasal approach which, in the past, would have required a more aggressive open approach or a transnasal approach with limited visibility.

Figure 5 A 16-year-old female who presented with fever, nuchal rigidity, and seizures 3 days after dental extractions: T1-weighted, contrast-enhanced coronal (a) and parasagittal (b) MRI sections demonstrate opacification of the left antrum and pathological enhancement of the left maxillary (double white arrowheads) and ethmoid (white arrowhead) mucosa. There is a left frontal lobe brain abscess (arrow) and abnormal enhancement of the meninges (black arrowhead).

Table 1   Equipment for Nasal Endoscopy

Flexible endoscope or rigid endoscope (preferably 2.7 mm diameter)
Light source appropriate to endoscope
Topical anesthetic (may not be necessary in all cases)
Topical vasoconstrictor (may not be necessary in all cases)
  1% Xylocaine with 1:100,000 epinephrine nicely fulfills both functions
  Afrin or neo synephrin, mixed with plain xylocaine will also work
Atomizer to spray the vasconstrictors into the nasal cavity
Additional instruments may be necessary if a procedure (e.g., biopsy) is to be
  performed

C. Features of Endoscopes

Rigid endoscopes are made by a wide variety of manufacturers and are all of a very high quality. Most importantly to office diagnosis is that they are available in a variety of diameters and optical angles. For office use, smaller endoscopes (2.7 mm diameter) are most useful. The optical angles may vary from 0 to 120°. Most useful to the outpatient clinic are the 0° and either 5 or 30° scope angles, depending on the manufacturer. The systematic use of these endoscopes will allow the physician to thoroughly examine the nasal cavity and sinus outflow areas.

Flexible endoscopes were primarily designed for examination of the larynx and hypopharynx; however, they can also be used to examine the nasal airway. With practice, their articulating end can be used to thoroughly examine the nasal cavity and lateral nasal wall. However, it is difficult to rotate a flexible scope into the average middle meatus. In addition, since it takes two hands to operate a flexible scope, it is not possible to perform other procedures (e.g., suctioning) while performing flexible endoscopy.

D. Conducting an Endoscopic Examination

The nasal cavities should be examined in a systematic manner. For the novice nasal endoscopist, the mucous membrane should first be sprayed with a decongestant mixed with a topical anesthetic. After gaining considerable experience in manipulating these endoscopes within the nasal cavity, one can usually perform the examination in a cooperative patient without these drugs, which do alter somewhat the appearance of the nasal mucosa. One should first pass the endoscope along the floor of the nasal cavity to examine the inferior turbinate, septum, the inferior meatus, and the nasopharynx. If one is using the 25 or 30° angled telescope, simple rotation of the instrument will allow examination of both sides of the nasopharynx in one pass. The next pass of the endoscope should be above the inferior turbinate to examine the middle turbinate and the very important area of the middle meatus (Fig. 6). This is the area, as well as the sphenoethmoidal recess, where the sinuses drain, and where early polyp formation would be expected (Fig. 7). The third pass should be slightly above the inferior end of the middle turbinate (Figure 8) to examine the superior turbinate and cribriform plate area.

A skilled endoscopist can inspect the area of the middle meatus directly to see the outflow tracks of the anterior ethmoid, frontal, and maxillary sinuses directly. This is particularly important in attempting to diagnose subtle cases of sinusitis. In more florid cases, gross purulence coming out of the middle meatus will be obvious on the first or second pass, as described earlier (Fig. 9).

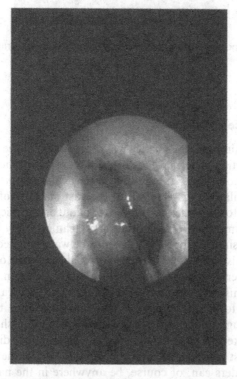

Figure 6 Normal anatomy of the middle meatus, as seen through the endoscope. The septum is to the far left. The middle turbinate is being pushed medially by a Freer elevator, seen at approximately 5 o'clock. Both the uncinate process and the bulla ethmoidalis can be seen, superior to the Freer elevator.

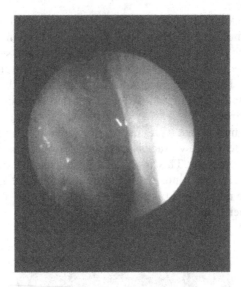

Figure 7 Small polyps visible in the middle meatus, photographed through an endoscope.

E. Endoscopic Diagnosis

Prior to the examination, the history will generally point the physician in the appropriate direction, in terms of the likely diagnosis and where to focus extra energy in the endoscopic examination. Of particular importance is whether the process is unilateral or bilateral. In the vast majority of cases, bilateral symptoms point toward allergic rhinitis, or acute or chronic bacterial sinusitis. Unilateral symptoms, on the other hand, can certainly be secondary to acute or chronic sinusitis, but one must also be wary of a neoplastic etiology for the process. Also important in the history is the duration of the symptoms, as well as the severity and previous attempts at management, if any.

From the history, the physician should have an idea of whether the process is likely to be inflammatory or neoplastic. While the examination should be thorough and systematic, particular attention should be paid to the areas most likely to yield a diagnosis. In inflammatory disorders, such as sinusitis, the most common area of abnormality will be the middle meatus. Neoplastic disorders can, of course, be anywhere in the nasal cavity or in the sinuses. If the examination reveals mucopurulent drainage from the middle meatus, one can confidently diagnose bacterial sinusitis. If this is an acute process, radiographic examination is probably not worthwhile, and one should merely institute appropriate antibiotic therapy.

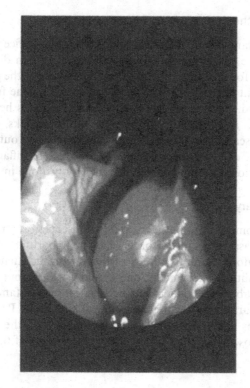

Figure 8 Widened middle turbinate from pneumatization—the so-called concha bullosa.

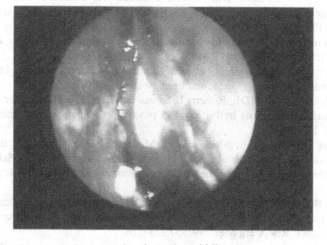

Figure 9 Gross purulence coming from the middle meatus.

F. Use of the Endoscope in Postoperative Care

A second important use of the nasal endoscope in an office setting is the postoperative care of the patient. Again, the same 2.7 mm diameter endoscope works well for this. For a variable amount of time in the postoperative period, the patient needs to be seen in the office with some frequency and carefully observed. Part of the utility of the endoscope is helping remove obstructing crusts and mucus from the sinus outflow tracks. One needs to also observe for scar tissue formation that might result in outflow obstruction. In addition, one can check for persistent areas of inflammation that might need additional therapy, which can usually be done in the office.

G. Summary

With the development of the modern rigid endoscopes, any physician who wishes to treat nasal and sinus disorders has the opportunity to become an expert in the anatomy and physiology of this region. In attempting to gain the maximum utility of instruments, one should use them routinely to examine normal and abnormal patients to become intimately familiar with the endoscopic appearance in a variety of clinical situations. Practiced use of these endoscopes will greatly enhance the ability of the physician to accurately diagnose and treat a wide variety of disorders of the nasal cavity and sinuses.

References

1. Williams JW Jr, Simel DL, Roberts L, Samsa GP. Clinical evaluation for sinusitis: making the diagnosis by history and physical examination. Ann Intern Med 1991; 117:705–710.
2. Shapiro GG, Rachelefsky GR. Introduction and definition of sinusitis. J Allergy Clin Immunol 1992; 90:417–418.
3. Spectro SL. Relationship between rhinitis/sinusitis and asthma. In Grand Rounds in Allergy, Asthma, and Immunology, Part 6 in a series.
4. Williams JW, Simel DL, Roberts L, Samsa GP. Clinical evaluation for sinusitis: making the diagnosis by history and physical examination. Ann Intern Med 1992; 117:705–710.
5. Evans FO, Sydnor E, Moore WEC, Moore GR, Manwaring JL, Brill AH, Jackson RT, Hanna S, Skaar JS, Holderman LV, Fitz-Hugh GS, Sande Ma, Gwaltney JM. Sinusitis of the maxillary antrum. N Engl J Med 1975; 293:735–739.
6. Lara Becerra A, Gonzalez Diaz SN, Gonzalez Morales JE, Canseco Gonzalez C. Determination of the eosinophil count in nasal mucus. Comparison of two techniques. Rev Alerg Mex 1990; 37:123–126.

7. Kohler C, Stringini R, Moneret DA, Grignon G. Study of cells harvested in nasal secretions after lavage. Improvement of the cytologic technique and application to ORL and bronchial pathology. Bul Assoc Anat 1992; 76:34–36.
8. Calderon-Gaciduenas L, Roy-Ocotia G. Nasal cytology in southwest metropolitan Mexico City inhabitants: a pilot intervention study. Environ Health Perspect 1993; 101:138–144.
9. Davidson AE, Miller SD, Settinpane RJ, Ricci AR, Klein DE, Settipane GA. Delayed nasal mucociliary clearance in patients with nonallergic rhinitis and nasal eosinophilia. Allergy Proc 1992; 13:81–84.
10. Cohen GA, MacPherson GA, Golembesky HE, Jalowayski AA, O'Connor RD. Normal nasal cytology in infancy. Ann Allergy 1985; 54:112–114.
11. Wilson NW, Jalowayski AA, Hamburger RN. A comparison of nasal cytology with sinus x-rays for the diagnosis of sinusitis. Am J Rhinol 1988; 2:55–59.
12. Gill FF, Neiburger JB. The role of nasal cytology in the diagnosis of chronic sinusitis. Am J Rhinol 1989; 3:13–15.
13. Jong CN, Olson NY, Nadel GL, Phillips PS, Gill FF, Neiburger JB. Use of nasal cytology in the diagnosis of occult chronic sinusitis in asthmatic children. Ann Allergy 1994; 73:509–514.
14. Gwaltney JM, Phillps CD, Miller RD, Riker DK. Computed tomographic study of the common cold. N Eng J Med 1994; 330:25–30.
15. Meltzer EO, Bronsky EA, Findlay SR, Georgitis JW, Grossman J, Ratner P, Wood CC. Ipratropium bromide aqueous nasal spray for patients with perennial allergic rhinitis. A study of its effect on their symptoms, quality of life, and nasal cytology. J Allergy Clin Immunol 1992; 90:242–249.
16. Metzer EO, Orgel Ha, Bronsky EA, Furukawa CT, Grossman J, LaForce CF, Lemanske RT, Paul BD, Pearlman DS, Ratner PH, et al. A dose-ranging study of fluticasone propionate aqueous nasal spray for seasonal allergic rhinitis assessed by symptoms, rhinomanometry, and nasal cytology. J Allergy Clin Immunol 1990; 66:221–230.
17. Rohr AS, Spector SL, Siegel SC, Katz RM, Rachelfsky GS. Correlation between A-mode ultrasound and radiography in the diagnosis of maxillary sinusitis. J Allergy Clin Immunol 1986; 68:58–61.
18. Pfister R, Lutolf M, Schapowal A, Giatte B, Schmitz M, Menz G. Screening for sinus disease in patients with asthma: a computed tomography–controlled comparison of A-mode ultrasonography and standard radiography. J Allergy Clin Immunol 1994; 94:804–809.
19. Berger W, Weiss J. A comparison of A-mode ultrasound and x-ray for the screening of maxillary sinus disease. J Allergy Clin Immunol 1985; 75:330.
20. Shapiro G, Furukawa CT, Pierson WE, Gilbertson E, Bierman CW. Ultrasound versus radiography for diagnosis of sinusitis. J Allergy Clin Immunol 1985; 75:330.
21. Pfeiederer AG, Drake-Lee AB, Lowe D. Ultrasound of the sinuses: a worthwhile procedure? A comparison of ultrasound and radiography in predicting the findings of proof puncture on the maxillary sinuses. Clin Otolaryngol 1984; 9:335–339.

22. Otten FW, Engberts GE, Grott JJ. Ultrasonography as a method of examination of the frontal sinuses. Clin Otolaryngol June 1991; 16(3):285–287.
23. Zinreich SJ. Imaging of chronic sinusitis in adults: x-ray, computed tomography, and magnetic resonance imaging. J Allergy Clin Immunol 1992; 90:445–451.
24. Unger JM, Shaffer K, Duncavage JA. Computed tomography in nasal and paranasal sinus disease. Laryngoscope 1984; 94:1319–1324.
25. Som PM. CT of the paranasal sinuses. Neuroradiology 1985; 27:189–201.
26. Beahm E, Teresi L, Lufkin R, Hanafee W. MR of the paranasal sinuses. Surg Radiol Anat 1990; 12:203–208.
27. McAlister WH, Lusk R, Muntz HR. Comparison of plain radiographs and coronal CT scans in infants and children with recurrent sinusitis. AJR Am J Roentgenol 1989; 153:1259–1264.
28. Babbel RW, Harnsberger HR. A contemporary look at the imaging issues of sinusitis: sinonasal anatomy, physiology, and computed tomography techniques. Semin Ultrasound Comput Tomogr Magn Reson 1991; 12:526–540.
29. Bonetti MG, Salvolini U, Scarabino T, Giannatempo GM, Casillo A, Cammisa M. Diagnostic yield in rhino-sinusal inflammatory pathology: comparison of projective radiology, CT and MR. Radiol Med (Torino) 1991; 82:260–264.
30. Burke TF, Guertler AT, Timmons JH. Comparison of sinus x-rays with computed tomography scans in acute sinusitis. Acad Emerg Med 1994; 1:235–239.
31. Lufkin RB, Hanafee W. Magnetic resonance imaging of head and neck tumors. Cancer Metastasis Rev 1988; 7:19–38.
32. Hunink MG, de Slegte RG, Gerritsen GJ, Speelman H. CT and MR assessment of tumors of the nose and paranasal sinuses, the nasopharynx and the parapharyngeal space using ROC methodology. Neuroradiology 1990; 32:220–225.
33. Lanzieri CF, Shah M, Krauss D, Lavertu P. Use of gadolinium-enhanced MR imaging for differentiating mucoceles from neoplasms in the paranasal sinuses. Radiology 1991; 178:425–428.
34. Brown JH, DeLuca SA. Imaging of sinonasal tumors. Am Fam Physician 1992; 45:1653–1656.
35. Kraus DH, Lanzieri CF, Wanamaker JR, Little JR, Lavertu P. Complementary use of computed tomography and magnetic resonance imaging in assessing skull base lesions. Laryngoscope 1992; 102:623–629.
36. Konen E, Faibel M, Kleinbaum Y, et al. The value of the occipitomental (Waters') view in diagnosis of sinusitis: a comparative study with computed tomography. Clin Radiol 2000; 55:856–860.
37. Kenny TJ, Duncavage J, Bracikowski J, Yildirim A, Murray JJ, Tanner SB. Prospective analysis of sinus symptoms and correlation with paranasal computed tomography scan. Otolaryngol Head Neck Surg 2001; 125:40–43.
38. Bilaniuk LT, Zimmerman RA. Computed tomography in evaluation of the paranasal sinuses. Radiol Clin North Am 1982; 20:51–66.

39. Sataloff RT, Grossman CB, Gonzales C, Naheedy MH. Computed tomography of the face and paranasal sinuses: I. Normal anatomy. Head Neck Surg 1984; 7:110–122.
40. Schatz CJ, Becker TS. Normal CT anatomy of the paranasal sinuses. Radiol Clin North Am 1984; 22:107–118.
41. Babbel R, Harnsberger HR, Nelson B, Sonkens J, Hunt S. Optimization of techniques in screening CT of the sinuses. AJNR Am J Neuroradiol 1991; 12:849–854.
42. Harnsberger HR, Babbel RW, Davis WL. The major obstructive inflammatory patterns of the sinonasal region seen on screening sinus computed tomography. Semin Ultrasound Comput Tomogr Magn Reson 1991; 12:541–560.
43. Melhem ER, Oliverio PJ, Benson ML, Leopold DA, Zinreich SJ. Optimal CT evaluation for functional endoscopic sinus surgery. AJNR Am J Neuroradiol 1996; 17:181–188.
44. Diament MJ, Senac MO Jr, Gilsanz V, Baker S, Gillespie T, Larsson S. Prevalence of incidental paranasal sinuses opacification in pediatric patients: a CT study. J Comput Assist Tomogr 1987; 11:426–431.
45. Calhoun KH, Waggenspack GA, Simpson CB, Hokanson JA, Bailey BJ. CT evaluation of the paranasal sinuses in symptomatic and asymptomatic populations. Otolaryngol Head Neck Surg 1991; 104:480–483.
46. Glasier CM, Ascher DP, Williams KD. Incidental paranasal sinus abnormalities on CT of children: clinical correlation. AJNR Am J Neuroradiol 1986; 7:861–864.
47. Cooke LD, Hadley DM. MRI of the paranasal sinuses: incidental abnormalities and their relationship to symptoms. J Laryngol Otol 1991; 105:278–281.
48. Moser FG, Panush D, Rubin JS, Honigsberg RM, Sprayregen S, Eisig SB. Incidental paranasal sinus abnormalities on MRI of the brain. Clin Radiol 1991; 43:252–254.
49. Rak KM, Newell JD 2nd, Yakes WF, Damiano MA, Luethke JM. Paranasal sinuses on MR images of the brain: significance of mucosal thickening. AJR Am J Roentgenol 1991; 156:381–384.
50. Ashraf N, Bhattacharyya N. Determination of the "incidental" Lund score for the staging of chronic rhinosinusitis. Otolaryngol Head Neck Surg 2001; 125:483–486.
51. Gwaltney JM Jr, Phillips CD, Miller RD, Riker DK. Computed tomographic study of the common cold. N Engl J Med 1994; 330:25–30.
52. Turner BW, Cail WS, Hendley JO, et al. Physiologic abnormalities in the paranasal sinuses during experimental rhinovirus colds. J Allergy Clin Immunol 1992; 90:474–478.
53. Goodman GM, Martin DS, Klein J, Awwad E, Druce HM, Sharafuddin M. Comparison of a screening coronal CT versus a contiguous coronal CT for the evaluation of patients with presumptive sinusitis. Ann Allergy Asthma Immunol 1995; 74:178–182.
54. Wippold FJ II, Levitt RG, Evens RG, Korenblat PE, Hodges FJ III, Jost RG.

Limited coronal CT: an alternative screening examination for sinonasal inflammatory disease. Allergy Proc 1995; 16:165–169.

55. Witte RJ, Heurter JV, Orton DF, Hahn FJ. Limited axial CT of the paranasal sinuses in screening for sinusitis. AJR Am J Roentgenol 1996; 167:1313–1315.

56. Mafee MF. Modern imaging of paranasal sinuses and the role of limited sinus computerized tomography; considerations of time, cost and radiation. Ear Nose Throat J 1994; 73:532–534, 536–538, 540–542 passim.

57. Stringer SP, Mancuso AA, Avino AJ. Effect of a topical vasoconstrictor on computed tomography of paranasal sinus disease. Laryngoscope 1993; 103:6–9.

58. MacLennan AC. Radiation dose to the lens from coronal CT scanning of the sinuses. Clin Radiol 1995; 50:265–267.

59. Sillers MJ, Kuhn FA, Vickery CL. Radiation exposure in paranasal sinus imaging. Otolaryngol Head Neck Surg 1995; 112:248–251.

60. Spencer DH. Radiation dose to the eye lens from coronal CT scanning of the sinuses. Clin Radiol 1996; 51:666.

61. Moulin G, Chagnaud C, Waultier S, et al. Radiation dose to the lenses in CT of the paranasal sinuses. Neuroradiology 1996; 38 suppl 1:S127–S129.

62. Kearney SE, Jones P, Meakin K, Garvey CJ. CT scanning of the paranasal sinuses—the effect of reducing mAs. Br J Radiol 1997; 70:1071–1074.

63. Cohnen M, Cohnen B, Ewen K, Teubert G, Modder U. Dosage measurements in spiral CT examinations of the head and neck region. Rofo Fortschr Geb Roentgenstr Neuen Bildgeb Verfahr 1998; 168:474–479.

64. Damilakis J, Prassopoulos P, Mazonakis M, Bizakis J, Papadaki E, Gourtsoyiannis N. Tailored low dose three-dimensional CT of paranasal sinuses. Clin Imaging 1998; 22:235–239.

65. Luntz M, Malatskey S, Tan M, Bar-Meir E, Ruimi D. Volume of mastoid pneumatization: three-dimensional reconstruction with ultrahigh-resolution computed tomography. Ann Otol Rhinol Laryngol 2001; 110:486–490.

66. Endo M, Tsunoo T, Nakamori N, Yoshida K. Effect of scattered radiation on image noise in cone beam CT. Med Phys 2001; 28:469–474.

67. Hasso AN, Lambert D. Magnetic resonance imaging of the paranasal sinuses and nasal cavities. Top Magn Reson Imaging 1994; 6:209–223.

68. Hahnel S, Ertl-Wagner B, Tasman AJ, Forsting M, Jansen O. Relative value of MR imaging as compared with CT in the diagnosis of inflammatory paranasal sinus disease. Radiology 1999; 210:171–176.

69. Weiss F, Habermann CR, Welger J, et al. MRI in the preoperative diagnosis of chronic sinusitis: comparison with CT. Rofo Fortschr Geb Roentgenstr Neuen Bildgeb Verfahr 2001; 173:319–324.

70. Terk MR, Underwood DJ, Zee CS, Colletti PM. MR imaging in rhinocerebral and intracranial mucormycosis with CT and pathologic correlation. Magn Reson Imaging 1992; 10:81–87.

71. Ashdown BC, Tien RD, Felsberg GJ. Aspergillosis of the brain and paranasal sinuses in immunocompromised patients: CT and MR imaging findings. AJR Am J Roentgenol 1994; 162:155–159.

72. Held P, Breit A. Comparison of CT and MRI in diagnosis of tumors of the

nasopharynx, the inner nose and the paranasal sinuses. Bildgebung 1994; 61:187–196.

73. Hussain S, Salahuddin N, Ahmad I, Salahuddin I, Jooma R. Rhinocerebral invasive mycosis: occurrence in immunocompetent individuals. Eur J Radiol 1995; 20:151–155.

74. Som PM, Dillon WP, Fullerton GD, Zimmerman RA, Rajagopalan B, Marom Z. Chronically obstructed sinonasal secretions: observations on T1 and T2 shortening. Radiology 1989; 172:515–520.

75. Yamada K, Zoarski GH, Rothman MI, Zagardo MT, Nishimura T, Sun CC. An intracranial aspergilloma with low signal on T2-weighted images corresponding to iron accumulation. Neuroradiology 2001; 43:559–561.

76. Metson R, Gliklich RE, Stankiewicz JA, et al. Comparison of sinus computed tomography staging systems. Otolaryngol Head Neck Surg 1997; 117:372–379.

77. Stoney P, Probst L, Shankar L, Hawke M. CT scanning for functional endoscopic sinus surgery: analysis of 200 cases with reporting scheme. J Otolaryngol 1993; 22:72–78.

78. Laine FJ, Smoker WR. The osteomeatal unit and endoscopic surgery: anatomy, variations, and imaging findings in inflammatory diseases. AJR Am J Roentgenol 1992; 159:849–857.

79. Chong VF, Fan YF, Lau D, Sethi DS. Functional endoscopic sinus surgery (FESS): what radiologists need to know. Clin Radiol 1998; 53:650–658.

80. Zinreich SJ. Functional anatomy and computed tomography imaging of the paranasal sinuses. Am J Med Sci 1998; 316:2–12.

81. Earwaker J. Anatomic variants in sinonasal CT. Radiographics 1993; 13:381–415.

82. Jones NS, Strobl A, Holland I. A study of the CT findings in 100 patients with rhinosinusitis and 100 controls. Clin Otolaryngol 1997; 22:47–51.

83. Kayalioglu G, Oyar O, Govsa F. Nasal cavity and paranasal sinus bony variations: a computed tomographic study. Rhinology 2000; 38:108–113.

84. Albritton FD, Kingdom TT, DelGaudio JM. Malleable registration mask: application of a novel registration method in image guided sinus surgery. Am J Rhinol 2001; 15:219–224.

85. Hopper KD, Iyriboz AT, Wise SW, Fornadley JA. The feasibility of surgical site tagging with CT virtual reality of the paranasal sinuses. J Comput Assist Tomogr 1999; 23:529–533.

86. Casiano RR, Numa WA Jr. Efficacy of computed tomographic image—guided endoscopic sinus surgery in residency training programs. Laryngoscope 2000; 110:1277–1282.

87. Messerklinger W. Endoscopische diagnose und chirurgie des residivierdes sinusitis. In: Krajina Z, ed. Advances in Nose and Sinus Surgery. Zagreb: Zagreb University, 1985.

88. Wigand ME, Steiner W, Jaumann MP. Endonasal sinus surgery with endoscopical control: from radical operation to rehabilitation of the mucosa. Endoscopy 1978; 10:255–260.

89. Draf W. Endoscopy of the Paranasal Sinuses. New York: Springer-Verlag, 1983.

10

Management of Allergic Rhinitis in Patients with Asthma

JONATHAN CORREN

Allergy Research Foundation
Los Angeles, California, U.S.A.

JEAN BOUSQUET

Hopital Arnaud de Villeneuve
Montpellier, France

The treatment of allergic rhinitis has evolved and improved markedly over the past two decades. Validation of environmental control strategies and the development of multiple new medications have made it possible to reduce significantly symptoms of rhinitis with minimal adverse effects. In addition, many of the therapies now employed for upper airway disease have also been shown to provide benefits to the lower airway.

In this chapter, we will review allergen avoidance measures; pharmacotherapy, including emerging new therapies; specific allergen immunotherapy; and discuss the effects of selected treatments on bronchial asthma.

I. Allergen Avoidance Measures

In patients with perennial symptoms attributable to indoor allergens (e.g., dust mites, furry animals, indoor molds, cockroaches), avoidance of the allergen is a critical first step in treatment. Environmental control programs should always be based on accurate assessments of both sensitization (by skin or in vitro testing) and exposure. These strategies are particularly helpful to patients who are sensitized only to indoor allergens, with no evidence of allergy to pollens or outdoor molds.

A. Dust Mites

House dust mites (*Dermatophagoides farinae* and *D. pteronyssinus*) are ubiquitous throughout the world (except in dry or alpine regions), and approximately 30–40% of patients with allergic rhinitis are allergic to allergens produced by these mite species (1). A large number of clinical trials have examined the efficacy of mite avoidance measures in patients with allergic asthma. In general, these studies have included encasement of pillows and mattresses in impermeable covers, washing of all bedding in hot (> 130°F) water, and elimination of carpeting in favor of tile or hardwood floors (2–4). A recent meta-analysis determined that encasing of pillows and mattresses was the single most effective measure in reducing symptoms of asthma and rhinitis caused by dust mite exposure (5). Frequent cleaning of floors with vacuum cleaners equipped with double-thickness reservoir bags and/or a high-efficiency particulate air (HEPA) filter attached to the exhaust port has also been suggested to help reduce the amount of settled dust (6). The application of acaricidal and denaturing solutions (7) and the installation of free-standing HEPA filters (8) in bedrooms have not proved effective in reducing symptoms caused by mite exposure.

B. Pets

Virtually any furry pet may result in allergic sensitization and ultimately symptoms of rhinitis and asthma. However, most of the available clinical data regarding the efficacy of animal avoidance measures come from studies of indoor cats and their major allergen, Fel d I. Contrary to patients' wishes, effective avoidance of cat allergen requires removal of the pet from the inside of the home. Even after this is accomplished, it may take several months or longer for the indoor concentration of Fel d I to return to low levels; this process is markedly expedited by the removal of indoor carpeting and aggressive cleaning (9). One study suggested that a combination of noncarpeted floors, plastic or leather furniture, frequent vacuuming, high-flow air filtration, and frequent washing of the cat substantially reduced indoor levels of Fel d I (10). However, long-term studies with clinical end points are needed before this approach can be advocated. One recent study that examined the effects of the removal of the cat from the bedroom (but not from the house) plus the use of a HEPA filter in the bedroom failed to demonstrate any clinical benefits (11).

C. Indoor Mold

Identification of homes with mold growth is often difficult. Indoor mold spores from species of *Aspergillus* and *Penicillium* are most likely to emanate from potentially damp areas such as crawl spaces (because of defective plumbing or poor drainage), attics (due to roof leaks), and under sinks (12). Following a thorough inspection of the house, attic, and crawl space, the visual presence of mold confirms the problem (13). Occasionally, however, wall spaces, carpet backing, and other areas with limited access may harbor mold growth, and identification of the mold may be delayed or even missed. Wallboard infested with mold will need to be replaced and wood framing cleaned thoroughly with a solution of bleach. Complete correction of all plumbing, drainage, and construction defects also must be undertaken to prevent future water intrusion and perpetuation of mold growth.

D. Cockroach

Cockroach allergy has recently been most implicated as a pathogenic factor in patients with asthma and allergic rhinitis (14). The best indicator of a significant cockroach infestation is the presence of emanations on the floor or in cabinetry. Cockroach exposure is usually not limited to the kitchen or dining room, but may occur in all living areas because allergen is passively transferred on shoes and clothing. Pesticide application is only temporarily effective, and problems will recur unless food and garbage are appropriately packaged and handled (15).

E. Outdoor Seasonal Allergens

Plant pollens and outdoor molds (e.g., species of *Alternaria* and *Cladosporium*) are responsible for the symptoms of seasonal allergic rhinitis, and are generally very difficult to avoid completely. During indoor activities, keeping all windows and doors shut and the use of an air conditioner eliminate most pollen from the inside of the house. Because outdoor pollen counts are highest between 11:00 a.m. and 3:00 p.m., especially on hot, sunny days, avoidance of outdoor activities during those times may be helpful. Certain mold spore counts tend to be highest late in the evening or early in the morning, especially in damp climates, and this may be a consideration for patients who are mold allergic. However, altering schedule and activities is undesirable for most patients, and, for this reason, avoidance measures play a limited role in allergic rhinitis caused by outdoor allergens.

II. Pharmacological Therapy

Patients with significant symptoms of seasonal allergic rhinitis will usually require medication to relieve their symptoms. Whereas environmental control measures may reduce the intensity of perennial rhinitis caused by indoor allergens, in most cases supplemental medical therapy will also be needed. Several different classes of medication are now available for the treatment of allergic rhinitis.

A. H₁ Antihistamines

General

H_1 antihistamines are the most commonly prescribed class of medication for allergic rhinitis. Although these drugs act primarily by blocking the H_1-histamine receptor, many of the agents have also been shown to have mild anti-inflammatory properties (e.g., reduction in expression of adhesion molecules). As a general rule, H_1 antihistamines reduce symptoms of sneezing, itching, rhinorrhea, and ocular injection but have little effect on nasal congestion (16). Because most antihistamines have a relatively rapid onset of action (1–3 h), these agents are frequently and effectively used on an intermittent, as-needed basis. Whereas chronic use of these drugs was once thought to result in therapeutic subsensitivity, recent studies have failed to support this contention (17).

First-Generation Antihistamines

First-generation antihistaminic compounds were the first to be developed, and most are available over the counter (OTC), either alone or in combination with a decongestant (Table 1). These drugs readily cross the blood–brain barrier and bind not only to the H_1-histamine receptor but in many cases to dopaminergic, serotonergic, and cholinergic receptors (18). These characteristics help to account for the adverse effects of these agents, which include both central nervous system (CNS) effects (e.g., sedation, fatigue, dizziness, impairment of cognition and performance) and anticholinergic effects (e.g., dryness of the mouth and eyes, constipation, inhibition of micturition, potential precipitation of narrow-angle glaucoma). Although tolerance to sedation may occur over a period of several days, substantial effects on intellectual functioning and performance may persist without the patient's knowledge (19). This is well-exemplified in studies of driving performance, which have demonstrated marked impairment with the use of single doses of triprolidine 50 mg (20). It may also help explain why serious workplace

Table 1 H1 Antihistamines

Compound	Dosage	Sedating[a]	Anticholinergic
First generation			
Chlorpheniramine	4–12 mg BID	Yes	Yes
Diphenhydramine	25–50 mg QID	Yes	Yes
Clemastine	1.25 mg BID	Yes	Yes
Second generation			
Loratadine	10 mg QD	No	No
Cetirizine	10 mg QD	Yes	No
Azelastine[b]	0.5 mg BID	Yes	No
Third generation			
Fexofenadine	60 mg BID or 180 mg QD	No	No
Desloratadine	5 mg	No	No

[a] Refers to sedation rate > placebo (from product insert).
[b] Administered topically.
QD, once daily; BID, twice daily; QID, four times daily.

accidents are more closely associated with first-generation antihistamines than any other class of medication (21).

A number of case reports from the 1970s and 1980s suggested that first-generation antihistamines, such as brompheniramine, induced broncho-spasm in a small number of patients (22). There were also theoretic concerns that these agents might cause drying and inspissation of mucus in the lower airways and, ultimately, lead to atelectasis. Large studies have demonstrated that these agents are safe to use in patients with asthma (23).

Because of the strong CNS effects of these agents, first-generation antihistamines should be prescribed with caution in all patients, but should be absolutely avoided in patients who are airplane pilots, drive extensively, or operate heavy or dangerous machinery; who have pre-existing intellectual impairment; who have benign prostatic hypertrophy or other forms of bladder outlet obstruction; or who have elevated intraocular pressure.

Although alternative forms of therapy for allergic rhinitis are preferable in many situations, patients who do not have medical insurance or formulary coverage often resort to self-medication with over-the-counter first-generation antihistamines. A recent strategy to avoid drug side effects, and to contain costs, has been to use a potentially sedating, first-generation antihistamine at night, coupled with a short-acting, nonsedating antihistamine in the morning. However, one study has demonstrated that adverse

CNS effects occur with this regimen as well, even after several days of administration (24).

Newer Antihistamines

Second-generation antihistamines have been shown to be at least as clinically effective as first-generation agents for the treatment of allergic rhinitis (16) (Table 1). They are larger and more lipophobic than first-generation drugs and, therefore, do not readily cross the blood–brain barrier. In addition, they bind specifically to the H_1-histamine receptor and have little affinity for other receptors. For these reasons, the second-generation agents cause little or no somnolence (19), do not affect performance (20), and have no anticholinergic effects (16).

Newer antihistamines have been developed that may offer some therapeutic or safety advantages over existing second-generation antihistamines. Because certain of these drugs represent metabolites of second-generation antihistamines, they have been termed third-generation antihistamines (25). Fexofenadine (terfenadine metabolite) (26) and desloratadine (loratadine metabolite) (27) are commercially available in the United States, while tecastemizole (astemizole metabolite) is currently in phase III clinical trials. All of these new agents will provide therapeutic efficacy equivalent to or greater to their parent compounds, along with excellent safety profiles.

A number of trials have examined the safety of these drugs in patients with allergic rhinitis and concomitant mild asthma, and found them to be safe and well tolerated (28).

B. Decongestants

A number of α-adrenergic agonists are available for oral use, including pseudoephedrine and phenylephrine (29). These drugs primarily reduce nasal congestion and, to some extent, rhinorrhea, but have no effect on sneezing, itching, or ocular symptoms. Therefore, they are most helpful in the treatment of allergic rhinitis when combined with an antihistamine. Most common side effects of oral decongestants include CNS (e.g., nervousness, insomnia, irritability, headache) and cardiovascular (e.g., palpitations, tachycardia) symptoms. In addition, these drugs may elevate blood pressure, raise intraocular pressure, and aggravate urinary obstruction. Their safety in asthma has been investigated, and there is no evidence that they induce drying of the airways or bronchospasm.

Largely owing to their effects on both the CNS and cardiovascular systems, this group of medications should be used very cautiously in elderly patients and should be avoided in patients with ischemic heart disease, glaucoma, and any form of bladder outlet obstruction. Although

clinical studies have demonstrated that short-term use of oral decongestants does not increase blood pressure in patients with controlled hypertension (30), other agents (e.g., intranasal corticosteroids) are preferable in
these individuals.

Topical intranasal decongestants continue to be widely used by patients
with allergic rhinitis and include phenylephrine, oxymetolazine, xylometo-
lazine, and naphazoline. When topical decongestants are used for longer
than 3–5 days, many patients will experience rebound congestion after
withdrawal of the drug (31). If patients continue to use these medications
over several months, a form of rhinitis (rhinitis medicamentosa) will develop
that can be difficult to treat effectively.

C. Antihistamine–Decongestant Combinations

The combination of an oral H_1 antihistamine and decongestant is one of
the most popular OTC remedies for allergic rhinitis. The second-generation
antihistamines loratadine and fexofenadine are both available in combination with long-acting pseudoephedrine and provide better symptom relief
than an antihistamine alone.

D. Intranasal Corticosteroids

Topical intranasal corticosteroids have made a significant impact on the
treatment of both seasonal and perennial allergic rhinitis. These drugs appear to exert their efforts through multiple mechanisms, including vasoconstriction and reduction of edema, suppression of cytokine production, and
inhibition of inflammatory cell influx (32). Prophylactic treatment before
nasal allergen challenge reduces both the early- and late-phase allergic
responses (33).

In a large number of clinical trials, intranasal corticosteroids have
been demonstrated to be the most effective class of therapy in treating nasal
allergy. When compared with oral H1 antihistamines, these drugs are more
effective at reducing most nasal symptoms, particularly nasal congestion.
An interesting finding is that, intranasal corticosteroids also appear to be
at least as effective in controlling concomitant symptoms of ocular allergy
as oral antihistamines.

Intranasal corticosteroids work best when taken regularly on a daily
basis. A number of investigations have demonstrated that this class of
agents may be most effective when started 1–2 weeks before the pollen
season. However, because of their rapid onset of action (within 12–24 h
for many agents), there is increasing evidence that they may also be
moderately effective when used intermittently following the start of the
pollen season (34).

A number of glucocorticoid compounds are now available for intra-nasal use in both aerosol and aqueous formulation (Table 2) (35). Although the topical potency of these agents varies widely, clinical trials have been unable to demonstrate significant differences in efficacy in patients with either seasonal or perennial allergic rhinitis (35). The most important pharmacological characteristic differentiating these agents is systemic bio-availability. After intranasal application, the majority of the dose of a glucocorticoid is swallowed. Most of the available compounds (including beclomethasone dipropionate, budesonide, flunisolide, and triamcinolone acetonide) are absorbed readily from the gastrointestinal tract into the systemic circulation and subsequently undergo significant first-pass hepatic metabolism (Table 2). The resulting bioavailabilities can be as high as 50%. However, neither fluticasone propionate nor mometasone furoate is well absorbed through the gastrointestinal tract, and the small amount of drug that reaches the portal circulation is rapidly and thoroughly metabolized (36,37). These low systemic drug levels may represent an advantage in adult patients who are prone to systemic effects of corticosteroids, such as those with developing cataracts or an elevation in intraocular pressure. The low systemic availabilities of these two newer agents may be most important in growing adolescents and in patients who are already using medium to high dosages of inhaled corticosteroids for bronchial asthma.

Table 2 Intranasal Corticosteroids

Medication	Dose per actuation (mg)	Formulation		Usual adult dosage	Systemic bioavailability (%)
		Aqueous	Aerosol		
Beclomethasone dipropionate	42	+	+	1–2 sprays each nostril, bid	Unknown
	84	+	0	2 sprays each nostril, qd	
Budesonide	32	0	+	2 sprays each nostril, bid, or	21
Flunisolide	25	+	0	2 sprays each nostril, bid	20–50
Fluticasone propionate	50	+	0	2 sprays each nostril, qd	<2
Mometasone furoate	50	+	0	2 sprays each nostril, qd	≤0.1
Triamcinolone acetonide	55	+	+	2 sprays each nostril, qd	Unknown

+, Available; 0, not available; bid, twice daily; qd, daily.

Patients using intranasal corticosteroids experience dryness and irritation of the nasal mucous membranes in 5–10% of cases, and mild epistaxis in approximately 5%. For mild symptoms, the dosage of corticosteroid may be reduced if tolerated, and/or saline nasal spray should be instilled before the drug is sprayed. Because there have been case reports of nasa septal perforation, patients who use these agents continuously for treatment of perennial rhinitis should be seen at yearly intervals. Evidence of superficial erosions or significant crusting or bleeding should prompt discontinuation of the drug.

E. Anticholinergics

Topical intranasal ipratropium bromide, 0.03% solution, reduces the volume of watery secretions but has little or no effect on other symptoms (38). Therefore, ipratropium is most helpful in the treatment of allergic rhinitis when rhinorrhea is refractory to topical intranasal corticosteroids and/or antihistamines. The most common side effects include nasal irritation, crusting, and occasional mild epistaxis.

F. Leukotriene Modifiers

Sulfidopeptide leukotrienes play an important role in the treatment of bronchial asthma. Leukotriene receptor antagonists have been demonstrated to be safe and efficacious in its treatment (39). These proinflammatory molecules are released into the nose after allergen challenge and it has been demonstrated that leukotrine C_4 contributes to nasal dysfunction in patients with allergic rhinitis (40). It is therefore not surprising that symptoms of allergic rhinitis are significantly reduced by administration of the leukotriene D_4 receptor antagonists zafirlukast and montelukast (39). A number of recent clinical trials have demonstrated that montelukast, 10 mg daily, provides relief of all nasal symptoms (congestion, sneezing, itching, and discharge), which is superior to placebo and equivalent to loratadine, 10 mg daily (41). The combination of montelukast plus loratadine has been demonstrated to offer no advantages over either agent used alone (42). Small trials in patients with seasonal allergic rhinitis have demonstrated that montelukast plus cetirizine was as effective as mometasone furoate nasal spray, 200 µg daily; these results await confirmation in large, well-controlled studies (43).

G. Cromolyn Sodium

Topical intranasal cromolyn sodium has an extensive record of use for treatment of allergic rhinitis (44). When given four to six times daily, it is as effective as antihistamines in controlling sneezing, rhinorrhea, and itching.

Although the drug has no significant side effects, the need for frequent administration limits its usefulness in adult patients with chronic, daily symptoms. Intranasal cromolyn is most useful as a prophylactic treatment before a known allergen exposure, when antihistamines are not tolerated.

III. Allergen Immunotherapy

Specific-allergen immunotherapy (allergy vaccine therapy) continues to be a useful and important treatment for many patients with moderate to severe allergic rhinitis. Immunotherapy attenuates airways inflammation in both the upper and lower airways. Research performed during the past decade has demonstrated that allergy immunotherapy induces a systemic state of allergen-specific T-lymphocyte tolerance with a subsequent reduction in mediator release and tissue inflammation (45). When administered to appropriately selected patients, allergy immunotherapy is effective in reducing nasal symptoms in approximately 85% of cases. In addition to these short-term benefits, recently published data suggest that the improvement in rhinitis symptoms persists for several years after the treatment is discontinued (46).

As allergy immunotherapy represents a systemic treatment, clinical observations from the 1950's suggested that early use of immunotherapy in patients with rhinitis might prevent the ultimate development of bronchial asthma (47). A recent large, prospective study in children with seasonal allergic rhinitis demonstrated that a 3 year course of immunotherapy reduced the development of asthma symptoms and improved bronchial hyperresponsiveness compared with an open control group (48). This observation suggests that allergy immunotherapy should be considered in patients with allergic rhinitis before lower airway symptoms become firmly established.

Global guidelines suggest that allergy immunotherapy should be strongly considered in patients who do not respond to a combination of environmental control measures and medications, experience substantial side effects with medications, have symptoms for a significant portion of the year that require daily therapy, or prefer long-term modulation of their allergic symptoms, particularly if asthma symptoms are becoming manifest (49).

IV. Treatment Considerations in Special Groups

A. Children

Infants may experience intermittent or persistent symptoms of rhinitis, most frequently consisting of nasal congestion and thick rhinorrhea. It is thought that these symptoms are due to persistent nasal inflammation following acute viral rhinosinusitis. Because the infant's nasal airway is small, clearance of secretions is difficult and may result in nasal obstruction. Allergic rhinitis in children younger than 1 year of age is unusual, and if present would most likely be due to a perennial allergen, such as an animal. Children do not usually experience symptoms of seasonal allergic rhinitis until after their third birthday, since repetitive exposure to seasonal pollens is required for the induction of sensitization.

First-line therapy for allergic rhinitis in children usually consists of an H1 antihistamine. Because older drugs, such as chlorpheniramine and diphenhydramine, have been implicated in altering cognitive functioning and school performance in young children, newer antihistamines may be more suitable in this population (50). Loratadine, 10 mg once daily given as a liquid or dissolvable tablet, has been shown to be efficacious in children as young as age 3 years and is without apparent CNS effects (38a). In children who have significant nasal congestion, the addition of pseudoephedrine at a dosage of 15–30 mg, three to four times daily as needed, may be helpful.

If oral antihistamines and/or pseudoephedrine are not sufficiently effective, an intranasal corticosteroid should be started. As noted above, intranasal coricosteroids are the most effective available therapy for symptoms of allergic rhinitis, particularly nasal congestion. One study using intranasal beclomethasone dipropionate, 168 ucg twice daily, demonstrated significant reduction in linear growth velocity during 1 year of use in young children (51). However, in another study using intranasal mometasone furoate, 100 µg once daily, there was no suppression of growth (52). Children treated with mometasone nasal spray demonstrated a significant increase in height compared with children treated with placebo. It is uncertain to why active treatment resulted in enhanced growth, but such a finding is of potential importance and will need to be replicated in additional similar studies.

B. Elderly

As people grow older, structural changes in the nose result in increased nasal airflow resistance and dryness and atrophy of the mucous membranes (53). These normal changes in nasal anatomy and physiological condition contribute to the symptoms of pre-existing allergic rhinitis and may make treatment more difficult. Often, nasal saline solution helps to eliminate dryness and reduces the need for antiallergy drugs.

Patients older than 60 years of age frequently use a number of medications that can be primary or contributing factors in chronic rhinitis. Antihypertensive drugs are most commonly implicated, including angiotensin-converting enzyme inhibitors, β-blockers, methyldopa, prazosin, reserpine, guanethidine, and phentolamine. Nonsteroidal anti-inflammatory drugs have been noted to cause nasal congestion and rhinorrhea, often but not always associated with sinusitis, nasal polyps, and asthma. If any one of these drugs may be contributing to significant nasal symptoms, consideration should be made to switching the patient to an alternative agent.

As mentioned above, elderly patients are more likely to experience a number of comorbid conditions that contraindicate the use of first-generation antihistamines and oral decongestants. Second- or third-generation antihistamines and intranasal steroids or corticosteroids have fewer adverse effects and are better choices in this population.

C. Pregnancy

Allergic rhinitis can worsen considerably during pregnancy. For symptoms of rhinorrhea, sneezing, or itching, intranasal cromolyn has an excellent safety profile and should be considered as a first line of therapy. If cromolyn is ineffective for these symptoms or is poorly tolerated, an oral antihistamine should be given. Chlorpheniramine and tripelennamine have an extensive record of use in pregnant women and remain the antihistamines of choice during pregnancy (54). If nasal congestion is prominent, intranasal corticosteroids are both safe and effective (54). To date, the intranasal corticosteroid with the longest record of safety is beclomethasone dipropionate. If an oral decongestant is desired, pseudoephedrine is the drug of choice. However, patients should be advised to avoid oral and topical decongestants during the first trimester because of the risk of infant gastroschisis (abdominal wall defect) (55).

V. Future Therapies

As our understanding of allergic disease pathophysiology has improved over the past decade, a number of new molecular targets has emerged. These targets serve as the basis of potential new interventions in treating patients with both allergic rhinitis and asthma.

A. Monoclonal Anti-IgE Antibody Therapy

A recombinant, humanized monoclonal IgG antibody directed against the Fc portion of IgE has recently been demonstrated to cause substantial reductions in the circulation of IgE levels (56), immediate skin test reactivity (57), and the immediate nasal reaction to allergen challenge (58). In a recent large study, patients with seasonal allergic rhinitis experienced significant improvements in symptoms of seasonal allergic rhinitis compared with patients receiving placebo (59). Long-term studies have demonstrated the treatment to be safe and well tolerated, with fewer adverse events than currently available allergen-specific immunotherapy. Although this new treatment offers a safe and effective alternative to both pharmacotherapy and specific-allergen immunotherapy, it is unknown whether long-term administration will result in a lasting modulation of the immune system (58).

B. Cytokine Antagonists

A growing list of cytokines has been indentified as playing key roles in regulating the induction and perpetuation of allergic inflammation. Among these, interleukins (IL)-4, -5, -9, and -13 have stood out as the most important, and potential strategies to antagonize their effects have been sought. To date, initial results using an IL-4 antagonist (soluble IL-4 receptor) were initially encouraging in patients with allergic asthma (60), but subsequent studies proved negative. Studies with a monoclonal antibody directed against IL-5 were likewise successful in reducing blood and sputum eosinophilia, but had no significant effects on lower airway physiology (61) or chronic symptoms of asthma. Future studies may focus on antagonizing multiple cytokines simultaneously, which may help to overcome the significant redundancy noted in human immune responses.

VI. Effects of Rhinitis Therapy on Asthma

Physicians often note anecdotally that treatment of allergic nasal disease results in improvements in asthma symptoms and pulmonary function. However, there have been relatively few well-controlled, large-scale clinical trials that have attempted to quantify this effect.

A. Intranasal Corticosteroids

Several small studies have examined the efficacy of topical intranasal corticosteroids in patients with allergic rhinitis and mild asthma. Two of these trials addressed the role of prophylactic, preseasonal treatment with nasal corticosteroids in patients with primarily seasonal symptoms. Welsh and co-workers compared the effects of intranasal beclomethasone dipropionate, flunisolide, and cromolyn with placebo in patients with ragweed-induced rhinitis (62). Both of the topical corticosteroids were significantly more effective in reducing nasal symptoms than either cromolyn or placebo. An unexpected finding was that in 58 of the subjects who also had mild ragweed asthma, lower airway symptoms were also significantly improved in the patients receiving intranasal corticosteroids. Corren and co-workers later examined the effects of seasonal administration of intranasal beclomethasone dipropionate on bronchial hyperresponsiveness in patients with fall rhinitis and mild asthma (63). Compared with baseline values, bronchial responsiveness to inhaled methacholine worsened significantly in the placebo group but did not change in the group using active treatment. Together, these two small trials suggest that prevention of seasonal nasal inflammation with topical corticosteroids reduces subsequent exacerbations of allergic asthma.

Other studies have examined the effects of intranasal corticosteroids on patients with chronic, perennial allergic rhinitis and mild asthma. The first study to document these effects used intranasal budesonide in children with severe allergic rhinitis and concomitant asthma (64). Four weeks of active therapy significantly reduced the objective measures of nasal obstruction as well as daily asthma symptoms and exercise-induced bronchospasm. In a subsequent study of patients with perennial rhinitis and asthma, Watson et al. evaluated the effects of intranasal beclomethasone dipropionate on chest symptoms and bronchial responsiveness to methacholine (65). Following 4 weeks of active treatment, asthma symptoms were significantly reduced, as was airway reactivity to methacholine. As an adjunct to this study, the investigators performed a radiolabeled deposition study of the beclomethasone aerosol and found that less than 2% of the drug was deposited into the chest area. These studies demonstrate that intranasal corticosteroids are effective in improving lower airway symptoms and bronchial hyperresponsiveness in patients with chronic, established nasal disease and asthma. In view of the fact that the corticosteroid spray did not penetrate into the lungs, the study by Watson et al. also asserts that the reduction observed in asthma was due to improvements in nasal function rather than direct effects of the medication on the lower airways.

B. Antihistamines

The presence of histamine in the lower airways has been correlated with bronchial obstruction (66), and histamine has long thought to play a role in bronchial asthma. However, early studies of first-generation antihistamines showed minimal improvements in bronchial asthma (67) and initial small trials of second-generation antihistamines yielded mixed results (68–72). However, two large-scale clinical studies using an antihistamine alone and an antihistamine–decongestant combination both resulted in significant improvements in asthma control. Grant et al. demonstated that seasonal symptoms of rhinitis and asthma were significantly attenuated in patients treated with cetirizine, 10 mg once daily (73). In a second study using loratadine 5 mg plus pseudoephedrine 120 mg, twice daily, in patients with seasonal allergic rhinitis and asthma, Corren et al. demonstrated that asthma symptoms, peak expiratory flow rates, and forced expiratory volume in 1s (FEV1) were all significantly improved in patients taking active therapy (74). In reviewing data from these and similar trials, it is difficult to determine whether the salutary effects of antihistamines in asthma can be attributed to direct effects on lower airway physiology or are due to improvements in rhinitis. Since many of the currently available agents appear to have weak or transient effects on resting airway tone, benefits to the lower airway may in fact be due to modulation of upper airway function (75).

Oral antihistamines have also been considered a potential treatments to prevent the development of asthma. In one long-term study of infants with atopic dermatitis and hypersensitivity to house dust mites and/or grass pollen, early treatment with cetirizine resulted in a significant reduction in the development of asthma symptoms (76). This finding suggests a possible role of oral antihistamine therapy in modulating the natural history of asthma.

C. Population-Based Studies

A number of recent epidemiological analyses have sought to determine the effects of rhinitis treatment on emergency room visits and hospitalizations for asthma. One retrospective cohort study demonstrated that either intranasal corticosteroids or oral antihistamines reduced hospital (emergency room and in-patient) care for asthma in patients with asthma and concomitant allergic rhinitis (77). In a second study utilizing a similar study design, the authors noted that either intranasal corticosteroids or antihistamines reduced the rate of emergency room care for asthma among patients with asthma and concomitant rhinitis (78). The most recent study utilized a nested case–control design and demonstrated that treatment with intranasal corticosteroids had a significantly lower risk of both asthma-related emergency room treatment and hospitalization while there was a trend toward lower risk of emergency room treatment and hospitalization in patients using second-generation antihistamines. Combined treatment with both medications was associated with a further lowering of the risk of both emergency room treatment and hospitalization (79).

The above studies have shown that treatment of rhinitis may result in improvements in mild asthma symptoms, pulmonary function, and bronchial hyperresponsiveness. Recent epidemiological studies also suggest that effective therapy of allergic rhinitis in patients with both asthma and rhinitis may reduce serious asthma exacerbations requiring hospital care. All of the above data provide an ample basis for aggressively seeking and treating allergic rhinitis in patients with bronchial asthma.

VII. Summary

In adults with allergic rhinitis, physicians should be alert to the frequency and severity of specific symptoms and how those symptoms affect the daily functioning of their patients. A stepped-care approach that involves environmental control measures, drug therapy, and possible immunotherapy should be considered and used in all patients with nasal allergy.

References

1. Galant S, Berger W, Gillman S, Goldsobel A, Incaudo G, Kanter L, et al. Prevalence of sensitization to aeroallergens in California patients with respiratory allergy: Allergy Skin Test Project Team. Ann Allergy Asthma Immunol 1998; 81:203–210.
2. Gøtzsche PC, Johansen HK, Burr ML, Hammarquist C. House dust mite control measures for asthma. Cochrane Database Syst Rev 2001; (3):CD001187.
3. Chapman MD, Heymann PW, Sporik RB, Platts-Mills TA. Monitoring allergen exposure in asthma: new treatment strategies. Allergy 1995; 50(25 suppl):29–33.
4. Hill DJ, Thompson PJ, Stewart GA, Carlin JB, Nolan TM, Kemp AS, et al. The Melbourne House Dust Mite Study: eliminating house dust mites in the domestic environment. J Allergy Clin Immunol 1997; 99:323–329.
5. Sheikh A, Hurwitz B. House dust mite avoidance measures for perennial allergic rhinitis. Cochrane Database Syst Rev 2002; (3):CD000247.
6. Munir AK, Einarsson R, Dreborg SK. Vacuum cleaning decreases the levels of mite allergens in house dust. Pediatr Allergy Immunol 1993; 4:136–143.
7. Sporik R, Hill DJ, Thompson PJ, Stewart GA, Carlin JB, Nolan TM, et al. The Melbourne House Dust Mite Study: long-term efficacy of house dust mite reduction strategies. J Allergy Clin Immunol 1998; 101:451–456.
8. Reisman RE, Mauriello PM, Davis GB, Georgitis JW, DeMasi JM. A double-blind study of the effectiveness of a high-efficiency particulate air (HEPA) filter in the treatment of patients with perennial allergic rhinitis and asthma. J Allergy Clin Immunol 1990; 85:1050–1057.
9. Wood RA, Chapman MD, Adkinson NF Jr, Eggleston PA. The effect of cat removal on allergen content in household-dust samples. J Allergy Clin Immunol 1989; 83:730–734.
10. deBlay F, Chapman MD, Platts-Mills TA. Airborne cat allergen (Fel d I): environmental control with the cat in situ. Am Rev Respir Dis 1991; 143:1334–1339.
11. Wood RA, Johnson EF, Van Natta ML, Chen PH, Eggleston PA. A placebo-controlled trial of a HEPA air cleaner in the treatment of cat allergy. Am J Respir Crit Care Med 1998; 158:115–120.
12. Jaakkola JJ, Jaakkola N, Ruotsalainen R. Home dampness and molds as determinants of respiratory symptoms and asthma in pre-school children. J Exp Anal Environ Epidemiol 1993; 1(suppl):129–142.

13. Chapman JA. Update on airborne mold and mold allergy. Allergy Asthma Proc. 1999; 20(5):289–292.
14. Kivity S, Struhar D, Greif J, Schwartz Y, Topilsky M. Cockroach allergen: an important cause of perennial rhinitis. Allergy 1989; 44:291–293.
15. Gergen PJ, Mortimer KM, Eggleston PA, Rosenstreich D, Mitchell H, Owenby D, et al. Results of the National Cooperative Inner-City Asthma Study (NCICAS) environmental intervention to reduce cockroach allergen exposure in inner-city homes. J Allergy Clin Immunol 1999; 103:501–506.
16. Howarth PH. Assessment of antihistamine efficacy and potency. Clin Exp Allergy 1999; 29:87–97.
17. Bousquet J, Chanal I, Skassa-Brociek W, Lemonier C, Michel FB. Lack of subsensitivity to loratadine during long-term dosing during 12 weeks. J Allergy Clin Immunol 1990; 86:248–253.
18. Yanai K, Ryu JH, Watanabe T, Iwata R, Ido T, Sawai Y, et al. Histamine H_1 receptor occupancy in human brains after single oral doses of histamine H_1 antagonists measured by positron emission tomography. Br J Pharmacol 1995; 116:1649–1655.
19. Kay GG, Berman B, Harris A. Self-reported sedation doesn't predict impaired CNS functioning after dose of sedating antihistamine [abstr]. J Allergy Clin Immunol 1999; 103:A975.
20. O'Hanlon JF, Ramaekers JG. Antihistamine effects on actual driving performance in a standard test: a summary of Dutch experience, 1989–1994. Allergy 1995; 50:234–242.
21. Gilmore TM, Alexander BH, Mueller BA, Rivara FP. Occupational injuries and medication use. Am J Indust Med 1996; 30:234–239.
22. Schuller DE. Adverse effects of brompheniramine on pulmonary function in a subset of asthmatic children. J Allergy Clin Immunol 1983; 72:175–179.
23. Popa VT. Bronchodilating activity of an H1 blocker, chlorpheniramine. J Allergy Clin Immunol 1977 Jan; 59(1):54–63.
24. Kay GG, Plotkin KE, Quig MB, Starbuck VN, Yasuda S. Sedating effects of AM/PM antihistamine dosing with evening chlorpheniramine and morning terfenadine. Am J Managed Care 1997; 3:1843–1848.
25. Caballero R, Delpon E, Valenzuela C, Longobardo M, Franqueza L, Tamargo J. Effect of descarboethoxyloratadine, the major metabolite of loratadine, on the human cardiac potassium channel Kv1.5. Br J Pharmacol 1997; 122:796–798.
26. Casale TB, Andrade C, Qu R. Safety and efficacy of once-daily fexofenadine HCl in the treatment of autumn seasonal allergic rhinitis. Allergy Asthma Proc 1999; 20:193–198.
27. Geha RS, Meltzer EO. Desloratadine: a new, nonsedating, oral antihistamine. J Allergy Clin Immunol 2001; 107(4):751–762.
28. Lordan JL, Holgate ST. H1-antihistamines in asthma. Clin Allergy Immunol 2002; 17:221–248.
29. Kanfer I, Dowse R, Vuma V. Pharmacokinetics of oral decongestants. Pharmacotherapy 1993; 13:116S–128S.
30. Petrulis AS, Imperiale TF, Speroff T. The acute effect of phenylpropanolamine and brompheniramine on blood pressure in controlled hypertension:

a randomized double-blind crossover trial. J Gen Intern Med 1991; 6:503–506.

31. Graf P. Rhinitis medicamentosa: aspects of pathophysiology and treatment. Allergy 1997; 52:28–34.

32. Meltzer EO. The pharmacological basis for the treatment of perennial allergic rhinitis and non-allergic rhinitis with topical corticosteroids. Allergy 1997; 52:33–40.

33. Pipkorn U, Proud D, Lichtenstein LM, Kagey-Sobotka A, Norman PS, Naclerio RM. Inhibition of mediator release in allergic rhinitis by pretreatment with topical glucocorticosteroids. N Engl J Med 1987; 316:1506–1510.

34. Juniper EF, Guyatt GH, Archer B, Ferrie PJ. Aqueous beclomethasone dipropionate in the treatment of ragweed pollen-induced rhinitis: further exploration of "as needed" use. J Allergy Clin Immunol 1993; 92:66–72.

35. Corren J. Intranasal corticosteroids for allergic rhinitis: comparing the available agents. J Allergy Clin Immunol 1999; 104:S144–S149.

36. Wiseman LR, Benfield P. Intranasal fluticasone propionate: a reappraisal of its pharmacology and clinical efficacy in the treatment of rhinitis. Drugs 1997; 53:885–907.

37. Onrust SV, Lamb HM. Mometasone furoate: a review of its intranasal use in allergic rhinitis. Drugs 1998; 56:725–745.

38. Grossman J, Banov C, Boggs P, Bronsky EA, Dockhorn RJ, Druce H, et al. Use of ipratropium bromide nasal spray in chronic treatment of nonallergic perennial rhinitis, alone and in combination with other perennial rhinitis medications. J Allergy Clin Immunol 1995; 95:1123–1127.

39. Horwitz RJ, McGill KA, Busse WW. The role of leukotriene modifiers in the treatment of asthma. Am J Respir Crit Care Med 1998; 157:1363–1371.

40. Creticos PS, Peters SP, Adkinson NF Jr, Naclerio RM, Hayes EC, Norman PS, et al. Peptide leukotrine release after antigen challenge in patients sensitive to ragweed. N Engl J Med 1984; 310:1626–1630.

41. Philip G, Malmstrom K, Hampel FC, et al. Montelukast for treating seasonal allergic rhinitis: a randomized, double-blind, placebo-controlled trial performed in the spring. Clin Exp Allergy 2002; 32:1020–1028.

42. Nayak AS, Philip G, Lu S, et al. Efficacy and tolerability of montelukast alone or in combination with loratadine in seasonal allergic rhinitis: a multicenter, randomized, double-blind, placebo-controlled trial performed in the fall. Ann Allergy Asthma Immunol 2002; 88:592–600.

43. Wilson AM, Orr LC, Sims EJ, et al. Effects of monotherapy with intra-nasal corticosteroid or combined oral histamine and leukotriene receptor antagonists in seasonal allergic rhinitis. Clin Exp Allergy 2001; 31:61–68.

44. Knight A, Underdown BJ, Demanuele F, Hargreave FE. Disodium cromoglycate in ragweed-allergic rhinitis. J Allergy Clin Immunol 1976; 58:278–283.

45. van Neerven RJ, Wikborg T, Lund G, Jacobsen B, Brinch-Nielsen A, Arnved J, et al. Blocking antibodies induced by specific allergy vaccination prevent the activation of CD4+ T cells by inhibiting serum-IgE-facilitated allergen presentation. J Immunol 1999; 163:2944–2952.

46. Durham SR, Walker SM, Varga EM, Jacobson MR, O'Brien F, Noble W,

et al. Long-term clinical efficacy of grass-pollen immunotherapy. N Engl J Med 1999; 341:468–475.

47. Johnstone DE, Dutlon A. The value of hyposensitization therapy for bronchial asthma in children—a 14-year study. Pediatrics 1968; 42(5):793–802.

48. Moller C, Dreborg S, Ferdosi HA, et al. Pollen immunotherapy reduces the development of asthma in children with seasonal rhinoconjunctivitis (the PAT-study). J Allergy Clin Immunol 2002; 109:251–256.

49. Bousquet J, Lockey R, Malling HJ. Allergen immunotherapy: therapeutic vaccines for allergic diseases. A WHO position paper. J Allergy Clin Immunol 1998; 102:558–562.

50. Vuurman EF, van Veggel LM, Uiterwijk MM, Leutner D, O'Hanlon JF. Seasonal allergic rhinitis and antihistamine effects on children's learning. Ann Allergy 1993; 71:121–126.

51. Skoner DP, Rachelefsky GS, Meltzer EO. Detection of growth suppression in children during treatment with intranasal beclomethasone. Pediatrics 2000; 105:E23.

52. Schenkel E, Skoner D, Bronsky E, et al. Absence of growth retardation in children with perennial allergic rhinitis following 1 year of treatment with mometasone furoate aqueous nasal spray. Pediatrics 2000; 105:E22.

53. Tan R, Corren J. Optimum treatment of rhinitis in the elderly. Drugs Aging 1995; 7:168–175.

54. Mazzotta P, Loebstein R, Koren G. Treating allergic rhinitis in pregnancy: safety considerations. Drug Safety 1999; 20:361–375.

55. Torfs CP, Katz EA, Gateson TF, Lam PK, Curry CJ. Maternal medications and environmental exposures as risk factors for gastroschisis. Teratology 1996; 54:84–92.

56. Corren J, Froehlich J, Schoenhoff M, Spector S, Rachelefsky G, Schanker H, et al. Phase I study of anti-IgE recombinant humanized monoclonal antibody rhuMAB-E25 (E25) in adults with moderate to severe asthma [abstr]. J Allergy Clin Immunol 1996; 97:A251.

57. Togias A, Corren J, Shapiro G, Reimann JD, von Schlegell A, Wighton TG, et al. Anti-IgE treatment reduces skin test (ST) reactivity [abstr]. J Allergy Clin Immunol 1998; 101:A706.

58. Corren J, Diaz-Sanchez D, Reimann J, Saxon A, Adelman D. Effects of anti-IgE antibody therapy on nasal reactivity to allergen and IgE synthesis in-vivo [abstract]. J Allergy Clin Immunol 1998; 101:A436.

59. Casale TB, Condemi J, LaForce C, et al. Effect of omalizumab on symptoms of seasonal allergic rhinitis: a randomized, controlled trial. JAMA 2001; 286: 2956–2967.

60. Borish LC, Nelson HS, Corren J, et al. Efficacy of soluble interleukin-4 receptor for the treatment of adults with asthma. J Allergy Clin Immunol 2001; 107: 963–970.

61. Leckie MJ, ten Brinke A, Khan J, et al. Efficacy of interleukin-5 blocking antibody on eosinophils, airway hyperresponsiveness, and the late asthmatic response. Lancet 2000; 356:2144–2148.

62. Welsh PW, Stricker EW, Chu-Pin C, et al. Efficacy of beclomethasone nasal

solution, flunisolide and cromolyn in relieving symptoms of ragweed allergy. Mayo Clin Proc 1987; 62:125–134.

63. Corren J, Adinoff AD, Buchmeier AD, Irvin CG. Nasal beclomethasone prevents the seasonal increase in bronchial responsiveness in patients with allergic rhinitis and asthma. J Allergy Clin Immunol 1992; 90:250–256.

64. Henriksen JW, Wenzel A. Effect of an intranasally administered corticosteroid (budesonide) on nasal obstruction, mouth breathing and asthma. Am Rev Respir Dis 1984; 130:1014–1018.

65. Watson WTA, Becker AB, Simons FER. Treatment of allergic rhinitis with intranasal corticosteroids in patients with mild asthma: effect on lower airway responsiveness. J Allergy Clin Immunol 1993; 91:97–101.

66. Casale TB, Wood D, Richerson HB, et al. Elevated bronchoalveolar lavage fluid histamine levels in allergic asthmatics are associated with methacholine bronchial hyperresponsiveness. J Clin Invest 1987; 79:1197–1203.

67. Karlin JM. The use of antihistamines in asthma. Ann Allergy 1972; 30:342–347.

68. Taytard A, Beaumont D, Pujet JC, Sapene M, Lewis PJ. Treatment of bronchial asthma with terfenadine; a randomized controlled trial. Br J Clin Pharmacol 1987; 24:743–746.

69. Rafferty P, Jackson L, Smith R, Holgate ST. Terfenadine, a potent H1-receptor antagonist in the treatment of grass pollen sensitive asthma. Br J Clin Pharmacol 1990; 30:229–235.

70. Wood-Baker R, Smith R, Holgate ST. A double-blind, placebo-controlled study of the effect of the specific histamine H1-antagonist, terfenadine, in chronic severe asthma. Br J Clin Pharmacol 1995; 39:671–675.

71. Bruttman G, Pedraii P, Arendt C, Rihoux JP. Protective effect of cetirizine in patients suffering from pollen asthma. Ann Allergy 1990; 64:224–228.

72. Dijkman JH, Hekking PRM, Molkenboer JF, et al. Prophylactic treatment of grass pollen-induced asthma with cetirizine. Clin Exp Allergy 1990; 20:483–490.

73. Grant JA, Nicodemus CF, Findlay SR, et al. Cetirizine in patients with seasonal allergic rhinitis and concomitant asthma: prospective, randomized, placebo-controlled trial. J Allergy Clin Immunol 1995; 95:923–932.

74. Corren J, Harris A, Aaronson D, et al. Efficacy and safety of loratadine plus pseudoephedrine in patients with seasonal allergic rhinitis and mild asthma. J Allergy Clin Immunol. In press.

75. Spector S, Lee N, McNutt B, et al. Effect of terfenadine in asthmatic patients. Ann Allergy 1992; 69:212–216.

76. Warner JO. A double-blinded, randomized, placebo-controlled trial of cetirizine in preventing the onset of asthma in children with atopic dermatitis: 18 months' treatment and 18 months' posttreatment follow-up. J Allergy Clin Immunol 2001; 108:929–937.

77. Crystal-Peters J, Neslusen C, Crown WH, et al. Treating allergic rhinitis in patients with comorbid asthma: the risk of asthma-related hospitalizations and emergency department visits. J Allergy Clin Immunol 2002; 109:57–62.

78. Adams RJ, Fuhlbrigge AL, Finkelstein JA, et al. Intranasal steroids and the risk of emergency department visits for asthma. J Allergy Clin Immunol 2002; 109:636–642.
79. Corren J, Strom BL, Manning BE, and Thompson SF, Hennessy S, Strom BL. Intranasal corticosteroids reduce risk of hospitalizations for asthma in patients with asthma and concomitant allergic rhinitis. J Allergy Clin Immunol 2003; 111:abstract

11

Medical Management of Sinusitis in Patients with Asthma

LARRY BORISH

University of Virginia Health System
Charlottesville, Virginia, U.S.A.

RAY SLAVIN

St Louis University
St Louis, Missouri, U.S.A.

**JAMES A. WILDE,
WILLIAM K. DOLEN, and
CHESTER STAFFORD**

Medical College of Georgia
Augusta, Georgia, U.S.A.

The term "sinusitis" refers to the presence of inflammation of the mucosa within the paranasal sinuses. Chronic symptoms referable to the sinuses are among the most common health care problems in the United States, affecting about 31 million Americans and accounting for approximately 16 million patient visits per year (1). In addition, rhinosinusitis is the fifth most common condition leading to an antibiotic prescription (2). Sinus disease is a common condition in patients with asthma, and treatment of concomitant sinusitis appears to have salutory effects upon the lower airways. Unfortunately, medical management of chronic sinusitis remains a challenge to all clinicians. This chapter outlines an approach to medical management of sinusitis and reviews existing data regarding the connection between sinus pathology and asthma.

I. Definitions and Pathophysiology

Sinusitis is typically divided into three categories: acute sinusitis, which is characterized by the presence of symptoms for 3 weeks or less; subacute sinusitis, defined as symptoms for a duration of 3 to 12 weeks; and, chronic sinusitis, with symptoms persisting beyond 12 weeks.

Usually, the acute and subacute forms of sinusitis represent infectious processes, most likely due to bacteria. Chronic sinusitis may also be due to infection, in which case it is usually associated with an anatomical obstruction of the sinus ostia. In patients with asthma, however, chronic sinusitis usually represents a noninfectious inflammatory process that has been termed chronic hyperplastic sinusitis (CHS). CHS is a disorder characterized by the accumulation of eosinophils, goblet cells, mast cells, fibroblasts, and TH2-like lymphocytes in the sinus mucosa (3–5). It is the prominent accumulation of eosinophils, however, which is most characterisitic of this disease (Fig. 1), and in the virtual absence of neutrophils this provides strong support for the concept that CHS is not caused by bacterial infection. CHS tissue demonstrates increased numbers of cells (including lymphocytes, eosinophils, and fibroblasts) expressing mRNA for granulocyte–macrophage colony-stimutating factor (GM-CSF), interleukins 3 and 5 (IL-3, IL-5), tumor necrosis factor (TNF), and C-C chemokines such as eotaxin (CCL11) (Fig. 2) (6). Thus, the hyperplastic tissue and eosinophils themselves are producing the cytokines and other growth factors necessary for eosinophil differentiation, recruitment, activation, survival, and proliferation. Activation and recruitment of eosinophils in such an autocrine fashion suggests that chronic hyperplastic

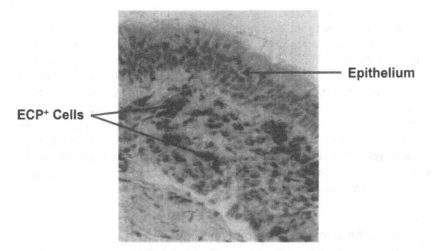

Figure 1 Immunohistochemical analysis of a biopsy from a patient with chronic hyperplastic sinusitis. Eosinophils were labeled with EG1, an anti–eosinophil catonic protein antibody. [Reproduced with permission from Demoly P, et al. J Allergy Clin Immunol 1994; 94:95 (Fig 2; Ref. 3a).]

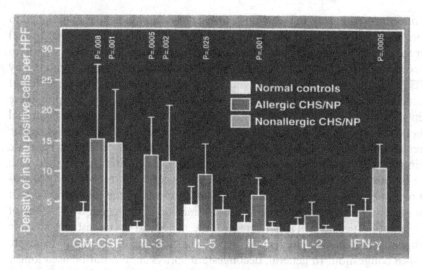

Figure 2 Cytokine expression in chronic hyperplastic sinusitis. Tissue was obtained from the nasal turbinates of healthy controls or from subjects with nasal polyposis without or with allergies. Comparison of the density of cells positive by in situ hybridization for the cytokines GM-CSF, IL-3, IL-5, IL-4, IL-2, and interferon (IFN-γ) is shown. Statistically significant differences in comparison with normal controls are illustrated. HPF, high power field. [Reproduced with permission from Hamilos DL, et al. J Allergy Clin Immunol 1995; 96:537 (Fig. 2) (Ref. 6a).]

eosinophilic sinusitis is a benign but uncontrolled proliferative disorder. CHS is frequently associated with nasal polyposis, which represents evagination of the hyperplastic mucosa into the nasal airway. Patients with CHS may experience recurrent bacterial infections superimposed upon the chronically diseased mucosa.

II. Approach to Treatment

Effective medical management of acute sinusitis in patients with asthma does not differ from treating this condition in the general population. Measures to reduce swelling, remove secretions, and treat the bacterial infection form the cornerstones of therapy. Therapy for chronic sinusitis is far more challenging and is directed toward the reduction of mucosal inflammation.

A. Decongestants

Sinus mucosal edema and reduction of ostial diameter are pathological events that occur early in the development of infectious sinusitis. Since the condition represents an infection within a closed space, measures designed to promote drainage such as topical nasal decongestants (e.g., oxymetazoline) may help facilitate recovery. Topical decongestants have been shown to reduce inferior turbinate swelling as measured by computed tomography (CT) (7). This same class of agents has been shown to improve rates of mucociliary clearance in patients with acute sinusitis (8). Despite these encouraging reports, a large clinical trial of oxymetazoline delivered by nasal bellows was unable to demonstrate that treatment with oxymetazoline resulted in improvements in radiological or clinical outcomes in acute sinusitis (9). In another trial, patients with acute sinusitis were treated with antibiotics plus topical oxymetazolone and a combination of phenylpropanolamine with brompheniramine (10). In that study, the adjunctive use of topical and oral decongestant–antihistamine added no benefit over the use of oral antibiotics alone (10). Therefore, use of topical decongestants in acute sinusitis should be reserved for symptomatic relief of moderate-to-severe nasal congestion. In general, decongestant sprays should not be used longer than 3 to 5 days, to minimize the risk of rebound congestion and rhinitis medicamentosa. Their value in chronic sinusitis has not been evaluated, but short-term use may be of help in selected cases to facilitate entry of topical intranasal anti-inflammatory therapies (e.g., corticosteroids).

Oral decongestants (e.g., pseudoephedrine) may be active in areas not reached by topical agents. This group of medications has been shown to increase the functional diameter of the maxillary sinus ostia in normal, healthy individuals (11). However, few studies have evaluated the efficacy of these agents in acute sinusitis. As noted earlier, in one of the few controlled trials performed to date, the combination of topical plus oral decongestants did not speed recovery from acute sinusitis (10). Important side effects of decongestants include central nervous system stimulation, cardiac irritability, and inhibition of micturition. While hypertension has long been a concern when oral decongestants are used, controlled trials of patients with stable hypertension have supported the safety of these agents when taken in appropriate dosages (12). However, recent reports of previously unsuspected adverse outcomes with use of phenylpropanolamine suggest the need for caution with the use of these agents.

B. Mucolytic Agents

Guaifenesin and potassium iodide can theoretically reduce the viscosity of thick mucous secretions. Support for the use of mucolytic agents in the treatment of sinusitis is primarily anecdotal, however, since few controlled studies have been performed to prove their efficacy. In a double-blind, placebo-controlled study of adults with acute rhinosinusitis, patients treated with guaifenesin (2400 mg daily) reported significantly less nasal congestion and less viscous nasal secretions (13). While further studies are needed, the data suggest that guaifenesin may provide some symptomatic relief in patients with acute sinusitis.

C. Corticosteroids

Corticosteroids, which reduce mucosal edema and inflammation, would be expected to be of potential benefit in both acute infectious sinusitis and chronic noninfectious sinusitis. Evidence suggests that topical corticosteroid sprays are distributed throughout the nasal airway by ciliary transport and that these topical agents can suppress inflammation near the sinus ostia. However, these agents do not generally penetrate into the sinus cavity and therefore have little ability to directly affect the sinus mucosa.

Intranasal corticosteroids have been examined in a number of clinical trials of patients with acute and recurrent acute sinusitis (14–19). All these trials demonstrated that treatment with intranasal corticosteroids resulted in significant improvement in symptoms of sinusitis, including nasal discharge and facial discomfort. In a carefully designed study examining patients with well-defined acute rhinosinusitis associated with chronic rhinitis, symptoms were significantly improved and the time to symptom improvement was shortened (19). Despite these salutary effects in acute sinusitis, none of the available formulations of intranasal corticosteroids has been approved for use in acute bacterial sinusitis. Based on these considerations, intranasal corticosteroids will probably be most effective in treating acute sinusitis in patients who have concomitant chronic rhinitis.

The case for using corticosteroids in patients with chronic hyperplastic sinusitis is theoretically a stronger one. The pathological similarity between CHS and asthma, particularly the prominent role of TH2 lymphocytes and eosinophils, supports the concept that corticosteroids should be useful in the treatment of both diseases (3–6). Unfortunately, intranasal corticosteroids do not readily penetrate into the sinus cavities, particularly in the presence of ostial occlusion. To date there has been very little study of topical nasal corticosteroids in patients with CHS. In one small clinical pilot study of patients with chronic sinus disease, intranasal corticosteroids were compared with placebo during 16 weeks of administration (20). In that study, there was a strong statistical trend toward reductions in sinus-related symptoms. Other end points, such as appearance of nasal tissue during endoscopy and nasal patency measured by acoustic rhinometry, were not affected by active treatment. Other investigators have suggested that corticosteroids might be more effective if delivered in an irrigating solution (21). Administration of nasal corticosteroids via conventional aqueous delivery systems as well as by means of irrigating systems will need to be examined in large, well-designed clinical trials using a number of relevant end points.

Nasal polyposis associated with CHS often responds well to consistent use of an intranasal corticosteroid. As many as half of the cases of nasal polyposis resolve with intranasal corticosteroids, and one recent study suggests that this medical approach may be at least as successful as surgical polypectomy at one-year follow-up (22). In patients with large, obstructing polyps who do not respond to a topical agent, a 7- to 10-day course of prednisone (0.5 mg/kg body weight) may be very helpful. Based on these observations, aggressive medical management with oral and topical corticosteroids should always be tried before surgical treatment is considered. If a 4- to 8-week trial of medical therapy has not been successful in reducing symptoms, a surgical consultation should be undertaken.

D. Saline Irrigation

The use of saline irrigation has been widely used as an adjunctive measure in patients with sinusitis, particularly in chronic sinus disease. Nasal irrigation has been proposed as a means of removing obstructing mucus and pathogens from the airway and sinuses, preventing nasal crusting, liquefying secretions, improving mucociliary clearance, and reducing the presence of inflammatory mediators and other irritants. In one physiological study, irrigation was shown to reduce nasal blood flow, resulting in a mild decongestant effect (23), while in another study nasal irrigations caused an increase in mucociliary clearance (24). A number of uncontrolled studies have demonstrated that nasal irrigation, using either isotonic or hypertonic solutions, resulted in significant improvements in symptoms, quality of life, and sinus radiography (24–27). In one study that compared an alkaline nasal douche with a saline spray, the douche proved superior in improving both endoscopic appearance of the inflamed mucosa and patient quality of life (28).

Various methods and devices have been used to irrigate the nasal airway. These include the following:

1. Nasal spray. Buffered sterile saline solution is commercially available as an over-the-counter preparation or can be made by the patient; it is sprayed into the nasal passages several times while gently sniffing in.
2. Bulb syringe. Saline is flushed into the nasal airway while the patient bends down over the sink. Typically, 1 teaspoon of salt is added to 800 mL of water.
3. Nasal Douche Cup. This commercially available plastic device (Alkolol Co., Taunton, MA 02780) allows saline to flow under gravity into the nasal passage.

4. Water Pik. This commercially available device is outfitted with a special nasal adapter (Nasal Irrigation Tip, from Hydro Med Inc., P.O. Box 91273, World Way Postal Center, Los Angeles, CA 90009) and is often used by patients after sinus surgery. The Water Pik is used at the lowest pressure and, with the patient leaning over the sink, the saline is allowed to flow down the back of the throat or out the other nostril.

E. Antibiotics

Acute Sinusitis

Antibiotic therapy has traditionally been considered to be the cornerstone of medical management for acute bacterial sinusitis. Appropriate antimicrobial therapy usually is selected empirically based on knowledge of the usual sinus pathogens. The efficacy of antibiotics in the treatment of acute sinusitis has been the subject of controversy (29–31). While some studies have shown that patients benefit from antibiotic treatment, a number of studies in both the adult and pediatric literature have failed to show a significant benefit from the use of these agents, in part because of spontaneous cure rates of 45 to 60% in both groups (32–34). Analysis of the available data shows that there is probably a real but limited benefit; approximately seven adult patients must be treated with antibiotics for every one who truly needs them (35). Several recently published articles propose practice guidelines for practitioners in various specialties who diagnose and treat sinusitis (32,33,35–37). The guidelines are unanimous in recommending antibiotic treatment for patients who fulfill well-defined clinical criteria. They are also unanimous in emphasizing that antibiotics should not be used indiscriminately, especially in light of the burgeoning problem of antimicrobial resistance. Despite warnings such as these, many practitioners continue to prescribe antibiotics when the indication is questionable (35,38–41).

With these concerns in mind, physicians who see patients with possible acute sinusitis should consider an important series of questions. First, do the patient's symptoms truly fulfill current recommended criteria for the diagnosis of bacterial sinusitis? Second, what are the likely target pathogens, and what antibiotics are effective against them? Third, are there any individual demographic factors, including recent antibiotic use, that need to be considered? Fourth, what is the narrowest spectrum antibiotic that can be used to treat the infection? Each of these questions warrants examination in detail when the use of antibiotics for possible acute sinusitis is under consideration.

As a crucial first step, physicians must first identify patients who likely suffer from acute sinusitis caused by a bacterial pathogen as opposed to other cause. Acute infectious rhinosinusitis is usually caused by viruses such as rhinovirus, adenovirus, coronavirus, respiratory syncytial virus, and influenza virus (32,42). Viral rhinosinusitis resolves spontaneously, and antibiotics do not change the natural course of these infections. The rate of bacterial involvement in rhinosinusitis is very low, with approximately 2% of adults and 0.5 to 5% of children demonstrating bacterial infection (32,43).

An understanding of the natural history of viral upper respiratory infections (URIs) can help to clarify the basis for recommendations regarding the use of antibiotics. Several recent studies in adults with experimentally induced rhinovirus URI have helped to distinguish the clinical profiles of viral URI versus acute bacterial sinusitis. First, fever is a common symptom of viral URI, particularly in children, and is not present in most cases of acute bacterial sinusitis. While most viral causes of URI in adults do not commonly cause fever, a major exception is influenza (44). Fever in viral URI can be expected to last 2 to 5 days for most viruses, and up to 7 or 8 days in influenza infections (45). Second, the presence of a mucopurulent discharge is not diagnostic of bacterial sinusitis (46). Nasal secretions change from clear to purulent during the first few days of viral upper respiratory illnesses, and the color does not predict whether a bacterial pathogen will be isolated. Third, symptoms of stuffiness, discharge, and cough generally persist in children for 2 to 3 weeks, although there should be improvement in those symptoms by day 10 (33). Adults generally show improvement within a week. Finally, radiographic evidence of mucosal thickening and fluid accumulation within the paranasal sinuses is quite common with viral rhinosinusitis and is not a specific indicator of bacterial involvement (46).

It can be difficult to differentiate between bacterial sinusitis and viral rhinosinusitis on clinical grounds alone, but several recent recommendations from the American College of Physicians, the American Academy of Pediatrics, and the Centers for Disease Control and Prevention (CDC) provide a framework for the intelligent management of these illnesses. A common theme from all these groups is that it is rarely necessary to treat symptoms of acute rhinosinusitis with antibiotics because the likelihood of acute bacterial infection is so low and the frequency of a spontaneous resolution is high even when a bacterial infection is present. A practice parameter regarding the diagnosis and treatment of acute rhinosinusitis in adults has been developed by the American College of Physicians (35), and the principles outlined in this parameter have been endorsed by the CDC, the American Academy of Family Physicians, the American Society of Internal Medicine, and the Infectious Diseases Society of America. The parameter states that the clinical diagnosis of acute bacterial sinusitis should be reserved for patients with symptoms lasting 7 days or longer who have maxillary pain or tenderness in the face or teeth (especially when unilateral) with purulent nasal secretions (2). A similar parameter, developed for children, states that the clinical diagnosis of bacterial sinusitis should be considered if symptoms of rhinosinusitis, particularly purulent nasal discharge or postnasal drip and cough, have been present without improvement for more than 10 to 14 days (33). The diagnosis should also be considered if more severe upper respiratory tract signs and symptoms, including fever of 39°C or higher, facial swelling, and/or facial pain, occur acutely. In general, the classic signs of bacterial sinusitis, such as pain in the teeth or frontal headache, are quite rare in children.

An understanding of antimicrobial resistance mechanisms and knowledge of recent trends is also crucial to understanding the rational selection of antibiotics. *Streptococcus pneumoniae* was almost uniformly sensitive to penicillin prior to 1980. However, by 1990 resistance rates began to climb significantly, and by the end of the 1990s penicillin resistance rates reached 50% in some parts of the United States. About half of this resistance is intermediate and half is high level (47). Importantly, pneumococcal penicillin resistance is not mediated by bacterial β-lactamase production. The mechanism of resistance is bacterial alteration of penicillin binding proteins, specifically involving the transpeptidases that catalyze cell wall production. When penicillin binds to these proteins, the normal enzymatic function is lost and cell wall production ceases, leading to cell death. Alteration of these proteins decreases the affinity of binding by penicillin, resulting in a resistant organism. Importantly, in the case of intermediate level penicillin resistance, an increase in the concentration of the antibiotic can partially overcome this resistance mechanism. This is the basis for the use of high dose amoxicillin for otitis or sinusitis in which pneumococcal resistance is suspected (48).

The mechanism of resistance among *Hemophilus influenzae* and *Moraxella catarrhalis* isolates is based on the production of a number of β-lactamases. More than 170 β-lactamases have been described, with widely varying characteristics (49). They all share the ability to hydrolyze the β-lactam ring on penicillins, cephalosporins, and monobactams. Once the β-lactam ring has been hydrolyzed, the molecule loses its normal three-dimensional conformational structure, which alters its ability to bind to the penicillin binding proteins that catalyze cell wall production. Prior to 1980 *M. catarrhalis* was mostly sensitive to penicillin. By 2000 it was almost uniformly resistant (36,50). Likewise, *H. influenzae* was highly sensitive to penicillin prior to 1980, but the resistance rate today is approximate 30% (36,50).

The likely pathogens in acute and persistent sinusitis are similar, they include *S. pneumoniae*, *H. influenzae*, and *M. catarrhalis*, with *S. pneumoniae* being the predominant organism. *Moraxella catarrhalis* demonstrates penicillin resistance in close to 100% of cases, *H. influenzae* demonstrates resistance in approximately 50% of cases, and *S. pneumoniae* is resistant to penicillin in approximately 20% of cases (51). If a patient has failed to improve on amoxicillin therapy, and considering the rates of both resistance and frequency of these organisms in infections, resistant *S. pneumoniae* is more likely to be present than either of the two β-lactamase producers (51).

It is known that resistance genes are often carried on plasmids or transposons, sequences of DNA that can be transferred via conjugation from one organism to another or propagated through normal cell division (47). It is also known that these DNA sequences often contain multiple resistance genes to several different antibiotics (52,53). Recent work has shown that pneumococci that are penicillin resistant are also likely to be resistant to sulfamethoxazole and to macrolides owing to this clustering of resistance genes (48). A patient who has failed to respond to amoxicillin is likely to also fail to respond to sulfamethoxazole–trimethoprim and erythromycin. Further, organisms that are resistant to erythromycin are also highly likely to be resistant to azithromycin and clarithromycin (54). Based on these data, it is probably not advisable to prescribe sulfamethoxazole–trimethoprim or any of the macrolide antibiotics in sinus infections caused by *Pneumococcus*.

One of the more common misconceptions among both patients and physicians is that when therapy for a bacterial infection is necessary, a "more powerful" antibiotic is better than one that is not so powerful. "Power" has no meaning in discussing the efficacy of an antibiotic in killing a specific organism. Either an antibiotic kills a target organism at the recommended dose or it does not. If it does, the organism is sensitive to the antibiotic; if it does not, the organism is resistant. When the word "power" is used to describe an antibiotic, generally it is used in reference to the spectrum of the antibiotic. Broad-spectrum antibiotics kill a wide array of organisms, while narrow-spectrum antibiotics kill a relatively narrow band of organisms. When therapy for an infection with a known pathogen(s) is chosen, there is no additional benefit to be derived by prescribing an antibiotic that kills non targets as well as the target(s). Thus, imipenim is no better than penicillin in killing group A streptococci. Along this same line of reasoning, an important principle in the selection of antibiotics for bacterial infections is that the narrowest spectrum antibiotic appropriate for the suspected infection should always be chosen. The indiscriminate use of broad-spectrum antibiotics only hastens the development of resistant organisms and should be avoided (47). Another concern is that broad-spectrum antibiotics significantly alter the normal flora of the upper respiratory tract. The nonpathogenic bacteria that are normally present may serve as a means to interfere with the growth of pathogenic bacteria. If these nonpathogenic strains are killed, resistant pathogens may be in a better position to remain as persistent or chronic infections (36).

Algorithms for the treatment of acute bacterial sinusitis in children have been published by the American Academy of Pediatrics alone and jointly by the AAP and the CDC (35,37). In spite of the growing proportion of bacterial sinusitis that is due to resistant pneumococci, the recommendation for amoxicillin as first-line therapy still stands. This is due to its proven efficacy for bacterial sinusitis and the high rate of spontaneous resolution. The high rate of spontaneous resolution also explains why many studies show a variety of antibiotics to be beneficial in the treatment of bacterial sinusitis (55). Amoxicillin should be prescribed at the conventional dose of 40 mg/kg/day for those at low risk for penicillin-resistant pneumococci or at the higher dose (80–90 mg/kg/day) for those at significant risk for resistant pneumococci. Those at high risk include children under the age of 2, children attending day care, and children who have received any antibiotics in the preceding 6 weeks. Alternative therapy for patients who are allergic to penicillin includes sulfamethoxazole–trimethoprim, a macrolide, cefuroxime axetil, cefdinir, or clindamycin. It should be noted that clindamycin has good activity against *S. pneumoniae* but has poor activity against *H. influenzae* and *M. catarrhalis*. Therapy is recommended for 7 to 10 days after substantial improvement in symptoms, usually for a total of 10 to 14 days (33). If there is no improvement in the symptoms within 72 h, a change in antibiotics may be warranted.

Second-line therapy includes high dose amoxicillin, amoxicillin–clavulanate, cefdinir, or cefuroxime axetil. Cefixime, cefaclor, and loracarbef should be avoided owing to their limited efficacy against pneumococci (48). Another alternative for second-line therapy is to use amoxicillin–clavulanate in its high dose amoxicillin formulation, such that the amoxicillin is taken at a dose of 80 to 90 mg/kg/day. If the symptoms still persist after another 72 h, further investigation may be warranted. It is at this point that imaging studies may be helpful (33). It also may be helpful to aspirate pus from the involved sinus to better ascertain the bacterial cause of the therapeutic failure. Surface swabs of the nasal mucosa in the region of the paranasal sinuses are of little value.

With regard to treating acute sinusitis in adults, amoxicillin is a good, inexpensive first-line therapy, with trimethoprim–sulfamethoxazole as an alternative in penicillin-allergic patients (36). Penicillin, erythromycin, cephalexin, tetracycline, and cefixime should be avoided as first-line antibiotics in adults with acute sinusitis because of the inadequacy of their spectrum of activity. For second-line therapy, amoxicillin–clavulenate or one of several cephalosporins, including cefprozil, cefuroxime axetil, and cefpodoxime proxetil, is suggested. These cephalosporins all provide the most reliable pharmacodynamic profiles against both penicillin-susceptible *S. pneumoniae* and strains that have an intermediate level of penicillin resistance. These agents also have excellent activity against beta lactamase producing *H.*

influenzae and *M. catarrhalis*. For third-line therapy, levofloxacin, gatifloxacin, and moxifloxacin offer excellent activity against both penicillin-resistant strains of *Pneumococcus* and strains of *H. influenzae* and *M. catarrhalis* that produce β-lactamase. Ciprofloxacin, on the other hand, does not offer adequate activity against penicillin-resistant strains of *Pneumococcus* (36). Caution is urged in the use of quinolones as first-line agents, since resistance among pneumococci is increasing, and two decades of quinolone use has resulted in the rapid emergence of resistance among other organisms (47).

Chronic Sinusitis

In children with chronic sinusitis and associated asthma, sinus involvement is often limited to a single sinus, particularly the maxillary sinus. The responsible bacteria are generally the same as those which cause acute sinusitis, including *S. pneumoniae*, *H. influenzae*, and *M. catarrhalis* (49,56,57). There are few published data regarding the efficacy of antibiotic treatment in these patients, although open-label trials suggest that the infection may be cleared, at least temporarily, with appropriate antimicrobials. Many physicians treat chronic sinusitis in children with 3 to 4 weeks of antibiotics (58,59), although there again are few data from well-designed studies to support this recommendation.

As already described, adult patients with asthma and concomitant chronic sinusitis usually have hyperplastic mucosal disease of the sinuses characterized by eosinophilic inflammation. While these patients may experience recurrent episodes of bacterial sinusitis, for the most part infectious organisms do not play a principal causative role in their sinus disease. Few microbiological studies of CHS have utilized proper techniques to assess the role of infection in this disorder. Investigative studies that have been appropriately performed suggest that CHS most likely involves the loss of the usual sterility of the sinuses and colonization with noninvasive flora. Because of the frequency of colonization of the sinuses, quantitative cultures must be performed, with infection defined as the recovery of a bacterial species in high density ($\geq 10^4$ cfu/mL). Many of these improperly performed studies have identified *Staphylococcus*, anaerobes (including gram-positive streptococci (*Peptococcus and Peptostreptococcus*) but also *Bacteroides* and *Fusobacterium* species) (60–62), and other *nonvirulent* organisms (*Propionibacterium acnes, Staphlococcus epdermidis, Streptococcus pyogenes, Streptococcus viridans, Corynebacterium,* and *Neisseria*) (56,63). The presence of multiple organisms, non- or minimally virulent organisms, organisms at low titers, and discordances between the species of organisms cultured from different sinuses all demonstrate evidence of colonization, not infection (61,63). In addition, these cultures often identify bacteria that are sensitive to an antimicrobial being administered at the time of the culture, additional evidence that these represent colonization, not an infectious process (61). Few controlled studies of antibiotics have been performed in adults with CHS and asthma, and none has shown a clearly defined benefit in chronic sinusitis (64). The historic failure of antimicrobial therapy in chronic sinus-itis—including long-term courses of rotating broad-spectrum antibiotics—further reflects the likelihood that this is not an infectious disorder (61). The absence of an infectious etiology in most subjects with CHS and associated asthma similarly raises questions regarding the benefits of surgical proce-dures designed to promote drainage of a presumed "closed-space" infection. The surgical literature acknowledges that asthmatic patients who have extensive mucosal disease involving multiple sinuses and nasal polyposis generally have poor outcomes with surgical therapy (65–68).

F. Aspirin Desensitization

A subset of chronic sinusitis subjects demonstrate the spectrum of asthma and aspirin intolerance. These subjects tend to have particularly severe sinusitis with panopacification of their sinuses observed on CT scans and nasal polyposis occurring in association with severe persistent asthma and aggressive airway remodeling. In these subjects, severe, often life-threatening attacks of asthma can occur in response to aspirin and other nonsteroidal anti-inflammatory drugs (NSAIDs) that suppress cyclooxygenase 1 (COX-1). Selective COX-2 inhibitors can be safely administered to individuals with aspirin-sensitive asthma and sinusitis (69,70). This condition of so-called triad asthma is associated with constitutive overproduction of cysteinyl leukotrienes, which is associated with an additional increase in leukotriene production following the ingestion of these agents (71). This overproduction of cysteinyl leukotrienes appears to reflect their overexpression of the enzyme leukotriene C4 synthase (71).

Aspirin desensitization has been shown to be remarkably effective in these subjects in mitigating the severity of the hyperplastic sinusitis and polyposis as well as the associated asthma. This technique, which must be used cautiously, involves successive ingestion of increasing doses of aspirin over several days until a therapeutic dose is achieved (325–650 mg, 1 or 2 times per day) (72). Successful aspirin desensitization succeeds in part through its ability to decrease basal and aspirin-stimulated leukotriene syn-thesis (73) as well as decreasing sensitivity to cysteinyl leukotrienes (74).

In the initial long-term study of aspirin desensitization conducted at the Scripps Clinic, approximately 100 aspirin-intolerant patients with asthma and CHS were evaluated (75). Approximately one-third of the group were desensitized to aspirin and treated with daily aspirin treatment for as long as 8 years (mean, 3.75 years). Patients undergoing desensitization demonstrated statistically significant reduction in the annual number of hospitalizations, emergency room visits, outpatient visits, episodes of acute sinusitis, need for nasal polypectomies and additional sinus operations, and improvement in sense of smell compared with the control group. Simultaneously, the aspirin treatment groups were able to significantly reduce systemic corticosteroid dosages, corticosteroid bursts per year, and doses of inhaled corticosteroids. These data have been confirmed (76) and further extended by the Scripps researchers in their more recent follow-up studies (77). These investigations have confirmed the ability of aspirin desensitization to improve important outcomes measures for both sinus disease and asthma, including frequency of acute bacterial superinfection and the need for repeat polypectomy as well as restoration of sense of smell (Table 1).

G. Leukotriene Modifiers

Cysteinyl leukotrienes were originally identified through their ability to mediate sustained and profound broncoconstriction, while more recent studies have established the potent proinflammatory influences of these

Table 1 Aspirin-Sensitive Patients with Rhinosinusitis-Asthma

	Baseline		ASA Rx		
	Median	Range	Median	Range	p Values[a]
Sinusitis	6	(1–12)	2	(0–12)	<0.0001
Sinus surgery/yr	0.2	(0–0.75)	0	(0–2)	0.09
Hospitalizations/yr	0.2	(0–0.54)	0	(0–1)	0.005
ED visits/yr	0	(0–1.22)	0	(0–1.5)	0.2
Olfaction score	0	(0–1)	3	(1–5)	<0.0001

	Baseline		ASA Rx		
	Mean	SEM	Mean	SEM	p Values[b]
Prednisone (mg/day)	7.9	±2.0	1.8	±0.7	0.01
Nasal steroid (µg/day)	137	±25.6	90	±22.3	0.09
Inhaled steroid (µg/day)	640	±146.2	885	±6.0	0.1

Patients treated 1–3 years. ASA Rx, aspirin therapy; ED, emergency department.
[a]Values were determined with Wilcoxon signed rank statistic. Two side p values were reported.
[b]Values were determined with paired t-test.
Adapted with permission from: Stevenson DD, et al. J Allergy Clin Immunol 1996; 98:751.

mediators. Leukotrienes are particulary important in activating eosinophils and contribute to their generation in the bone marrow, recruitment, adhesion and egress from the circulation, and activation at sites of inflammation, while concomitantly inhibiting their apoptosis. In addition, leukotrienes stimulate mucus secretion and may contribute to fibrotic and other tissue remodeling pathways through their abilities to promote epithelial and myofibroblast proliferation. These mechanisms suggest an important role for cysteinyl leukotrienes in contributing to the development and severity of CHS. Recent studies have demonstrated the presence of leukotrienes in CHS (78). These observations support the concept that insofar as CHS is mediated by eosinophilic inflammation, leukotriene modifiers may analogously be useful in this disorder.

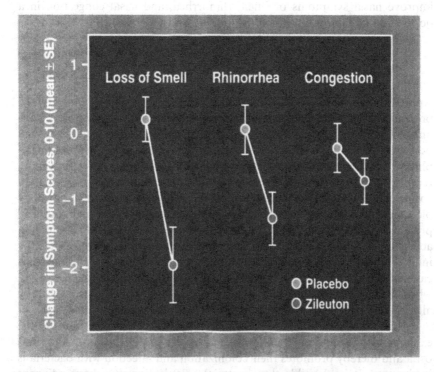

Figure 3 Nasal symptom score improvement on zileuton. Patients with aspirin-intolerant asthma with chronic sinusitis and nasal polyposis were randomized to received either zileuton or a placebo. Nasal symptom scores showed a significant reduction in loss of smell and rhinorrhea. [Reproduced with permission from Dahlen B, et al. Am J Resp Crit Care Med 1997; 157:1187 (Fig. 4) (Ref. 81).]

While extensively studied primarily in asthma, leukotriene modifiers have been less well studied in rhinitis and sinusitis; increasing evidence, however, suggests a role for these agents in at least some patients (79). Leukotriene modifiers include agents that inhibit the enzyme 5-lipoxygenase (zileuton) and those that block the cysteinyl leukotriene type 1 receptor (montelukast and zafirlukast). In contrast to topical intranasal corticosteroids, these orally administered anti-inflammatory medications can gain access to the sinuses. As previously noted, aspirin-intolerant asthma with CHS is associated with particularly elevated production of cysteinyl leukotrienes, and these subjects may represent a uniquely relevant potential target for anti-leukotriene therapy. Leukotriene modifiers in uncontrolled studies have been shown to improve symptoms of sinusitis, restore olfaction, and alleviate nasal polyposis in 50% of the patients (80). In one placebo-controlled, double-blind study, the 5-lipoxygenase inhibitor zileuton was shown to improve nasal symptoms of smell, rhinorrhea, and nasal congestion in a population of aspirin-intolerant asthmatics with CHS (81) (Fig. 3).

III. Allergy Evaluation

Approximately 40 to 75% of subjects with CHS are atopic, as defined by the presence of IgE specific to inhaled aeroallergens (82). Some studies have linked CHS to allergy and have shown that nasal allergen challenges may exacerbate sinusitis, as shown by changes observed on sinus x-ray and single-photon emission computed tomography (SPECT) scanning (83–85). A more recent study demonstrated the ability of nasal allergen challenge to elicit an eosinophilic inflammatory response in the maxillary sinus, as shown by placement of a catheter and lavage of the sinus cavity (86). Although routinely present in the nose and lungs, however, aeroallergens are not likely to gain access to the sinus mucosa. This has been confirmed in studies on healthy individuals in which no radiolabeled pollen grains accumulated in the sinus cavities. Such accumulation is even less likely to occur in subjects with CHS whose sinus ostia are likely to be occluded (87). The mechanism whereby allergy may contribute to the development of CHS is therefore unclear.

Insofar as infection is not related to most cases of chronic sinusitis, the explanation that underlying allergic rhinitis leads to occlusion of the sinus ostia and thereby promotes their colonization and infection with bacteria is inadequate. It is plausible that bacterial colonization may have adjuvant influences promoting the breakdown of tolerance and immune nonreactivity in the sinuses or may provide "intrinsic" antigens or even superantigens that could activate a TH2-like disorder. These mechanisms would not explain the rapid changes in sinus tissue observed in the allergen challenges studies. An alternative hypothesis is that nasal allergy can contribute to CHS through the intranasal activation of TH2-like lymphocytes and eosinophil precursors. These cells can then migrate both systemically and through nasal lymphatic tissue. These activated lymphocytes and eosinophil precursors, as well as newly generated bone marrow–derived eosinophils and basophils are characterized by their expression of VLA-4. It is then plausible that after an allergen challenge and in the presence of vascular cell adhesion molecule 1 (VCAM-1) and other adhesion molecules expressed in CHS tissue, these cells will localize in the sinus tissue, where they will exacerbate allergic inflammation.

The data regarding the linkage of allergen sensitization and allergic mechanisms to the presence of chronic sinusitis support the concept that interventions designed to attenuate allergic inflammation in this disorder may be beneficial. Despite their effectiveness in allergic rhinitis, however, no study of allergen avoidance, allergic rhinitis pharmacotherapy, or immunotherapy has ever addressed the efficacy of these measures in the treatment of sinusitis. Reasonable recommendations at present would be to utilize all these measures as appropriate to treat patients with asthma, CHS, and documented sensitivities to aeroallergens.

Food allergy has not been shown to play a contributing role in either recurrent acute or chronic sinusitis.

IV. Medical Treatment of Sinusitis: Effects on Concomitant Asthma

An association between sinus disease and bronchial asthma is well established, and acute sinusitis often accompanies asthma flares and may contribute to asthma severity. Up to 75 to 90% of asthmatic patients have abnormal findings on sinus imaging (87–94). Aggressive therapy for sinusitis is considered to be a component of the treatment of patients with difficult-to-control asthma. However, reports that treatment of sinusitis has beneficial influences on asthma are tempered by the absence of properly controlled studies. For example, one study demonstrated that children with combined sinusitis and lower airway hyperreactivity showed significant improvement of the asthmatic state when they receive medical treatment for sinusitis (91). Indeed, 79% of the children were able to discontinue bronchodilator therapy after resolution of the sinusitis, and pulmonary function tests showed normal result in 67% of those with pretreatment abnormalities. Similar results were reported in another group of children with asthma and sinusitis from the University of Pittsburgh (92). Since, however, there was no control group, and all the subjects also received interventions to improve their asthma, it is impossible to interpret these studies (91,92). Thus, the possibility must be entertained that there is no salutary effect of sinus therapy on the underlying asthma and that these studies merely report coincidental but not causally related improvement in asthma.

Several mechanisms have been suggested to explain the apparent relationship between sinusitis and asthma. Earlier theories including direct aspiration of mediators from the upper to lower airway are considered unlikely given the absence of evidence of aspiration in radionuclide studies in humans (95). A sinobronchial neurological reflex mediated by the cholinergic pathway is supported by some data but is unlikely to explain what is predominantly an inflammatory disease of the lower airway. A more plausible explanation for the influence of sinus disease on asthma is that this linkage is mediated through the circulation. Thus, patients with CHS have an intense immunologically mediated inflammatory process of the upper airways. The generation of cytokines, allergen-specific T-helper lymphocytes, eosinophil precursors, and inflammatory mediators in the sinuses leads to increased production of eosinophils, mast cells, and basophils in the bone marrow. This is consistent with the reported association of CHS with circulating eosinophilia (78,90,96). These processes will ultimately lead to the selective recruitment of these eosinophils, mast cell precursors, T-helper lymphocytes, and other cells and mediators into the lungs, where they exacerbate the airways inflammation characteristic of asthma. This mechanism is consistent with the common histological picture of patients with chronic hyperplastic sinusitis with asthma.

Finally, it must be recognized that sinusitis may be an important and underappreciated precipitant of vocal cord dysfunction (97). This induction of variable extrathoracic airway obstruction by chronic postnasal drip may represent another important way in which sinus disease is connected to respiratory symptoms.

V. Conclusions

Carefully selected and individualized therapy and commitment to an ongoing patient–physician relationship can lead to improved well-being for individuals with sinusitis. The task for clinicians is to optimize therapy by rational and combined use of available drugs. It is incumbent upon every physician to become much more selective and appropriate in the use of antibiotics for both acute and chronic sinusitis. Nasal saline irrigation, intranasal corticosteroids, aspirin desensitization, and possibly leukotriene modifiers may all be beneficial in appropriately selected patients. Since chronic hyperplastic sinusitis mirrors the pathophysiology of asthma, it seems plausible that the next generation of asthma therapies may also prove helpful in improving chronic sinus disease.

References

1. Bolger WE, Kennedy DW. Guidelines for diagnosis, medical therapy, and surgery, current prospects on sinusitis in adults. J Respir Dis 1992; 13(3):421–445.
2. Snow V, Mottur-Pilson C, Hickner JM. Principles of appropriate antibiotic use for acute sinusitis in adults. Ann Intern Med 2001; 134:495–497.
3. Harlin BL, Ansel DG, Lane SR, et al. A clinical and pathologic study of chronic sinusitis: the role of the eosinophil. J Allergy Clin Immunol 1988; 81:867–875.
4. Hamilos DL, Leung DYM, Wood R, et al. Chronic hyperplastic sinusitis: association of tissue eosinophilia and mRNA expression of granulocyte–macrophage colony-stimulating factor and interleukin-3. J Allergy Clin Immunol 1993; 92:39–47.
5. Hamilos DL, Leung DYM, Wood R, et al. Eosinophil infiltration in nonallergic chronic hyperplastic sinusitis with nasal polyposis (CHS/NP) is associated with endothelial VCAM-1 upregulation and expression of TNF-α. Am J Respir Cell Mol Biol 1996; 15:443–450.
6. Hamilos DL, Leung DYM, Wood R, Cunningham L, Bean DK, Yasruel Z, Schotman E, Hamid Q. Evidence for distinct cytokine expression in.allergic versus nonallergic chronic sinusitis. J Allergy Clin Immunol 1995; 96:537–544.
7. Stringer SP, Mancuso AA, Avino AJ. Effect of a topical vasoconstrictor on computed tomography of paranasal sinus disease. Laryngoscope 1993; 103:6–9.
8. Inanli S, Ozturk O, Korkmaz M, Tutkun A, Batman C. The effects of topical agents of fluticasone propionate, oxymetazoline, and 3% and 0.9% sodium chloride solutions on mucociliary clearance in the therapy of acute bacterial rhinosinusitis in vivo. Laryngoscope 2002; 112:320–325.
9. Wiklund L, Stierna P, Berglund R, Westrin KM, Tonnesson M. The efficacy of oxymetazoline administered with a nasal bellows container and combined with oral phenoxymethyl–penicillin in the treatment of acute maxillary sinusitis. Acta Otolaryngol Suppl 1994; 515:57–64.
10. McCormick DP, John SD, Swischuk LE, Uchida T. A double-blind, placebo-controlled trial of decongestant–antihistamine for the treatment of sinusitis in children. Clin Pediatr 1996; 35:457–460.
11. Melen I, Andreasson L, Ivarsson A, Jannert M, Johansson CJ. Effects of phenylpropanolamine on ostial and nasal airway resistance in healthy individuals. Acta Otolaryngol (Stockh) 1986; 102:99–105.
12. Radack K, Deck CC. Are oral decongestants safe in hypertension? An evaluation of the evidence and a framework for assessing clinical trials. Ann Allergy 1986; 56(5):396–401.
13. Wawrose SF, Tami TA, Amoils CP. The role of guaifenesin in the treatment of sinonasal disease in patients infected with the human immunodeficiency virus (HIV). Laryngoscope 1992; 102(11):1225–1228.
14. Qvarnberg Y, Kantola O, Salo J, Toivanen M, Valtonen H, Vuori E. Influence of topical steroid treatment on maxillary sinusitis. Rhinology 1992; 30(2):103–112.

15. Meltzer EO, Orgel HA, Backhaus JW, Busse WW, Druce HM, Metzger WJ, Mitchell DQ, Selner JC, Shapiro GG, Van Bavel JH. Intranasal flunisolilde spray as an adjunct to oral antibiotic therapy for sinusitis. J Allergy Clin Immunol 1993; 92:812–823.

16. Barlan IB, Erkan E, Bakir M, Berrak S, Basaran MM. Intranasal budesonide spray as an adjunct to oral antibiotic therapy for acute sinusitis in children. Ann Allergy Asthma Immunol 1997; 78:598–601.

17. Yilmaz G, Varan B, Yilmaz T, Gurakan B. Intranasal budesonide spray as an adjunct to oral antibiotic therapy for acute sinusitis in children. Eur Arch Otorhinolaryngol 2000; 257:256–259.

18. Meltzer EO, Charous BL, Busse WW, Zinreich SJ, Lorber RR, Danzig MR. Added relief in the treatment of acute recurrent sinusitis with adjunctive mometasone furoate nasal spray. The Nasonex Sinusitis Group. J Allergy Clin Immunol 2000; 106:630–637.

19. Dodor RJ, Witsell DL, Hellkamp AS, Williams JW Jr, Califf RM, Simel EL, Ceftin and Flonase for Sinusitis (CAFFS) Investigators. Comparison of cefuroxime with or without intranasal fluticasone for the treatment of rhinosinusitis. The CAFFS Trial: a randomized controlled trial. JAMA 2001; 286:3097–3105.

20. Parikh A, Scadding GK, Darby Y, Baker RC. Topical corticosteroids in chronic rhinosinusitis: a randomized, double-blind, placebo-controlled trial using fluticasone propionate aqueous nasal spray. Rhinology 2001; 39:75–79.

21. Cuenant GJ, Stipon JP, Plante-Longchamp G, Baudoin C, Guerrier Y. Efficacy of endonasal neomycin–tixocortol pivalate irrigation in the treatment of chronic allergic and bacterial sinusitis. 1 ORL. J Otorhinolaryngol Relat Spec 1986; 48:226–232.

22. Blomqvist EH, Lundblad L, Anggard A, Haraldsson P-O, Stjarne P. A randomized controlled study evaluating medical treatment versus surgical treatment in addition to medical treatment of nasal polyposis. J Allergy Clin Immunol 2001; 107:224–228.

23. Druce HM, Bonner RF, Patow C, Choo P, Summers RJ, Kaliner MA. Response of nasal blood flow to neurohormones measured by laser–Doppler velocimetry. J Appl Physiol 1984; 57(4):1276–1283.

24. Talbot AR, Herr TM, Parsons DS. Mucociliary clearance and buffered hypertonic saline solutions. Laryngoscope 1997; 107:500–503.

25. Tomooka LT, Murphy C, Davidson TM. Clinical study and literature review of nasal irrigation. Laryngoscope 2000; 110:1189–1193.

26. Heatley DG, McConnell KE, Kille TL, Leverson GE. Nasal irrigation for the alleviation of sinonasal symptoms. Otolaryngol Head Neck Surg 2001; 125:44–48.

27. Bachmann G, Hommel G, Michel O. Effect of irrigation of the nose with isotonic salt solution on adult patients with chronic paranasal sinus disease. Eur Arch Otorhinolaryngol 2000; 257:537–541.

28. Taccarrielo M, Parkh A, Darby Y, Scadding G. Nasal douching as a valuable adjunct in the management of chronic rhinosinusitis. Rhinology 1999; 37:29–32.

29. Harris SJ. The sinusitis debate (letter). Pediatrics 2002; 109:166–167.

30. Hirschmann JV. Antibiotics for common respiratory tract infections in adults. Arch Intern Med 2002; 162:256–264.
31. Ioannidis JP, Lau J. Technical report: evidence for the diagnosis and treatment of acute uncomplicated sinusitis in children: a systematic overview. Pediatrics 2001; 107:electronic abstracts e57.
32. Sinus and Allergy Health Partnership. Antimicrobial treatment guidelines for acute bacterial rhinosinusitis. Executive summary. Otolaryngology-Head and Neck Surgery 2000; 123:S1–S31.
33. O'Brien KL, Dowell SF, Schwartz B, et al. Acute sinusitis—principles of judicious use of antimicrobial agents. Pediatrics 1998; 101:174–177.
34. Garbutt JM, Goldstein M, Gellman E, Shannon W, Littenberg B. A randomized, placebo-controlled trial of antimicrobial treatment for children with clinically diagnosed acute sinusitis. Pediatrics 2001; 107:619–625.
35. Hickner JM, Bartlett JG, Besser RE, et al. Principles of appropriate antibiotic use for acute rhinosinusitis in adults: background. Ann Intern Med 2001; 134:498–505.
36. Brook I, Gooch WM, Jenkins SG. Medical management of acute bacterial sinusitis: recommendations of a clinical advisory committee on pediatric and adult sinusitis. Ann Otol Rhinol Laryngol 2000; 109:2–20.
37. American Academy of Pediatrics Subcommittee on Management of Sinusitis and Committee on Quality Improvement. Clinical Practice Guideline: Management of Sinusitis. Pediatrics 2001; 108:798–808.
38. Nyquist AC, Gonzalez R, Steiner JF. Antibiotic prescribing for children with colds, upper respiratory tract infections, and bronchitis. JAMA 1998; 279:875–877.
39. Hamm RM, Hicks RJ, Bemben DA. Antibiotics and respiratory infections: are patients more satisfied when expectations are met? J Fam Pract 1996; 43:56–62.
40. Mainous AG, Hueston WJ, Clark JR. Antibiotics and upper respiratory infection: do some folks think there is a cure for the common cold? J Fam Pract 1996; 42:357–361.
41. Gonzales R, Steiner JF, Sande MA. Antibiotic prescribing for adults with colds, upper respiratory tract infections, and bronchitis by ambulatory care physicians. JAMA 1997; 278:901–904.
42. Chonmaitree T, Heikkinen T. Viruses and acute otitis media. Concise Rev Pediatr Infec Dis October 2000; 1005–1007.
43. Wald E, Guerra N, Byers C. Upper respiratory tract infections in young children: duration of and frequency of complications. Pediatrics 1991; 87:129–133.
44. Glezen WP, Cherry JD. Influenza Viruses. In: Feigin RD, Cherry JD, eds. Textbook of Pediatric Infectious Diseases. 3d ed. Philadelphia: WB Saunders Company, 1992:1688–1704.
45. Gwaltney JM, Hendley JO, Phillips CD, et al. Rhinovirus infections in an industrial population. II. Characteristics of illness and antibody response. JAMA 1967; 202:494–500.
46. Wald ER. Purulent nasal discharge. Pediatr Infect Dis J 1991; 10:329–333.
47. Wilde JA. Antibiotic resistance and the problem of antibiotic overuse. Pediatr Emerg Med Rep 2001; 6:45–56.

48. Dowell SF, Butler JC, Giebink GS. Acute otitis media: management and surveillance in an era of pneumococcal resistance—a report from the Drug-Resistant *Streptococcus pneumoniae* Therapeutic Working Group. Pediatr Infect Dis J 1999; 18:1–9.

49. Medeiros AA. Evolution and dissemination of beta-lactamases accelerated by enerations of beta-lactam antibiotics. Clin Infect Dis 1997; 24(suppl 1):S19–S45.

50. Doern GV, Jones RN, Pfaller MA, et al. *Haemophilus influenzae* and *Moraxella catarrhalis* from patients with community-acquired respiratory tract infections: antimicrobial susceptibility patterns from the SENTRY antimicrobial surveillance program (United States and Canada, 1997). Antimicrob Agents Chemother 1999; 43:385–389.

51. Klein JO. Otitis media: state of the art clinical article. Clin Infect Dis 1994; 19:823–833.

52. Levin BR, Lipsitch M, Perrot V, et al. The population genetics of antibiotic resistance. Clin Infect Dis 1997; 24(suppl 1):S9–S16.

53. Tomasz A. Antibiotic resistance in *Streptococcus pneumoniae*. Clin Infect Dis 1997; 24(suppl 1):S85–S88.

54. Reed MD, Blumer JL. Azithromycin: a critical review of the first azilide antibiotic and its role in pediatric practice. Pediatr Infect Dis J 1997; 16:1069–1083.

55. Marchant C, Carlin S, Johnson C, et al. Measuring the comparative efficacy of antibacterial agents for acute otitis media: the "Pollyanna phenomenon". J Pediatr 1992; 120:72–77.

56. Muntz HR, Lusk RP. Bacteriology of the ethmoid bullae in children with chronic sinusitis. Arch Otolaryngol Head Neck Surg 1991; 117:179–181.

57. Tinkelman DG, Silk HJ. Clinical and bacteriologic features of chronic sinusitis in children. Am J Dis Child 1989; 143:938–941.

58. Businco L, Fiore L, Frediani T, et al. Clinical and therapeutic aspects of sinusitis in children with bronchial asthma. Int J Pediatr Otorhinolaryngol 1981; 3:287.

59. Cummings NP, Wood RW, Lere JL, et al. Effect of treatment of rhinitis/sinusitis on asthma: results of a double-blind study. Pediatr Res 1983; 17:373.

60. Gwaltney JM, Philips CD, Miller RD, et al. Computed tomographic study of the common cold. N Engl J Med 1994; 330:25–30.

61. Wald ER. Microbiology of acute and chronic sinusitis in children and adults. Am J Med Sci 1998; 316:13–20.

62. Brook I. Bacteriologic features of chronic sinusitis in children. J Am Med Assoc 1981; 246:967–969.

63. Orobello PW Jr, Park RI, Belcher LJ, Eggleston P, Lederman HM, Banks JR, Modlin JF, Naclerio RM. Microbiology of chronic sinusitis in children. Arch Otolaryngol Head Neck Surg 1991; 117:980–983.

64. Otten FWA, Grote JJ. Treatment of chronic maxillary sinusitis in children. Int J Pediatr Otorhinolaryngol 1988; 15:269–278.

65. Matthews BL, Smith LE, Jones R, Miller C, Brookschmidt JK. Endoscopic sinus surgery: outcome in 155 cases. Otolaryngol Head Nec Surg 1991; 104:244–246.

66. Kennedy DW. Prognostic factors, outcomes and staging in ethmoid sinus surgery. Laryngoscope 1992; 102:1–17.
67. Orlandi RR, Kennedy DW. Surgical management of rhinosinusitis. Am J Med Sci 1998; 316:29–38.
68. Lavigne F, Nguyen CT, Cameron L, Hamid Q, Renzi PM. Prognosis and prediction of response to surgery in allergic patients with chronic sinusitis. J Allergy Clin Immunol 2000; 105:746–751.
69. Szczeklik A, Nizankowska E, Bochenek G, Nagraba K, Mejza F, Swierczynska M. Safety of a specific COX-2 inhibitor in aspirin-induced asthma. Clin Exp Allergy 2000; 31:219–225.
70. Stevenson DD, Simon RA. Lack of cross-reactivity between rofecoxib and aspirin in aspirin-sensitive patients with asthma. J Allergy Clin Immunol 2001; 108:47–51.
71. Cowburn AS, Sladek K, Soja J, Adamek L, Nizankowska E, Szczeklik A, Lam BK, et al. Overexpression of leukotriene C4 synthase in bronchial biopsies from patients with aspirin-intolerant asthma. J Clin Invest 1998; 101:834–846.
72. Kowalski ML. Management of aspirin-sensitive rhinosinusitis–asthma syndrome: what role for aspirin desensitization? Allergy Proc 1992; 13(4):175–184.
73. Juergens UR, Christiansen SC, Stevenson DD, Zuraw BL. Inhibition of monocyte leukotriene B4 production after aspirin desensitization. J Allergy Clin Immunol 1995; 96:148–156.
74. Arm JP, O'Hickey SP, Spur BW, Lee TH. Airway responsiveness to histamine and leukotriene B4 in subjects with aspirin-induced asthma. Am Rev Respir Dis 1989; 140:148–153.
75. Sweet JM, Stevenson DD, Simon RA, Mathison DA. Long-term effects of aspirin desensitization—treatment for aspirin–sensitive rhinosinusitis–asthma. J Allergy Clin Immunol 1990; 85(1 pt 1):59–65.
76. Mardiney M, Borish L. Aspirin desensitization for chronic hyperplastic sinusitis, nasal polyposis, and asthma triad. Arch. Otolaryngol Head Neck Surg 2001; 127:1287.
77. Stevenson DD, Hankammer MA, Mathison DA, Christiansen SC, Simon RA. Aspirin desensitization treatment of aspirin-sensitive patients with rhinosinusitis–asthma: long-term outcomes. J Allergy Clin Immunol 1996; 98:751–758.
78. Steinke JW, Bradley D, Arango P, Crouse D, Frierson H, Kountakis SE, Kraft M, Borish L. Cysteinyl leukotriene expression in chronic hyperplastic sinusitis/ nasal polyposis: Importance to eosinophilia and asthma. J Allergy Clin Immunol 2003; 111:342–349.
79. Borish L. The role of leukotrienes in upper and lower airway inflammation and the implications for treatment. Ann Allergy Asthma Immunol 2002; 88:16–22.
80. Parnes SM, Churna AV. Acute effects of antileukotrienes on sinonasal polyposis and sinusitis. Ear Nose Throat 2000; 79:18–21.
81. Dahlen B, Nizankowska E, Szczeklik A, et al. Benefits from adding the 5-lipoxygenase inhibitor zileuton to conventional therapy in aspirin-intolerant asthmatics. Am J Respir Critic Care Med 1998; 157:1187–1194.
82. Rachelefsky GS. National guidelines needed to manage rhinitis and prevent complications. Ann Allergy Asthma Immunol 1999; 82:296–305.

83. Pelikan Z, Pelikan-Filipek M. Role of nasal allergy in chronic maxillary sinusitis—diagnostic value of nasal challenge with allergen. J Allergy Clin Immunol 1990; 86:484–491.

84. Borts MR, Slavin RG, et al. Further studies in allergic sinusitis utilizing single photon emission computerized tomography (SPECT). J Allergy Clin Immunol 1989; 83:302A.

85. Slavin RG, et al. Is there such an entity as allergic sinusitis? J Allergy Clin Immunol 1988; 81:284A.

86. Baroody FM, Saengpanich S, Detineo M, Haney L, Votypka V, Naclerio RM. Nasal allergen challenge leads to bilateral maxillary sinus eosinophil influx. J Allergy Clin Immunol 2002; 109:S84.

87. Pfister R, Lutolf M, Schapowal A, Glatte B, Schmitz M, Menz G. Screening for sinus disease in patients with asthma: a computed tomography-controlled comparison of A-mode ultrasongraphy and standard radiography. J Allergy Clin Immunol 1994; 94:804–809.

88. Fuller C, Richards W, Gilsanz V, Schoettler J, Church JA. Sinusitis in status asthmaticus [abstr]. J Allergy Clin Immunol 1990; 85:222.

89. Rossi OVJ, Pirila T, Laitinen J, et al. Sinus aspirates and radiographic abnormalities in severe attacks of asthma. Int Arch Allergy Immunol 1994; 103:209–216.

90. Newman LJ, Platts-Mills TAE, Phillips CD, et al. Chronic sinusitis: relationship of computed tomography findings in allergy, asthma and eosinophilia. JAMA 1994; 271:363–367.

91. Rachelefsky GS, Katz RM, Siegel SC. Chronic sinus disease with associated reactive airway disease in children. Pediatrics 1984; 783:526–529.

92. Friedman R, Ackerman M, Wald E. Asthma and bacterial sinusitis in children. J Allergy Clin Immunol 1984; 74:185–189.

93. Slavin RG, Cannon RE, Friedman WH. Sinusitis and bronchial asthma. J Allergy Clin Immunol 1980; 66:250–257.

94. Bresciani M, Paradis L, Des Rouches A, et al. Rhinosinusitis in severe asthma. J Allergy Clin Immunol 2001; 107:73–80.

95. Bardin PG, Van Heerden BB, Joubert FR. Absence of pulmonary aspiration of sinus contents in patients with asthma and sinusitis. J Allergy Clin Immunol 1990; 86:82–88.

96. ten Brinke A, Grootendorst DC, Schmidt JT, De Bruine FT, van Buchem MA, Sterk PJ, Rabe KF, Bel EH. Chronic sinusitis in severe asthma is related to sputum eosinophilia. J Allergy Clin Immunol 2002; 109:621–626.

97. Bucca C, Rolla G, Scappaticci E, Chiampo F, Bugiani M, Magnano M, D'Alberto M. Extrathoracic and intrathoracic airway responsiveness in sinusitis. J Allergy Clin Immunol 1995; 95:52–59.

12

Surgical Management of Rhinitis, Sinusitis, and Nasal Polyposis in Patients with Asthma

R. JANKOWSKI

Henri Poincaré University
Nancy, France

There is the consistent observation that control of asthma remains difficult in many patients when their sinus disease is not treated, and it has been observed that treatment of sinusitis may improve the course of asthma. However, treatment of sinusitis in asthmatic patients is more empirical than determined by prospective clinical studies.

Sinusitis is one of the most commonly diagnosed chronic diseases in the world, yet there is no universally accepted definition of the syndrome. Although it appears that obstruction of the ostiomeatal complex is a significant factor in the development of the disorder, it is clearly not the only component in the development of the disease, perhaps especially not in the asthmatic patient. Asthma is associated with inflammation in the lower airways, and the same inflammation might involve the sinuses in a parallel fashion. In many asthmatics, sinusitis could represent the intervening stage between rhinitis and nasal polyposis.

How nose and sinus surgery can help to manage patients with asthma remains a challenging question. Nasal polyposis certainly is the upper respiratory tract disease associated to asthma for which the role of surgery has the most been studied. In light of this model, the role of surgery in sinusitis and rhinitis associated to asthma can thereafter be discussed.

I. Definition and Preliminary Remarks

Patients with chronic nose complaints can easily be classified into three groups by the means of noninvasive tools (i.e., nasal endoscopy and computed tomography). The diagnosis of nasal polyposis is easy and is exclusively based on nasal endoscopic identification of bilateral polyp formations. Whereas nasal polyps can occur in isolation and unilaterally, nasal polyposis refers to a bilateral, more or less diffuse, edematous disease of the mucosa, essentially the mucosa of the middle meatus and the ethmoid sinuses, that leads to the protrusion of polyps into the nasal cavity (1). Differential diagnoses to be kept in mind are fungal allergic sinusitis and, in case of unilateral polyps, such tumors as inverted papillomas and carcinomas.

Consensus documents have defined sinusitis as inflammation of the paranasal sinus mucosa (2). In practice, the diagnosis of sinusitis is based on radiographic findings. Computed tomography (CT) has dramatically improved the imaging of the paranasal sinuses. Its ability to display bone, soft tissue, and air optimally facilitates accurate definition of regional anatomy and degree of mucosal hyperplasia and/or accumulation of secretion in each sinus cavity. Chronic sinusitis can be defined by persistent opacities, whereas between two episodes of recurrent sinusitis, CT scans can clear up.

Rhinitis is a confusing term, used as a diagnosis for patients of different kinds showing nasal symptoms. It would be preferable to restrict the diagnosis of rhinitis to symptomatic patients having no nasal polyposis or sinus opacities on CT scans. Differential diagnoses to be kept in mind are noninflammatory diseases such as obstructive septal deviations, obstructive turbinates, and cholinergic rhinorhea. CT scans can hardly be performed in all patients with nose complaints but can certainly be justified for asthmatic patients with chronic nose complaints that cannot be explained by endo-scopic and standard radiographic findings.

II. Surgical Management of Nasal Polyposis in Patients with Asthma

Most studies report on how surgery has influenced the course of asthma, but no one has analyzed the phenomenon on a prospective controlled basis. Sinus surgery techniques have dramatically improved since surgical vision with a headlight was replaced first by the microscope and more recently by the endoscope (3,4). Medical therapy for both nasal polyposis and asthma has also changed over the years and has gained in efficacy. The literature is therefore very difficult to analyze. However, opinions regarding the surgical management of nasal polyposis in patients with asthma have slowly changed over the last decades and are becoming more and more favorable.

A. Conflicting Opinions Regarding the Effects of Surgery

Van der Veer, (5), in 1920, was the first author to report that polypectomy might aggravate asthma, and this viewpoint was supported in 1929 by Francis (6), who reported that asthma was worse after polypectomy in 9 of his 13 patients.

Decades after the pioneering work, some authors also reported that polypectomy can cause the first attack of asthma. In 1958 Samter and Lederer (7) reported on 17 patients, all of whom had an increased reactivity of the bronchial tree after polypectomy. Later Samter and Beers (8) found that 18 of 182 patients developed the first attack of asthma within 9 months after polypectomy. Then in 1977 Moloney and Collins (9) reported the development of asthma after polypectomy in a ratio of 1:2.5, and in 1986 English (10) found a ratio of 1:6.25.

Most studies published before the 1980s report highly variable results of surgery on the course of asthma. Weille and Richards (11) reported the results of nasal and sinus surgery in 216 adult asthmatics, 128 of whom had nasal polyps. There were 120 patients (56%) in whom the severity of asthma was diminished, 59 patients (27%) in whom the asthma was unchanged, and 37 patients (17%) in whom the asthma was worse. Without making a parallel between sinus and lung results, however, the investigators reported that the nasal polyps and sinusitis were cured in 63 patients (32%), improved in 69 patients (35%), unchanged in 53 patients (27%), and worse in 7 patients (3.5%). In Schenck's 1974 study of 18 patients (12), there were 5 patients who had less severe asthma, 7 in whom there were no change in the asthma, and 6 with increased asthma after surgery. Five years later, Brown et al. (13) reported the results of polypectomy on 101 patients: the asthma was improved in 30 patients, worse in 14 patients, and unchanged in 56 patients. These authors reported a median of three polypectomies per patient. Interestingly, they noted that of 39 patients with unstable asthma before the operation, despite immediate preoperative hospitalization to control active asthma, 19 had wheezing postoperatively, whereas of the 62 patients with inactive asthma, only 3 had wheezing postoperatively.

B. Studies Suggesting a Positive Effect of Surgery on Asthma

English's 1986 paper (10) was the first to highlight the importance of medical preparation to improve the results of surgery. Before deciding on surgery, medical therapy that included theophyllin at maximally tolerated serum levels, antihistamines, decongestants, and antibiotics was given to adjust the steroid doses to the smallest quantity that controlled the patient's broncho-spasm. Whenever it became apparent that the patient had already received maximum benefit from medical treatment and that the polyps and sinusitis were irreversible, surgery was recommended and was performed at what appeared to be the optimal time for the particular clinical situation. An asthma classification system, based upon the quantity of corticosteroid needed to control bronchospasm, was used: class I, no steroids; class II, need only for burst of steroids; class III, good response to chronic use of steroids; class IV, poor response to all treatment + steroid dependent. Before surgery, there were no patients in class I, 72 patients in class II, 71 in class III, and 62 in class IV; that is, all patients in this study were steroid dependent. After surgery, there were 82 patients in class I, 93 in class II, 24 in class III, and 6 in class IV; that is, a total of 173 patients (84%) benefited enough either to discontinue steroids or to use them in burst or on alternate days, 28 patients (14%) who were able to decrease the dose but required steroid therapy daily, and 4 patients (2%) who had no change in steroid therapy. All patients were encouraged to return for follow-up examinations as long as possible. The length of follow-up ranged from 6 months to 13 years. The best results were obtained in patients who were able to discontinue steroids after surgery. Patients with the most severely disabling asthma were the least likely to benefit from surgery. The effect in this study was remarkable, in as much as asthma improved in 98% of cases, and did not worsen in a single patient, following surgery. However, a control group was not included, and there were no measurements of airflow limitation or bronchial reactivity.

We have performed radical endoscopic ethmoidectomy in 30 patients with nasal polyposis and asthma, and we measured lung function and bronchial reactivity to carbachol before and after surgery (14). Surgery was always performed after medical therapy had been adjusted to attain maximum pulmonary function. Patients were controlled in a range of 12 to 40 months (mean of 18 months) after surgery. Most patients stated that their asthma had improved, reporting a lower frequency of attacks, a distinct decrease of respiratory difficulty, less need for antiasthmatic medication, and especially less reliance on steroids. Only three patients reported no improvement, but no patient's asthma was worse after surgery. There was a clear tendency of decreased bronchial obstruction (increased FEV_1) and reduced sensitivity to carbachol after surgery. However, during the observation period, most patients received nasal steroids, and the number of patients on inhaled steroids increased from 34% to 50%. Hosemann et al. (15) found similar results. Lung function tests of 13 asthmatics and 4 patients with only bronchial hyper-reactivity were performed before and on an average of 12 months after endonasal sinus surgery. In the four subjects, bronchial hyperreactivity disappeared. Ten asthmatics were able to reduce medications. Lung function and medication were unchanged in two patients, and one needed to increase medications. A decreasing need for antiasthmatic medication after surgery has also been documented by Nishioka et al. (16). In spite of the difficulties and uncertainties in interpreting studies of this type, we have the clear impression that surgery for nasal polyposis improves the asthma condition.

It seems now clear that surgery for nasal polyposis does not induce bronchial hyperreactivity or cause asthma. We have reported (14) on 20 patients with nasal polyposis and normal preoperative bronchial reactivity to carbachol. No one developed asthma or bronchial hyperreactivity 12 to 40 months (mean of 18 months) after surgery. Downing et al. (17), in a series of 13 patients tested before and 6 months after polypectomy, found also no difference in bronchial reactivity. Lambling et al. (18), however, found in a 4-year follow-up study that nonreversible airflow obstruction appears in topical steroid nonresponders with nasal polyposis requiring nasal surgery, despite no change in pulmonary symptoms and/or severity of asthma. The authors' conclusion is that the long-term contribution of these changes to the development of respiratory symptoms remains to be documented.

The lack of controlled studies definitely does not allow one to conclude that nasal polyposis surgery has demonstrated its efficacy in the management of the asthma disease. It seems, however, that asthmatic patients can nowadays undergo surgery for their nasal polyposis without risk of inducing or aggravating asthma. Our experience is that effective surgery for nasal polyposis has the potential for improving the asthma condition. However, the type of sinus surgery that is performed may have some importance in the outcome of both the nose and bronchus functions.

C. What Type of Surgical Procedure?

In 1997 we recently addressed the question of surgical procedure (19) by taking advantage of a natural experimental situation. Specifically, we compared the results after functional ethmoidectomy (29 patients, 9 asthmatics) and nasalization (34 patients, 20 asthmatics). The principles that guided functional ethmoidectomy were to remove only the diseased mucosa and restore ventilation and drainage of the diseased sinuses. So the extent of surgery was different from one procedure to another and was determined by the extent of the disease predicted on CT scans and the disease found at the time of surgery. The principles that guided nasalization were a systematic and radical exenteration of the ethmoid structures and mucosa, with large antrostomy, sphenoidotomy, frontotomy, and resection of the middle turbinate, so that the restructured sinuses largely open into the nose. Functional results were evaluated by using visual analogue scales on a questionnaire mailed at the same time to all patients. Both groups reported improvement after surgery, but with the following differences. The overall nasal improvement was 8.8 ± 0.2 (mean ± SEM) after nasalization and 5.9 ± 0.6 after ethmoidectomy ($p = 0.0001$). Olfaction improvement was similar in both groups 6 months after surgery, remained at the same level 36 months after nasalization (6.9 ± 0.7), but decreased to 4.2 ± 1 after ethmoidectomy ($p = 0.02$). Asthma improvement remained significantly better after nasalization ($p < 0.05$). After 3 years of follow-up after nasalization ($n = 16$), still 8 asthmatics were reporting real improvement since surgery (score 7–10), with 5 of them scoring 10 (complete disappearance of asthma symptoms), 4 a mild improvement (score 1–7), and 3 no improvement (score 0–1). Only one reported a worsening of his asthma, which started during the third postoperative year (score –6). By contrast, in the ethmoidectomy group ($n = 7$ asthmatics), none reported a complete disappearance of asthma, 1 scored 8, 1 scored 4, 3 scored 0 or 1, and 2 reported a worsening of their asthma, one being severe (–10). After 5 years of follow-up (unpublished data), only 2 out of 34 patients of the nasalization group (1 out of the 20 asthmatics) had nasal polyps calling for reoperation, whereas 7 out of 29 patients (4 out of the 9 asthmatics) in the ethmoidectomy group needed surgery again.

The results obviously must be confirmed by further studies and moreover must be interpreted with great care, in as much as patients were not randomly assigned to the groups. However, many factors could explain the difference in outcomes. First, applying the concept of tailoring the extent of the surgical procedure to the extent of the disease (functional ethmoidectomy) calls for great expertise and exposes one to the risk of performing incomplete procedures. Second, from what we know about the pathophysiology (20), nasal polyposis might be considered to be more the expression of an irreversible disease of the mucosa than a reversible diseased mucosa. Third, the nasalization procedure considerably reduces the surface of the sinus mucosa, which also becomes largely accessible to local drugs such as topical steroids.

In sum, surgery can safely be proposed to asthmatic patients suffering from nasal polyposis. At least these patients will improve their level of nasal comfort. There is, however, a definite need for further controlled studies both to define the type of surgery that should be performed in nasal polyposis and to evaluate the impact of effective surgery for nasal polyposis on the management of asthma.

III. Surgical Management of Sinusitis in Patients with Asthma

Chronic symptoms of sinusitis often are neglected in patients with asthma, possibly because the symptoms are mild in comparison to those of the bronchial component of the disease. Persistent nasal congestion, hyposmia, intermittent postnasal drip, or frequent need to blow the nose, pressure, sore throat, cough, and recurent infections are banal. Sinusitis is usually discovered on radiographs performed either in a systematic way or in case of acute exacerbation of either sinusitis or asthma.

A. Sinus X-Ray Abnormalities and Asthma

Several studies have documented the association between abnormal sinuses and asthma ranging from about 30 to 80% of patients. In the prospective study by De Cleyn et al. (21) on 270 patients, the taking of x-rays of the sinuses was not dependent on or related to temporarily occurring symptoms that could be attributed to acute sinusitis. Asthma was significantly more often associated with sinus x-ray abnormalities (65.1%) than was rhinitis and/or chronic cough (44.4%). Zimmermann et al. (22) also found that in children the prevalence of abnormalities found by sinus x-rays was significantly greater in the patients with asthma (43 of 138), than in control patients with dental problems (0 of 50). They could not find, however, a relation between sinus x-ray abnormalities and severity of asthma. In work of Schwartz et al. (23), 47% of 217 patients with flare-ups of asthma had abnormal sinus roentgengrams, a highly significant difference from the 29% prevalence in 120 patients presenting with complaints of rhinitis. A smaller, parallel group of 23 patients with urticaria and no rhnitis or asthma had sinus radiographs in which only 4 (17%) demonstrated any radiological abnormality. Rossi et al. (24) detected abnormalities in the paranasal sinuses in 85% of patients admitted to the hospital for acute asthma.

The prevalence of sinus abnormalities would probably have been greater in all the studies just cited if computed tomography had been used (25). Newman et al. (26) found, for instance, in a survey of 104 patients undergoing surgery for chronic sinusitis, that the 39 patients with asthma had significantly more extensive disease discernible on CT scans than the nonasthmatics.

B. Significance of Sinus Radiographic Abnormalities in Asthmatics

Infectious Theory

Several studies have shown that in acute sinusitis, in which clinical symptoms are accompanied by abnormal sinus radiographs, bacteria are found in most of the sinus aspirations. Cultures revealed aeraobic bacteria, primarily *Streptococcus pneumoniae, Hemophilus influenzae*, and *Branhamella catarrhalis* (27–30).

In patients with sinusitis and asthma, the bacteriology of sinus aspirates has not routinely been studied. Friedman et al. (31) found organisms
in sinus aspirate cultures of five asthmatic children with acute sinusitis that
were similar to those found in children with acute sinusitis without
asthma. The situation is much less clear in *chronic sinusitis*. Berman et
al. (32) found bacteria in only 5 of 25 sinus aspirates, Adinoff and
Cummings (33) in only 4 aspirates of 42 asthmatics with abnormal sinus
radiographs. In a series of 110 consecutive patients admitted to a hospital
for severe attack of asthma, Rossi et al. (34) detected 87% patients with
abnormal sinus radiographs, but a positive bacteriological culture was
obtained from only 23 out of 70 aspirates; there were 7 aspirates in which
both a bacterium and a virus could be detected. However, in Newman's
study (26) of 104 patients with chronic sinusitis, in which surgically
specimens were obtained from 60 persons and cultured, all cultures grew
at least one aerobic organism. Coagulase-negative staphylococci was the
most common, then *Corynebacterium* species, α-hemolytic streptococci,
Staphylococcus aureus, and *Enterobacter aerogenes*. Unfortunately the
authors do not give detailed results for the 39 asthmatics included in the
study, especially how many samples from asthmatics were included in the 60
cultured specimens.

At the present time, the reasons for discrepancies in bacteriological
results are not clear, but patient selection, sampling, or microbiological
techniques may be involved.

Inflammation Theory

The discrepancies in bacteriological results led other authors (33,35) to
suggest that radiographic abnormalities represent the noninfectious inflammation that is the cause of asthma, with this inflammation occurring in both
upper and lower airways.

Support for this hypothesis comes from studies of tissue from paranasal sinuses in patients with asthma. Hansel (36) was the first to call
attention to the histopathological similarity of nasal, sinus, and bronchial
tissues in subjects with asthma, finding the most outstanding feature of these
tissues to be their infiltration by eosinophils. Harlin et al. (37) confirmed this
observation and additionally demonstrated a striking association between
the presence of extracellular deposition of major basic protein and damage
to the mucosa of the sinus. This effect was not observed in tissue obtained
from chronic sinusitis in the absence of asthma. Thus, these authors
concluded that sinus disease in patients with asthma may be due to the
same mechanisms that cause damage to bronchial epithelium. In the work of
Newman (26), too, the presence of tissue eosinophilia in the mucosa of the

sinus was significantly associated with a history of wheezing, and extensive disease appeared in CT images. However, in all these studies, chronic sinusitis is used as a generic name, and despite descriptions of thorough otolaryngologic examinations, especially for the presence of nasal polyposis, no one states how many patients with nasal polyposis were in the study. A precise answer to this question may, however, be of importance, since tissue eosinophilia is a major characteristic of nasal polyps, independently of their association with asthma (19,38). Whether the histopathology of chronic sinusitis associated with asthma is similar to the pathology seen in asthmatic bronchi remains to be demonstrated. Actually, the reality probably is that the mechanisms of chronic sinusitis in patients with asthma are similar to those of bronchial asthma in some patients, but very different, and similar to those of common chronic sinusitis, in a few others.

Pathophysiology of Common Chronic Sinusitis and Principles of Functional Endoscopic Sinus Surgery

Although the underlying causes of chronic inflammatory sinus disease require further elucidation, obstruction in the ostiomeatal complex is today thought to be a significant factor in the final development of chronic and recurrent sinusitis (3,39). Sinuses are air-filled spaces connected to the rest of the nasal mucosa by narrow orifices. Obstruction of a sinus orifice by any of a legion of causes leads to retention of mucosal secretions within the sinus. Inoculation of microorganisms into such culture media leads to infection. Functional sinus surgery principles are based on opening the obstructed orifice(s), draining the obstructed viscus, permitting mucoliliary clearance of secretions, eliminating microbiological overgrowth, and addressing the underlying cause of the ostial obstruction. The ethmoid labyrinth, which is rich in anatomical variations, is the main target of functional sinus surgery. The extent of the surgical procedure is determined by the extent of the disease present. Ethmoidectomy is continued until all disease identified by CT imaging has been exenterated or marsupialized, and ethmoidal cells with normal mucosa have been opened. The maxillary, or frontal, or sphenoid ostia are opened only if they are narrowed and when there is significant maxillary, or frontal, or sphenoid sinus disease. As much as possible of the mucosa is preserved, and resection of the middle turbinate is avoided.

C. Surgical Management of Chronic Sinusitis in Patients with Asthma

The data linking sinusitis to asthma are mainly associative, and causality has not been proved. It is clear that well-designed, blinded, prospective studies with standardized diagnostic and therapeutic regimens are necessary to clarify the relationship between chronic sinusitis and asthma. Therefore, at the present time, any recommendation for the surgical treatment of sinusitis in asthmatic patients can be based only on our understanding of the pathogenic processes that lead to sinusitis, the mechanisms by which sinus surgery might improve asthmatic symptoms, and our clinical experience.

We select patients for surgery only if, despite correct medical treatment, the sinus disease continues uncontrolled and the asthmatic symptoms are extremely labile or dependent on unacceptable doses of oral corticosteroids. It is not clear whether surgery should be limited to restoring ventilation and drainage of the diseased sinus cavities or, rather, should be more extensive, to largely marsupialize the sinuses into the nose, so that topical drugs can easily reach a reduced surface and volume of mucosa to be treated postoperatively on a long-term basis. A majority of surgeons are defenders of functional surgery, following the opinion of authorities who mention that asthma symptoms in their patients are significantly improved, and a reduction in medication is often achieved. It is our experience that extensive surgery is more effective than functional surgery, especially in patients whose surgically removed mucosa, is found to contain large numbers of eosinophils. Actually, we consider patients having chronic sinusitis with eosinophilia as patients who potentially could develop an authentic nasal polyposis (40). Since, however, it has been shown that topical nasal steroids can markedly decrease bronchial hyperresponsiveness associated with allergic rhinitis, this result could be due to the postoperative use of topical steroids (41,42).

IV. Surgical Management of Rhinitis in Patients with Asthma

When the diagnosis of rhinitis is reserved for patients without evidence of nasal polyposis or chronic sinusitis, there is no place for surgery in the management of rhinitis. In such patients, however, chronic nose obstruction may not be the consequence of rhinitis alone and surgery can be helpful by correcting a deviated septum or reducing the volume of hypertrophied turbinates. Gottlieb (43) postulated that nasal obstruction that leads to increased mouth breathing of relatively cold and dry air could be one of the pathogenic factors explaining how upper airways dysfunction could worsen asthma. This could explain the positive effects of inferior turbinectomy on the evolution of asthma, which have been presented in many recent meetings and were first reported by Ophir et al. (44). Among 186 patients who were interviewed and examined 10 to 15 years after inferior turbinectomy, 32 had suffered from bronchial asthma. Postoperatively, there was an improvement in 16, no change in 13, and an exacerbation of asthmatic attacks in 3 patients. However, as for nasal polyposis and chronic sinusitis, there is a definite need for controlled studies.

V. Conclusion

There is no well-designed, controlled study proving that nose or sinus surgery improves the course of asthma. However, the evidence that upper airway disease worsens asthma is circumstantial, and it is our clinical impression that when medical therapies have failed, nose or sinus surgery can result in significant improvement of asthma in these patients. At least, we can state that when well indicated and properly performed, nose or sinus surgery does not aggravate asthma. To clarify the impact of upper airways surgery on the course of asthma, if surgery is indicated for polyposis, sinusitis, or structural abnormalities associated to rhinitis, it seems necessary to clearly state this, and to clearly describe the surgical procedure being performed.

References

1. Lildholdt T. Position statement on nasal polyps. Rhinology 1994; 32:126.
2. Shapiro GG, Rachelefsky GS. Introduction and definition of sinusitis. J Allergy Clin Immunol 1992; 90:518–520.
3. Stammberger H. Endoscopic endonasal surgery. Concepts in treatment of recurring rhinosinusitis. Otolaryngol Head Neck Surg 1986; 94:143–156.
4. Kennedy DW. Functional endoscopic sinus surgery. Arch Otolaryngol 1985; 111:643–649.
5. Van Der Veer A Jr. The asthma problem. N Y Med J 1920; 112:392–399.
6. Francis C. Prognosis of operations for removal of nasal polyps in asthma. Practitioner 1929; 123:272–278.
7. Samter M, Lederer FL. Nasal polyps: their relationship to allergy, particularly bronchial asthma. Med Clin North Am 1958; 42:175–179.
8. Samter M, Beers RF Jr. Concerning the nature of intolerance to aspirin. J Allergy 1967; 40:281–293.
9. Moloney JT, Collins J. Nasal polyps and bronchial asthma. Br J Dis Chest 1977; 71:1–6.
10. Englisch GM. Nasal polypectomy and sinus surgery in patients with asthma and aspirin idiosyncrasy. Laryngoscope 1986; 96:374–380.
11. Weill FL, Richards AB. Influence of fundamental concepts in allergy upon special problems in otolaryngology. Arch Otolaryngol 1951; 54:231.
12. Schenck NL. Nasal polypectomy in the aspirin sensitive asthmatic. Trans Am Acad Ophthalmol Otolaryngol 1974; 78:109–119.
13. Brown BL, Harner SG, Van Delen RG. Nasal polypectomy in patients with asthma plus sensitivity to aspirin. Arch Otolaryngol 1979; 105:413–416.

14. Jankowski R, Moneret-Vautrin DA, Goetz R, Wayoff M. Incidence of medicosurgical treatment for nasal polyps on the development of associated asthma. Rhinology 1992; 30:249–258.

15. Hosemann W, Michelson A, Weindler J, Mang H, Wigand ME. The effect of endonasal paranasal sinus surgery on lung function of patients with bronchial asthma. Laryngorhinootologie 1990; 69:521–526.

16. Nishioka GJ, Look PR, Davis WE, Mc Kinsey JP. Functional endoscopic sinus surgery in patients with chronic sinusitis and asthma. Otolaryngol Head Neck Surg 1994; 110:494–500.

17. Dowing E, Bramah S, Settipane G. Bronchial reactivity in patients with nasal polyps before and after polypectomy. J Allergy Clin Immunol 1982; 69:102.

18. Lambling C, Brichet A, Perez T, Darras J, Tonnel AB, Wallaert B. Long-term follow-up of pulmonary function in patients with nasal polyposis. Am J Respir Crit Care Med 2000; 161:406–413.

19. Jankowski R, Pigret D, Decroocq F. Comparison of functional results after ethmoidectomy and nasalization for diffuse and severe nasal polyposis. Acta Otolaryngol (Stockh) 1997; 117:601–608.

20. Jankowski R. Eosinophils in the pathophysiology of nasal polyposis. Acta Otolaryngol (Stockh) 1996; 116:160–163.

21. De Cleyn KM, Kersshot EA, De Clerk LS, Ortmanns PM, De Schepper AM, Van Bever HP, Stewens WJ. Paranasal sinus pathology in allergic and nonallergic respiratory tract diseases. Allergy 1986; 41:313–318.

22. Zimmermann B, Stringer D, Feanny S, Reisman J, Hak H, Rashed N, Debenedictis F, McLaughlin J. Prevalence of abnormalities found by sinus x-rays in childhood asthma: lack of relation to severity of asthma. J Allergy Clin Immunol 1987; 80:268–273.

23. Schwartz HJ, Thompson JS, Sher TH, Ross RJ. Occult sinus abnormalities in the asthmatic patient. Arch Intern Med 1987; 147:2194–2196.

24. Rossi OVJ, Lahde S, Laitinen J, Huhti E. Contribution of chest and paranasal sinus radiographs to the management of acute asthma. Int Arch Allergy Immunol 194; 105:96–100.

25. Pfister R, Lutolf M, Schapowal A, Glatte B, Schmitz M, Menz G. Screening for sinus disease in patients with asthma: a computed tomography-controlled comparison of A-mode ultrasonagraphy and standard radiography. J Allergy Clin Immunol 1994; 94:804–809.

26. Newman LJ, Platt-Mills TAE, Phillips CD, Hazen KC, Gross CW. Chronic sinusitis. Relation of computed tomographic findings to allergy, asthma and eosinophilia. JAMA 1994; 271:363–367.

27. Wald ER, Mildoe GJ, Bowen AD. Acute maxillary sinusitis in children. N Engl J Med 1981; 304:749–754.

28. Evans FO, Syonor JB, Moore WEL. Sinusitis of the maxillary antrum. N Engl J Med 1981; 304:749–754.

29. Hamory BH, Sande MA, Sydnor AJ. Etiology and antimicrobial therapy of acute sinusitis. J Infect Dis 1979; 132:197.

30. Wald ER. Management of sinusitis in infants and children. Pediatr Infect Dis J 1988; 7:449–452.

31. Friedmann R, Ackerman M, Wald ER. Bacterial sinusitis exacerbating asthma. J Allergy Clin Immunol 1984; 74:185–189.
32. Berman JZ, Mathison DA, Stevenson DD. Maxillary sinusitis and bronchial asthma: correlations of recent roentgengrams, cultures and thermograms. J Allergy Clin Immunol 1974; 53:311–317.
33. Adinoff AD, Cummings NP. Sinusitis and its relationship to asthma. Pediatr Ann 1989; 18:785–790.
34. Rossi OUJ, Pirila T, Laitinen J, Huhti H. Sinus aspirates and radiographic abnormalities in severe attacks of asthma. Int Arch Allergy Immunol 1994; 103:209–213.
35. Zimmermann B, Gold M. Role of sinusitis in asthma. Pediatrician 1991; 18:312–316.
36. Hansel FK. Clinical and histopathologic studies of the nose and sinuses in allergy. J Allergy 1929; 1:43.
37. Harlin SL, Ansel LDG, Lane SR, Myers J, Kephart GM, Gleich GJ. A clinical and pathologic study of chronic sinusitis: the role of the eosinophil. J Allergy Clin Immunol 1988; 81:867–875.
38. Jankowski R, Bene MC, Haas F, Faure G, Simon C, Wayoff M. Immunohistologic characteristics of nasal polyps. A comparison with healthy mucosa and chronic sinusitis. Rhinology 1989; 8(suppl):51–58.
39. Kennedy DW. Prognostic factors, outcomes and staging in ethmoid sinus surgery. Laryngoscope 1992; 102:1–17.
40. Moneret-Vautrin DA, Jankowski R, Bene MC, Kanny G, Hsieh V, Faure G, Wayoff M. NARES: a model of inflammation caused by activated eosinophils? Rhinology 1992; 30:161–168.
41. Aubier M, Levy J, Clerici C, Neukirch F, Herman D. Different effects of nasal and bronchial glucocorticosteroid administration on bronchial hyperresponsiveness in patients with allergic rhinitis. Am Rev Respir Dis 1992; 146:122–126.
42. Reed CE, Marcoux JP, Welsch PW. Effects of topical nasal treatment on asthma symptoms. J Allergy Clin Immunol 1988; 81:1042–1047.
43. Gottlieb MJ. Relation of intranasal disease in the production of bronchial asthma. JAMA 1925; 85:105–107.
44. Ophir D, Schindel LD, Halperin D, Marshak G. Long-term follow-up of the effectiveness and safety of inferior turbinectomy. Plast Reconstr Surg 1992; 90:980–984.

13

Manifestations of Aspirin Sensitivity in the Upper and Lower Airways

DONALD D. STEVENSON

Scripps Clinic and The Scripps Research Institute
La Jolla, California, U.S.A.

Aspirin (ASA) and nonsteroidal anti-inflammatory drugs (NSAID) induce a number of different adverse reactions. These include cross-reacting respiratory reactions, cross-reacting urticarial reactions, single-drug-induced urticaria or anaphylaxis, and single-drug-induced aseptic meningitis or hypersensitivity pneumonitis. Generally, individual patients react in the same manner to each exposure of the same drug(s).

A subset of asthmatic patients experience adverse respiratory reactions to ASA and NSAIDs characterized by nasal and ocular mucosal swelling and bronchospasm. Such asthmatic patients have been classified as ASA sensitive (1) and ASA intolerant (2), as idiosyncratic (3), and as having aspirin-induced asthma (4) and, recently, aspirin-exacerbated respiratory disease (AERD) (5). All five descriptors refer to the same population of asthmatics. This chapter focuses on the clinical setting in which ASA/NSAID respiratory reactions occur, the clinical features of ASA respiratory disease, methods available for diagnosis, ASA desensitization, and cross-reactions between NSAIDs and ASA, as well as some insights into pathogenesis and treatment.

I. Clinical Entity

ASA-exacerbated respiratory disease occurs in patients with chronic rhinitis, sinusitis, nasal polyps, and asthma (4,6). Patients are identified as ASA sensitive only after a respiratory reaction to ASA or an NSAID has occurred. Except for their sensitivity to ASA/NSAIDs, such patients cannot be distinguished from others with clinically similar patterns of respiratory inflammation (7). AERD is the result of progressive inflammation in the respiratory tract that continues in the absence of exposure to ASA/NSAIDs. Once the respiratory mucosal inflammation is under way, exposure to ASA or any cross-reacting drug temporarily exacerbates the underlying inflammation and bronchospasm, resulting in the clinically recognized respiratory reactions (4,8).

A. Clinical Features of AERD

Typically, ASA disease is acquired in adulthood, with rare onset during early childhood (9). ASA disease is found in all ethnic groups and in both sexes, with a slight preponderance in females. Without any prior history of respiratory disease or having experienced unrelated hay fever and/or asthma during childhood, ASA-sensitive patients usually develop upper respiratory viral infections (URIs) as the sentinel event in the onset of their ASA disease. However, unlike prior viral respiratory illnesses, inflammation in the nasal and sinus membranes persists, worsens, and eventually evolves into chronic rhinosinusitis, with aggressive formation of nasal polyps and secondary hypertrophic and/or purulent pansinusitis (8). Inflammation may appear only in the upper airway (10), leading to a condition called ASA-sensitive rhinosinusitis. However, more commonly nasal polyps, sinusitis, and asthma occur together (11). This "intrinsic" type of asthma progresses and persists, irrespective of environmental exposures. Asthma activity increases, coincident with bouts of purulent sinusitis. Their clinical course is usually complicated by intractable pansinusitis (8). Table 1 summarizes the clinical features of aspirin respiratory disease. The clinical setting in which the clinician should be most suspicious of ASA/NSAID sensitivity is an asthmatic patient with relentless re-formation of nasal polyps, recurrent need for sinus and polyp surgery, and secondary acute and then chronic pansinusitis, with increasing asthma activity.

Without a past history of ASA-associated asthmatic exacerbations, it is virtually impossible to differentiate between ASA sensitive and insensitive asthmatics. In fact, two-thirds of patients who fit the clinical description provided in Table 1 are not sensitive to ASA or NSAIDs (1). Most ASA-insensitive patients have IgE-mediated rhinitis with nasal polyps; a few

Table 1 Clinical Characteristics of Patients with Aspirin Disease

Category	Characteristic
Age of onset	After age 10 to age 40
Rhinitis	Vasomotor instability (>90%); associated allergies (40–60%)
Nasal symptoms	Congestion, rhinorrhea, anosmia, paranasal headache, sleep deprivation
Nasal examination	Pale, congested membranes, polypoid tissue to polyps
Nasal smear	Eosinophils: variable[a]; mast cells: variable[a]; many polymorphonuclear cells
Sinus imaging (CT)	Abnormal, with any pattern pansinusitis most common
Sinusitis	Intermittent evolving to chronic
Asthma	Intermittent and usually in remission when sinuses not infected
	Chronic; particularly severe when associated with chronic sinusitis

[a] Topical and systemic corticosteroids substantially decrease numbers of eosinophils.

are sulfite sensitive, but others have idiopathic rhinosinusitis with nasal polyps, sinusitis, and asthma. Some of the "idiopathic" asthmatic patients will eventually "convert" to ASA sensitivity, upon subsequent experience of an ASA/NSAID-induced respiratory reaction (12). Many asthmatics have been advised to avoid ASA. As the numbers of asthmatics avoiding ASA and NSAIDs grows, the population of potential ASA-sensitive asthmatics expands, with most asthmatic patients falling into a category of "unknown" with respect to ASA sensitivity, since they have never been exposed to ASA/NSAIDs during the course of their illness.

II. Sinusitis and Asthma in ASA-Sensitive Asthmatics

Clinically, it is apparent that active sinusitis in ASA-sensitive asthmatics is a powerful stimulus for lower airway inflammation and bronchospasm. Indeed, the typical course of ASA-sensitive asthmatics is to have predominant and ongoing nasal obstruction and anosmia, with relatively good control of associated asthma, while using inhaled corticosteroids and β-adrenergic agonist inhalers. However, when the patient develops a viral respiratory illness, it is usually followed by purulent sinusitis, which in turn further activates asthma. Control of asthma then changes dramatically with substantial requirements for systemic corticosteroids, antibiotics, and β-adrenergic agonists. Most hospitalizations for asthma in ASA-sensitive asthmatic patients are the result of sinusitis-provoked asthma episodes or accidental ingestion of ASA or one of the NSAIDs.

Other chapters in this book document the relationships between the upper and lower regions of the respiratory tract. Suffice it say here that abnormal sinus x-rays and computed tomography (CT) scans of the sinuses are found in most ASA-sensitive asthmatics. In one study by McDonald et al. (13) in 1972, sinus radiographs were reviewed in all new asthmatic patients evaluated in the allergy division of the authors' institution for one year. Of the 282 patients, 38% had abnormal sinus x-rays. These were compared to the 22 asthmatic patients having documented ASA-sensitive asthma, where the incidence of abnormal sinus x-rays was 86%. Despite the small sample size of ASA-sensitive asthmatics, the results were significantly different by chi square (p = 0.001). In a more recent sample of our AERD patients (1991–1997), 198 ASA patients were evaluated for sinus disease. Including both plain roentgenograms and CT images of the sinuses, 189 of the 198 had available records to indicate whether abnormal sinuses had been documented by imaging methods in the course of the patients' illness. In only 6 of the 189 patients (3%) were sinus x-ray or CT images found to be normal. Although the matter is difficult to study, my impression is that early in ASA disease, the patient may have abnormal sinus x-rays only during acute respiratory infections. Over time, with increasing and aggressive formation of nasal and sinus polypoid tissues, the roentgen findings evolve into a picture of pansinusitis in most, if not all, AERD patients. Patients who are referred to our institution for ASA desensitization tend to have long-standing and severe ASA disease (averaging 13 years). Therefore they are more likely to already have pansinusitis.

III. Identification of ASA Sensitivity

Currently, an acceptable in vitro biochemical or immunological test for identification of patients with ASA sensitivity does not exist. Therefore, the gold standard for making the diagnosis is ASA challenge. There are a number of challenge protocols, but all testing depends on the dose dependence of ASA-induced respiratory reactions.

A. Oral ASA Challenges

In the United States, oral ASA challenges are available (14). Physicians conducting these challenges should be experienced in the proper use and performance of this test and should be prepared to treat severe asthma attacks, up to and including intubation and ventilator support. Therefore, these challenges should be performed in an environment offering physicians rapid access to emergency resuscitative equipment, an intensive care unit, and skilled chest and critical care specialists.

Several important observations regarding the safe and accurate performance of oral ASA challenges might be helpful. First, the more unstable or irritable the tracheobronchial tree at the time of challenge, the more severe the bronchospastic response to ASA will be. Therefore, before starting challenges, oral and inhaled corticosteroids, intranasal corticosteroids, theophylline, and leukotriene modifier drugs should be continued if the patient is already requiring these medications. The reactions induced by ASA and NSAIDs routinely occur while the patients are taking their regular doses of theophylline and inhaled corticosteroids (12). Weber et al. (15) demonstrated that discontinuing theophylline on the day of oral challenges allowed a "spontaneous" (anti–asthmatic drug deprivation) 20% decline in FEV_1 values unrelated to challenge substances. Nizankowska and Szczeklik (16) demonstrated that systemic corticosteroids provide partial protection to the bronchi during oral ASA challenges and shift the dose response to ASA upward. Thus pretreatment with systemic corticosteroids may be responsible for a few false-negative oral ASA challenges. However, for the majority of asthmatic patients, particularly those afflicted with chronic sinusitis, discontinuing corticosteroids allows bronchial inflammation to return and hyperirritability of the bronchi to increase to such a degree that ASA challenges cannot be accurately or safely performed.

More recently, leukotriene-modifying drugs (LTMDs) have been available to treat AERD. Despite early reports that LTMDs blocked ASA-induced respiratory reactions (17), we now know that if the doses of ASA are increased above the baseline ASA-provoking dose, LTMDs do not block naso-ocular reactions and block only about half of the bronchospastic reactions (18,19). Therefore, much as with systemic corticosteroids, the use of LTMDs as controller medications helps to stabilize bronchial airways to such a degree that oral ASA challenges can be safely and accurately performed. Only AERD patients with pure lower respiratory tract reactions are at risk for experiencing false-negative challenge results, in the face of treatment with an LTMD. Fortunately it is very unusual to have a pure asthmatic response, without upper airway involvement.

Some medications should be discontinued 24 h prior to oral ASA challenges; these include anticholinergics, antihistamines, cromolyn, and short-acting β-adrenergic agonists. Antihistamines can block the upper respiratory tract reaction, which is largely mediated by histamine (20,21). Cromolyn probably has minor effects on the severity of ASA, induced respiratory reaction (22), but there is evidence that cromolyn delays the onset of oral ASA-induced reactions (23), potentially risking exposure to the next highest challenge dose of ASA when the prior dose of ASA has not yet

induced all its effects. Anticholinergics and short-acting β-adrenergic agonists falsely elevate the baseline lung function values, producing pseudo-
reactions as the bronchodilator effects of the drugs wear off (14).

Following ASA ingestion, the onset of asthmatic reactions (elapsed
times) usually occurs between 15 min and 3 h. The mean elapsed time was 50
min in one study (13). There is a refractory period lasting 2 to 5 days after an
ASA-induced respiratory reaction, during which time the patient becomes
tolerant to ASA or NSAID (24).

Table 2 presents our standard 3-day oral ASA challenge protocol. An
intravenous access line should be in place. Spirometry values, including
expiratory and inspiratory loops, are recorded every hour, and the baseline
or first morning FEV_1 value should be > 60% of that predicted. On the first
day the patient ingests placebo capsules every 3 h, and FEV_1 values should
not vary by more than 10% from baseline during this full day of placebo
challenges. Laryngospasm can sometimes be identified by the flat and
notched inspiratory loop seen in the flow–volume curves.

Assuming that the second day's baseline FEV_1 values are within 10%
of the placebo day baseline, oral administration of ASA begins, starting
with 30 mg of ASA, depending on the patient's history of prior ASA
reactions. Very few patients react to 30 mg, and essentially no one reacts
to doses below 30 mg. A maximum of three doses of ASA are given per day
(7 a.m. to 4 p.m.) with a full 3 h between doses. As soon as signs and
symptoms of reactions occur (> 15% decrease in FEV_1, rhinorrhea, ocular
injection, periorbital edema, stridor and rarely flushing, urticaria, gastrointestinal cramps, or explosive diarrhea), subsequent ASA challenges are
suspended for that day and the reaction is reversed by means of the
following: five breaths of an inhaled bronchodilator (albuterol or terbuta-
line) delivered by a nebulizer aerosol device every 15 to 10 min until the
reaction subsides; racemic epinephrine by nebulizer for laryngospasm; top-

Table 2 Single-Blind 3-day Oral ASA Challenge Conducted at
Scripps Clinic[a]

	ASA (mg)		
Time	Day 1	Day 2	Day 3
7:00 A.M.	Placebo	30	100–150
10:00 A.M.	Placebo	45–60	150–325
1:00 P.M.	Placebo	60–100	325–650

[a] Individualized doses of ASA: second dose may be reduced and timing may
be altered, depending upon the severity of the historical reaction to ASA.
During placebo day, baseline FEV_1 values > 70% predicted and changes
should be <10%.

ical nasal decongestants (oxymetazoline); topical opthalmic antihistamine/decongestants; and/or adrenaline administered intramuscularly. For gastrointestinal symptoms, 50 mg of intravenous ranitidine is very effective, as is 50 mg of intravenous diphenhydramine for hives and angioedema.

The different types of respiratory reaction that are observed during oral ASA challenges are listed in Table 3. Such a reaction identifies patients who are ASA sensitive. If the patient can ingest 650 mg of ASA without any reaction, the oral challenge test is negative and the patient does not, at that time, have ASA respiratory disease, assuming the person was not taking prednisone or a leukotriene modifier drug. If prednisone and LTMD treatment was essential to prepare the respiratory tract for challenge and the challenge was negative, rechallenge at a later date, assuming prednisone or LTMDs could be withdrawn, might be an option for confirming that the challenge results were truly negative.

B. Inhalation Challenge with ASA-Lysine

In Europe and other parts of the world, inhalation challenges with ASA-lysine are routinely performed (25,26), but since the U.S. Food and Drug Administration (FDA) has not approved use of ASA-lysine in humans it cannot be used in the United States. After inhalation of ASA-lysine, the elapsed time until induced bronchospasm is under 30 min, and the prompt relief of such bronchospasm with inhaled β-adrenergic agonist is routinely observed. Extrabronchial symptoms, such as naso-ocular, cutaneous, or other systemic events, are uncommon during ASA-lysine inhalation challenges. Since the elapsed time from inhalation to onset of bronchospasm is under 30 min, each subsequent increase in concentration of inhaled ASA-

Table 3 Respiratory Reactions During Oral ASA and NSAID Challenges

Types of Reaction	Features of Reactions
No reaction	No respiratory symptoms; changes in $FEV_1 < 15\%$
Classic	Decrease in $FEV_1 > 20\%$ associated with naso-ocular reactions
Pure asthma	Decrease in FEV_1 values $> 20\%$; no naso-ocular signs or symptoms
Pure rhinitis	Naso-ocular reaction alone
Partial asthma, naso-ocular	Decline of 15–20% in FEV_1 values combined with naso-ocular reaction
Laryngospasm	Stridor; flow–volume curve: inspiratory loop flat and notched
Extrapulmonary	Flush, cramping gastrointestinal pain, explosive diarrhea, rarely mild urticaria, rarely hypotension

lysine can be delivered at 30 min intervals. Thus an ASA-lysine inhalation challenge can be completed within 5 h and performed in the outpatient clinic. There is some controversy about whether ASA-lysine inhalation can induce late asthmatic reactions, resembling those seen in IgE-mediated bronchospasm. During 26 positive bronchial responses to lysine-ASA, Kuna et al. (27) found isolated immediate bronchospastic responses in 16, immediate and late responses in 8, and late responses in only 2 ASA-sensitive asthmatic individuals. There is also controversy about how high the concentration of ASA-lysine should be advanced, because of concern that concentrations above 50 mg/mL may be too acidic and irritating to the bronchial tree, thus producing nonspecific bronchospasm (25,26).

C. Comparing Inhalation Challenge with ASA-Lysine to Oral ASA Challenge

A study comparing the diagnostic accuracy and safety of the two types of ASA challenge was conducted by Dahlen and Zetterstrom (28). In summary, both challenges accurately detected ASA-induced bronchospastic reactions and thus provided evidence that the patient has ASA respiratory disease. By definition, bronchial challenge is not directed at the nasal or ocular mucosa and therefore does not detect ASA-induced naso-ocular reactions.

D. ASA Nasal Challenges with ASA-Lysine

ASA-lysine by nasal insufflation induced local swelling of the nasal membranes in ASA-sensitive rhinosinusitis patients (29,30). Accuracy of nasal inhalation challenges can be further enhanced by simultaneous rhinometry measurements.

To be confident that both upper and lower airway challenges were negative, ASA-lysine challenge would need to be performed twice, once by bronchial inhalation and once by nasal insufflation.

IV. ASA Desensitization Procedures

All ASA-sensitive asthmatics can be successfully desensitized to ASA (8,24). After oral challenges with increasing doses of ASA, sensitive patients eventually experience respiratory reactions. As shown in Table 3, these reactions vary from the pure upper respiratory tract type to bronchospasm and various combinations in between. Desensitization is accomplished by reintroducing the provoking dose of ASA that initiated the first ASA-induced reaction. As soon as a reaction dissipates, after reexposure to the same dose of ASA, the next highest dose of ASA is given and repeated until further reactions cease. When a reaction occurs, ASA doses are suspended for that day. The process of escalating ASA doses continues on successive days until the patient can tolerate 650 mg of ASA without any reactions. At this point, the patient can safely take any dose of ASA or NSAID (31). After ASA desensitization, in the absence of further exposure to ASA, the desensitized state persist for 2 to 5 days, with full sensitivity returning after 7 days (24). Table 4 displays relevant data on a patient undergoing oral ASA challenge, followed by ASA desensitization.

A. Other Procedures to Conduct ASA Desensitization

Inhalation challenges with ASA-lysine are used extensively throughout the world to induce bronchospasm and to prove that ASA sensitivity exists in the patient under investigation (32,33). Following repeated inhalation challenges, patients have been shown to become refractory to further inhalation of ASA-lysine (32). At that point, ASA in oral doses can be introduced without inducing reactions, usually in doses between 150 and 325 mg. Continued daily treatment with ASA can then be started.

Table 4 Example of Aspirin Desensitization

| | | | Respiratory/responses | |
| | | | Nasal | Decline in FEV_1 (%) |
Day	Hour	Substance (dose)		
1	8:00 A.M.	Placebo	+	0
	11:00 A.M.	Placebo	+	0
	2:00 P.M.	Placebo	+	4
	Baseline airway stability demonstrated on day 1.			
2	8:00 A.M.	ASA (30 mg)	+ +	10
	11:00 A.M.	ASA (60 mg)	+ + + +	32
	Classic upper and lower respiratory reaction to ASA (60 mg).			
3	8:30 A.M.	ASA (60 mg)	+ +	10
	11:30 A.M.	ASA (100 mg)	+ + +	27
	Second reaction but to the next highest dose, 100 mg.			
4	8:00 A.M.	ASA (100 mg)	0	0
	11:00 A.M.	ASA (150 mg)	0	7
	2:00 P.M.	ASA (325 mg)	0	0
	Rapid desensitization after ingesting ASA (100 mg)			
5	7:00 A.M.	ASA (650 mg)	0	0
	Acute ASA desensitization completed; nasal congestions clears up.			

In most known ASA-sensitive asthmatics, pretreatment with sodium salicylate, which does not induce respiratory reactions in ASA-sensitive asthmatics, attenuates the respiratory reactions during oral ASA challenges and in many cases allowed "silent desensitization" (34). Induced tolerance (desensitization) was achieved in 10 known ASA-sensitive asthmatics by introducing subthreshold doses of ASA orally without inducing respiratory reactions (35). Patients were instructed to start with ingestion of 20 mg of ASA, and each day increase the dose by 20 mg until reaching 300 mg of ASA. None of the patients reacted to the increasing doses of ASA. Therefore, assuming one knows that the patient is ASA sensitive on the basis of a prior oral or inhalation ASA challenge, it is not necessary to induce a respiratory reaction to achieve ASA desensitization. However, failure to establish the diagnosis of ASA-sensitive respiratory sensitivity could result in silent "non-desensitization" in a patient who never was ASA sensitive in the first place. From a practical standpoint, an ASA-sensitive asthmatic with concomitant arthritis or need for antiplatelet therapy can be desensitized to ASA and then take daily ASA (at least 81 mg of ASA daily) indefinitely or switch to any cross-sensitizing NSAID as long as ASA or NSAID is continued daily.

V. ASA Cross-Sensitivity and Cross-Desensitization

A. Cyclooxygenase 1 and 2 (COX-1 and -2)

In 1971 Vane (36) discovered the shared pharmacological effects of ASA and NSAIDs on cyclooxygenase (COX) enzymes. We now know there are at least two isoforms of COX: COX-1 constitutively expressed in most mammalian cells, including respiratory and gut epithelial cells and most inflammatory cells; and COX-2, which is 60% homologous with COX-1 and is highly inducible by proinflammatory mediators, such as cytokines, growth factors, and tissue injury. ASA and most NSAIDs are nonspecific COX inhibitors, although they are far more potent inhibitors of COX-1 than COX-2. By contrast, the new selective COX-2 inhibitors are potent and specific inhibitors of the COX-2 enzyme, having no effect on COX-1 (37).

B. Efficient Inhibitors of Cyclooxygenase

All NSAIDs, which inhibit cyclooxygenase in vitro, cross-react with ASA, producing respiratory reactions (36,38,39). Furthermore, cross-reactions occur upon first exposure to the new NSAID in ASA-sensitive asthmatics (39). Six years after Vane's report (36) that ASA and NSAIDs inhibit formation of prostaglandins, Szczeklik et al. (38) reported in vitro and in vivo experiments demonstrating that ASA and NSAIDs inhibit COX (prostaglandin synthetase) in vitro. Furthermore, they showed that those

NSAIDs, which inhibited COX in vitro, with the least concentration of drug, were the most potent NSAIDs in cross-reacting with ASA. In addition, these potent cross-reacting NSAIDs produced large reactions after very small challenge doses. The reverse was also true. Table 5 lists NSAIDs that cross-react and cross-desensitize with ASA. Cross-desensitization occurs between all drugs that inhibit COX-1 (24). Thus, NSAIDs and ASA not only share the pharmacological effect of cross-reactivity but also participate in the phenomenon of cross-desensitization.

C. Weak Inhibitors of Cyclooxygenase

Based on the study by Szczeklik et al. (38), one would assume that weak inhibitors of COX either would not cross-react with ASA or would cross-react poorly and only after challenges with large doses of the suspected analgesic. Based on this reasoning, one would predict that cross-desensitization with weak COX inhibitors, after establishing an ASA-desensitized state with ASA, would be relatively easy to accomplish.

Settipane and Stevenson (40) studied three ASA-sensitive asthmatics who also gave an associated history of respiratory reactions occurring 2 h after ingestion of 500 to 1000 mg of acetaminophen. All three patients reacted to provoking doses of 60 mg of ASA. None reacted to 500 mg of acetaminophen, but all experienced bronchospastic reactions (FEV_1 values declined by > 20%) after ingesting 1000 mg of acetaminophen. Two patients were temporarily desensitized to 1000 and 1500 mg of acetaminophen, but desensitization to 2000 mg could not be sustained. Two patients were then desensitized to ASA (650 mg) and were able to immediately ingest 1000 mg of acetaminophen without adverse effect, demonstrating cross-desensitization. In a prospective study of 50 ASA-sensitive asthmatic subjects, Settipane and colleagues demonstrated that only 34% of the patients reacted to oral challenges with acetaminophen, even when the challenge doses were advanced to 1500 mg (41).

Salsalate is also a weak COX inhibitor with some anti-inflammatory effects and is used in the treatment of arthritis. Stevenson et al. (42) challenged 10 ASA-sensitive asthmatic patients with salsalate. After ingesting 2 g of salsalate, 2 of 10 patients experienced bronchospastic reactions. Repeated challenges with 2 g of salsalate reproduced the same bronchospastic reactions, demonstrating that a weak inhibitor of COX could not elicit desensitization at threshold provoking doses and suggested that much larger doses of the drug would be needed to achieve desensitization. Both patients then underwent ASA challenge and desensitization to ASA. Once desensitized to ASA (650 mg), both patients were able to immediately ingest 2 g of salsalate without adverse reactions, demonstrating cross-desensitiza-

Table 5 Nonsteroidal Anti-inflammatory Drugs (NSAIDs)
That Inhibit COX-1 and Induce Other Reactions to Other
Drugs

NSAIDs That Inhibit COX-1 and Cross-React and Cross-
Desensitize with Aspirin

Generic	Brand names
Piroxicam	Feldene
Indomethacin	Indocin
Sulindac	Clinoril
Tolmetin	Tolectin
Ibuprofen	Motrin, Rufen, Advil
Naproxen	Naprosyn
Naproxen sodium	Anaprox, Aleve
Fenoprofen	Nalfon
Meclofenamate	Meclomen
Mefenamic acid	Ponstel
Flurbiprofen	Ansaid
Diflunisal	Dolobid
Ketoprofen	Orudis, Oruval
Diclofenac	Voltaren
Ketoralac	Toradol
Etodolac	Lodine
Nabumetone	Relafen
Oxaprozin	Daypro

NSAIDS that weakly inhibit COX-1 and cross-react with
aspirin, only with high doses of these drugs:

Acetaminophen	Tylenol
Salsalate	Disalcid

NSAIDs that preferentially inhibit COX-2 but in higher
doses partially inhibit COX-1 also; they cross-react at high
doses:

Nimsulide	Not available in the United State
Meloxicam	Mobic

NSAIDs that selectively inhibit COX-2 and do not cross-
react with aspirin in the respiratory reaction and rarely
induce cutaneous reactions:

Celecoxib	Celebrex
Refecoxib	Vioxx

tion. Compared with acetaminophen, the same principles seemed to apply. Both acetaminophen and salsalate have sufficient inhibitory effects on COX-1 to induce mild respiratory reactions, particularly when supertherapeutic doses of the drugs are used in challenges. The cross-desensitization that occurs between ASA/NSAIDs and acetaminophen and salsalate proves that the mechanisms of reactions and desensitization are the same (Table 5).

D. Selective COX-2 Inhibitors

Highly selective COX-2 inhibitors, such as rofecoxib and celecoxib, do not appear to cross-react in AERD (43–45) or in acute/chronic urticaria (46). Both drugs can induce IgE-mediated reactions after prior sensitization, and it is important to distinguish IgE-mediated reactions from COX-1-inhibited cross-reactions. One large study by Sanchez-Borges et al. (47) showed that patients with urticarial reactions to ASA and NSAIDs also rarely reacted to COX-2 inhibitors.

Partial Inhibitors of COX-2

Less selective COX-2 inhibitors, such as nimsulide and meloxicam, do not cross-react when small doses of these drugs are given. However, cross-reactivity occurs, with either cutaneous or respiratory reactions, as the doses of nimesulide (48,49) or meloxicam (50,51) are increased. This pattern of reactions is consistent with predominant inhibition of COX-2 at low doses and increasing inhibition of COX-1 as the doses were increased (52) (Table 5).

E. Ineffective Inhibitors of Either COX-1 or COX-2

Azo and nonazo dyes, dextropropoxyphene, hydrocortisone, and sulfites do not cross-react with ASA/NSAID. Stevenson et al. (53,54) challenged 194 known ASA-sensitive asthmatic with tartrazine, and no reactions occurred. Documentation of a lack of cross-sensitivity between ASA and other dyes and chemicals, nonacetylated salicylates, sulfites, and dextropropoxyphene has been extensively studied and reviewed (55–58). Reports of severe asthma attacks within minutes of receiving hydrocortisone, but not dexamethasone intravenously have been published (59–61). Feigenbaum et al. (62) reported that 44 of 45 known ASA-sensitive asthmatics did not react to intravenous hydrocortisone succinate. One ASA-sensitive asthmatic patient experienced respiratory reactions to both hydrocortisone succinate and methylprednisolone sodium succinate, suggesting an IgE-mediated reaction to the succinate. After ASA desensitization, cross-desensitization to hydrocortisone succinate did not occur, showing that this ASA-sensitive asthmatic did not experience cross-reactions (or cross-desensitization) between ASA and succinate. The investigators concluded that reported reactions to intravenous corticosteroids in AERD patients were due to true allergic reactions to succinate, in a population that was likely to have been excessively exposed to this antigen.

VI. Pathogenesis

In 1967 Vanselow and Smith (63) reported cross-reactions between ASA and an NSAID (indomethacin). This fact is important in understanding the pathogenesis of reactions to ASA and NSAIDs because simultaneous immune recognition of ASA and the different NSAIDs is virtually impossible. Furthermore, first-exposure reactions to NSAIDs, in known ASA-sensitive asthmatics, occur routinely, clearly eliminating the possibility of prior immune recognition and sensitization to these NSAIDs. In 1971 Vane (36) discovered that ASA and NSAIDs shared the pharmacological effect of disabling the essential constitutive enzyme COX-1 (originally named prostaglandin synthetase). Since then, many investigators have focused research efforts on the products of arachidonic acid metabolism, as well as the identity of cells present in the respiratory tract, which might be capable of synthesizing arachidonic acid products (Table 6).

In the early 1980s, Samuelsson et al. (64,65) reported a second metabolic pathway for arachidonate metabolism, the 5-lipoxygenase (5-LO) pathway, through which leukotrienes (LTs) LTA_4, LTB_4, LTC_4, LTD_4, and LTE_4 are formed. These molecules, originally called slow-reacting substance of anaphylaxis (SRS-A), are potent mediators of chemotaxis for eosinophils, increased vascular permeability, mucus secretion, and prolonged constriction

Table 6 Cellular and Pathophysiological Events Characteristic of ASA-Exacerbated Respiratory Disease

Infiltration of respiratory mucosa with PMNs, eosinophils, and mast cells.

Eosinophils and mast cells preferentially increased in bronchial biopsy samples.

Peripheral monocytes synthesize excessive arachidonate products.

Urinary LTE_4 concentrations are increased.

Urinary TXB_2 concentrations are increased.

Bronchial lavage fluid contains increased number of eosinophils and increased concentrations of LTs, PGE_2, PGD_2, $PGE_{2\alpha}$ and TXB_2.

Bronchial *CysLT1* receptors highly sensitive to LTE_4. Histamine bronchial sensitivity same as for ASA- insensitive asthmatics.

of bronchial smooth muscles via stimulation of cysteinyl leukotriene (CysLT1 and CysLT2) receptors present on effector cells.

In understanding ASA disease and the respiratory reactions to ASA/NSAID, several attractive hypotheses have evolved. First, LTs are overproduced and participate in the inflammation, which causes ASA respiratory disease. Second, arachidonate is allowed to proceed down the 5-LO pathway, when the blocking effect of prostaglandin E_2 (PGE_2) is removed. ASA/NSAIDs stop PGE_2 synthesis by disabling or blocking COX-1. When this occurs, 5-LO is no longer inhibited by PGE_2, and synthesis of LTs proceeds at a brisk pace, inducing part of the reaction (66). Third, *CysLT1* receptors in bronchial smooth muscle are thought to be upregulated, such that small molecular stimulation by LTs induces larger bronchial responses than occur in nonsensitive asthmatics (67). Histamine release from mast cells does play some role in the ASA-induced reactions, particularly upper respiratory tract reactions, flushing and laryngospasm.

A. Pathogenesis of ASA Respiratory Disease

What is the evidence that ASA disease is caused by continued and relentless formation of arachidonate products? Clinically, this concept is intuitively acceptable. In fact, the inflammatory features of ASA disease, with infiltration of inflammatory cells, including neutrophils, eosinophils, and mast cells, has been observed in nasal cytograms and tissue biopsy samples (69). In other words, cells capable of generating arachidonate products are available in the inflamed tissues of the upper respiratory tract. Similarly, when compared with specimens from ASA-insensitive asthmatics, bronchial biopsy specimens from ASA-sensitive asthmatics contain increased numbers of mast cells and eosinophils, both of which stain for high concentrations of 5-LO (69).

In ASA-sensitive patients before exposure to ASA/NSAIDs, there is compelling evidence that excess arachidonate products are continually synthesized. In comparison to normal controls and ASA-tolerant asthmatics, Christie and colleagues (70) and Smith et al. (71) reported high baseline or prechallenge LTE_4 and thromboxane B_2 (TXB_2) concentrations in the urine of ASA-sensitive asthmatics. These findings have been confirmed by all investigators (72–75). Since LTE_4 is the final leukotriene in the 5-LO pathway, urinary concentrations of LTE_4 reflect systemic synthesis of all LTs, and high levels of TXB_2 are a reflection of excess and simultaneous synthesis of COX products. Continuous and excessive synthesis of arachidonate products appears to be either the cause of ASA disease or a prominent feature of that condition.

Yamashita et al. (68) compared polyps from ASA-sensitive asthmatics with those from patients with IgE-mediated rhinitis and chronic sinusitis and found significantly greater LTs in polyps from ASA-sensitive asthmatics than from the controls. Sladeck et al. (76) compared ASA-sensitive and ASA-insensitive asthmatics and counted increased numbers of eosinophils and measured elevated levels of PGE_2, PGD_2, $PGF_{2\alpha}$, and TXB_2 in the bronchial lavage fluid taken from 10 ASA-sensitive asthmatics prior to challenge with ASA-lysine.

These findings all support the notion that in patients with AERD, bronchial inflammation is well under way prior to exposure to ASA/NSAIDs and probably is caused in part by archidonate products. Table 6 summarizes the cellular and the pathophysiological features of ASA-exacerbated respiratory disease.

B. Pathogenesis of ASA-Induced Respiratory Reactions

Ferreri et al. (77) measured LTC_4, histamine, and PGE_2 in nasal lavage fluid after oral ASA challenges in ASA-sensitive and -insensitive asthmatics, as well as in normal controls. Patients experienced naso-ocular and asthmatic responses to ASA challenges, and following oral doses of ASA between 60 and 100 mg, histamine and LTC_4 concentrations in the nasal lavage fluid increased significantly in comparison to those in baseline and control subjects. Furthermore, both histamine and LTC_4 appeared in the nasal secretions slightly before the onset of naso-ocular reactions, indicating that both mediators were available to induce profound nasal congestion and rhinorrhea. During the same ASA-induced reactions, PGE_2 concentrations rapidly declined to undetectable levels in all subjects. Thus, ASA inhibited COX-1, immediately reducing PGE_2 and allowing increased activation of 5-LO. We concluded that histamine and LTC_4 were preferentially released/synthesized in ASA-sensitive asthmatics and rhinitics and at least contributed to, perhaps caused, the ASA-induced nasal reactions. Whether histamine is the predominant mediator cannot be stated with certainty, but pretreatment with antihistamines substantially blocked upper airway reactions to ASA in AERD patients (20). Similar findings of increased histamine and LTC_4 in nasal secretions during oral challenges with ASA have been reported by other investigators (21,78) and, after intranasal challenges with ASA-lysine, by Picado et al. (79).

In a study by Sladek et al. (76), bronchoalveolar lavage fluid (BALF) was obtained 30 min after ASA-lysine inhalation in 10 patients with ASA-sensitive asthma. The BALF contained increased concentrations of LTE_4 and decreased concentrations of PGE_2, PGD_2, $PGF_{2\alpha}$, and TXB_2. Tryptase declined sharply in 3 of 10 patients, increased in 3 of 10 patients, and remained unchanged in the remaining 4 patients. This important study confirmed that both upper and lower respiratory airways of ASA-sensitive asthmatics behave in a similar manner when challenged with ASA. Such an exposure to ASA, a potent inhibitor of COX-1, resulted in reduced formation of prostaglandins and enhanced formation of 5-LO products, presumably utilizing available intracellular arachidonic acid as substrate. After obtaining baseline bronchial biopsies, Nasser et al. (80) performed ASA-lysine inhalation challenges in 7 ASA-sensitive and 8 ASA-insensitive asthmatic subjects. Twenty minutes later, a second biopsy was performed on all study subjects. Biopsy specimens from the ASA-sensitive asthmatics revealed a decrease in mast cells (presumably degranulated) and an increase in activated eosinophils. These data strongly suggest that mast cells and eosinophils are important sources of LTs and preformed granular mediators, which appear to mediate ASA-induced respiratory reactions.

Christie et al. (70) measured urinary LTE_4 in ASA-sensitive and -insensitive asthmatics during oral ASA challenges. In the ASA-sensitive asthmatics, a significant increase in urinary LTE_4 was measured after ASA-induced bronchospasm, with values peaking at 6 h postreaction. In ASA-sensitive asthmatics, after oral challenged with ASA, or challenge with placebo in ASA-sensitive asthmatics, there were no changes in levels of urinary LTE_4. These observations have been confirmed by other investigators (71–73,75). Using ASA-lysine by inhalation to provoke asthma, Kumlin et al. (72) and Christie and associates (81) reported significant increases in urinary LTE_4 in ASA-sensitive asthmatics. Therefore, whether bronchospasm was induced locally with ASA-lysine or systemically during oral ASA challenges, a rise in urinary LTE_4 always followed ASA-induced bronchospasm and was specific for ASA-sensitive asthmatic patients. Daffern et al. (75) correlated the degree of rise in urine LTE_4 levels with the severity of the asthmatic reactions to oral ASA challenges. They found that the greater the drop in FEV_1 values, the higher the rise in LTE_4 in the urine. For naso-ocular reactors, a minimal rise in urinary LTE_4 values occurred. Thus, LTs appear to be the main mediators of lower respiratory tract reactions, and histamine appears to be the main mediator of upper respiratory tract reactions during ASA challenge studies.

Sladek et al. (74) demonstrated a simultaneous sharp decline in thromboxane B_2 in the urine of ASA-sensitive asthmatics during oral-ASA-induced bronchospastic reactions. Thus, during ASA-induced bronchospasm, simultaneously, TXB_2, representing a COX product, rapidly declined, while LTE_4, the terminal LT in the 5-LO pathway, was increasing. These data all point to the conclusion that 5-LO products are preferentially available during ASA-induced respiratory reactions, whereas COX products diminish rapidly and become unavailable.

In an elegant study by Sestini et al. (82), pretreatment with PGE_2 by inhalation preceded ASA-lysine inhalation challenges in seven ASA-sensitive asthmatic subjects. Despite challenges with ASA-lysine, at previously established provoking doses, no bronchospastic reactions occurred. Simultaneously, urinary LTE_4 concentrations did not increase from baseline levels after ASA challenge, once PGE_2 pretreatment was in effect. Thus, the presence of inhaled PGE_2 in the bronchial tissues protected them from ASA-induced reactions by artificially replacing endogenous PGE, and blocking 5-LO. Thus, the elimination of PGE_2 and its artificial restoration appear to cause or protect tissues from ASA-induced reactions and are probably the central event in the respiratory-induced reaction.

If LTs are preferentially synthesized during ASA-induced respiratory reactions and are mediators of bronchospasm under such circumstances, blockade of LTs should prevent or modify subsequent ASA-induced reactions. When the LTD_4 receptor antagonist SK&F 104353 was used to pretreat known ASA-sensitive asthmatic subjects, four of five patients experienced markedly attenuated responses to oral ASA challenges (83). Another potent LTD_4 receptor antagonist (MK-0679) was also shown to inhibit ASA-induced reactions when ASA-lysine by inhalation was the provoking stimulus (84). Using an inhibitor of 5-LO (Zileuton), Israel and associates (17) showed that inhibition of 5-LO by pretreatment with zileuton prevented ASA-induced respiratory reactions after previously established ASA oral provoking doses (mean 90 and range 20–300 mg of ASA) had been given during oral challenges. Nasser and associates (85) using another 5-LO inhibitor, ZD2138, were also able to block oral challenges with ASA in known ASA-sensitive asthmatics. Such data showed that either inhibition of formation or antagonism of effects of 5-LO products strongly implicate LTs as the agents responsible for ASA reactions in the respiratory tract.

Evidence for mast cell activation during ASA-induced reactions has also been published. Stevenson et al. (86) measured increased levels of histamine in the plasma of ASA-sensitive asthmatics during oral-ASA-induced bronchospastic reactions. Bosso et al. (87) measured serum tryptase and plasma histamine levels in 17 ASA-sensitive rhinosinusitis asthmatic patients during oral ASA challenges. Two of 17 patients, experiencing both naso-ocular and bronchospastic reactions, were found to have marked elevations of histamine and serum tryptase levels postreaction, and one other patient had moderate elevation of tryptase and histamine. Of note, these three patients had the same magnitude of respiratory reactions experienced by the remaining 14 patients; in addition to their respiratory reactions, however, they experienced systemic symptoms, consisting of flushing and either nausea or diarrhea.

Sladek and Szczeklik (74) measured increased serum tryptase levels and simultaneously increased urine LTE_4 concentrations during ASA-provoked bronchospastic reactions. Their studies implicated mast cells as the source of preformed mediators and possibly synthesis of LTs. These data suggest that mast cells may be directly activated by ASA/NSAIDs through a mechanism currently not understood. Such activation could be at multiple sites, inhibition of COX-1 (decreasing synthesis of PGE_2) with rapid formation of 5-LO products as well as release of preformed mediators from their cytoplasmic granules. ASA may primarily activate other cells (monocytes, macrophages, eosnophils, or neutrophils), a process that also generates 5-LO products and, in the case of eosinophils, major basic proteins and eosinophilic cationic proteins as the initiating or sustaining mechanisms. These products, in turn, could secondarily stimulate mast cells to release stored mediators and perhaps to synthesize additional archidonate products.

In addition to the mast cell, there is strong evidence that eosinophils are activated during ASA-induced reactions (69). Although alveolar macrophages have not been studied in this manner, their precursor cells, peripheral blood monocytes, are preferentially stimulated by ASA during ASA-induced reactions. Juergens et al. (88) obtained peripheral monocytes from ASA-sensitive asthmatics before and during ASA-induced bronchospastic reactions and stimulated the cells with calcium ionophore. After inducing reactions during oral challenges with 60 mg of ASA, COX products were profoundly inhibited in monocytes. By contrast, peripheral blood monocytes from normal controls and ASA-insensitive asthmatics did not demonstrate inhibition of COX after ingestion of 60 mg of ASA. Only after oral challenges with 650 mg of ASA did COX inhibition occur in the control monocytes. This suggested that COX in the monocytes of ASA-sensitive asthmatics is peculiarly susceptible to acetylation by ASA. Such susceptibility could represent an inborn error of metabolism, which distinguishes ASA-sensitive asthmatics from those able to tolerate ASA/NSAIDs.

Arm et al. (67) evaluated airway responsiveness to histamine and LTE_4 in 5 ASA-sensitive asthmatics and found a 13-fold increase in airway responsiveness to inhaled LTE_4 in comparison to 15 non-ASA-sensitive asthmatics. There were no differences between the two groups in their response to inhaled histamine. The implications of this study are substantial. Not only are LTs formed during ASA-induced reactions, but ASA-sensitive asthmatics have an unusual and marked sensitivity to the effects of the terminal LTs on their bronchial smooth muscle receptors, thus further magnifying the degree of bronchospasm that occurs after ASA stimulation. Whether similar upregulation of *CysLT1* or *CysLT2* receptors occurs in the upper airway would be of considerable interest (Table 7).

C. Pathogenesis of ASA Desensitization

Juergens et al. (89) studied peripheral blood monocytes from 10 ASA-sensitive asthmatics who had been successfully desensitized to ASA (acute

Table 7 Pathophysiological Events During ASA-Induced Respiratory Reactions

Nasal lavage fluid contains increased concentrations of histamine and LTC_4 and decreased concentrations of PGE_2.

Bronchial lavage fluid contains increased LTC_4, LTE_4, and tryptase (inconstant), and decreased concentrations of PGE_2 and TXB_2.

Urine concentrations of LTE_4 are increased, peaking at 6 h.

Urine concentrations of TXB_2 diminished.

Prechallenge inhalation of PGE_2 prevents ASA- lysine-induced bronchospasm.

$CysLT_1$ bronchial receptors demonstrate a heightened (13-fold) bronchospastic response to inhaled LTE_4.

Tryptase and histamine are released into the blood in some patients, with systemic reactions.

Antagonists for $CysLT_1$ receptors or inhibitors of 5-LO prevent ASA-induced bronchospastic reactions when threshold doses of ASA are reintroduced.

desensitization) and treated with 650 of mg ASA twice a day for a number of months (long-term ASA desensitization treatment). During acute desensitization, peripheral monocytes synthesized significantly less thromboxane B_2 but only slightly less LTB_4, the preferential 5-LO product of peripheral monocytes. By contrast, peripheral monocytes from ASA respiratory patients undergoing chronic desensitization showed marked reduction in LTB_4 synthesis after stimulation by means of calcium ionophore. Indeed, LTB_4 synthesis declined to the same level found in normal controls.

Nasser et al. (90) recorded a slight reduction in urinary LTE_4 values when samples were taken at acute ASA desensitization. However, when ASA-sensitive asthmatic patients were desensitized to ASA and then treated with daily ASA (600 mg/day) over a number of months, urine LTE_4 levels declined, but not to the levels found in normal controls. This suggests that long-term desensitization is associated with diminished synthesis of LTs, and at the same time *CysLT1* receptors are less responsive to the available LTs. In the study by Arm et al. (67), beginning on the first day following ASA desensitization and only in ASA-sensitive asthmatics, there was a 20-fold decrease in responsiveness of bronchial *CysLT1* receptors. ASA-insensitive asthmatics did not experience a change in bronchial responsiveness to histamine or LTE_4 after ASA challenge. Bronchial hyperresponsiveness to LTE_4 returned in the ASA-sensitive asthmatics after discontinuation of ASA ingestion a week later. Such findings are compatible with the hypothesis that in ASA desensitization, ASA binds to *CysLT1* and *CysLT2* receptors on smooth muscles and eosinophils, decreasing responses to both end organs but possibly interrupting chemotaxis of new activated eosinophils into the respiratory tissues. This would account for a slow reduction in formation of LTs by the diminishing pool of activated eosinophils (Table 8).

Table 8 Changes in Pathophysiological Events During Acute and Chronic ASA
Desensitization Treatment

Nasal lavage fluid no longer contains measurable LTC_4, PGE_2, or histamine.
Urinary LTE_4 diminishes during acute desensitization, and mean concentrations
    decrease to levels found in normal controls during long- term, high dose
    ASA desensitization.
Urinary TXB_2 disappears immediately after ASA- induced respiratory reactions
    and is unmeasurable during chronic ASA desensitization.
Histamine and tryptase are no longer measured in blood samples at acute
    desensitization.
Peripheral blood monocytes synthesize less LTB_4/LTC_4 at acute desensitization,
    and synthesis decreases during chronic desensitization to levels found in
    monocytes of normal controls.
CysLT1 bronchial receptors are no longer supersensitive to LTE_4 by inhalation
    and respond in the same manner as those of ASA-insensitive asthmatics.

VII. Treatment

A. Prevention and Treatment of ASA/NSAID-Induced Respiratory Reactions

Avoidance of ASA and all cross-reacting NSAIDs is essential in preventing
respiratory reactions to these medications in unprotected ASA-sensitive
asthmatic patients. Patient education should include a discussion of the
adverse effects that reexposure to ASA/NSAIDs might induce and emphasis
on cross-reactivity between ASA and all COX-1-inhibiting NSAIDs. In
addition ASA-sensitive asthmatics should research any new drugs for potential of cross-reactivity before them. These patients' doctors should provide
appropriate warnings to patients, other physicians and nurses (chart and
electronic database), and pharmacists (pharmacy computers). Only with
continued vigilance, particularly on the part of the patient for over-the-
counter ASA or NSAIDs, obvious or hidden, can future disasters be avoided.

B. Treatment of ASA/NSAID-Induced Respiratory Reactions

Treatment of ASA-induced reactions in the emergency room or physician's
office should include the following. For bronchospasm, inhalation from
nebulizers of β-adrenergic agonists, delivering no more than five inhalations
every 5 to 10 min is generally effective in providing bronchodilation, while
ASA-induced reaction gradually subsides over a number of hours. For
laryngospasm, racemic epinephrine by inhalation or subcutaneous epinephrine is usually effective treatment. For nasal congestion with paranasal
headache, topical nasal application of oxymetazoline is an effective, rapidly

acting decongestant. Topical antihistamine/decongestant solutions can also be instilled in the conjunctivae. Flush or gastrointestinal reactions, for which histamine is the mediator, can be treated effectively by intravenous administration of 50 mg of diphenhydramine and 50 mg of ranitidine. If a patient fails to respond to these measures in the emergency room, transportation to an intensive care unit may be necessary, as well as intubation followed by mechanical ventilation.

C. Treatment of ASA Disease

A major goal in controlling ASA disease, and its component of corticosteroid-dependent asthma, is the development of strategies to reduce mucosal inflammation (Table 9). Only in this manner is it possible to prevent nasal polyp formation, secondary sinusitis, and worsening asthma. There is irrefutable evidence that a major contributor to mucosal inflammation is overproduction of archidonate products. It should not be a surprise that corticosteroids, because they stimulate synthesis of phospholipase A_2 (PLA_2) inhibitor protein (lipocortin) (91,92) and through blocking effects on transcription of mRNA synthesis (93), offer significant therapeutic benefits to ASA-sensitive asthmatic patients. High dose topical corticosteroids, by both nasal insufflations and oral inhalation, are mainstays in reducing inflammation and retarding nasal polyp formation (94). Unfortunately, in some ASA-sensitive asthmatic patients, inflammation cannot be adequately controlled with topical corticosteroids alone. This is particularly the case when patients experience viral respiratory illnesses, which usually progress to secondary bacterial sinus infections. Because of the degree of inflammatory obstruction in the nose and sinus ostia, topical corticosteroids may not, under these circumstances, penetrate sufficiently into the areas of inflammation. Therefore, bursts of systemic corticosteroids are usually required during such infectious episodes. Bursts of systemic corticosteroids are also helpful in shrinking nasal polyps and the swollen mucosae around sinus ostia, reestablishing temporary sinus drainage. An unhappy feature of ASA respiratory disease is the requirement for increasing doses of daily systemic corticosteroids. At such a point, the side effects of corticosteroids may become more devastating than the disease.

Antibiotic treatment is also important, and long courses of broad-spectrum antibiotics are usually required to clear purulent nasal secretions. If medical treatment fails, patients should undergo sinus CT scans and be referred to an ear, nose, and throat surgeon for consideration of operative intervention. The purpose of such surgery is to debulk sinuses and nasal passages of excessive and hypertrophic inflammatory mucosa, reestablish drainage for sinus ostia, and remove as much infected mucosa as possible

Table 9 Treatment of ASA-Exacerbated Respiratory Disease

Avoid ASA and other NSAIDs that inhibit COX-1.
Treat with selective COX-2 inhibitors, if needed.
Primary pharmacological intervention (daily)
    Topical nasal corticosteroids
    Topical bronchial corticosteroids
    Antihistamines and decongestants
    Montelukast (10 mg at bedtime)
Intervention for expected bouts of acute sinusitis
    Broad-spectrum antibiotics (2–3 weeks)
    Systemic corticosteroids (40–60 mg of prednisone tapering over 2–3 weeks)
Intervention for chronic pansinusitis
    Alternate-day prednisone
    Surgical intervention with cultures and pathology stains for fungi
    Appropriate antimicrobial treatment
    ASA desensitization and treatment with daily ASA
Intervention for difficult-to-control asthma
    Add zileuton (600 mg, four to two times a day)
    Add long-acting β-adrenergic agonists
    Add theophylline.
    Add ipratropium by inhalation.
    Bursts and alternate-day prednisone.
Intervention for aggressive re-formation of nasal polyps
    Bursts of systemic corticosteroids
    Alternate-day systemic corticosteroids
    Surgical polypectomies
    ASA desensitization and daily treatment

without injuring essential structures (95–98). Patients with ASA sensitivity have a poorer outcome with respect to long-term remissions after sinus surgery than ASA-insensitive patients (96). This may be due to the sheer mass of polypoid tissue at the time of surgery, as well as the aggressive re-formation of additional polypoid tissues after surgery (99). Nevertheless, the role of sinusitis in provoking asthma is generally accepted (100), and good surgical results after extensive sinus surgery in ASA-sensitive asthmatics have been reported (98,100,101). The fundamental issues surrounding the indications for sinus surgery in ASA-sensitive asthmatics are not related to effectiveness of these procedures in removing masses of hypertrophic and infected nasal and sinus tissues. In fact, rapid improvement in both upper and lower airways is observed in most patients shortly after surgery (98,101). Rather, because of re-formation of polypoid tissues, the indications for repeated surgical procedures provide difficult dilemmas. In point of fact, it is impossible to safely remove enough of the inflamed and infected mucosal tissues to prevent reoccurrence. Furthermore, surgery does not influence the fundamental biochemical features of ASA disease, namely, continued overproduction of arachidonate products and perhaps other mediators of inflammation.

D. Treatment with ASA Desensitization

In 1980 Stevenson et al. (101a) reported two ASA-sensitive asthmatic subjects who were successfully desensitized to ASA and then treated with daily ASA continuously. Both patients rapidly experienced improvement in nasal patency and one regained her sense of smell. Furthermore, when daily ASA treatment was continued over a number of months, nasal airway patency was maintained, regrowth of nasal polyps ceased, and asthma activity diminished.

Taking into consideration variations in study design, doses of ASA employed, length of treatment with ASA, and criteria for successful clinical outcomes, efficacy has been reported in most studies of ASA desensitization treatment (102–106). One study by Naeije et al. (107) did not show efficacy of ASA treatment in 10 ASA-sensitive asthmatic subjects. Lumry et al. (10) demonstrated that ASA treatment of patients with ASA-sensitive rhinosinusitis without asthma, after ASA desensitization, was associated with clearing of hypertrophic rhinitis in 77% of the patients studied.

Stevenson et al. (108) conducted the only double-blind crossover study of treatment with ASA, after ASA desensitization, in 25 ASA-sensitive asthmatics. During the 3-month treatment arm with daily ASA therapy, patients experienced significant improvement in nasal symptom scores and a reduced use of nasal beclomethasone. However, only half the patients experienced improvement in asthma symptom scores, and systemic corticosteroid doses could not be significantly reduced during the ASA treatment period. This short-term study employed variable doses of ASA, fewer study subjects than had been projected were recruited. Thus the multiple-dose patient samples were of insufficient size to permit comparison of subgroups based on treatment doses and outcomes. Retrospectively, it would have been preferable if all 25 patients had been treated with the daily dose of ASA (1300 mg/day) rather than dividing the 25 patients into treatment subgroups, particularly for only 325 mg/day, now known to be below therapeutic threshold dose of ASA. Furthermore, the time frame of 3 months was insufficient to assess rate of polyp regrowth or need for additional sinus or nasal polyp surgery.

Between 1986 and 1988, we attempted to conduct a long-term, double-blind, placebo-controlled study of ASA desensitization treatment. After 2 years of recruitment, only two patients had volunteered to participate. Both underwent ASA oral challenges, followed by successful ASA desensitization. As usually occurs, they immediately noted improvement in their nasal patency at the completion of ASA desensitization. Both started daily treatment with the study drug but disenrolled from the study several weeks later, when nasal congestion returned. In both patients, placebo treatment had been randomly assigned. Thus, patients could distinguish between placebo and ASA therapy because nasal congestion recurred while they were taking placebo. Furthermore, ASA as a "study drug" is available over the counter and not controlled by the investigators, allowing patients the option of not enrolling in a study where placebo treatment would be expected 50% of the time. Finally, the human subjects committee at our institution required full disclosure of therapeutic options, including the opportunity for these patients to enroll in open treatment with ASA in adjusted dosages. Essentially all patients elected this last option.

In 1990 our research group (102) reported the clinical courses of 107 known ASA-sensitive rhinosinusitis asthmatic patients treated with ASA between 1975 and 1988. Forty-two patients avoided aspirin and served as the control group. Thirty-five patients were desensitized to ASA and treated continuously with ASA daily for as long as 8 years. Thirty patients were initially desensitized to ASA and treated with ASA but discontinued ASA after a mean of 2 years, usually because of gastric side effects. Retrospective analysis of the three groups showed that the patients treated with ASA enjoyed statistically significant reductions in hospitalizations, emergency room visits, outpatient visits, need for additional sinus surgery, need for additional nasal polypectomies, number of upper respiratory infections/ sinusitis requiring antibiotics, and improved sense of smell. ASA-desensitized and treated patients were also able to significantly reduce systemic corticosteroid maintenance doses and corticosteroid bursts per year and, in the group treated continuously, were able to reduce inhaled corticosteroids in comparison to the control group. In the patients who had to discontinue ASA treatment after several years, symptoms lessened while being treated with daily ASA but reverted toward pretreatment status after ASA treatment was discontinued. This study showed that ASA desensitization followed by long-term ASA treatment improved the clinical courses of ASA-sensitive asthma rhinosinusitis and prevented regrowth of nasal polyps, while at the same time allowing significant reduction in systemic and inhaled corticosteroids. Side effects from gastritis occurred in 20% patients treated with ASA. Unfortunately, 30 of 65 patients who started ASA desensitization therapy discontinued ASA, largely for misperceived reasons, reducing the active treatment group to only 35 patients. This made it impossible to subdivide the patient population into short- and long-term treatment groups to determine whether therapeutic effects were concentrated in a particular phase of treatment and whether escape of treatment effect was observed in a long-term treatment group.

In 1996 Stevenson, et al. (103) analyzed the clinical courses of an additional 65 ASA-sensitive asthmatics who underwent oral ASA challenges followed by ASA desensitization between 1988 and 1994. These patients, after ASA oral challenges and standard oral desensitization to ASA, were then treated with twice daily doses of ASA (650 mg) and followed for an average of 3.3 years (range 1–6 years). The following clinical parameters were significantly improved after long-term ASA desensitization treatment: number of sinus infections per year, number of hospitalizations for asthma per year, number of sinus operations per year, improvement in sense of smell, and reduction in use of both nasal topical corticosteroids and systemic corticosteroids. Unchanged after ASA desensitization treatment were number of emergency room visits for asthma per year and use of inhaled corticosteroids. This study showed that the main components of ASA disease, namely, aggressive nasal polyp formation and sinusitis, were significantly reduced during long-term ASA desensitization treatment. Concomitantly, nasal and systemic corticosteroids could be successfully reduced or discontinued without the expected increase in inflammation. Also important, when the 65 patients were subdivided into an early and a late treatment group, the results were essentially the same, indicating that therapeutic escape did not occur during long-term treatment with ASA. These data further showed that early reduction in systemic corticosteroids during the first year of ASA treatment was not associated with escape of disease activity. For the total group of 65 patients, the need for sinus surgery declined from a pretreatment interval of one operation every 3 years to one every 9 years during treatment with daily ASA.

In our most recent study (106), 110/126 AERD patients, who were treated with ASA 1300 mg/day for 1 or more years, had significant improvement in their clinical courses.

E. Leukotriene Inhibitors and Antagonists

At least 8 antagonists for LTB_4 and another 10 antagonists for *CysLT1* receptors have proceeded through various stages of pharmacological development (109,110). However, LTB_4 antagonists have not reached the market, and only three *CysLT1* antagonists have been marketed: montelukast and zafirlukast (in the United States and Europe) and pranlukast (in Japan). Drugs that disable 5-LO activating protein (FLAP) have not been developed, and one 5-LO inhibitor, zileuton, has reached the U.S. market. Theoretically, all members of this class of drugs have potential to significantly help patients with AERD, since they prevent formation of LTs or block the effects of LTs on one CysLT receptor (111). Dahlen et al. (112) conducted a double-blind, placebo-controlled, short-term study of treatment effects of zileuton in ASA-sensitive asthmatics in Sweden and Poland. The treatments were efficacious both by decreasing asthma activity as well as effecting a return of smell in some patients. One *CysLT1* receptor antagonist, Montelukast was also studied for efficacy in the treatment of 80 ASA-sensitive asthmatics. In a one-month, randomized double-blind study, a remarkable improvement in all measures of asthma activity was recorded (113).

F. Combination Treatment

Evolution of clinical management of AERD patients has now reached the point where most physicians are using combination treatment. This makes sense because multiple mechanisms are involved in the disease. A first-line treatment program is topical corticosteroids, an antihistamine–decongestant and montelukast. When sinusitis episodes occur, add broad-spectrum antibiotics and bursts of systemic corticosteroids. If control of asthma is difficult, add zileuton. If control of hypertrophic rhinitis and sinusitis is difficult, or requires excessive systemic corticosteroids, activate ASA desensitization and treatment with aspirin (Table 9).

In the future, cytokine inhibitors, particularly inhibitors of interleukins 2 to 5, might also provide opportunities to interrupt cell signals before synthetic activities begin. Additional knowledge about the fundamental defects or excesses in ASA-sensitive asthmatics will be necessary to understand the disease and guide us in selecting therapeutic interventions.

References

1. Stevenson DD, Simon RA. Sensitivity to aspirin and non-steroidal anti-inflammatory drugs. In: Middleton EJ, Reed CE, Ellis EF, Adkinson NFJr, Yunginger JW, Busse WW, eds. Allergy: Principles and Practice. Vol. 2. St. Louis, MD: Mosby, 1993:1747–1767.
2. Samter M, Beers R Jr. Intolerance to aspirin: clinical studies and consideration of its pathogenesis. Ann Intern Med 1968; 68:975–983.
3. Spector SL, Wangaard CH, Farr RS. Aspirin and concomitant idiosyncrasies in adult asthmatic patients. J Allergy Clin Immunol 1979; 64(6 pt 1): 500–506.
4. Szczeklik A. Aspirin-induced asthma: pathogenesis and clinical presentation [review]. Allergy Proc 1992; 13:163–173.
5. Stevenson D, Sanchez-Borges M, Szczeklik A. Classification of allergic and pseudoallergic reactions to drugs that inhibit cyclooxygenase enzymes. Ann Allergy, Asthma, Immunol 2001; 87:1–4.

6. Stevenson DD. Diagnosis, prevention, and treatment of adverse reactions to aspirin and nonsteroidal anti-inflammatory drugs. J Allergy Clin Immunol 1984; 74:617–622.

7. Mathison DA, Stevenson DD, Tan EM, Vaughn JH. Clinical profiles in asthma. JAMA 1973; 224:1134.

8. Stevenson D, Simon RA. Sensitivity to aspirin and nonsteroidal antiinflammatory drugs. In: Middleton E Jr, Ellis EF, Yunginger JW, Reed CE, Adkinson NF Jr, Busse WW, eds. Allergy: Principles and Practice. Vol. 2. St. Louis, MD: Mosby, 1998:1225–1234.

9. Szczekik A, Nizankowska E, Duplaga M. Natural history of aspirin-induced asthma. AIANE Investigators. European Network on Aspirin-Induced Asthma. Eur Respir J 2000; 16:432–436.

10. Lumry WR, Curd JG, Zieger RS, Pleskow WW, Stevenson DD. Aspirin-sensitive rhinosinusitis: the clinical syndrome and effects of aspirin administration. J Allergy Clin Immunol 1983; 71:580–587.

11. Stevenson DD. Aspirin and nonsteroidal anti-inflammatory drugs. Immunol Allergy Clin North Am 1995; 15:529–549.

12. Pleskow WW, Stevenson DD, Mathison DA, Simon RA, Schatz M, Zieger RS. Aspirin-sensitive rhinosinusitis/asthma: spectrum of adverse reactions to aspirin. J Allergy Clin Immunol 1983; 71:574–579.

13. McDonald J, Mathison DA, Stevenson DD. Aspirin intolerance in asthma—detection by challenge. J Allergy Clin Immunol 1972; 50:198–207.

14. Stevenson DD. Oral challenges to detect aspirin and sulfite sensitivity in asthma. N Engl Reg Allergy Proc 1988; 9:135–142.

15. Weber RW, Hoffman M, Raine DA, Nelson HS. Incidence of bronchoconstriction due to aspirin, azo dyes, non-azo dyes, and preservatives in a population of perennial asthmatics. J Allergy Clin Immunol 1979; 64:32–37.

16. Nizankowska E, Szczeklik A. Glucocorticosteroids attenuate aspirin-precipitated adverse reactions in aspirin-intolerant patients with asthma. Ann Allergy 1989; 63:159–162.

17. Israel E, Fischer AR, Rosenberg MA, et al. The pivotal role of 5-lipoxygenase products in the reaction of aspirin-sensitive asthmatics to aspirin. Am Rev Respir Dis 1993; 148:1447–1451.

18. Pauls JD, Simon RA, Daffern PJ, Stevenson DD. Lack of effect of the 5-lipoxygenase inhibitor zileuton in blocking oral aspirin challenges in aspirin-sensitive asthmatics. Ann Allergy Asthma Immunol 2000; 85:40–45.

19. Stevenson D, Simon RA, Mathison DA, Christiansen SC. Montelukast is only partially effective in inhibiting aspirin responses in aspirin-sensitive asthmatics. Ann Allergy Asthma Immunol 2000; 85:477–482.

20. Szczeklik A, Serwonska M. Inhibition of idiosyncratic reactions to aspirin in asthmatic patients by clemastine. Thorax 1979; 34:654–658.

21. Fischer AR, Rosenberg MA, Lilly CM, et al. Direct evidence for a role of the mast cell in the nasal response to aspirin in aspirin-sensitive asthma. J Allergy Clin Immunol 1994; 94:1046–1056.

22. Dahl R. Oral and inhaled sodium cromoglycate in challenge tests with food allergens and acetylsalicylic acid. Allergy 1981; 36:161–172.

23. Stevenson DD, Simon RA, Mathison DA. Cromolyn pretreatment delays onset of aspirin (ASA) induced asthmatic reactions. J Allergy Clin Immunol 1984; 73:162.

24. Pleskow WW, Stevenson DD, Mathison DA, Simon RA, Schatz M, Zieger RS. Aspirin desensitization in aspirin-sensitive asthmatic patients: clinical manifestations and characterization of the refractory period. J Allergy Clin Immunol 1982; 69:11–19.

25. Phillips GD, Foord R, Holgate ST. Inhaled lysine–aspirin as a bronchoprovocation procedure with aspirin in aspirin-sensitive asthma. J Allergy Clin Immunol 1989; 84:232–241.

26. Melillo G, Podovano A, Cocco G, Masi C. Dosimeter inhalation test with lysine acetylsalicylate for the detection of aspirin-induced asthma. Ann Allergy 1993; 71:61–65.

27. Kuna P, Zielinska E, Bpchenska-Marciniak M, Rozniecki J. Early and late asthmatic response after inhalation challenge with lysine-ASA in subjects with aspirin-induced asthma. J Allergy Clin Immunol 1997; 99:S 11, (Abstract 1669).

28. Dahlen B, Zetterstrom O. Comparison of bronchial and peroral provocation with aspirin in aspirin-sensitive asthmatics. Eur Respir J 1990; 3:527–534.

29. Pawlowicz A, Williams WR, Davies BH. Inhalation and nasal challenge in the diagnosis of aspirin-induced asthma. Allergy 1991; 46:405–409.

30. Patriarca G, Nucera E, Di Rienzo V. Nasal provocation test with lysine acetylsalicylate (LAS) in aspirin-sensitive patients. Ann Allergy 1991; 67:60–62.

31. Stevenson DD, Simon RA, Mathison DA. Aspirin-sensitive asthma: tolerance to aspirin after positive oral aspirin challenges. J Allergy Clin Immunol 1980; 66:82–88.

32. Bianco SR, Petrini MG. Aspirin-induced tolerance in aspirin-asthma detected by a new challenge test. IRCS J Med Sci 1977; 5:129–136.

33. Schmitz-Schumann VM, Juhl E, Costabel U. Analgesic asthma-provocation challenge with acetylsalicylic acid. Atemw Lungenkrkh Jahrgang 1985; 10:479–485.

34. Nizankowska E, Dworski R, Soja J, Szczeklik A. Salicylate pre-treatment attenuates intensity of bronchial and nasal symptoms precipitated by aspirin in aspirin-intolerant patients. Clin Exp Allergy 1990; 20:647–652.

35. Szmidt M, Grzelewska-Rzymowska I, Rozniecki J. Tolerance to aspirin in aspirin-sensitive asthmatics. Methods of inducing the tolerance state and its influence on the course of asthma and rhinosinusitis [review]. J Invest Allergol Clin Immunol 1993; 3:156–159.

36. Vane JR. Inhibition of prostaglandin synthesis as a mechanism of action for aspirin-like drugs. Nat New Biol 1971; 231:232–235.

37. Hawley C. COX-2 inhibitors. Lancet 1999; 353:307–314.

38. Szczeklik A, Gryglewski RJ, Czerniawska-Mysik G. Clinical patterns of hypersensitivity to nonsteroidal anti-inflammatory drugs and their pathogenesis. J Allergy Clin Immunol 1977; 60(5):276–284.

39. Mathison DA, Stevenson DD. Hypersensitivity to nonsteroidal anti-inflam-

matory drugs: Indications and methods for oral challenge. J Allergy Clin Immunol 1979; 64:669–674.
40. Settipane RA, Stevenson DD. Cross-sensitivity with acetaminophen in aspirin-sensitive asthmatics. J Allergy Clin Immunol 1989; 84:26–33.
41. Settipane RA, Shrank PJ, Simon RA, Mathison DA, Christensen SC, Stevenson DD. Prevalence of cross-sensitivity with acetaminophen in aspirin-sensitive asthmatic subjects. J Allergy Clin Immunol 1995; 96:480–485.
42. Stevenson DD, Hougham A, Schrank P, Goldlust B, Wilson R. Disalcid cross-sensitivity in aspirin-sensitive asthmatics. J Allergy Clin Immunol 1990; 86:749–758.
43. Dahlen B, Szczeklik A, Murray JJ. Celecoxib in patients with asthma and aspirin intolerance. N Engl J Med 2001; 344:142.
44. Szczeklik A, Nizankowska E, Bochenek G, Nagraba K, Mejza F, Swierczynska M. Safety of a specific COX-2 inhibitor in aspirin-induced asthma. Clin Exp Allergy 2001; 31:219–225.
45. Stevenson D, Simon RA. Lack of cross-reactivity between rofecoxib and aspirin in aspirin-sensitive asthmatic patients. J Allergy Clin Immunol 2001; 108:47–51.
46. Berges-Gimeno M, Camacho-Garrido E, Garcia-Rodriguez RM, Martin-Garcia C, Alfaya T, Hinojosa M. Rofecoxib: Safe in NSAID intolerant patients. Eur J Allergy Clin Immunol 2001; 56:1017–1018.
47. Sanchez-Borges M, Capriles-Hulett A, Caballero-Fonseca F, Ramon-Perez C. Tolerability to new COX-2 inhibitors in NSAID-sensitive patients with cutaneous reactions. Ann Allergy Asthma Immunol 2001; 87:201–204.
48. Asero R. Aspirin and paracetamol tolerance in patients with nimesulide-induced urticaria. Ann Allergy Asthma Immunol 1998; 81:237–238.
49. Bavbek S, Celik G, Ediger D, Mungan D, Demirel YS, Misirligil Z. The use of nimesulide in patients with acetylsalicylic acid and nonsteroidal anti-inflammatory drug intolerance. J Asthma 1999; 36:657–663.
50. Quaratino D, Romano A, Di Fonso M, et al. Tolerability of meloxicam in patients with histories of adverse reactions to nonsteroidal anti-inflammatory drugs. Ann Allergy Asthma Immunol 2000; 84:613–617.
51. Vaghi A. Tolerance of meloxicam in aspirin-sensitive asthmatics. Am J Respir Crit Care Med 1998; 157:715(A).
52. Sampson A, Holgate S, Austen KF, Szczeklik A. Cyclo-oxygenase. Thorax 1998; 53:719–720.
53. Stevenson DD, Simon RA, Lumry WR, Mathison DA. Adverse reactions to tartrazine. J Allergy Clin Immunol 1986; 78:182–191.
54. Stevenson DD, Simon RA, Lumry WR, Mathison DA. Pulmonary reactions to tartrazine. Pediatr Allergy Immunol 1992; 3:222–227.
55. Stevenson DD. Cross-reactivity between aspirin and other drugs/dietary chemicals: a critical review. In: Pichler WJ, Stadler MM, Dahinden CA, Pecoud AR, Frei P, Schneider CH, deWeck AL, eds. Progress in Allergy and Clinical Immunology. Vol. 1. Lewiston, NY: Hogrefe and Huber, 1989:462–473.
56. Simon RA. Adverse reactions to drug additives. J Allergy Clin Immunol 1984; 74:623–630.

57. Simon RA, Stevenson DD. Lack of cross-reactivity between aspirin and sulfite in sensitive asthmatic patients. Aspen Allergy Conference 1986; July: 23–26.

58. Manning ME, Stevenson DD. Pseudoallergic drug reactions: aspirin, nonsteroidal anti-inflammatory drugs, dyes, additives and preservatives. In: Van Arsdel P Jr, ed. Immunology and Allergy Clinics of North America. Vol. 11:3. Philadelphia: WB Saunders Co, 1991:659–678.

59. Partridge MR, Gibson GJ. Adverse bronchial reactions to intravenous hydrocortisone in 2 aspirin-sensitive patients. Br Med J 1978; 1:1521–1523.

60. Szczeklik A, Nizankowska E, Czerniawska-Mysik G, Sek S. Hydrocortisone and airflow impairment in aspirin-induced asthma. J Allergy Clin Immunol 1985; 76:530–536.

61. Dajani BM, Sliman NA, Shubair KS. Bronchospasm caused by intravenous hydrocortisone sodium succinate (Solu-Cortef) in aspirin-sensitive asthmatics. J Allergy Clin Immunol 1981; 68:201–204.

62. Feigenbaum BA, Stevenson DD, Simon RA. Lack of cross-sensitivity to IV hydrocortisone in aspirin-sensitive subjects with asthma. J Allergy Clin Immunol 1995; 96:545–548.

63. Vanselow NA, Smith JR. Bronchial asthma induced by indomethacin. Ann Intern Med 1967; 66:568–573.

64. Samuelsson B, Hammarstroem S, Murphy RC, Borgeat P. Leukotrienes and slow reacting substance of anaphylaxis (SRS-A). Allergy 1980; 35:375–381.

65. Samuelsson B. Leukotrienes; mediators of hypersensitivity reactions and inflammation. Science 1983; 220:568–570.

66. Szczeklik A, Stevenson DD. Aspirin-induced asthma: advances in pathogenesis and management. J Allergy Clin Immunol 1999; 104:5–13.

67. Arm JP, O'Hickey SP, Spur BW, Lee TH. Airway responsiveness to histamine and leukotriene E4 in subjects with aspirin-induced asthma. Am Rev Respir Dis 1989; 140:148–153.

68. Yamashita T, Tsuyi H, Maeda N, Tomoda K, Kumazawa T. Etiology of nasal polyps associated with aspirin-sensitive asthma. Rhinology 1989; 8:15–24.

69. Nasser SM, Pfister R, Christie PE, Sousa AR, Barker J, Schmitz-Schumann M, Lee TH. Inflammatory cell populations in bronchial biopsies from aspirin-sensitive asthmatic subjects. Am J Respir Crit Care Med 1996; 153:90–96.

70. Christie PE, Tagari P, Ford-Hutchinson AW, et al. Urinary leukotriene E4 concentrations increase after aspirin challenge in aspirin-sensitive asthmatic subjects. Am Rev Respir Dis 1991; 143:1025–1029.

71. Smith CM, Hawksworth RJ, Thien FC, Christie PE, Lee TH. Urinary leukotriene E4 in bronchial asthma. Eur Respir J 1992; 5:693–699.

72. Kumlin M, Dahlen B, Bjorck T, Zetterstrom O, Granstrom E, Dahlen SE. Urinary excretion of leukotriene E4 and 11-dehydro-thromboxane B2 in response to bronchial provocations with allergen, aspirin, leukotriene D4, and histamine in asthmatics. Am Rev Respir Dis 1992; 146:96–103.

73. Knapp HR, Sladek K, Fitzgerald GA. Increased excretion of leukotriene E4 during aspirin-induced asthma. J Lab Clin Med 1992; 119:48–51.

74. Sladek K, Szczeklik A. Cysteinyl leukotriene overproduction and mast cell

activation in aspirin-provoked bronchospasm in asthma. Eur Respir J 1993; 6:391–399.

75. Daffern P, Muilenburg D, Hugli TE, Stevenson DD. Association of urinary leukotriene E4 excretion during aspirin challenges with severity of respiratory responses. J Allergy Clin Immunol 1999; 104:559–564.

76. Sladek K, Dworski R, Soja J, et al. Eicosanoids in bronchoalveolar lavage fluid of aspirin-intolerant patients with asthma after aspirin challenge. Am J Respir Crit Care Med 1994; 149:940–946.

77. Ferreri NR, Howland WC, Stevenson DD, Spiegelberg HL. Release of leukotrienes, prostaglandins, and histamine into nasal secretions of aspirin-sensitive asthmatics during reaction to aspirin. Am Rev Respir Dis 1988; 137: 847–854.

78. Kowalski ML, Sliwinska-Kowalska M, Igarashi Y, et al. Nasal secretions in response to acetylsalicylic acid. J Allergy Clin Immunol 1993; 91:580–598.

79. Picado C, Ramis I, Rosello J, et al. Release of peptide leukotriene into nasal secretions after local instillation of aspirin in aspirin-sensitive asthmatic patients. Am Rev Respir Dis 1992; 145:65–69.

80. Nasser S, Christie PE, Pfister R, et al. Effect of endobronchial aspirin challenge on inflammatory cells in bronchial biopsy samples from aspirin-sensitive asthmatic subjects. Thorax 1996; 51:64–70.

81. Christie PE, Tagari P, Ford-Hutchinson AW, et al. Urinary leukotriene E4 after lysine-aspirin inhalation in asthmatic subjects. Am Rev Respir Dis 1992; 146:1531–1534.

82. Sestini P, Armetti L, Gambaro G, et al. Inhaled PGE2 prevents aspirin-induced bronchoconstriction and urinary LTE4 excretion in aspirin-sensitive asthma. Am J Respir Crit Care Med 1996; 153:572–575.

83. Christie PE, Smith CM, Lee TH. The potent and selective sulfidopeptide leukotriene antagonist, SK&F 104353, inhibits aspirin-induced asthma. Am Rev Respir Dis 1991; 144:957–958.

84. Dahlen BJ, Kumlin M, Margolskee D, et al. The leukotriene receptor antagonist MK-0679 blocks airway obstruction induced by bronchial provocation with lysine-aspirin in aspirin-sensitive asthmatics. Eur Respir J 1993; 6:1018–1026.

85. Nasser SM, Bell GS, Foster S, et al. Effect of the 5-lipoxygenase inhibitor ZD2138 on aspirin-induced asthma. Thorax 1994; 49:749–756.

86. Stevenson DD, Arroyave CM, Bhat KN, Tan EM. Oral aspirin challenges in asthmatic patients: a study of plasma histamine. Clin Allergy 1976; 6:493–505.

87. Bosso JV, Schwartz LB, Stevenson DD. Tryptase and histamine release during aspirin-induced respiratory reactions. J Allergy Clin Immunol 1991; 88:830–837.

88. Juergens UR, Christiansen SC, Stevenson DD, Zuraw BL. Arachidonic acid metabolism in monocytes of aspirin-sensitive asthmatic patients before and after oral aspirin challenge. J Allergy Clin Immunol 1992; 90:636–645.

89. Juergens UR, Christiansen SC, Stevenson DD, Zuraw BL. Inhibition of

monocyte leukotriene B4 production following aspirin desensitization. J Allergy Clin Immunol 1995; 96:148–156.

90. Nasser SMS, Patel M, Bell GS, Lee TH. The effect of aspirin desensitization on urinary leukotriene E4 concentration in aspirin-sensitive asthma. Am J Respir Crit Care Med 1995; 115:1326–1330.
91. Peers SH, Flower RJ. The role of lipocortin in corticosteroid actions. Am Rev Respir Dis 1990; 141:18–21.
92. Ambrose MP, Hunninghake GW. Corticosteroids increase lipocortin I in BAL fluid from normal individuals and patients with lung disease. J Appl Physiol 1990; 68:1668–1671.
93. Nakano T, Ohara O, Teraoka H, Arita H. Glucocorticoids suppress group II phospholipase A2 production by blocking mRNA synthesis and post-transcriptional expression. J Biol Chem 1990; 265:12745–12748.
94. Mastalerz L, Milewski M, Duplaga M, Nizankowska E, Szczeklik A. Intranasal fluticasone propionate for chronic eosinophilic rhinitis in patients with aspirin-induced asthma. Allergy 1997; 52:895–900.
95. Nishioka GJ, Cook PR, Davis WE, McKinsey JP. Functional endoscopic sinus surgery in patients with chronic sinusitis and asthma. Otolaryngol Head Neck Surg 1994; 110:494–500.
96. Schaitkin B, May M, Shapiro A, Fucci M, Mester SJ. Endoscopic sinus surgery: 4-year follow-up on the first 100 patients. Laryngoscope 1993; 103: 1117–1120.
97. Nakamura H, Kawasaki M, Higuchi Y, Takahashi S. Effects of sinus surgery on asthma in aspirin triad patients. Acta Otolaryngol 1999; 119:592–598.
98. McFadden EA, Woodson BT, Fink JN, Toohill RJ. Surgical treatment of aspirin triad sinusitis. Am J Rhinol 1997; 11:263–270.
99. Kennedy DW. Prognostic factors, outcomes and staging in ethmoid sinus surgery. Laryngoscope 1992; 102:1–18.
100. Mings R, Friedman WH, Linford PA, Slavin RG. Five-year follow-up of the effects of bilateral intranasal sphenoidethmoidectomy in patients with sinusitis and asthma. Am J Rhinology 1988; 2:13–16.
101. McFadden EA, Kany RJ, Fink JN. Surgery for sinusitis and aspirin triad. Laryngoscope 1990; 100:1043–1050.
101a. Stevenson DD, Simon RA, Mathison DA. Aspirin sensitive asthma: Tolerance to aspirin after positive oral aspirin challenges. J. Allergy Clin Immunol 1980; 66:82–88.
102. Sweet JA, Stevenson DD, Simon RA, Mathison DA. Long-term effects of aspirin desensitization treatment for aspirin-sensitive rhinosinusitis asthma. J Allergy Clin Immunol 1990; 86:59–65.
103. Stevenson DD, Hankammer MA, Mathison DA, Christensen SC, Simon RA. Long-term ASA desensitization-treatment of aspirin-sensitive asthmatic patients: clinical outcome studies. J Allergy Clin Immunol 1996; 98:751–758.
104. Chiu JT. Improvement in aspirin-sensitive asthmatic subjects after rapid aspirin desensitization and aspirin maintenance (ADAM) treatment. J Allergy Clin Immunol 1983; 71(6):560–567.

105. Nelson RP, Stablein JJ, Lockey RF. Asthma improved by acetylsalicylic acid and other nonsteroidal anti- inflammatory agents. N Engl Reg Allergy Proc 1986; 7:117–121.

106. Berges-Gimeno MP, Simon RA, Stevenson DD. Treatment with aspirin desensitization in patients with aspirin exacerbated respiratory disease. J Allergy Clin Immunol 2003; 111:180–186.

107. Naeije N, Bracamonte M, Michel O, et al. Effects of chronic aspirin ingestion in aspirin-intolerant asthmatic patients. Ann Allergy 1984; 53(3):262–264.

108. Stevenson DD, Pleskow WW, Simon RA, et al. Aspirin-sensitive rhinosinusitis asthma: A double-blind cross-over study of treatment with aspirin. J Allergy Clin Immunol 1984; 73:500–507.

109. Henderson W. New modalities for the pharmocotherapy of asthma: leukotriene inhibitors and antagonists. Immunol Allergy Clin North Am 1996; 16:797–808.

110. Holgate ST, Bradding P, Sampson AP. Leukotriene antagonists and synthesis inhibitors: new directions in asthma therapy. J Allergy Clin Immunol 1996; 98:1–13.

111. Henderson WR. The role of leukotrienes in inflammation. Ann Intern Med 1994; 121:684–697.

112. Dahlen SE, Nizankowska E, Dahlen B. The Swedish–Polish treatment study with the 5-lipoxygenase inhibitor zileuton in aspirin-intolerant asthmatics. Am J Respir Crit Care Med 1995; 151:A 376.

113. Dahlen S, Malstrom K, Nizankowska E, Dahlen B, Kuna P, Kowalski M, Lumry WR, Picado C, Stevenson DD, Bousquet J, Pauwels R, Holgate ST, Shahane A, Zhang J, Reiss TF, Szczeklik A. Improvement of aspirin-intolerant asthma by montelukast, a leukotriene antagonist. A randomized, double blind, placebo-controlled trial. Am J Respir Crit Care Med 2002; 165:9–14.

14

Effects of Sleep on Upper and Lower Airways

ROBERT D. BALLARD

National Jewish Medical and Research Center
and University of Colorado Health Sciences Center
Denver, Colorado, U.S.A.

Introduction

During the last three decades interest in the interactions between sleep and breathing has focused on the syndrome of obstructive sleep apnea. However, it is also clear that sleep can alter breathing in a variety of ways independent of frank sleep apnea. Edward Smith reported in 1860 that ventilation is reduced during sleep in apparently healthy subjects (1). This has been confirmed multiple times in recent years, with the decrement in ventilation commonly resulting from a sleep-associated reduction in tidal volume (2,3).

Although such changes are usually of minimal importance in subjects with normal respiratory function during wakefulness, this is often not the case in patients with lung disease. Nocturnal bronchoconstriction has been observed in the majority of patients with asthma (4,5), a pattern that appears to disrupt sleep in affected patients (6) and may explain earlier reports of an excessive nocturnal death rate from asthma (7). Patients with chronic obstructive pulmonary disease (COPD) often demonstrate nocturnal worsening manifested by hypoxemia (8), disrupted sleep (9), and increased airflow obstruction (10). Sleep-associated hypoxemia is also commonly observed in patients with cystic fibrosis and is thought to contribute to neurocognitive dysfunction and daytime sleepiness (11).

Although it is clear that these nocturnal patterns of respiratory dysfunction are both common and clinically important, there continues to be no unifying hypothesis that fully explains these phenomena. One likely area of relevance is the effect of sleep on interactions between upper and lower airway function. Although knowledge of this area remains limited, in this chapter we review what is known about potential interactions between the sleep-associated alterations in upper and lower airway function.

I. Sleep and Upper Airway Function

Sleep onset leads to upper airway narrowing that occurs even in persons without sleep apnea (3,12,13). This narrowing apparently results from a combination of sleeping in the supine posture and a sleep-associated reduction in pharyngeal dilator muscle activity (14,15). Such narrowing of the upper airway constitutes an intrinsic resistive load to breathing (16). As compensatory responses to resistive loading are decreased during sleep (17,18), upper airway narrowing may be an important contributor to the sleep-associated reduction in ventilation.

Although the effects of this narrowing appear to be insignificant in the majority of people, some have upper airways that are anatomically narrowed at one or more levels between the nasal choanae and the epiglottis. A number of factors can contribute to such narrowing, including craniofacial characteristics (19), increased size and fat content of the soft palate and uvula (20,21), a large or posterior-lying tongue (22), and vascular congestion or edema of the pharyngeal mucosa (23). Affected persons can compensate for this anatomical narrowing during wakefulness by increasing upper airway dilator muscle activity (24). With sleep onset this compensatory response is reduced or lost, creating an imbalance between forces that promote collapse of the pharynx and opposing forces that support upper airway patency (25). This imbalance may lead to closure or critical narrowing of the airway, typically posterior to the palate and/or the tongue (26,27).

A subsequent reduction or loss of ventilation may result from this limitation of flow, causing hypercapnia and hypoxia, which in turn lead to a progressive increase in inspiratory effort that eventually triggers arousal or awakening. Return to wakefulness restores the compensatory increase in upper airway dilator activity (14), opening the airway and allowing resumption of normal ventilation until a return to sleep again allows airway narrowing or closure. This cycle can repeat itself hundreds of times during a

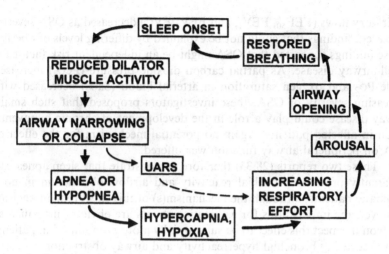

Figure 1 Pathophysiologic sequence of repetitive obstructive apneas and hypopneas during sleep in OSA. UARS = upper airway resistance syndrome.

single night, resulting in the syndrome of obstructive sleep apnea (OSA) (Figure 1).

II. Obstructive Sleep Apnea and Airway Function in Patients Without Other Airways Disease

At least two reports have suggested that OSA can lead to altered lower airway function in otherwise healthy patients. Lin and Lin (28) observed that 4 of 16 patients with OSA had bronchial hyperreactivity demonstrated by a positive methacholine challenge, while none of 32 subjects with snoring alone had an abnormal methacholine challenge. Bronchial hyperreactivity was subsequently eliminated after a 2- to 3-month trial with nasal continuous positive airway pressure (nCPAP). These investigators speculated on several mechanisms by which OSA could induce reflex bronchoconstriction, including hypoxia-induced bronchoconstriction (29,30), the stimulation of glottic inlet and laryngeal mechanoreceptors by snoring (31) (although none of the snoring-only patients demonstrated bronchial hyperreactivity), and vagal "hyperfunction" induced by repetitive Müller maneuvers during obstructive apneas (32). However, no specific mechanism by which OSA could increase bronchial reactivity was offered.

In 1997 Zerah-Lancner and colleagues (33) evaluated pulmonary function in 170 obese snorers with and without OSA. They observed that forced expiratory flows (FEF_{50}, FEV_1, and FEV_1/FVC) decreased as OSA severity increased, findings that could not be explained by differing levels of obesity. These findings suggested that OSA might be an independent risk factor for small-airway disease. As partial carbon dioxide pressure (PCO_2) increased while PO_2 and oxygen saturation in arterial blood (SaO_2) decreased with increasing severity of OSA, these investigators proposed that such small-airway disease could play a role in the development of chronic hypoventilation in affected patients. Again no potential mechanism for the effect of OSA on peripheral airway function was offered.

These two reports (28,33) therefore demonstrate that sleep apnea can apparently promote bronchial reactivity and airflow obstruction in non-asthmatic patients, although the mechanism(s) of this effect remain unclear. However, the implications for asthmatic patients are obvious, inasmuch as one would expect this effect to be substantially more pronounced in patients with preexisting bronchial hyperreactivity and airway obstruction.

III. Obstructive Sleep Apnea and Asthma

Hudgel and Shucard (34) published the initial report of an asthmatic patient with coexisting OSA. Their patient presented with nocturnal worsening of his dyspnea that evidently led to hourly awakenings, despite what was described as well-controlled asthma during the day. A subsequent sleep study confirmed severe OSA, with oxygen desaturation to as low as 40%. Therapy with supplemental oxygen and medroxyprogesterone was ineffective, leading eventually to the performance of a tracheotomy. The tracheotomy resolved all symptoms of sleep apnea, although there was no mention of its effect on asthma severity.

Chan and colleagues (35) made the subsequent observation that OSA and snoring could be important triggers of nocturnal asthma attacks. They reported nine patients with asthma and concurrent OSA, noting that all patients had frequent nocturnal exacerbations of their asthma. When treated with nasal continuous positive airway pressure for OSA, these patients demonstrated marked improvement in their asthma, manifested by decreased symptoms, improved peak expiratory flow rate (PEFR) (Fig. 2), a reduced need for bronchodilator therapy, and resolution of their patterns of nocturnal worsening. Although no specific mechanism for this effect was established, it was suggested that OSA might provoke asthma via apnea-associated hypoxemia, which could then induce reflex bronchoconstriction via the carotid bodies (29,30). However, review of Chan's patient data reveals that hypoxemia was actually quite mild in these patients, with only one of nine patients demonstrating transient desaturation to under 85%. It

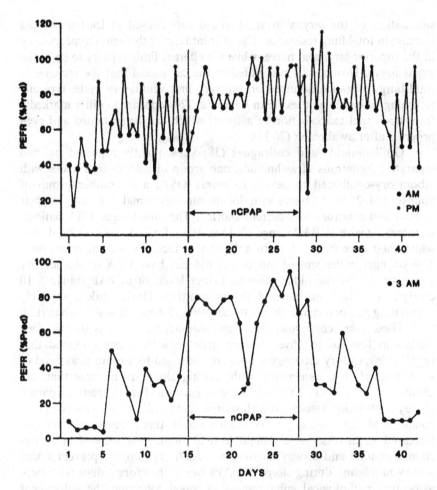

Figure 2 PEFR recordings in an individual patient who showed improvement in asthma during nCPAP therapy (upper panel). Greatest improvement was observed at 3 a.m. (lower panel), but the arrow indicates a single night in which the patient did not use nCPAP. From Ref. 35, with permission.

also had been noted by Hudgel and Shucard that supplemental oxygen was ineffective therapy for nocturnal dyspnea in their asthmatic patient with sleep apnea (34).

Chan and colleagues subsequently proposed that snoring and repetitive upper airway closures stimulate neural receptors at the glottic inlet and in the laryngeal region, triggering reflex-induced bronchoconstriction. As early as 1962, Nadel and Widdicombe (31) had demonstrated that mechanical stimulation of the larynx in anesthetized cats caused at least a twofold increase in total lung resistance. The afferent limb of this reflex appears to be in the superior laryngeal nerve, while the efferent limb appears to be in the vagus nerve. However, it was noted in the cat model that the increase in total lung resistance occurred on the very first ventilatory cycle, typically returning to baseline in less than a minute. This appears to differ markedly from nocturnal exacerbation of asthma, which can be sustained and even progress after awakening (36,37).

Guilleminault and colleagues (38) subsequently reported on two separate populations of asthmatics: one group of middle-aged males with laboratory-confirmed moderate to severe OSA, and another group of younger (14–21 years) males with documented nocturnal worsening of their asthma and a history of recurrent snoring. The middle-aged OSA patients were treated with nCPAP (range 10–15 cmH_2O) for 12 to 14 months, during which their once frequent nocturnal asthma exacerbations totally resolved. The younger males snored loudly but did not have OSA of the severity demonstrated by the older patients. Lower levels of nCPAP (range 5–10 cmH_2O) resolved snoring and the intermittent OSA, while completely eliminating all nocturnal asthma attacks during a 6-month follow-up period.

These researchers also positioned esophageal balloons during sleep studies in four of the five younger male patients. They observed that negative inspiratory esophageal pressure increased to a mean peak level of 47 ± 8 cmH_2O in association with snoring alone, an increase that was eliminated by nCPAP. This led to the suggestion that complete or partial airway obstruction associated with snoring can result in repetitive partial or complete Müller maneuvers. As already noted, this process may result in increased vagal tone, which might lead to subsequent increases in bronchomotor tone and airway narrowing (32,39). Therapy to prevent upper airway narrowing during sleep (nCPAP) would therefore reduce this sleep-associated pathological enhancement of vagal tone and the subsequent worsening of asthma. However, one would again expect any reflex-induced increase in bronchomotor tone to improve or resolve with arousal, whereas nocturnal exacerbations of asthma are often persistent or even progressive after awakening.

Martin and Pak (40) subsequently investigated the role of nCPAP in asthmatic patients with nocturnal worsening, but no snoring or OSA. They observed that two of seven patients demonstrated marked improvement in their nocturnal asthma when treated overnight with nCPAP at 10 cmH_2O. For the entire group there was no significant difference between overnight falls in FEV_1 on control and nCPAP nights (mean decrements of $29.3 \pm 5.0\%$ and $21.4 \pm 5.1\%$, respectively, $p > 0.05$), but given the small sample size, a type 2 error seems likely. These investigators did report that the two patients who improved in response to nCPAP had more pronounced nocturnal oxygen desaturation than the other five patients, although it did not appear that the nocturnal asthma of the former was any more severe. These two patients could, therefore, have had an undetected upper airway resistance syndrome (41), which would also have responded to nCPAP. Martin and Pak also pointed out that these two patients improved in response to nocturnal supplemental oxygen, suggesting that hypoxemia could induce bronchoconstriction via a reflex mediated by the carotid body (29), augmented bronchial responsiveness (42), a direct action on bronchial smooth muscle (30), or the release of bronchoconstricting mediators (43). Whatever the potential mechanism(s) for their pattern of nocturnal asthma, these investigators emphasized that nCPAP was not well tolerated by this group of patients, who demonstrated reduced sleep efficiency and decreased REM sleep when treated with nCPAP.

Several population-based studies have suggested that asthma is commonly associated with symptoms suggestive of concurrent OSA. Janson and colleagues reported from 98 asthmatic patients that 44% complained of daytime sleepiness and 44% had difficulty maintaining sleep (44). The same investigators more recently reported from a multinational study of over 2000 subjects that the diagnosis of asthma was an independent risk factor for difficulty initating sleep, early morning awakening, daytime sleepiness, snoring, and self-reported apneas (45). Fitzpatrick and coinvestigators studied a random sample of 1478 subjects, noting that young asthmatics were more likely to report frequent snoring than young nonasthmatics (46). Most recently Larsson and colleagues randomly surveyed 5425 subjects from the Swedish population, noting that problem snoring, witnessed apneas, and daytime sleepiness were all more common in patients with physician-diagnosed asthma (47). These reports all suggest that OSA might be more prevalent in the asthmatic population, possibly contributing to asthma severity and nocturnal worsening. However, we presently lack a definitive polysomnographic assessment of the association between asthma and sleep-disordered breathing.

IV. Sleep, Lung Volumes, and Intrapulmonary Blood Volume in Asthmatics with Nocturnal Worsening: A Potential Role for the Upper Airway

To better assess the effect of sleep on airflow resistance in asthmatics with nocturnal worsening, we initially performed overnight studies on five patients while monitoring esophageal pressure and airflow via a facemask with an attached pneumotachygraph (48). Using these data to calculate pulmonary resistance (R_L) on a breath-by-breath basis, we observed that R_L increased during sleep in all five patients, leading to a 51.8 ± 10.7% increase ($p < 0.01$) from bedtime to morning awakening.

In a subsequent study of six asthmatics selected for having nocturnal worsening but no snoring or known sleep apnea, we combined these methods with the addition of a supraglottic pressure catheter (37). This allowed us to also measure the contribution of the upper airway (supraglottic resistance — R_{sg}) to sleep-associated changes in R_L. Lower airway resistance ($R_{la} = R_L - R_{sg}$) increased overnight whether patients were allowed to sleep or were kept awake throughout the night, although the rate of increase was twofold greater while both mean and peak R_{la} were higher when patients were allowed to sleep (Fig. 3). Although we intentionally selected patients without known snoring or sleep apnea, R_{sg} was also significantly greater when the patients slept. Given the earlier reports of an association between snoring/OSA and nocturnal worsening of asthma, one can hypothesize that simple upper airway narrowing during sleep could by itself play a role. However, earlier observations clearly do not confirm a cause-and-effect relationship between sleep-associated changes in upper and lower airway resistance.

Another sleep-related change that could possibly serve as an intermediary step between sleep-associated changes in upper and lower airway resistance is the intrapulmonary pooling of blood. Using a horizontal body plethysmograph to study sleeping subjects, we reported in 1990 that sleep was associated with an impressive reduction in functional residual capacity (FRC) in asthmatics with nocturnal worsening (49). Although in 1993 we found evidence that reductions in inspiratory muscle tonic activity could contribute to sleep-associated changes in lung volume (50), several observations led us to suspect that sleep could promote intrapulmonary pooling of blood and thereby contribute to the observed reduction in FRC. First, it had been documented in 1932 that moving from the upright to the supine posture (the usual sleeping posture) increases venous return from peripheral vascular beds and augments pulmonary blood volume, an effect felt likely to contribute to the supine-posture-dependent reduction in FRC (51). Additional findings from studies of the effects of general anesthesia (52) and submaximal paralysis (53) (two conditions that mimic many physiological changes of sleep) also suggest that additional pulmonary blood pooling can occur during sleep.

The intrapulmonary pooling of blood could then worsen asthma by at least three mechanisms: (1) reflex brochoconstriction triggered by the activation of intrapulmonary C-fiber nerve endings (54), (2) bronchial wall edema (55), and (3) an increase in bronchial responsiveness, as has been observed with the pulmonary vascular congestion associated with left ventricular dysfunction (56).

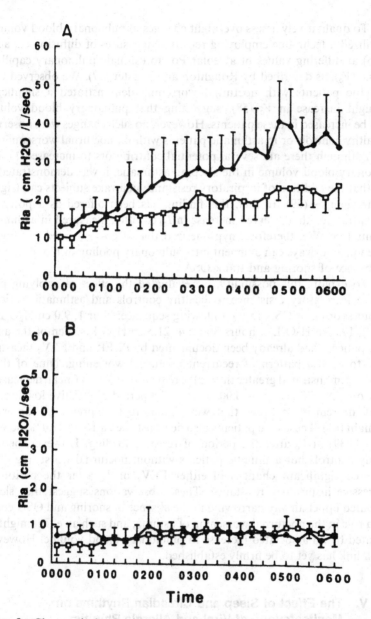

Figure 3 Changes in lower airway resistance (R1a) in asthmatics (panel A) and healthy controls (panel B) overnight during normal sleep (closed triangles) and during enforced wakefulness (open squares). Adapted from Ref. 37, with permission.

To qualitatively assess overnight changes in pulmonary blood volume, we utilized a technique employing repetitive measures of diffusion capacity ($D_L$co) at differing values of alveolar Po_2 to estimate pulmonary capillary volume (V_c), as described by Roughton and Forster (57). We observed that asthmatic patients with nocturnal worsening demonstrated a significant overnight increase in V_c (58), suggesting that pulmonary blood volume could be increased in these patients. However, no such changes were observed in healthy controls or in asthmatic patients without nocturnal worsening.

Although there are several potential contributors to increased V_c and pulmonary blood volume in the sleeping asthmatic, it was demonstrated in 1965 that the addition of inspiratory resistance in awake subjects can trigger similar changes (59). In fact, this finding has been offered as a potential explanation for the observed increase in $D_L$co often measured in asthmatic patients (60). We, therefore, hypothesized that sleep-associated narrowing of the upper airways can augment intrapulmonary pooling of blood, even in the absence of snoring and frank OSA.

To explore this possibility, we evaluated the effect of applying progressive inspiratory resistance to healthy controls and asthmatic patients without snoring or OSA in the following sequence: hour 1, 9.0 cmH$_2$O/L/s; hour 2, 17.0 cmH$_2$O/L/s; hours 3 and 4, 21.5 cmH$_2$O/L/s. Ten of the asthmatic patients had already been documented by PEFR and FEV$_1$ measurements to have a pattern of recurrent nocturnal worsening. Nine of these patients demonstrated greater than 20% reduction in FEV$_1$ (mean decrease in FEV$_1$ of $29.9 \pm 5.7\%$, $p = 0.0025$) after the period of resistive loading, an overall decrement in FEV$_1$ that was similar to that previously observed overnight (61). These nine patients also demonstrated a $16.0 \pm 7.0\%$ increase ($p = 0.039$) in V_c after the period of resistive loading. However, neither healthy controls nor asthmatic patients without nocturnal worsening demonstrated significant changes in either FEV$_1$ or V_c after the period of progressive inspiratory resistance. These observations suggest that sleep-associated upper airway narrowing in the absence of snoring and OSA could play a role in the nocturnal worsening of asthma, and such an effect might be mediated by an associated increase in pulmonary blood volume. However, such a link has yet to be firmly established.

V.   The Effect of Sleep and Circadian Rhythms on Manifestations of Viral and Allergic Rhinitis: Potential Implications for Asthmatic Patients

There is substantial evidence of a link between rhinitis and asthma. Allergic rhinitis has been reported in up to 57% of asthmatic adults (62), while up to

38% of patients with allergic rhinitis may have asthma (63). The onsets of rhinitis and asthma symptoms are also often temporally linked (62,64). Finally, bronchial hyperreactivity to methacholine and histamine can often be demonstrated in patients with allergic rhinitis, with up to 32% of these patients demonstrating responses that are in the range of those observed in asthmatic patients (65).

Other studies have assessed the effects of therapy with rhinitis-specific anti-inflammatory medications upon asthma severity. Corren and colleagues (66) found that intranasal administration of beclomethasone to patients with seasonal allergic rhinitis and asthma blocked their usual seasonal increase in methacholine responsiveness. In a similar study, Watson and associates (67) observed that 4 weeks of intranasal therapy with beclomethasone significantly reduced bronchial responsiveness in patients with concurrent allergic rhinitis and asthma. Aubier and colleagues (68) demonstrated that intranasal administration of beclomethasone to asthmatic patients with rhinitis improved bronchial responsiveness, whereas intrabronchial administration of the same steroid had no effect on reactivity.

These studies suggest that nasal inflammation associated with allergic rhinitis may play a significant role in modulating lower airway responsiveness in asthmatic patients. Several potential mechanisms for this relationship have been suggested. The existence of a nasal–bronchial reflex is supported by observations that application of silica particles to the nasal mucosa can trigger immediate and marked increases in lower airway resistance (69). This effect can be blocked by systemic atropine (69) or upon resection of the trigeminal nerve (70). Corren and associates (71) reported that nasal allergen challenge in patients with seasonal allergic rhinitis and asthma triggered an immediate increase in nonspecific bronchial responsiveness to methacholine. The rapidity of these changes also supports the involvement of a neural reflex.

It has also been proposed that nasal obstruction resulting from mucosal swelling and secretions promotes mouth breathing, which has been demonstrated to aggravate exercise-induced bronchospasm (72). Even if patients continue to breathe transnasally, the subsequent narrowing of the nasal passages would still constitute an additional intrinsic resistive load to breathing, which could also contribute to OSA during sleep (73,74) and lead to nocturnal worsening of asthma. Finally, it also has been suggested that the postnasal drainage of cellular and biochemical inflammatory mediators with subsequent pulmonary aspiration enhances lower airway responsiveness (75). Regardless of which of these mechanisms might most closely link nasal inflammation to lower airway function, there is substantial evidence that symptoms of allergic rhinitis increase at night and during the early morning. One study of "hay fever" sufferers suggested that in 75% of those sampled, symptoms (sneezing, nasal stuffiness, wheeze, and cough) were most severe while in bed at night or with morning awakening (76). Another study of nearly 1000 patients with perennial or seasonal rhinitis reported that 56% of those with seasonal rhinitis and 66% of those with perennial rhinitis claimed that their most severe symptoms (sneezing, nasal stuffiness, postnasal drainage) occurred with morning awakening (77). These findings are supported by those of Reinberg and associates (78), who studied the day–night variation of allergic rhinitis symptoms in 765 patients. They observed that sneezing, nasal stuffiness, and rhinorrhea were all most severe in the early morning after awakening.

These studies all suggest that allergic rhinitis can increase in severity during the night and early morning hours. This may signify a nocturnal intranasal increase in inflammation, such as has been observed in the joints of patients with rheumatoid arthritis (79) and in the airways of asthmatic patients (80). As already discussed, evidence supports a link between nasal inflammation and lower airway function, and it is possible that a nocturnal or early morning increase in nasal inflammation could trigger worsening of asthma. One can therefore speculate that a sleep-induced or circadian-rhythm-dependent early morning increase in nasal inflammation may contribute to patterns of nocturnal worsening or "morning dipping" that are typical of asthma.

VI. Inflammatory Changes Associated with Obstructive Sleep Apnea: Potential Implications for Asthma

Several recent studies have linked OSA with changes in indicators of inflammation. Brander and colleagues (81) evaluated 49 consecutive OSA patients, finding symptoms of rhinitis to be quite common: recurrent sneezing was reported in 53% of patients, post-nasal drip in 51%, nasal congestion in 45%, and rhinorrhea in 37% of all patients. These patients also commonly demonstrated inflammatory changes during rhinoscopy, with 71% of them also demonstrating nasal turbinate swelling by sinus X-ray. In a similar study, Massie and associates (82) evaluated 38 OSA patients, finding chronic nasal congestion in 61% and post-nasal drip in 34% of all patients. Clinical evidence of nasal inflammation therefore appears to be quite common in OSA patients.

There is also evidence that biochemical markers of upper airway inflammation are increased by OSA. Olopade and colleagues (83) measured exhaled pentane (an indicator of oxidative stress) and nitric oxide as indicators of inflammation in 20 OSA patients and 8 healthy controls. They reported that exhaled nasal pentane and nitric oxide were increased after sleep only in the OSA patients. Carpagnano and co-investigators (84) more recently reported elevated levels of 8-isoprostane (another indicator of oxidative stress) and interleukin-6 (IL-6) in breath condensate from 18 OSA patients (Fig. 4), changes that correlated with apnea/hypopnea index. Thus, there is now convincing evidence of increased nasal/upper airway inflammation in OSA patients. Given the previously discussed links between inflammatory rhinitis and asthma severity, it seems likely that OSA can enhance asthma severity via its effect upon nasal inflammation.

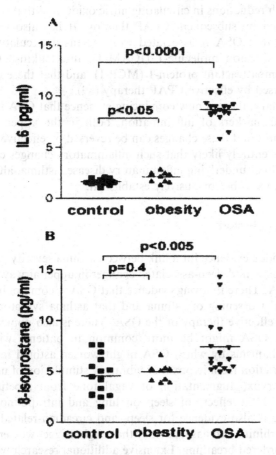

Figure 4 Interleukin-6 (IL-6) and 8-isoprostane concentrations in breath condensate from OSA patients, obese control subjects, and healthy control subjects. From Ref. 84, with permission.

Evidence is also accumulating that OSA is associated with changes in systemic indicators of inflammatory function. Schulz and colleagues (85) reported from 18 OSA patients that neutrophil superoxide generation was markedly enhanced in comparison to controls, and that this enhancement was immediately blunted by effective CPAP therapy. Dyugovskaya and associates (86) similarly demonstrated increased reactive oxygen species production from monocytes and granulocytes in 18 OSA patients, an effect that was again blunted by subsequent CPAP therapy. Such studies lend support for the role of hypoxia/reoxygenation typical of OSA in promoting injury and inflammatory responses in OSA patients. This concept is further supported by observations from 2 separate laboratories (87,88) that OSA is associated with reductions in circulating nitric oxide, and that these changes can be reversed by subsequent CPAP therapy. It has also recently been demonstrated that OSA is associated with increased circulating levels of intercellular adhesion molecule-1 (ICAM-1), interleukin-8 (IL-8), and monocyte chemoattractant protein-1 (MCP-1), and that these changes can again be reversed by effective CPAP therapy (89).

In summary, there is now convincing evidence that OSA is associated with increased markers of inflammation, both in the upper airway and systemically, and that these changes can be reversed by effective therapy for OSA. It seems entirely likely that such inflammatory changes can alter the activity of another underlying inflammatory disease, asthma, although such an effect remains to be conclusively established.

VII. Conclusion

We have provided evidence for a link between asthma severity, in particular nocturnal asthma, and sleep-associated changes in upper airway function, in particular OSA. There is strong evidence that OSA is commonly associated with nocturnal worsening of asthma and that asthma symptoms typically improve after effective therapy of the OSA. There is also population-based evidence that OSA might be more common in patients with asthma. Potential mechanisms by which OSA might worsen asthma include reflex bronchoconstriction from hypoxia or vibratory stimulation of neural receptors in the larynx, augmentation of vagal tone from repetitive Müller maneuvers, and the effects of sleep on lung and intrapulmonary blood volume. There is also evidence for sleep- and circadian-related changes in inflammatory rhinitis and nasal patency that might trigger worsening asthma and sleep-disordered breathing. Extensive additional research will be necessary at all levels to clarify the interactions between sleep, upper airway function, and asthma severity.

References

1. Smith E. Recherches experimentales sur la respiration. J Physiol Homme Anim 1860; 3:506–521.
2. Douglas NJ, White DP, Pickett CK, Weil J, Zwillich C. Respiration during sleep in normal man. Thorax 1982; 37:840–844.
3. Hudgel DW, Martin RJ, Johnson B, Hill P. Mechanics of the respiratory system and breathing pattern during sleep in normal humans. J Appl Physiol 1984; 56:133–137.
4. Turner-Warwick M. Epidemiology of nocturnal asthma. Am J Med 1988; 85:6–8.
5. Connolly CK. Diurnal rhythms in airway obstruction. Br J Dis Chest 1979; 73:357–366.
6. Montplaisir J, Walsh J, Malo JL. Nocturnal asthma: features of attacks, sleep, and breathing patterns. Am Rev Respi Dis 1982; 125:18–22.
7. Hetzel MR, Clark TJH, Branthwaite MA. Asthma: analysis of sudden deaths and ventilatory arrests in hospital. Br Med J 1977; 1:808–811.
8. Douglas NJ, Calverley PMA, Leggett RJE, Brash HM, Flenley DC, Brezinova V. Transient hypoxemia during sleep in chronic bronchitis and emphysema. Lancet 1979; 1:1–4.
9. Cormick W, Olsen LG, Hensley MJ, Saunders NA. Nocturnal hypoxemia and quality of sleep in patients with chronic obstructive lung disease. Thorax 1986; 41:846–854.
10. Ballard RD, Clover CW, Suh BY. Influence of sleep on respiratory function in emphysema. Am J Respir Crit Care Med 1995; 151:945–951.
11. Dancey DR, Tullis ED, Heslegrave R, Thornley K, Hanly PJ. Sleep quality and daytime function in adults with cystic fibrosis and severe lung disease. Eur Respir J 2002; 19:504–510.
12. Lopes JM, Tabachnik E, Muller NL, Levison H, Bryan AC. Total airway resistance and respiratory muscle activity during sleep. J Appl Physiol 1983; 54:773–777.
13. Hudgel DW, Hendricks C, Hamilton HB. Characteristics of the upper airway pressure–flow relationship during sleep. J Appl Physiol 1988; 64:1930–1935.
14. Remmers JE, de Groot WJ, Sauerland EK, Anch AM. Pathogenesis of upper airway occlusion during sleep. J Appl Physiol 1978; 44:931–938.
15. Tangel DJ, Mezzanotte WS, White DP. Influence of sleep on tensor palatini EMG and upper airway resistance in normal men. J Appl Physiol 1991; 70:2574–2581.
16. Skatrud JB, Jempsey JA. Airway resistance and respiratory muscle function in snorers during NREM sleep. J Appl Physiol 1985; 59:328–335.
17. Iber C, Berssenbrugge A, Skatrud JB, Dempsey JA. Ventilatory adaptations to resistive loading during wakefulness and non-REM sleep. J Appl Physiol 1982; 52:607–614.
18. Wiegand L, Zwillich CW, White DP. Sleep and the ventilatory response to resistive loading in normal men. J Appl Physiol 1988; 64:1186–1195.

19. Guilleminault C, Riley R, Powell N. Obstructive sleep apnea and abnormal cephalometric measurements. Implications for treatment. Chest 1984; 86:793–794.

20. Horner RL, Mohiaddin RH, Lowell DG, Shea SA, Burman ED, Longmore DB, Guz A. Sites and sizes of fat deposits around the pharynx in patients with obstructive sleep apnea and weight matched controls. Eur Respir J 1989; 2:613–622.

21. Shelton KE, Woodson H, Gay S, Suratt PM. Pharyngeal fat in obstructive sleep apnea. Am Rev Respir Dis 1993; 148:462–466.

22. Ryan CF, Lowe AA, Li D, Fleetham JA. Three-dimensional upper airway computed tomography in obstructive sleep apnea. Am Rev Respir Dis 1991; 144:428–432.

23. Shepard JW, Pevernagie DA, Stanson AW, Daniels BK, Sheedy PF. Effects of changes in central venous pressure on upper airway size in patients with obstructive sleep apnea. Am J Respir Crit Care Med 1996; 153:250–254.

24. Suratt PM, McTier FR, Wilhoit SC. Upper airway muscle activation is augmented in patients with obstructive sleep apnea compared to with that in normal subjects. Am Rev Respir Dis 1988; 137:889–894.

25. Mezzanotte WS, Tangel DJ, White DP. Waking genioglossal electromyogram in sleep apnea patients: aneuromuscular compensatory mechanism. J Clin Invest 1992; 89:1571–1579.

26. Stein MG, Gamsu G, de Geer G, Golden JA, Crumley RL, Webb WR. Cine CT in obstructive sleep apnea. AJR Am J Roentgenol 1987; 148:1069–1074.

27. Horner RL, Shea SA, McIvor J, Guz A. Pharyngeal size and shape during wakefulness and sleep in patients with obstructive sleep apnea. Q J Nucl Med 1989; 72:719–735.

28. Lin CC, Lin CY. Obstructive sleep apnea syndrome and bronchial hyperreactivity. Lung 1995; 173:117–126.

29. Nadel JA, Widdicombe JG. Effect of changes in blood gas tensions and carotid sinus pressure on tracheal volume and total lung resistance to airflow. J Physiol 1962; 163:13–33.

30. Stephens NL, Kroger EA. Effects of hypoxia on airway smooth muscle mechanics and electrophysiology. J Appl Physiol 1970; 28:630–635.

31. Nadel JA, Widdicombe JG. Reflex effects of upper airway irritation on total lung resistance and blood pressure. J Appl Physiol 1962; 17:861–865.

32. Guilleminault C, Tilkian A, Lehrman K, Forno L, Dement WC. Sleep apnea syndrome: states of sleep and autonomic dysfunction. J Neurol Neurosurg Psychphysiol 1977; 40:718–725.

33. Zerah-Lancner F, Lofaso F, Coste A, Ricolfi F, Goldenberg F, Harf A. Pulmonary function in obese snorers with or without sleep apnea syndrome. Am J Respir Crit Care Med 1997; 156:522–527.

34. Hudgel DW, Shucard DW. Coexistence of sleep apnea and asthma resulting in severe sleep hypoxemia. J Am Med Assoc 1979; 242:2789–2790.

35. Chan CS, Woolcock AJ, Sullivan CE. Nocturnal asthma: role of snoring and obstructive sleep apnea. Am Rev Respir Dis 1988; 137:1502–1504.

36. Hetzel MR, Clark TJH. Does sleep cause nocturnal asthma? Thorax 1979; 34:749–754.
37. Ballard RD, Saathoff MC, Patel DK, Kelly PL, Martin RJ. Effect of sleep on nocturnal bronchoconstriction and ventilatory patterns in asthmatics. J Appl Physiol 1989; 67:243–249.
38. Guilleminault C, Quera-Salva MA, Powell N, Riley R, Romaker A, Partinen M, Baldwin R, Nino-Murcia G. Nocturnal asthma: snoring, small pharynx and nasal CPAP. Eur Respir J 1988; 1:902–907.
39. Guilleminault C, Winkle R, Melvin K, Tilkian A. Cyclical variation of the heart rate in sleep apnea syndromes: mechanisms and usefulness of 24-hour electroencephalography as a screening technique. Lancet 1984; 1:126–136.
40. Martin RJ, Pak J. Nasal CPAP in nonapneic nocturnal asthma. Chest 1991; 100:1024–1027.
41. Guilleminault C, Stoohs R, Clerk A, Cetel M, Maistros P. A cause of excessive daytime sleepiness: the upper airway resistance syndrome. Chest 1993; 104:781–787.
42. Denjean A, Roux C, Herve P, Bonniot JP, Comoy E, Duroux P, Gaultier C. Mild isocapnic hypoxia enhances the bronchial response to methacholine in asthmatic subjects. Am Rev Respir Dis 1988; 138:789–79.
43. Peters SP, Lichtenstein LM, Adkinson NF. Mediator release from human lung under conditions of reduced oxygen tension. J Pharmacol Exp Ther 1986; 238:8–13.
44. Janson C, Gislason T, Boman G, Hetta J, Roos BE. Sleep disturbances in patients with asthma. Respir Med 1990; 84:37–42.
45. Janson C, De Backer W, Gislason T, Plaschke P, Bjornsson E, Hetta J, Kristbjarnarson, Vermiere P, Boman G. Increased prevalence of sleep disturbances in subjects with bronchial asthma: a population study of young adults in three European studies. Eur Respir J 1996; 9:2132–2138.
46. Fitzpatrick MF, Marin K, Fossey E, Shapiro CM, Elton RA, Douglas NJ. Snoring, asthma and sleep disturbance in Britain: a community-based survey. Eur Respir J 1993; 6:531–535.
47. Larsson LG, Lindberg A, Franklin KA, Lundback B. Symptoms related to obstructive sleep apnea are common in subjects with asthma, chronic bronchitis and rhinitis in a general population. Respir Med 2001; 95:423–429.
48. Ballard RD, Kelly PL, Martin RJ. Estimates of ventilation from inductance plethysmography in sleeping asthmatics. Chest 1988; 93:128–133.
49. Ballard RD, Irvin CG, Martin RJ, Pak J, Pandey R, White DP. Influence of sleep on lung volume in asthmatic patients and normal subjects. J Appl Physiol 1990; 68:2034–2041.
50. Ballard RD, Clover CW, White DP. Influence of non-REM sleep on inspiratory muscle activity and lung volume in asthmatic patients. Am Rev Respir Dis 1993; 147:880–886.
51. Hamilton WF, Morgan AB. Mechanism of the postural reduction in vital capacity in relation to orthopnea and storage of blood in the lungs. Am J Physiol 1932; 99:526–533.

52. Hedenstierna G, Lofstrom B, Lundh R. Thoracic gas volume and chest–abdomen dimensions during anesthesia and muscle paralysis. Anesthesiology 1981; 55:499–506.
53. Kimball WR, Loring SH, Basta SJ, DeTroyer A, Mead J. Effects of paralysis with pancuronium on chest wall statics in awake humans. J Appl Physiol 1985; 58:1638–1645.
54. Chung KF, Keyes SJ, Morgan BM, Jones PW, Snashall PD. Mechanisms of airway narrowing in acute pulmonary oedema in dogs: influence of vagus and lung volume. Clin Sci 1983; 65:289–296.
55. Regnard JP, Baudrillard P, Salah B, Dinh Xuan AT, Cabanes L, Lockhart A. Inflation of antishock trousers increases bronchial response to methacholine in healthy subjects. J Appl Physiol 1990; 68:1528–1533.
56. Cabanes LR, Weber S, Matran R, Regnard J, Richard MO, DeGeorges ME, Lockhard A. Bronchial hyperresponsiveness to methacholine in patients with impaired left ventricular function. N Engl J Med 1989; 320:1317–1322.
57. Roughton FJW, Forster RE. Relative importance of diffusion and chemical reaction rate in determining rate of exchange of gases in the human lung, with special reference to true diffusing capacity of pulmonary membrane and volume of blood in the lung capillaries. J Appl Physiol 1957; 11:290–302.
58. Desjardin JA, Sutarik JM, Suh BY, Ballard RD. Influence of sleep on pulmonary capillary volume in normal and asthmatic subjects. Am J Respir Crit Care Med 1995; 152:193–198.
59. Steiner SH, Frayser R, Ross JC. Alterations in pulmonary diffusing capacity and pulmonary capillary volume with negative pressure breathing. J Clin Invest 1965; 44:1623–1630.
60. Stewart RI. Carbon monoxide diffusing capacity in asthmatic patients with mild airflow limitation. Chest 1988; 94:332–336.
61. Sutarik JM, Suh BY, Ballard RD. Effect of flow-resistive load on airflow obstruction and capillary volume in asthmatics [abstr]. Am J Respir Crit Care Med 1994; 149(suppl 4):A222.
62. Peckham C, Butler N. A national study of asthma in childhood. J Epidemiol Community Health 1978; 32:79–85.
63. Blair H. Natural history of childhood asthma. Arch Dis Child 1977; 52:613–619.
64. Matternowski CJ, Mathews KP. The prevalence of ragweed pollinosis in foreign and native students at a midwestern university and its implications concerning methods for determining inheritance of atopy. J Allergy 1962; 33:130–140.
65. Ramsdale EH, Morris MM, Robers RS, Hargreave FE. Asymptomatic bronchial hyperresponsiveness in rhinitis. J Allergy Clin Immunol 1985; 75:573–577.
66. Corren J, Adinoff AD, Buchmeier AD, Irvin CG. Nasal beclomethasone prevents the seasonal increase in bronchial responsiveness in patients with allergic rhinitis and asthma. J Allergy Clin Immunol 1992; 90:250–256.
67. Watson WTA, Becker AB, Simons FER. Treatment of allergic rhinitis with intranasal corticosteroids in patients with mild asthma: effect on lower airway responsiveness. J Allergy Clin Immunol 1993; 91:97–101.

68. Aubier M, Clerici C, Neukirch F, Herman D. Different effects of nasal and bronchial glucocorticosteroid administration on bronchial hyperresponsiveness in patients with allergic rhinitis. Am Rev Respir Dis 1992; 146:122–126.

69. Kaufman J, Wright GW. The effect of nasal and oropharyngeal irritation on airway resistance in man. Am Rev Respir Dis 1969; 100:626–630.

70. Kaufman J, Chen JC, Wright GW. The effect of trigeminal resection on reflex bronchoconstriction after nasal and nasopharyngeal irritation in man. Am Rev Respir Dis 1970; 101:768–769.

71. Corren J, Adinoff AD, Irvin CG. Changes in bronchial responsiveness following nasal provocation with allergen. J Allergy Clin Immunol 1992; 89:611–618.

72. Shturman-Ellstein R, Zeballaos RJ, Buckley JM, Souhrada JF. The beneficial effect of nasal breathing on exercise-induced bronchoconstriction. Am Rev Respir Dis 1978; 118:65–73.

73. Young T, Finn L, Kim H. Nasal obstruction as a risk factor for sleep-disordered breathing. J Allergy Clin Immunol 1997; 99:S757–S762.

74. Scharf MB, Cohen AP. Diagnostic and treatment implications of nasal obstruction in snoring and obstructive sleep apnea. Ann Allergy Asthma Immunol 1998; 81:279–290.

75. Irvin CG. Sinusitis and asthma: an animal model. J Allergy Clin Immunol 1992; 90:521–533.

76. Nicholson PA, Bogie W. Diurnal variation in the symptoms of hay fever: implications for pharmaceutical development. Curr Med Res Opin 1973; 1:395–401.

77. Binder E, Holopainen E, Malmberg H, Salo O. Anamnestic data in allergic rhinitis. Allergy 1982; 37:389–396.

78. Reinberg A, Gervais P, Levi F, Smolensky M, Del Carro L, Ugolini C. Circadian and circannual rhythms of allergic rhinitis: an epidemiologic study involving chronobiologic methods. J Allergy Clin Immunol 1988; 81:51–62.

79. Labrecque G. Inflammatory reaction and disease. In: Touitou Y, Haus E, eds. Biological Rhythms in Clinical and Laboratory Medicine. Berlin: Springer-Verlag, 1992:483–492.

80. Martin RJ, Cicutto LC, Smith HR, Ballard RD, Szefler SJ. Airways inflammation in nocturnal asthma. Am Rev Respir Dis 1991; 143:351–357.

81. Brander PE, Soririnsuo M, Lohela P. Nasopharyngeal symptoms in patients with obstructive sleep apnea syndrome. Respiration 1999; 66:128–135.

82. Massie CA, Hart RW, Peralez K, Richards GN. Effects of humidification on nasal symptoms and compliance in sleep apnea patients using continuous positive airway pressure. Chest 1999; 116:403–408.

83. Olopade CO, Christon JA, Zakkar M, Hua C, Swedler WI, Scheff PA, Rubinstein I. Exhaled pentane and nitric oxide levels in patients with obstructive sleep apnea. Chest 1997; 111:1500–1504.

84. Carpagnano GE, Kharitonov SA, Resta O, Foschino-Barbaro MP, Gramiccioni E, Barnes PJ. Increased 8-isoprostane and interleukin-6 in breath condensate of obstructive sleep apnea patients. Chest 2002; 122:1162–1167.

85. Schulz R, Mahmoudi S, Hattar K, Sibelius U, Olschewski H, Mayer K, Seeger W, Grimminger F. Enhanced release of superoxide from polymorphonuclear neutrophils in obstructive sleep apnea. Am J Respir Crit Care Med 2000; 162: 566–570.

86. Dyugovskaya L, Lavie P, Lavie L. Increased adhesion molecules expression and production of reactive oxygen species in leukocytes of sleep apnea patients. Am J Respir Crit Care Med 2002; 165:934–939.

87. Ip MSM, Lam B, Chan L, Zheng L, Tsang KWT, Fung PCW, Lam W. Circulating nitric oxide is suppressed in obstructive sleep apnea and is reversed by nasal continuous positive airway pressure. Am J Respir Crit Care Med 2000; 162:2166–2171.

88. Schulz R, Schmidt D, Blum A, Lopes-Ribeiro X, Lucke C, Mayer K, Olschewski H, Seeger W, Grimminger F. Decreased plasma levels of nitric oxide derivatives in obstructive sleep apnea: response to CPAP therapy. Thorax 2000; 55:1046–1051.

89. Ohga E, Tomita T, Wada H, Yamamoto H, Nagase T, Ouchi Y. Effects of obstructive sleep apnea on circulating ICAM-1, IL-8, and MCP-1. J Appl Physiol 2003; 94:179–184.

15

Vocal Cord Dysfunction

KENNETH B. NEWMAN

Forest Laboratories, Inc.
New York, New York, U.S.A.

"Asthma is like love," it has been "tough to define, but you know it when it comes along." However, in the diagnosis of asthma, as in matters of love, we are sometimes mistaken. Many different etiologies of airway obstruction can produce wheezing or dyspnea and imitate asthma. One of the best imitators of asthma is the entity of vocal cord dysfunction (VCD). The term refers to a syndrome in which the vocal cords close, usually during inspiration, and can produce airflow obstruction and symptoms that can mimic asthma (1–10). Subjects with vocal cord dysfunction are usually misdiagnosed as having asthma and undergo inappropriate therapy—often with significant resulting morbidity (9,11).

Although we think of VCD as a recently described entity, there have been descriptions of patients who had conditions as least similar to VCD. Duglison described "hysteric croup" in his 1842 textbook of medicine (11). William Osler described a hysterical woman who had a "remarkable inspiratory cry" (12). In the past 30 years there have been numerous case reports and case series described in both the adult and pediatric literature. The prevalence of VCD has been shown to be surprisingly high in tertiary care centers, and it is almost certainly underdiagnosed in the community (13). The key to diagnosis is keeping a high degree of clinical suspicion.

The literature includes a number of different names for the condition, including laryngeal dyskinesia (14), vocal cord malfunction (15), and factitious asthma (1). However, there seems to be a growing consensus to simply name this condition vocal cord dysfunction.

I. Demographics

The description of the typical adult VCD patient is a young, obese, psychologically impaired woman, often a health care worker. In adults, patients usually are in their second or third decade of life and are predominantly female (9,11,14). In one large series of VCD patients, 41 of 42 with VCD were women. Of the patients with both VCD and asthma, 39 of 53 were women (9). Patients are usually overweight: on average they have almost 140% of ideal body weight. It is not clear whether this is just a result of prior oral steroid use or a predisposing factor (9). There is a high prevalence of psychological disease, as discussed shortly (9,17). Approximately one-quarter of the patients worked in the health care profession.

VCD has been reported in children as young as 6 months old, the mean age being 13 years (7). Females predominate, being 68% in one series of 37 child patients, but not as overwhelming as in adults. These children tend to be overachievers, either academically or athletically. Almost one-third had a history of diagnosed psychiatric illness (18).

II. Clinical History and Physical Examination

The two most common presentations of VCD are either wheezing, which is suggestive of asthma or stridor, suggestive of an upper airway obstruction. The vast majority of patients had been diagnosed with asthma, which has been refractory to medical therapy (3,9,14). They have been treated with numerous asthma medications without success, and often are on chronic steroid therapy. In our series, the average daily dose of prednisone was 29 mg/day (9). These patients have occasionally been placed on trials of steroid-sparing medications, such as methotrexate.

The symptoms of the VCD group are very difficult to distinguish from those of asthma. On sensitive symptom scales such as the asthma symptom checklist, the symptoms reported by the VCD group were as follows: likely to awaken during the night with dyspnea, and population (14). Asthmatics are more likely to awaken during the night with dyspnea and are more likely to respond to inhaled bronchodilators. However, nocturnal awakening is not a reliable differentiating factor between asthma and VCD (19). Somctimes the VCD patient will report that during an attack there is throat tightness and voice changes, and the neck is identified as the site where airflow stops. The symptoms can be quite sudden in onset, frightening to both patient and caregiver. Almost a third of the reported patients have been intubated or had a tracheostomy performed (9). Triggers for VCD attacks are very similar to those for asthma: exercise, strong smells, viruses, and irritants such as cigarette smoke (14). Sometimes the triggers are rather bizarre, such as the smell of cooked corn. A recent case series describes how VCD was misdiagnosed as exercise-induced bronchospasm in a series of seven patients, and the authors postulate that VCD was a cause of athletic "choking" (20). Another study highlighted the fact that some patients had been diagnosed as having multiple food allergies or chemical sensitivities (17). Perkner et al. reported a series of 11 cases of VCD occurring within 24 h of an exposure to a respiratory irritant, thereby imitating reactive airway dysfunction syndrome (RADS) (28). Attacks tend to have sudden onsets, to fail to respond to asthma therapy, and to resolve spontaneously.

The medical utilization of these patients can be overwhelming. Almost all the adults and half of the children had been hospitalized for presumed asthma attacks. The adults averaged 5.9 hospital admissions in the year prior to diagnosis, with almost 9.7 emergency room visits. There is high utilization of medications, with the average patient being on 4 to 10 different medications (9).

During acute attacks, patients with VCD may be able to hold their breath, which in an asthmatic may increase symptoms and wheezing (22). The symptoms may improve with panting, or with diverting the patient's attention. On physical exam, inspiratory wheezing may be loudest over the larynx (23,24). Since, however, the large airways are excellent transmitters of sound, this is an unreliable physical finding. Furthermore, stridor and wheezing produce the exact same sound frequencies and differ only in their timing within the respiratory cycle (25). Anecdotally, we have seen many patients who appeared to have laryngeal wheezing who, when the larynx was visualized with a fiberoptic scope, were completely normal. Likewise, we have tested the ability of medical house staff to distinguish between acute episode of VCD and asthma on exam. There were frequent errors. Therefore, the physical exam appears to be of limited usefulness in the diagnosis of VCD.

III. Laboratory Evaluation

There are several important clues to the diagnosis of VCD, although a definitive diagnosis is dependent on direct visualization of the vocal cords. During an acute attack, the alveolar–arterial oxygen difference is usually normal (26). Occasionally, a VCD patient can hypoventilate with carbon dioxide retention. There are a few case reports of patients developing hypoxemia unrelated to hypoventilation. The chest radiograph of an acute asthmatic typically shows hyperinflation and peribronchial thickening, whereas the VCD patient should have a normal chest radiograph. In terms of blood chemistries, most acute asthmatics have eosinophilia, which is not seen in VCD alone (9).

Pulmonary function testing is extremely important in the evaluation of VCD as well as in asthma. While an asthmatic may well have a normal spirogram between attacks, such a finding should raise the index of suspicion that VCD is a possible diagnosis. The one pulmonary function abnormality that persists in asthmatics, even between acute episodes, is an elevated residual volume (27). This is due to air trapping from the closure of small airways. Again, a normal study should raise the level of clinical suspicion. The most common physiological abnormality in VCD is a variable extra-

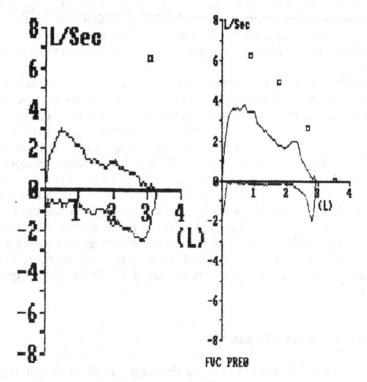

Figure 1 Two representative flow volume loops from symptomatic patients with VCD. Both had negative methacholine challenges.

thoracic obstruction shown on flow–volume loops. However, these decreased inspiratory flows are seen in only about 25% of VCD patients when they are asymptomatic, either spontaneously or after a bronchial challenge procedure (17). It is important to note that since the glottic orifice is dynamically determined, the flow–volume curve can take any appearance (21). If the vocal cord adduction continues into expiration, the flow–volume loop (Fig. 1) can mimic that seen with obstructive lung diseases and can therefore be misinterpreted (21). Thomas et al. point out that the most common expiratory pattern seen in flow–volume loops in their series of 14 patients was a transient airflow obstruction followed by an expiratory overshoot (21). This is suggestive of vocal cord closure early in expiration that artifactually lowers the FEV. VCD patients are often unable to reliably perform spirometry, and the inability of a patient with presumed severe asthma to perform reproducible spirometry should alert the physician to the possibility of VCD.

IV. Laryngoscopy

The diagnosis of VCD is best established from direct visualization of the vocal cords, preferably with a flexible fiberoptic rhinoscope (3,9). Normally, the vocal cords abduct widely during inspiration to decrease inspiratory resistance (29,30). In patients with VCD, the vocal cords adduct during inspiration. The classic appearance is that of closure of the anterior two-thirds of the vocal cords, with only a posterior "chink" remaining open (3). While this appearance is diagnostic, it is not uniformly found. There may also be mucus stranding across the cords. During expiration in individuals without lung disease, there is a minimal adduction of the cords. There is a 10 to 40% decrease in glottic area during expiration. In patients with obstructive lung diseases, there is exaggerated closure of the vocal cords—both during tidal breathing and with forced expirations such as in pulmonary function testing (31). It has been shown that the more severe the lung disease, the more pronounced the glottic closure (32,33). The theory is that by closing during expiration, the vocal cords act to prolong expiration and increase intrathoracic pressures, thereby preventing closure of small airways. This sequence has been called "laryngeal PEEP" and paralleled to physiological pursed-lip breathing.

At the time of laryngoscopy, the patient should be instructed to sequentially breath normally, as rapidly and deeply as possible, and then repeat a low- and a high-pitched "e" (34). However, in the asymptomatic patient, vocal cord motion is often normal. Therefore, it may be necessary to attempt to provoke the abnormal vocal cord motion. This can be done with methacholine, histamine, or exercise challenge studies. Sometimes it is necessary to reproduce the stimulant the patient reports as the trigger—such as the smell of cooked corn. How these stimulants can produce VCD remains unclear. Bronchial challenges in both normal subjects and asthmatics is associated with a decrease in expiratory glottic area, with the average fall in glottic area being 10% in normal subjects and 45% in asthmatics (31). These changes have been shown to be reversed by application of continuous positive airway pressure (CPAP). Therefore, one should not diagnose VCD based on expiratory closure of the vocal cords alone, as this can be seen in asthma. However, inspiratory closure, which can continue into expiratory, is clearly abnormal.

V. Prevalence

The prevalence of vocal cord dysfunction in the population is unknown; however, there is increasing evidence that this is not an uncommon disorder. At the National Jewish Center for Immunology and Respiratory Medicine, an 18-month study found that of the patients referred for inpatient evaluation of severe asthma, 13.6% had VCD without any evidence for asthma. An additional 16.7% of patients were found to have VCD in addition to asthma. In this study, all patients had videotaped laryngoscopies reviewed by independent reviewers to confirm the correct diagnosis of VCD (14). At Baylor, of 15 patients seen in the emergency department for acute asthma, 2 were found to have VCD alone, and an additional 4 had VCD and asthma (35). In a series of patients with recurrent attacks of wheezing, dyspnea, or cough in association with normal spirometry, 26.5% were found to have decreased inspiratory, but not expiratory flows, with histamine challenges. This effect was termed extrathoracic hyperresponsiveness (36), and it indicates that a significant percentage of "asthma-like symptoms" are associated with glottic inspiratory closure. The authors were also able to correlate chronic disease of the upper airway, such as sinusitis, with extrathoracic hyperreactivity. This suggests that chronic stimulation of irritant receptors in the upper airway may be associated with abnormal vocal cord function. Also noted has been decreased inspiratory flows during viral upper respiratory infections and with acute sinusitis. These studies indicate that abnormal vocal cord motion is probably a common event and may be a cause of asthma symptoms and inappropriate asthma diagnosis.

VI. Psychological Factor

There is a high incidence of psychological dysfunction in subjects with VCD, but there is no uniformity of diagnoses. In a case series of 41 adult patients with VCD, 9 had prior psychiatric hospitalizations; DSM-III-R Axis I (major psychiatric illness) disorders were diagnosed in 73% of subjects; and Axis II (personality disorder) disorders diagnosed in 37% (9). Therefore, the VCD group is a psychologically impaired group. Sensitive psychological tests show that the VCD patients have very dysfunctional intrapersonal and interpersonal behaviors that can be characterized as interpersonally exploitive and provocative. They also tend to have a vigilant mistrust of others, which can make their acceptance of the diagnosis of VCD difficult (14). There has also been reported a high incidence of sexual abuse in these patients, but the large case series have not found the rate of sexual or physical abuse higher than in the asthma control population (14,37). There appears to be a correlation between the severity of the underlying psychopathology and prognosis from the VCD. In adolescents, the only difference in psychological testing between patients with VCD or asthma was a higher level of anxiety and anxiety-related diagnoses in the VCD group (38). In children with VCD, Brugman et al. found a high percentage of patients to be overachievers and athletes; 70% of the patients were felt to have dysfunctional families (17). Psychiatric consultation is useful in discovering underlying psychological issues and in providing appropriate guidance and therapy.

VII. Therapy

The therapy for VCD starts with a careful explanation of the condition to the patient (2,40). Showing a videotape of the laryngoscopy may be useful (40). Unnecessary medications need to be discontinued. When discussing psychological factors, it is sometimes useful to draw an analogy to asthma, where emotions are seen as a common trigger of symptoms. It is important that the patient not draw the conclusion that he or she is being dismissed as a psychological case. However, psychological therapy does play an important role in the treatment of VCD.

Speech therapy is used to help abduct the vocal cords (9,22,41). Occasionally even simple panting is enough to break an attack. However, most techniques use relaxed throat breathing, similar to that used with functional voice disorders (such as vocal cord nodules). The concept is to decrease laryngeal muscle tone. One technique is inhaling with a relaxed throat, by laying the tongue on the floor of the mouth with the teeth slightly apart. During expiration, a gentle "s" sound is produced. The patient can be given a number to count to during expiration to help prevent concentration on inspiration (15,30). While there are no prospective clinical trials of speech therapy in VCD, it does appear to have a beneficial action.

During an acute attack, a helium–oxygen mixture, Heliox, can be used (9,24). Flow in the glottis and large airways is density dependent; therefore, using a light gas can increase flows around the adducted cords and may completely or partially ablate the VCD attack. The mixture can vary from 60 to 80% helium, with the remainder being oxygen. It is important to note that asthmatics may also note decreased dyspnea with Heliox, so that response to the gas does not necessarily indicate that the patient has VCD (42).

Treatment of any underlying gastroesophageal reflux and postnasal drip appears to be important, inasmuch as one or both of these factors is present in almost all patients with VCD (13,43). There does not appear to be an increased incidence of chronic sinusitis in patients with VCD (39). Other possible treatment modalities include biofeedback and relaxation training, although these have been described only anecdotally. Antidepressants or anxiolytics may be an important part of the patient's therapy. Several interventions have been described for severe cases of VCD that are unresponsive to speech, psychological, and medical therapy. Vocal cord injections of botulinum toxins have been described in case reports (45). This can cause a localized muscle weakness by blocking acetylcholine release. This technique has been successfully used for treatment of spasmatic dysphonia (43). Altman et al. reported a series of five patients who received botulinum toxin injections, with two of the patients having other signs of dystinias; all patients had at least a partial response to the injections (46). However, repeated injections may be necessary. In rare patients, a tracheostomy or sectioning of the laryngeal nerve may be necessary.

VIII. Conclusion

Vocal cord dysfunction is a close imitator of asthma. The keys to diagnosis are keeping a high index of suspicion and identifying the "red flags" that could indicate that asthma is not the correct diagnosis. Missing the diagnosis of VCD leads to significant morbidity, often from prescribed medications, and high medical utilization. The prevalence in presumed severe asthmatics appears to be high enough to suggest the usefulness of screening all these patients for VCD. This can probably be accomplished by a flow-volume loop while the patient is symptomatic. If there is evidence of inspiratory truncation in the loop, a laryngoscopy should be performed. The natural history of VCD patients needs to be better defined, but a majority, especially children, do appear to respond to medical and psychological management.

References

1. Downing ET, Braman SS, Fox MJ, et al. Factitious asthma: psychological approach to diagnosis. JAMA 1982; 248:2878–2881.

2. Rodenstein DO, Francis C, Stanescu DC. Emotional laryngeal wheezing: a new syndrome. Am Rev Respir Dis 1983; 127:354–356.
3. Christopher KL, Wood RP, Eckert RC, et al. Vocal cord dysfunction presenting as asthma. N Engl J Med 1983; 308:1566–1570.
4. Chawla SS, Upadhyay BK, MacDonnell KF. Laryngeal spasm mimicking bronchial asthma. Ann Allergy 1984; 53:319–321.
5. Appelblatt NH, Baker SR. Functional upper airway obstruction. Arch Otolaryngol 1981; 107:305–306.
6. Cormier YF, Camus P, Desmeules MJ. Non-organic acute upper airway obstruction: description and a diagnostic approach. Am Rev Respir Dis 1980; 121:147–150.
7. Kattan M, Ben-Zvi Z. Stridor caused by vocal cord malfunction associated with emotional factors. Clin Pediatr 1990; 24:158–160.
8. McFadden ER. Glottic function and dysfunction. J Allergy Clin Immunol 1987; 79:707–710.
9. Newman KB, Mason U, Schmaling K. Clinical features of vocal cord dysfunction. Am J Respir Crit Care Med 1995; 152:1382–1386.
10. Landwehr LP, Wood RP, Blager FB, Milgrom H. Vocal cord dysfunction mimicking exercise-induced bronchospasm in adolescents. Pediatrics 1996; 97: 971–974.
11. Duglison R. Practice of Medicine. Philadelphia: Lea and Blanchard, 1842.
12. Osler W. The Principles and Practice of Medicine. 6th ed. New York: D. Appleton, 1908:1081.
13. Newman KB, Schmaling KB, Mason UG. Prevalence of vocal cord dysfunction in patients with presumed asthma. Submitted manuscript.
14. Remirez J, Leon I, Rivera LM. Episodic laryngeal dyskinesia, clinical and psychiatric characterization. Chest 1986; 90:716–720.
15. Kattan M, Ben-Zvi Z. Stridor caused by vocal cord malfunction associated with emotional factors. Clinical Pediatr 1984; 24(3):158–160.
16. Selner JC, Staudenmayer H, Koepke JW, Harvey R, Christopher K. Vocal cord dysfunction: the importance of psychologic factors and provocation challenge testing. J Allergy Clin Immunmol 1987; 79:726–733.
17. Brugman SM, Howell JH, Rosenberg DM, Blager FB, Lack G. The spectrum of pediatric vocal cord dysfunction. Am J Respir Crit Care Med 1994; 149(4): A353.
18. McFadden ER Jr, Zawadski DK. Vocal cord dysfunction masquerading as exercise-induced asthma. A physiological cause for "choking" during athletic activities. Am J Respir Crit Care Med 1996; 153(3):942–947.
19. Reisner C, Nelson HS. Vocal cord dysfunction with nocturnal awakening. J Allergy Clin Immunol 1997; 99(1)(6).
20. Newman KB, Dubester SN. Vocal cord dysfunction: Masquerader of asthma. Semin Respir Crit Care Med 1994; 15:161–167.
21. Thomas PS, Duncan MG, Barnes PJ. Pseudo-steroid resistant asthma. Thorax 1999; 54:352–356.
22. McFadden ER. Glottic dysfunction, asthma, and factitious asthma. Airway Dis 1986; 15–18.
23. O'Connell MA, Sklarew PR, Goodman DL. Spectrum of presentation of

paradoxical vocal cord motion in ambulatory patients. Ann Allergy Asthma Immunol 1995; 74:341–344.

24. Martin RJ, Blager FB, Gay ML, et al. Paradoxic vocal cord motion in presumed asthmatics. Semin Respi Med 1987; 8:332–337.

25. Baugman RP, Loudon RG. Stridor: differentiation from asthma or upper airway noise. Am Rev Respir Dis 1989; 139:1407–1409.

26. Goldman J, Meurs M. Vocal cord dysfunction and wheezing. Thorax 1991; 46:401–404.

27. Orzalesi MM, Cood CD, Hart MC. Pulmonary function in symptom free asthmatic patients. Acta Paediatr Scand 1964; 53:401–401.

28. Perkner JJ, Fennelly KP, Balkissoon R, Bucher Bartelson B, Ruttenber AJ, Wood RP, Newman LS. Irritant-associated vocal cord dysfunction. JOEM 1998; 40(2):136–143.

29. Baier H, Wanner A, Zarseck S, et al. Relationships among glottis opening, respiratory flow, and upper airway resistance in humans. J Appl Physiol 1977; 43:603–611.

30. Brancatisano TP, Collett PW, Engel LA. Respiratory movements of the vocal cords. J Appl Physiol 1983; 54:1269–1276.

31. Collett PW, Branacatisano T, Engel LA. Changes in the glottic aperture during bronchial asthma. Am Rev Respir Dis 1983; 128:718–723.

32. Higgenbottam T, Payne M. Glottis narrowing in lung disease. Am Rev Respir Dis 1982; 125:746–750.

33. Wood RP, Jafek BW, Cherniak RM. Laryngeal dysfunction and pulmonary disorder. Arch Otolaryngol Head Neck Surg 1986; 94:374–378.

34. Wood RP, Milgrom H. Vocal cord dysfunction. J Allergy Clin Immunol 1996; 98:481–485.

35. Bandi V, Wolley M, Hanania N, Zimmerman J, Guntupalli K. Vocal cord dysfunction in patients presenting with asthma exacerbation. Chest 1996; 110(4):84S.

36. Bucca C, Rolla G, Brussino L, DeRose V, Bugiani M. Are asthma-like symptoms due to bronchial or extrathoracic airway dysfunction? Lancet 1995; 346:791–795.

37. Freedman MR, Rosenberg SJ, Schmaling KB. Childhood sexual abuse in patients with paradoxical vocal cord dysfunction. J Nerv Ment Dis 1991; 179:295–298.

38. Gavin LA, Wamboldt M, Brugman S, Roesler TA, Wamboldt F. Psychological and family characteristics of adolescents with vocal cord dysfunction. J Allergy 1998; 35(5):409–417.

39. Hatley T, Peters E, Crater S, McLoughlin T, Platts-Mills TAE, Borish L. Abstract of sinus CT and markers of inflammation in vocal cord dysfunction and asthma. J Allergy Clin Immunol 2002; 109(1):S253.

40. O'Hollaren MT. Dyspnea and the larynx. Ann Allergy Asthma Immunol 1995; 75:1–4.

41. Newman KB. Vocal cord dysfunction: an asthma mimic. Pulmon Perspect 1993; 10:3–5.

42. Manthous CA, Hall JB, Caputo MA, et al. Heliox improves pulsus paradokus and peak expiratory flow in nonintubated patients with severe asthma. Am J Respir Crit Care Med 1995; 151(2 pt 1):310–314.

43. Brin MF, Blitzer A, Braun N, Stewart C, Fahn S. Respiratory and obstructive laryngeal dysfunction: treatment with botulinum toxin (Botox). Neurology 1991; 41(suppl 1):291.

44. Andrianopoulos MV, Gallivan GJ, Gallivan KH. PVCM, PVCD, EPL, and irritable larynx syndrome: what are we talking about and how do we treat it? J Voice 2000; 14(4):607–618.

45. Garibaldi E, LaBlance G, Hibbett A, et al. Exercise-induced paradoxical vocal cord dysfunction: diagnosis with video-stroboscopic endoscopy and treatment with *Clostridium* toxin. J Allergy Clin Immunol 1992; 91–200.

46. Altman KW, Mirza N, Ruiz C, Sataloff RT. Paradoxical vocal fold motion: presentation and treatment options. J Voice 2000; 14(1):99–103.

16

Manifestations of Cystic Fibrosis in the Upper and Lower Airways

PETER MAGUIRE, ROBERT C. BOCIAN, JUDY PALMER, and DALE T. UMETSU

Stanford University
Stanford, California, U.S.A.
and Palo Alto Medical Foundation
Palo Alto, California, U.S.A.

Cystic fibrosis (CF), the most common lethal autosomal-recessive disease in Caucasians, is caused by mutations in the cystic fibrosis transmembrane conductance regulator (CFTR) gene on the long arm of chromosome 7. Clinical disease results from mutations in CFTR that lead to defective transmembrane conductance of chloride ions and, thereby, to impaired transport of water. As a consequence, the viscosity of all exocrine fluids increases substantially, principally in the lungs and in the gastrointestinal tract, but also in the upper-respiratory tract, including the paranasal sinuses. Therapeutic advances over the past 35 years have enhanced the survival of patients with CF from a mean of 4 years in 1960 to a mean of 30 years in 1991, according to the CF Foundation patient registry. This chapter reviews the clinical manifestations of cystic fibrosis in the upper and lower airways, focusing on the interaction of paranasal sinus disease on lower-respiratory tract symptoms.

401

I. Pathophysiology of Cystic Fibrosis

The CFTR gene, which was isolated in 1989, codes for a 1480 amino acid plasma membrane protein that is thought to function as an ATP-dependent regulator of transmembrane exchange of chloride ions and, perhaps, other solutes across the cell membrane (1). The most common of the more than 700 known CFTR gene mutations is a 3 base-pair deletion in exon 10, resulting in the removal of the phenylalanine residue at the 508th position. Approximately 49% of CF patients are homozygous for this deletion, known as ΔF508, which accounts for 70% of the mutant haplotypes (2). Considerable variation in clinical severity occurs even among siblings with CF who carry identical CFTR mutations. However, the ΔF508 mutation is associated with a small but statistically significant increase in the severity of clinical disease and carries a greater likelihood of pancreatic insufficiency, although this may hold true only in Caucasian and not in non-Caucasian individuals with CF (3,4). An increasing number of individuals who have minimal respiratory symptoms and no gastrointestinal symptoms, but do have chronic sinusitis and/or infertility due to congenital bilateral absence of the vas deferens, are being diagnosed by molecular analysis for CFTR mutations. Many of these individuals have non-ΔF508 mutations in the CFTR gene (e.g., R117H and 33849 + 10 kB C→T), suggesting the possibility that, in rare instances, chronic sinusitis in an otherwise healthy individual may represent a clinical variant of CF (5,6).

The abnormal function of chloride channels (abnormal CFTRs) in the respiratory epithelium of patients with CF leads to respiratory secretions of reduced volume but increased viscosity. Fluid volume depletion in secretions greatly affects mucociliary clearance function of the airway surface liquid (ASL) in the lungs by reducing the fluid volume in the periciliary liquid layer (PCL) (the fluid that surrounds the cilia of epithelial cells) and by increasing the concentration of solute in the mucus layer (7). These effects on the PCL and on the mucus layer result in greater adherence of mucus to the epithelial cell surface and greatly diminish mucociliary transport. In addition, the increase in sodium chloride concentration in the ASL limits the activity of the defensins (8). Derived from epithelial cells, defensins are "killing factors," components of the innate immune system that have broad antibiotic activity and are produced in normal quantities by respiratory epithelial cells in patients with CF. However, these factors, which have potent activity against *Pseudomonas aeruginosa* and *Staphylococcus aureus*, are inactivated by the high salt concentration in the respiratory secretions of patients with CF, and their inactivation contributes to the sensitivity of patients with CF to respiratory infection with the named pathogens. Much research is focused on defensins and on the possibility of modifying them to permit them to function in the high-salt conditions present in the respiratory secretions and lungs of patients with CF.

Other immunological factors contribute to the progressive lung damage in patients with CF. Recruitment and activation of neutrophils, often caused by exoproducts of *P. aeruginosa*, cause tissue damage that is due to the release of proteases such as neutrophil elastase and cathepsin G. Increased protease activity has been associated with cleavage and inactivation of opsonins, thus imparing immune activity against offending pathogens. Immune-complex formation may also lead to progressive pulmonary destruction by immunoinflammatory mechanisms (9). Additionally, increased osmolarity within the lungs in CF may lead to increased expression of exoproducts such as neuraminidase and alginate. These exoproducts may also contribute to airway damage. Elastase derived from *P. aeruginosa* is able to cleave IgG, releasing crystallizable fragments (Fc) that further block opsinization and phagocytosis.

II. Lower-Respiratory Tract Symptoms in Patients with Cystic Fibrosis

As a result of the abnormal respiratory secretions, chronic endobronchial infection, principally of the small bronchioles, occurs in most patients early in life, leading to inflammation and obstruction of the air-conducting bronchioles. Bronchilolitis and mucopurulent plugging of the airways occurs secondary to obstruction. In the presence of constant inflammation, bacterial colonization and infection cause progressive destruction of the airways and lung parenchyma. Initial sputum isolates in CF usually feature *Staphylococcus aureus* and *Hemophilus influenzae*. As the disease progresses, colonization with different types of *P. aeruginosa* occurs. Nonmucoid forms of *P. aeruginosa* usually colonize the airways prior to mucoid forms. Colonization with mucoid forms of *P. aeruginosa* often coincides with progressive lung disease and cellular destruction. CF patients may also be colonized and infected with other bacteria such as *Escherichia coli, Stenotrophomonas maltophilia, Alcaligenes (Achromobacter) xylosidans*, atypical mycobacteria (usually *Mycobacterium avium* complex), and *Burkholderia cepacia* (10,11). *Burkholderia cepacia* (formally *Pseudomonas cepacia*) is usually resistant to most antibiotics and may ultimately cause a rapid clinical deterioration after chronic colonization. Unlike *P. aeruginosa, B. cepacia* has been found occasionally in blood cultures of severely ill CF patients (12).

The primary lower-respiratory tract symptoms in patients with CF include chronic cough and wheeze, usually exacerbated by superimposed respiratory infection. The cough is often nonproductive in young children, but it becomes productive with progressive disease. Although there is evidence that, in heterozygotes, the ΔF508 CF allele protects against asthma in childhood and early adult life (13), wheezing is often prominent in patients with CF, perhaps in as many as 50% of these patients, owing to fixed bronchial obstruction, airway inflammation, and bronchial hyperreactivity. On pulmonary function testing, the earliest detectable changes are air trapping and decreased expiratory flow rates at low lung volumes, particularly in the small airways. Later in the disease course, airway obstruction, air trapping, and ventilation-perfusion inequalities are prominent findings on pulmonary function studies. This set of symptoms reflects a mixture of obstructive and restrictive lung disease due to fibrosis, which reduces lung volume and worsens flow limitation at low lung volumes. Patients with a forced expiratory volume in one second (FEV_1) of below 30% are predicted have a 2-year mortality rate greater than 50%. Irreversible pulmonary destruction often leads to abscess formation and hemoptysis. Cysts and blebs may rupture in advanced disease, causing pneumothorax. In patients with reversible obstructive airways disease, it is often unclear whether the reversible bronchospastic component is due to chronic bronchitis and inflammation in the bronchial mucosa or to upper-airway inflammation of the sinuses, particularly since both have been demonstrated to be causes of airway hyperreactiviy (see later).

III. Upper Respiratory Tract Symptoms in Patients with Cystic Fibrosis

A. Nasal Polyps and Mucoceles

The incidence of nasal polyposis in patients with CF ranges from 10 to 50%, with a higher frequency in older patients (11,14–18). Mucoceles, which are cyst-like, mucus-containing structures that can erode into surrounding bone, occur occasionally in patients with CF. However, mucoceles occur in non-CF patients with other forms of sinus disease as well. The two main risk factors for mucocele formation are ostial obstruction and chronic inflammation (19). Although the pathophysiology of nasal polyposis in CF is not completely understood, chronic inflammation secondary to infection probably plays a significant role. Conversely, nasal obstruction due to nasal polyps or mucoceles can predispose patients to chronic infection in the sinuses. CF polyps differ histopathologically from their non-CF counterparts in possessing thin (normal) epithelial basement membranes, hyperplastic mucous glands, mucous cysts, acidic rather than neutral mucins, and relative lack of eosinophilia in favor of a predominantly plasmacytic and mast cell infiltrate in the mucosa and submucosa (20). However, the extent to which there may be important distinctions in the pathogenesis of CF- versus non-CF polyps is unclear. Combined aggressive medical and surgical treatment of sinusitis and nasal polyposis appears to reduce the recurrence rate of nasal polyposis in these patients (21,22).

B. Middle-Ear Disease

Because the incidence of otitis media in children with chronic sinusitis but without CF is very high (23), the finding that middle-ear abnormalities are distinctly uncommon in patients with CF is unexpected (16). The basis for this difference is not fully known, but it may be related to the relative paucity of mucus-secreting goblet cells in the eustachian tube compared with the sinonasal mucosa (24). It has also been proposed that otitis media, compared with other respiratory tract infections, is more easily suppressible or preventable by the frequent courses of antibiotic therapy typically prescribed to CF patients (17).

C. Allergic Disease and Reactive Airways Disease

Although the prevalence of reactive airways disease is as high as 50% in patients with CF (25–28), the prevalence of atopic dermatitis, pollen-induced allergy, and positive skin tests to nonmold allergens in patients with CF is similar to that in the general population (approximately 15–20%) (18,25,26). This suggests that the high prevalence of airways hyperreactivity is due to chronic endobronchial infection rather than atopy. The presence of sinusitis may also contribute to reactive airways disease in patients with CF, as will be discussed. In addition, wheezing may be exacerbated by mold hypersensitivity, since the prevalence of skin-prick test reactivity to *Aspergillus* as high as 35 to 60% in CF patients. In patients with CF, the prevalence of allergic bronchopulmonary aspergillosis (ABPA) is 10 to 15%, and the condition appears to occur more frequently in CF patients who have IgE-mediated allergic responses to other inhaled allergens (29).

D. Sinus Disease

In the upper-respiratory tract, dehydration of mucosal fluids and increased sulfation of mucus glycoproteins results in retention of viscous, tenacious sinus secretions and predisposes to bacterial infection manifested in virtually all CF patients as chronic pansinusitis. Such infection further stimulates mucus production, perpetuating chronic sinusitis. In most instances the inspissated secretions are so viscous that perfusion of antibiotics into the secretions is limited, and removal of the secretions can occur only by surgical curettage (30).

Patients with CF are predisposed to develop chronic sinusitis not only as a consequence of inspissation of respiratory secretions and inactivation of defensin activity, but also due to the presence of nasal polyps, which occur with a high frequency in patients with CF. The ostiomeatal complex is often patent in patients with CF, whereas in non-CF patients ostiomeatal obstruction often occurs in conjunction with sinusitis (31). Thus, in CF, both the retention of viscous, tenacious sinus secretions and nasal obstruction due to the presence of polyps predispose patients to the development of mucosal infection.

Radiographic evidence of sinus disease is invariably present in patients with CF, with a prevalence of 92 to 100% in patients over 2 years of age (14,32–34). In the past, abnormal sinus radiographs were interpreted as reflecting the exocrinopathy of CF (i.e., inspissated mucus) rather than active infection. In addition, the bronchopulmonary ramifications of chronic sinus infection were underrecognized. Sinus disease thus received little attention in the past, since the potentially life-threatening pulmonary and gastrointestinal manifestations of CF have often overshadowed the less dramatic symptoms of sinusitis (e.g., nasal congestion and discharge, post-nasal drainage, and frequent cough). However, it has become apparent that abnormal sinus radiographs in patients with CF are in fact evidence of sinus disease. Sinusitis, as diagnosed microbiologically by maxillary–antral puncture and culture, is virtually universal in children and adults with CF and causes significant morbidity, as will be discussed (11,32,35).

IV. Symptoms and Signs of Sinusitis in Cystic Fibrosis

Patients with CF who have chronic sinusitis occasionally may have chronic purulent nasal discharge or maxillary tenderness. These symptoms are intensified by upper-respiratory viral infection. Headaches, most often frontotemporal, are not uncommon, especially in adolescent and adult patients. Many patients report symptoms related to nasal obstruction (e.g., rhinorrhea, mouth breathing, postnasal drainage, sleep disturbance, nocturnal cough, anosmia, and anorexia), all of which tend to worsen with upper respiratory infection. Lower-respiratory symptoms of cough and wheezing are also exacerbated by chronic and acute sinusitis in patients with CF (see later). Because patients often grow accustomed to sinusitis-related symptoms and often do not complain about them, it is incumbent upon the physician to elicit this information.

On physical exam, nasal findings may be surprisingly normal or may include mucosal edema and hyperemia, turbinate hypertrophy, and viscous, mucopurulent discharge, the last being of particular diagnostic importance when visualized in the middle meatus. Rarely, there is tenderness to palpation over the paranasal sinuses. Islands of lymphoid hyperplasia of the posterior pharyngeal wall, also known as "cobblestoning," result from chronic drainage of irritative sinonasal secretions. Nasal polyps, arising from maxillary and/or ethmoid sinuses and appearing as gelatinous, gray tissue with very fine blood vessels, may be present in the middle meatus and may partially or completely block the nasal passage.

V. Sinusitis and Reactive Airways Disease in Patients with Cystic Fibrosis

The recognition that sinusitis can cause airway hyperreactivity in patients with asthma and that sinusitis is present in virtually all patients with CF suggests that sinusitis may cause significant bronchial hyperreactivity and exacerbate lower-respiratory tract symptoms in patients with CF. This relationship was first proposed by our group in 1989, yet it has been difficult to prove causality because chronic bronchitis, itself a major cause of airway hyperreactivity, is also a serious problem in patients with CF. In a small series of patients, we showed that aggressive surgical therapy (Caldwell–Luc procedure) combined with pharmacotherapy (antibiotic lavage of sinuses) for sinus disease greatly reduced respiratory symptoms, the use of systemic corticosteroids (from a mean of 37 mg/day to 16 mg/day), and the length of hospitalization (from a mean of 58 days to 28 days), particularly in CF patients with a high degree of reactive airways (35). Wheeze, as documented by the examining physician, was also reduced substantially after surgery. Although this study could not demonstrate a direct causal link between sinusitis and lower-respiratory-tract disease in patients with CF, it showed parallel improvement in lower-respiratory-tract disease as sinus disease lessened. This result is analogous to that observed in asthmatic patients in whom a relationship between asthma and sinusitis has been strongly supported but not proven (36).

More recently, our group has extended the observations regarding sinusitis and CF respiratory disease by examining in a larger group of CF patients who were treated with functional endoscopic sinus surgery. Because we noted that patients who underwent sinus surgery improved in the immediate postoperative period but had recrudescence of sinus disease several months thereafter, a protocol involving serial antimicrobial lavage of the sinuses was also examined (see Sec. IX on treatment). The rationale for institution of dual therapy is based on our observations that despite endoscopic sinus surgery, sinus drainage remains compromised and, at best, infection persists subclinically. Therefore, to sustain the benefits following surgery, all patients received repeated lavage of the maxillary sinuses with antibiotics, usually tobramycin, 40 mg in 1 mL of solution instilled into each sinus, every 2 to 4 weeks. Tobramycin is usually chosen because *Pseudomonas aeruginosa*, the most prevalent organism causing sinusitis in CF, is usually sensitive to the very high topical concentrations of tobramycin.

Twenty-eight patients, average age of 23.7 years, ranging from 11 to 40 years, were evaluated for respiratory signs and symptoms before and after functional endoscopic sinus surgery with serial sinus antimicrobial lavage. Prior to surgery, the majority of these patients had symptoms of nasal congestion, postnasal drip, persistent headache, nasal obstruction, or nasal polyposis that failed to improve on pharmacotherapy, which included intravenous antibiotics and intranasal topical steroids. CT examination in all patients showed total opacification of at least one major sinus cavity. The 28 patients underwent endoscopic sinus surgery, involving ethmoidectomy and antrostomy. Polypectomy was performed in 68% of the patients. Following endoscopic sinus surgery and subsequent antibiotic lavage at regular intervals, symptoms related to the head and upper-respiratory tract improved substantially, with significant reduction of headache, nasal congestion, and nasal discharge. Although respiratory symptoms such as cough and wheeze, and the use of medications, decreased only marginally, hospitalization related to pulmonary exacerbation 6 months postsurgery (vs 6 months presurgery) decreased substantially, from an average of 21.4 days to 9.7 days. All but one of the patients in this study voluntarily continued with serial sinus antimicrobial lavage every 3 to 4 weeks for at least 12 additional months, attesting to the perceived clinical efficacy of the program. Some patients required repeat endoscopic sinus surgery to maintain the improvement in respiratory symptoms; however, the frequency of repeat surgical procedures was reduced substantially by serial sinus antimicrobial lavage (37).

Other centers have described their experience with functional endoscopic sinus surgery in patients with CF. A recent multicenter retrospective study of 112 endoscopic sinus surgery procedures in 66 patients demonstrated that endoscopic sinus surgery markedly reduced hospital days (by 9.5 days, $p = 0.001$) during the subsequent 6 months (38). There was no statistically significant change in oral or inhaled steroid use, or in pulmonary function. Investigators confirmed in another smaller study that sinus surgery had no effect on pulmonary function (39). However, sinus surgery significantly improved the quality of life (decreased nasal obstruction, discharge, and cough; improved olfactory function; improved activity level), even when there was no decrease in hospitalization (40–42). The lack of reduction in hospitalization may reflect either the possibility that surgical therapy without postoperative serial antimicrobial sinus lavage is only transiently effective (43) or the necessity of studying larger patient populations to observe improvements in hospitalization rates in patients with less severe disease (e.g., young patients, those who use only limited quantities of oral corticosteroids, those who are not hospitalized frequently).

VI. Interaction of Upper- and Lower-Respiratory Airways

Although our observations support a contributory role of the upper respiratory tract in lower-respiratory tract dysfunction, the specific physiological mechanisms that relate the two distinct anatomical areas are not yet clear. Since sinusitis has caused lower-respiratory-tract disease in CF patients who are recipients of lung allograft transplants, several mechanisms that explain how sinus disease may affect lower-airway function have been hypothesized (33). First, a neuronal connection (parasympathetic or C-fiber related) is highly unlikely because all neuronal connections are severed in the lung allograft. More likely is the possibility of direct seeding of the lungs with bacteria from infected sinuses, resulting in bronchitis and pneumonia, which then causes airway hyperreactivity and cough. In support of this idea is evidence that adults with CF and *Pseudomonas* lower-respiratory infection have *Pseudomonas* in the upper airways that is identical in genotype to bacteria isolated from the lungs (44).

Further support of this hypothesis is the observation that *Pseudomonas* species is a frequent cause of infection in the lung allograft (at the bronchial anastomosis or in the lung parenchyma) of recipients who have CF. Since non-CF recipients who undergo lung allograft transplantation do not normally develop infection with *Pseudomonas*, the sinuses are the most likely source of *Pseudomonas* in the lung allograft in CF recipients. This possibility has prompted the cardiothoracic/transplantation surgeons at Stanford University Medical Center to require all prospective lung-allograft recipients who have CF to undergo functional endoscopic sinus surgery and serial sinus antimicrobial lavage prior to transplantation, with antimicrobial lavage continued at regular intervals after transplantation (33). This regimen appears to significantly reduce the occurrence of lung infection and to promote lung-allograft survival in patients with CF thereby supporting the hypothesis that mechanical extension via postnasal drainage causes lower-respiratory-tract infection. This idea is also supported by animal studies of sinusitis, in which gravitational drainage is an important factor in development of airway hyperresponsiveness in the presence of experimentally induced sinusitis (45,46). Thus, although CF patients, including those receiving lung allografts, have medical problems more complex than most non-CF patients with asthma, much of what has been learned in patients with CF may be directly applicable to patients with asthma.

VII. Bacteriology of Sinusitis, Bronchitis, and Pneumonia in Patients with Cystic Fibrosis

As in lower-respiratory-tract disease, the bacterial pathogens that cause sinusitis in patients with CF include *Pseudomonas aeruginosa* most commonly, as well as *Hemophilus influenzae*, streptococci, *Escherichia coli*, *Staphylococcus aureus*, diphtheroids, and anaerobes (32). However, while the bacteria isolated from the sinuses and from the lungs of a given individual with CF have been shown to be similar, the species and antibiotic resistance patterns may be different (14). Fungi also have been isolated with increasing frequency from the sinuses of patients with CF. Isolation of *Aspergillus fumigatus* from the sinuses is associated with an allergic fungal disease similar immunopathologically to allergic bronchopulmonary aspergillosis; in ABPA and in CF patients, *A. fumigatus* is present as a saprophytic organism rather than as an invader.

VIII. Diagnostic Evaluation for Sinusitis in Cystic Fibrosis

As mentioned, roentgenographic examination of the sinuses of patients with CF commonly shows panopacification. Culture of the sinuses in adults indicates that these opacities indeed reflect active infection (11,32), although in young children the inspissated secretions in the sinuses may be sterile. Frontal sinuses of at least one-third of CF patients are not apparent on plain radiographs, a circumstance that may be related to the limited pneumatization and increased bony thickening that occur with chronic infection (14). Computed tomography is recognized increasingly as the diagnostic imaging standard for sinusitis, particularly in the preoperative evaluation for sinus surgery (36,41). Unlike plain radiography, computed tomography provides high specificity and sensitivity, and excellent detail of the ostiomeatal complex. Although magnetic resonance imaging is superior to computed tomography in its ability to demonstrate soft tissue characteristics (e.g., in the distinction between invasive fungal and bacterial sinusitis or between inflammation and neoplasia), computed tomography is superior in its ability to furnish good resolution of maxillofacial bony detail, soft tissue, fluid, and air (47). Other diagnostic modalities that have been suggested include ultrasonography and transillumination, both of which have relatively low sensitivity and specificity (48). Direct visualization by anterior rhinoscopy of mucopurulent secretions emanating from the middle meatus can confirm a diagnosis of sinusitis or monitor its response to therapy (49).

IX. Treatment of Lower-Respiratory-Tract Disease

Treatment of pulmonary disease in CF includes clearance of airway secretions, aggressive antimicrobial therapy, and suppression of excessive inflammation. Chest physiotherapy, also known as airway clearance, is accomplished by manual or mechanical percussion, by autogenic drainage (a practice mastered by some patients that enables expectoration of mucus through a sequence of special respiratory techniques), by vibration, or by use of intrapulmonary percussive ventilation (IPV, Percussionare Corporation, Sandpoint, ID). IPV employs patient-actuated or programmed bursts of aerosolized saline and bronchodilators that mobilize endobronchial secretions. A small handheld device called the Flutter Valve (ScandiPharm, Birmingham AL) mobilizes secretions in a similar manner. Upon blowing into this device, expiratory oscillations are created within the respiratory tract that dislodge adherent mucus. Mucolytic drugs can be valuable in aiding mobilization of particularly viscous and tenacious secretions. Newer medications in this class include recombinant human DNase (Pulmozyme; Genentech, South San Francisco), which enzymatically degrades the high-molecular-weight DNA that is abundant in purulent sputum, and gelsolin, which cleaves filamentous actin in sputum. In a large phase III clinical study of nebulized Pulmozyme (2.5 mg once or twice daily), there was a 28 to 37% reduction in the rate of pulmonary exacerbation and approximately a 6% sustained improvement in FEV_1 over 6 months (50).

Anti-inflammatory medications may also be effective in slowing or preventing permanent lung damage. Although oral corticosteroids may be used during acute pulmonary exacerbations in CF patients with severe disease, long-term use may be problematic owing to the well-recognized risks of systemic steroid therapy. Inhaled corticosteroids are now used commonly in CF, but their long-term potential benefit is still under investigation. In addition, nonsteroidal anti-inflammatory agents may be beneficial in CF. In one large study, it was found that CF patients with mild lung disease who were given high dose ibuprofen for 4 years had a slower progression of their lung disease than CF control patients (51).

In addition to anti-inflammatory agents, antibiotics, usually administered intravenously in synergistic combinations, are used to reduce endobronchial infection, which is the cause of inflammation. Usually, a β-lactam antibiotic (aminopenicillin, cephalosporin, or monobactam) and an aminoglycoside are given together, since the two are synergistic in terms of antimicrobial activity. Alternatively, oral quinolones (e.g., ciprofloxacin) and aerosolized aminoglycosides (e.g., tobramycin) may be used. Finally, aerosolized tobramycin (TOBI, Chiron Corp.), which achieves very high endobronchial concentrations of tobramycin, has been shown in extensive clinical studies to reduce the frequency and length of hospital stays, to decrease the use of intravenous antibiotics, and to improve lung function.

X. Experimental Therapies for CF

Aminoglycoside antibiotics (G418) recently have been shown to enhance production of the CFTR in one type of CF mutation. Some mutations, including the most common, ΔF508, disrupt the processing of the CFTR and prevent it from reaching the apical membrane of the mucosal and submucosal glandular cells, while other mutations disrupt the ability of the CFTR to function as a chloride channel. A third type of mutation (nonsense or stop mutation) causes a truncated, nonfunctional CFTR gene. Although this mutation accounts for only about 5% of all mutations, Howard et al. demonstrated that treatment with the aminoglycoside G418 resulted in the appearance of the full-length functional CFTR protein in a dose-dependent manner (52). Therefore, aminoglycosides have the potential to correct the basic biological defect in certain CF patients, particularly those in the Ashkenazic Jewish population. In this population, 60% of chromosomes bearing a CF mutation contain a single nonsense mutation that appears to respond to in vitro aminoglycoside therapy at the cellular level.

Improvement of antibody-mediated immunity against *Pseudomonas aeruginosa* has also been attempted in CF patients. Administration of immune globulin with a high titer against *P. aeruginosa* in CF patients has been found to be safe (53); however, additional clinical study demonstrating efficacy from this form of therapy is needed. Active vaccination against *P. aeruginosa* may enhance immunity against this organism and thereby reduce endobronchial infection, but clinical investigation of this potential form of therapy is also needed.

Another potential therapy for CF utilizes a method to improve the chloride-ion balance in the lungs of CF patients by using alternative chloride channels. The calcium-activated chloride ion channel can be stimulated by extracellular nucleotide triphosphates such as ATP or uridine triphosphate (UTP). It has been reported that aerosolized UTP enhances the ability of the airways of healthy volunteers and CF patients to clear inhaled radiolabeled particles the size of bacteria (54). These investigators have postulated that cultured cells that lack CFTR may overproduce the calcium-activated chloride-ion channel to compensate for the defect.

Although the exact mechanism by which UTP improves the clearance of particles in this model is still under examination, further study may yield promising results.

Gene therapy is another exciting potential therapy designed to directly incorporate normal CFTR genes within respiratory epithelial cells (55). It poses, however, many technical obstacles. Both viral and nonviral vectors have been successful at transfecting normal CFTR genes in vitro and in vivo. Although ion flux experiments suggest that only 6 to 10% of respiratory epithelial cells are required to physiologically correct the chloride ion abnormality within the lungs, penetration of the gene vectors through the thick mucus layer in CF patients is difficult to achieve. Additionally, efficient viral vector binding to cell receptors and internalization of gene products is difficult to accomplish. A further challenge is the prolongation of the vector's life such that successful transfection of desired products, and subsequent lasting biological effects, can be achieved prior to destruction of the virus-infected cells by the host's own immune system. The host's own immune system normally removes cells infected by viruses. The adeno-associated virus vector, which has altered biological properties, is being studied in the hope that long-term transfection can occur, while engendering reduced host immune response to viral antigens. Cationic liposomes are also being studied as nonviral alternative for CFTR gene delivery to the lungs.

A. Therapy for Sinusitis in Cystic Fibrosis

Medical Therapy

In young children who are not yet colonized by *Pseudomonas*, oral antibiotics appear to be efficacious in treating sinusitis, particularly when antibiotics effective against both *Staphylococcus aureus* and *Hemophilus influenzae* are used. However, large dosages and long courses (3–6 weeks) of antibiotics (such as cefaclor, amoxicillin-clavulanate, cefuroxime axetil, azithromycin, clarithromycin) appear to be required, presumably because penetration of the antibiotics into the sinus spaces and drainage of secretions is poor in CF patients. In older children who are colonized with *P. aeruginosa*, antipseudomonal antibiotics such as oral quinolones (ciprofloxacin, ofloxacin) can be used. Treatment failures are frequent, however, and intravenous antibiotics such as tobramycin and/or ceftazidime are often required to control acute exacerbations of chronic sinusitis. The symptoms of sinusitis can improve significantly with intravenous antibiotics; however, inasmuch as *Pseudomonas* can be grown from sinus aspirates even after patients have received 7 to 14 days of intravenous antipseudomonal antibiotics (35), it is not surprising that sinus symptoms recur frequently. Adjunctive therapy can be prescribed, including nasal administration of antibiotics (by lavage or by inhalation

[TOBI, tobramycin (300 mg, in 5 mL of saline)]), nasal corticosteroids, decongestants (oral, e.g., pseudephedrine, and/or topical, e.g., oxymetazoline), and mucoevacuants such as guaifenesin, although controlled studies showing the effectiveness of these medications have not been performed (56). If present, allergic disease must be treated, but antihistamines, particularly first-generation antihistamines, must be used cautiously because their anticholinergic properties may cause further inspissation of respiratory secretions, often compounding the desiccating effect of supplemental oxygen administered via nasal cannula.

Intranasal corticosteroid sprays may improve symptoms of allergic rhinitis and may cause short-term regression of nasal polyps (57,58). Since sinus secretions contain significant concentrations of DNA that increase their viscosity, instillation into the sinus cavities of human recombinant deoxyribonuclease (DNAse, Pulmozyme), currently being used to liquefy secretions in the lower respiratory tract of patients with CF (50), may prove to be beneficial by limiting the adherence, accumulation, and impaction of sinus secretions (intermittent irrigation of sinuses following endoscopic sinus surgery is discussed below).

Surgical Management of Sinus Disease

Polypectomy

If polyps are present, control of sinusitis is dependent on polyp-size reduction by means of nasal corticosteroids or surgical polypectomy. The recurrence rate of polyps is high unless efforts are made to control infection and inflammation with medical and/or surgical management.

Endoscopically Performed Sinus Surgery

The indications to proceed with sinus surgery in patients with CF include persistent headaches related to sinusitis that are unresponsive to pharmacotherapy, chronic drainage of purulent nasal secretions that is refractory to pharmacotherapy, chronic nasal obstruction with mouth breathing that is not due to allergic disease and is unresponsive to pharmacotherapy, and persistent reactive airways disease that is unresponsive to pharmacotherapy. These situations unfortunately occur regularly in patients with CF as a result of profound inspissation of secretions, particularly in older patients, and because the etiological bacteria in these patients are usually resistant to antibiotics. Thus, sinus surgery is common therapy for patients with CF.

Prior to sinus surgery, patients are evaluated with computed tomography in the coronal plane and usually receive 14 days of intravenous antibiotics and chest physiotherapy. Usually, under light general anesthesia in adults (and general anesthesia in children), endoscopically guided surgery is then performed, which usually includes creation of large middle-meatus antrostomies. This allows access to the maxillary sinus cavity so that the adherent, inspissated mucopurulent material can be effectively curettaged; in addition, subsequent drainage of the sinuses is enhanced. Occasionally, additional surgery is indicated, including bilateral transantral ethmoidectomy, limited resection of tissue in the region of the ostiomeatal complex (e.g., the uncinate process), and/or frontal sinus trephination. At our institution, the sinuses are often irrigated in the operating room with antipseudomonal antibiotics, and small plastic catheters (19–21 gauge flexible tubing: e.g., modified "butterfly" tubing without needles and with external Luer-lok ends) are inserted temporarily through the surgically created antrostomies so that the maxillary sinuses can be irrigated thrice daily with antipseudomonal antibiotics for 5 to 7 postoperative days (30). Postoperative care to limit adhesions is critical for ensuring successful surgical results, and debridement, if required, is usually performed one week after surgery.

Because thickened secretions continue to form in the sinuses, particularly during upper respiratory infection, and since oral or intravenous antibiotics rarely sterilize the sinuses of patients with CF, we have found that long-term benefit from endoscopic surgery requires intermittent irrigation of the sinuses with antipseudomonal antibiotics every 3 to 4 weeks (serial sinus antimicrobial lavage). The maxillary windows are catheterized under rhinoscopic guidance after topical anesthesia and decongestion with 4% lidocaine and 0.25% phenylephrine hydrochloride (NeoSynephrine). Antibiotic solution (e.g., tobramycin, 1 mL of 40 mg/mL solution) is then instilled into each maxillary sinus, and the catheters are withdrawn. The procedure usually requires about 20 min in the office setting. This program has resulted in prolonged improvement of respiratory symptoms (35) and improved control of nasal polyposis (22). For CF patients who may undergo heart–lung or lung transplantation at our institution, this program is mandatory as a means of reducing lower respiratory tract complications after transplantation (33). A similar pretransplantation protocol for CF patients has been established at University of California, San Diego, involving endoscopic sinus surgery followed by a rigorous regimen of nasal lavage and daily tobramycin irrigation (59).

XI. Conclusions

Beginning in late infancy, sinus disease is ubiquitous in patients with CF. While symptoms of sinusitis such as nasal congestion, headache, and postnasal drainage are not uncommon, sinusitis in patients with CF (as in non-CF patients with asthma), worsens lower-respiratory disease, particularly by aggravating reactive airways. Oral antibiotics and adjunctive decongestant, mucoevacuant, and anti-inflammatory therapy may be helpful, but because of the tenacious, inspissated sinus secretions present particularly in older patients with CF, sinusitis is usually resistant to pharmacological and even surgical management. Endoscopic sinus surgery, by resection of portions of the ostiomeatal complex, construction of generous antral windows, and removal of obstructing nasal polyps, endeavors to establish greater patency of drainage pathways to facilitate egression of inspissated mucopurulent secretions. Although such therapy can reduce the frequency of hospitalization in selected patients with a reactive airways component, our experience has shown that serial antibiotic lavage is also required to prolong symptomatic improvement and reduce the recurrence rate of nasal polyps. Further studies are in progress to optimize therapy for sinusitis in patients with CF and to assess accurately the long-term benefits of aggressive management of sinusitis with respect to the pulmonary course of cystic fibrosis.

References

1. Riordan JR, Rommens JM, Kerem B-S, Alon N, Collins FS, Tsui L-C. Identification of the cystic fibrosis gene: cloning and characterization of complementary DNA. Science 1989; 245:1066.
2. Lemna WK, Feldman GL, Kerem BS, Fembach SD, Zerkovich EP, O'Brien WE, Riordan JR, Collins FS, Tsui LC, Beadet AL. Mutation analysis for heterozygote detection and the prenatal diagnosis of cystic fibrosis. N Engl J Med 1990; 322:91.
3. Kerem E, Corey M, Kerem BS, Rommens J, Markiewicz D, Levison H, Tsui LC, Dune P. The relationship between genotype and phenotype in cystic fibrosis: analysis of the most common mutation (ΔF508). N Engl J Med 1990; 323:1517.
4. Wiatrak BJ, Myer CM, Cotton RT. Cystic fibrosis presenting with sinus disease in children. Am J Dis Child 1993; 147:258.
5. Welsh MJ, Smith AE. Molecular mechanisms of CFTR chloride channel dysfunction in cystic fibrosis. Cell 1993; 73:1251.
6. Kaplan D, Niv A, Avirman M, Parvari R, Leiberman A, Fliss D. The 3849 + 10 kB C→T mutation in a 21-year-old patient with cystic fibrosis. Ear Nose Throat 1996; 75:93.
7. Knowles MR, Boucher RC. Mucus clearance as a primary innate defense mechanism for mammalian airways. J Clin Invest 2002; 109:571.
8. Goldman MJ, Anderson GM, Stolzenberg ED, Kari UP, Zasloff M, Wilson JM. Human beta-defensin-1 is a salt-sensitive antibiotic in lung that is inactivated in cystic fibrosis. Cell 1997; 88:553.
9. Dasgupta MK, Zuberbuhler P, Abbi A, Harley FL, Brown NE, Lam K,

Dossetor JB, Costerton JW. Combined evaluation of circulating immune complexes and antibodies to *Pseudomonas aeruginosa* as an immunologic profile in relation to pulmonary function in cystic fibrosis. J Clin Immunol 1987; 7:51.

10. Bye MR, Ewig JM, Quittell LM. Cystic fibrosis. Lung 1994; 172:251.
11. Shapiro ED, Milmoe GJ, Wald ER, Rodnan JB, Bowen A. Bacteriology of the maxillary sinuses in patients with cystic fibrosis. J Infect Dis 1982; 146:589.
12. Goldmann DA, Klinger JD. *Pseudomonas cepacia*: biology, mechanisms of virulence, epidemiology. J Pediatr 1986; 2:806.
13. Schroeder SA, Gaughan DM, Swift M. Protection against bronchial asthma by CFTR delta F508 mutation: a heterozygote advantage in cystic fibrosis. Nat Med 1995; 1:703.
14. Ledesma-Medina J, Osman MZ, Girdany BR. Abnormal paranasal sinuses in patients with cystic fibrosis of the pancreas. Pediatr Radiol 1980; 9:61.
15. Cepero R, Smith RJH, Catlin FI, Bressler KL, Furuta GT, Shandera KC. Cystic fibrosis—an otolaryngologic perspective. Otolaryngol Head Neck Surg 1987; 97:356.
16. Neely JG, Harrison GM, Jerger JF, Greenberg SD, Presberg J. The otolaryngologic aspects of cystic fibrosis. Trans Am Acad Ophthalmol Otol 1972; 76:313.
17. Taylor B, Evans JN, Hope GA. Upper respiratory tract in cystic fibrosis. Ear–nose–throat survey of 50 children. Arch Dis Child 1974; 49:133.
18. Stern RC, Boat TF, Wood RE, Matthews LR, Doershuk CF. Treatment and diagnosis of nasal polyps in cystic fibrosis. Am J Dis Child 1982; 136:1067.
19. Lund VJ. Anatomical considerations in the aetiology of fronto-ethmoidal mucoceles. Rhinology 1987; 25:83.
20. Duplechain JK, White JA, Miller RH. Pediatric sinusitis: role of endoscopic sinus surgery in cystic fibrosis and other forms of sinonasal disease. Arch Otolaryngol Head Neck Surg 1991; 117:422.
21. Crockett DM, McGill TJ, Healy GB, Friedman EM, Salkeld LJ. Nasal and paranasal sinus surgery in children with cystic fibrosis. Ann Otol Rhinol Laryngol 1987; 96:367.
22. Moss RB, Umetsu DT, Wine JJ, King VV. A successful long-term approach to management of sinusitis in cystic fibrosis. Pediatr Pulmonol 1992; 8S:301.
23. Umetsu DT. Sinus disease in children. Am J Asthma Allergy Pediatr 1988; 1:85.
24. Tos M, Bak-Pederson K. Goblet cell population in the normal middle ear and eustachian tube of children and adults. Ann Otol Rhinol Laryngol 1976; 25:44.
25. Tobin MJ, Maguire O, Reen D, Tempany E, Fitzgerald MX. Atopy and bronchial reactivity in older patients with cystic fibrosis. Thorax 1980; 35:807.
26. Tepper RS, Eigen H. Airway reactivity in cystic fibrosis. Clin Rev Allergy 1991; 9:159.
27. Mitchell I, Corey M, Woenne R. Bronchial hyperreactivity in cystic fibrosis and asthma. J Pediatr 1978; 93:744.
28. Mellis CM, Levison H. Bronchial reactivity in cystic fibrosis. Pediatrics 1978; 61:446.
29. Becker JW, Burke W, McDonald G, Greenberger PA, Henderson WR, Aitken

ML. Prevalence of allergic bronchopulmonary aspergillosis and atopy in adult patients with cystic fibrosis. Chest 1996; 109:1536.

30. King VV. Upper respiratory disease, sinusitis, and polyposis. Clin Rev Allergy 1991; 9:143.

31. Babbel RW, Harnsberger HR, Sonkens J, Hunt S. Recurring patterns of inflammatory sinonasal disease demonstrated on screening sinus CT. Neuroradiology 1992; 13:903.

32. Jaffe BF, Strome M, Khaw K-T, Shwachman H. Nasal polypectomy and sinus surgery for cystic fibrosis—a 10-year review. Otolaryngol Clin N Am 1977; 10:81.

33. Lewiston NJ, King VV, Umetsu DT, Starnes V, Marshall S, Kramer M, Theodore J. Cystic fibrosis patients who have undergone heart-lung transplantation benefit from maxillary sinus antrostomy and repeated sinus lavage. Transplant Proc 1991; 23:1207.

34. Gharib R, Allen RP, Joos HA, Bravo LR. Paranasal sinuses in cystic fibrosis. Am J Dis Child 1964; 108:499.

35. Umetsu DT, Moss RB, King VV, Lewiston NJ. Sinus disease in patients with severe cystic fibrosis: relation to pulmonary exacerbation. Lancet 1990; 335: 1077.

36. Rachelefsky GS, Spector SL. Sinusitis and asthma. J Asthma 1990; 27:1.

37. Moss RB, King VV. Management of sinusitis in cystic fibrosis by endoscopic surgery and serial antimicrobial lavage. Arch Otolaryngol Head Neck Surg 1995; 121:566.

38. Rosbe KW, Jones DT, Rahbar R, Lahiri T, Auerbach AD. Endoscopic sinus surgery in cystic fibrosis: do patients benefit from surgery? Int J Pediatr Otorhinolaryngol 2001; 61:113.

39. Madonna D, Isaacson G, Rosenfeld RM, Panitch H. Effect of sinus surgery on pulmonary function in patients with cystic fibrosis. Laryngoscope 1997; 107: 328.

40. Jones JW, Parsons DS, Cuyler JP. The results of functional endoscopic sinus (FES) surgery on the symptoms of patients with cystic fibrosis. Am J Pediatr Otolaryngol 1993; 28:25.

41. Cuyler JP. Cystic fibrosis and sinusitis. J Otolaryngol 1989; 18:173.

42. Nishioka GJ, Barbero GJ, Konig P, Parsons DS, Cook PR, Davis WE. Symptom outcome after functional endoscopic sinus surgery in patients with cystic fibrosis: a prospective study. Otolaryngol Head Neck Surg 1995; 113:440.

43. Batsakis J, El-Naggar A. Cystic fibrosis and the sinonasal tract. Ann Otol Rhinol Laryngol 1996; 105:329.

44. Taylor RF, Morgan DW, Nicholson PS, Mackay IS, Hodson ME, Pitt TL. Extrapulmonary sites of *Pseudomonas aeruginosa* in adults with cystic fibrosis. Thorax 1992; 47:426.

45. Brugman SM, Larsen GL, Henson PM, Honor J, Irvin CG. Increased lower airways responsiveness associated with sinusitis in a rabbit model. Am Rev Respir Dis 1993; 147:314.

46. Bucca C, Rolla G, Scappaticci E, Chiampo F, Bugiani M, Magnano M,

D'Alberto M. Extrathoracic and intrathoracic airway responsiveness in sinusitis. J Allergy Clin Immunol 1995; 52:9.

47. Zinreich SJ. Radiologic diagnosis of the nasal cavity and paranasal sinuses. Clin Allergy Immunol 1994; 1:57.
48. Shapiro GG, Furukawa CT, Pierson WE, Gilbertson E, BCW. Blinded comparison of maxillary sinus radiography and ultrasound for diagnosis of sinusitis. J Allergy Clin Immunol 1986; 77:59.
49. Castellanos J, Axeirod D. Flexible fiberoptic rhinoscopy in the diagnosis of sinusitis. J Allergy Clin Immunol 1989; 83:91.
50. Fuchs HJ, Borowitz DS, Christiansen DH, Morris EM, Nash ML, Ramsey BW, Rosenstein BJ, Smith AL, Wohl ME. Effect of aerosolized recombinant human DNase on exacerbations of respiratory symptoms and on pulmonary function in patients with cystic fibrosis. N Engl J Med 1994; 331:638.
51. Konstan MW, Byard PJ, Hoppel CL, Davis PB. Effect of high-dose ibuprofen in patients with cystic fibrosis. N Engl J Med 1995; 332:848.
52. Howard M, Frizzell RA, Bedwell DM. Aminoglycoside antibiotics restore CFTR function by suppressing premature stop mutations. Nat Med 1996; 2: 467.
53. Van Wye JE, Collins MS, Baylor M, Pennington JE, Hsu YP, Sampanvejsopa V, Moss RB. *Pseudomonas* hyperimune globulin passive immunotherapy for pulmonary exacerbations in cystic fibrosis. Pediatric Pulmonol 1990; 9:7.
54. Bennett WD, Olivier K, Zeman KL, Hohneker KW, Boucher RC, Knowles MR. Effect of uridine 5'-triphosphate plus ameloride on mucociliary clearance in cystic fibrosis. Am J Respir Crit Care Med 1996; 153:1796.
55. Davies JC, Geddes DM, Alton EW. Gene therapy for cystic fibrosis. J Gene Med 2001; 3:409.
56. Zeiger R. Prospects for ancillary treatment of sinusitis in the 1990s. J Allergy Clin Immunol 1992; 90:478.
57. Berman JM, Colman BH. Nasal aspects of cystic fibrosis in children. J Laryngol Otol 1977; 91:133.
58. Donaldson JD, Gillespie CT. Observations on the efficacy of intranasal beclomethasone dipropionate in cystic fibrosis patients. J Otolaryngol 1988; 17: 43.
59. Davidson TM, Murphy C, Mitchell M, Smith C, Light M. Management of chronic sinusitis in cystic fibrosis. Laryngoscope 1995; 105:354.

17

The Sinobronchial Syndrome and Diffuse Panbronchiolitis

YUKIHIKO SUGIYAMA

Jichi Medical School
Tochigi, Japan

SHOJI KUDOH

Nihon Medical School
Tokyo, Japan

I. Sinobronchial Syndrome

A. Historic Background

A condition characterized by chronic paranasal sinusitis and simultaneous chronic pulmonary infection was recognized and reported as long ago as the early 1900s. Thomson suggested that persistent bronchorrhea and chronic bronchitis might be due to chronic infection of the paranasal sinuses in 1914 (1), and Wasson reported such cases as "bronchosinusitis disease" in 1929 (2). Thereafter, other investigators reported the interrelationship of sinus disease and bronchiectasis (3,4). Greenberg used the term "sinobronchial syndrome" (SBS) in 1966 (5).

The main question in the early years was whether the paranasal sinusitis and lower respiratory tract infection developed first. Quinn and Meyer reported that when iodized oil was placed in the nose of a sleeping person without known disease of the upper respiratory tract, 50% of the contrast medium could be shown by x-ray to have reached the lower tracheobronchial tree by the following morning (6). This experiment suggested that suppurative nasal discharge containing many bacteria could reach the lower respiratory tract by tracheal aspiration and cause infection and inflammation there. In addition to this tracheal aspiration route, lymphatic pathways and lymphatic–hematogenous routes were considered to be the probable routes of infection in SBS (7).

In later years, Chew and Burnsed advocated the position that chronic nasal obstruction altered pulmonary function in a reflex manner and that this might be the cause of sinobronchial syndrome (8). None of these hypotheses, however, has been confirmed.

SBS is also found in Japan. These conditions exclude bronchial asthma with chronic sinusitis and/or nasal polyp. Mikami classified SBS, according to the condition of the lower respiratory tract, into three types: chronic bronchitis, bronchiectasis, and diffuse panbronchiolitis (DPB) (9). Among the types of SBS in Japan and elsewhere in East Asia, the most important is DPB.

B. Subtypes of Sinobronchial Syndrome

Many types of sinobronchial syndrome are reported (Table 1). Kartagener's syndrome/immotile cilia syndrome is a well-known disease having a pattern of sinobronchial syndrome. In this syndrome it is recognized that the pathogenesis is due to the congenital dysfunction of the mucociliary transport system, which is important as a defense mechanism in the upper and lower respiratory tract. Another important subtype of SBS is that in various immunoglobulin deficiencies, which include IgA deficiency (10,11), IgG subclass deficiency (12,13), and familial IgE deficiency (14).

Bare lymphocyte syndrome characteristically shows lack the expression of HLA class I antigen on the surface of lymphocytes. The adult type of this syndrome is also SBS (15–17). Additionally, cystic fibrosis, common variable immunodeficiency, and Young's syndrome are subtypes of SBS.

C. Pathogenesis of the Sinobronchial Syndrome

The various types of SBS show certain common characteristic features. Most of these diseases are associated with deficiencies of various types involving

Table 1 Subtypes of Sinobronchial Syndrome

---

1. Diffuse panbronchiolitis
2. Cystic fibrosis
3. Dyskinetic cilia syndrome (immotile cilia syndrome/Kartagener's syndrome)
4. Immunoglobulin deficiency (IgA, IgG subclass)
5. Common variable immunodeficiency
6. Young's syndrome
7. Bare lymphocyte syndrome
8. Yellow nail syndrome

---

the defense mechanism of upper and lower respiratory tracts, and many of them are inherited diseases. Thus, it is speculated that the pathogenesis of sinobronchial syndrome might involve inherited predisposition, probably accompanied by deficiencies in the host defense of the respiratory system.

II. Diffuse Panbronchiolitis

A. Disease Entity

A disease condition with severe recurrent sinopulmonary infection and chronic airflow limitation has received increasing attention in Japan since the late 1950s. This disease differs from bronchial asthma, chronic bronchitis, pulmonary emphysema, and pulmonary fibrosis in both clinical and pathological aspects. In 1960 Yamanaka pointed out the pathological importance of bronchiolitis and bronchiolectasis in this disease condition (18). Yamanaka et al. termed this condition diffuse panbronchiolitis (DPB) in their 1969 report regarding autopsy cases (19). The lesions are diffusely scattered throughout the lung, and the main pathological changes encompass the entire wall in the respiratory bronchioles.

In 1983 Homma et al. (20), having conducted a nationwide survey, reported 82 cases, and this disease condition became established as a definite clinical entity, specifically a sinobronchial syndrome characterized by chronic sinusitis and bronchial inflammation accompanied by chronic bronchiolitis as the characteristic pathological feature in the lung and chronic airflow limitation. This disease is not rare in Japan; according to Izumi's report regarding the pattern at Kyoto University Hospital (21), the incidence of DPB appears to be comparable to that of pulmonary emphysema, making it a disease of great significance in respiratory clinics in Japan. However, incidence of DPB has significantly decreased in recent years.

B. Clinical Findings

Clinical Manifestations

Almost all affected patients have a history of chronic paranasal sinusitis, usually with onset before adolescence. They often undergo sinus surgery, but the surgery usually has no significant effect. Chronic cough and copious sputum are frequent complicating symptoms that may appear at the onset or following several years of sinus disease, usually occurring in the second to fifth decade (average age, 39.5 years) (22), although the patients' ages are distributed from the first to the seventh decade. In the advanced stage, patients produce large amounts of purulent sputum and complain of progressive dyspnea.

In the early and middle phases of the disease, we find mainly *Hemophilus influenzae* or, less frequently, *Streptococcus pneumoniae* in the patients' sputum. In the advanced stages, the patients develop lung destruction and/or bronchiectasis, and chronic respiratory failure and cor pulmonale progressively exacerbated by the recurrent infection and inflammation. In that phase, *Pseudomonas aeruginosa* can invariably be found. The prognosis in this disease had been very poor. Two-thirds of the patients are nonsmokers, and there is no sexual predominance. Auscultation of the chest reveals coarse crackles throughout, but more strongly in the middle and lower lung fields. Sometimes one can hear wheezes, rhonchi, and/or squawks.

Blood and Serological Studies

Leukocytosis is common, but anemia usually is not found. The level of C-reactive protein and the erythrocyte sedimentation rate also are increased. In the serum, increased titers of IgG and IgA are found (23). The rheumatoid arthritis test often is positive, but the rheumatoid arthritis hemagglutination test is negative. The most characteristic feature is persistent elevation of cold agglutinin. The titer is often elevated 4- to 16-fold ($\times$512 to $\times$2048; normal, $< \times$128) (23,24). It has been reported that cold agglutinin in DPB is polyclonal, containing IgG and, in some cases, IgA as well as IgM, and has anti-I specificity (25). These findings are similar to those found in infections, such as those caused by *Mycoplasma* species. In DPB, however, tests for antibody against *Mycoplasma pneumoniae* are negative.

The percentage of activated (HLA-DR positive) CD4$^+$ and CD8$^+$ lymphocytes in peripheral blood is increased, and both percentages return to the normal levels after erythromycin therapy (26). No consistent decrease or defect of serum immunoglobulins (IgG, IgA, IgM, IgD, and IgE) is found, although the levels of IgG and IgA reactively increase because of the chronic pulmonary infection.

Lung Imaging Studies

Chest Roentgenography

The chest roentgenogram is characteristic and is very helpful in arriving at a diagnosis. Typical radiographic findings are diffusely disseminated small nodular shadows up to 2 mm in diameter with unclear margin, most prominent over both lung bases, and lung hyperinflation caused by air trapping (Fig. 1). Slight bronchiectasis usually develops at the middle lobe and lingula, appearing as tramlines on the chest roentgenograph. With the progression of disease, some patients show cystic changes and/or diffuse bronchiectasis (Fig. 2).

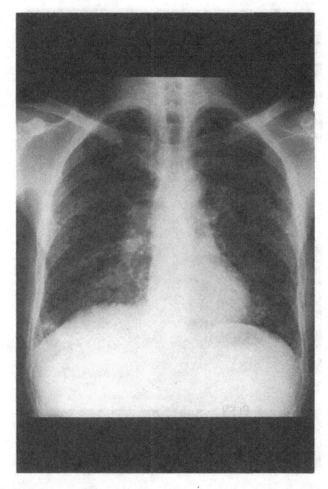

Figure 1 Diffuse panbronchiolitis in a 40-year-old male whose radiographic films show diffusely disseminated nodular shadows and slight lung hyperinflation.

Nakata and Tanimoto have identified five chest roentgenographic patterns (27): exclusively overinflation of both lungs (type I); overinflation with bilateral nodular shadows whose combined area does not exceed the area of one lung (type II); overinflation with bilateral nodular shadows throughout the lungs (type III); the type III pattern plus tramlines (type IV); and the type IV pattern plus cystic shadows and/or pneumonia (type V).

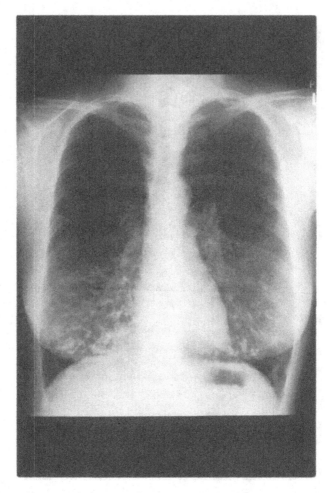

Figure 2 Progressive diffuse panbronchiolitis in a 50-year-old female with chronic respiratory failure showing extensive cystic bronchiectasis.

Computed Tomography

Computed tomography (CT), especially high resolution computed tomography (HR-CT), is useful in the diagnosis of DPB and in evaluating its progression (Fig. 3). The CT findings of DPB are diffuse, small nodular shadows located in the centrilobular regions, dilatation of small bronchi and bronchioles, and bronchial and bronchiolar wall thickening. The small nodular and linear opacities represent dilated bronchioles filed with

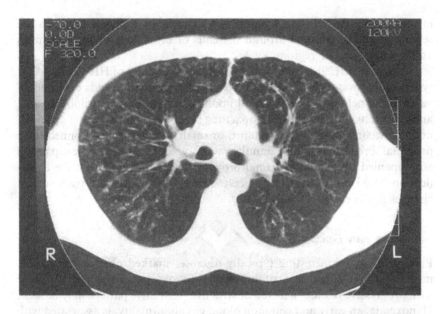

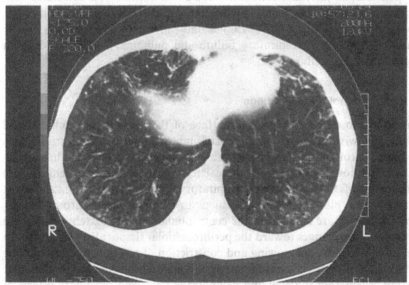

Figure 3 CT images of diffuse panbronchiolitis showing small nodular shadows located in the centrilobular regions.

intrabronchial fibrosis or secretion (28). The small rounded opacities are separated and distributed around the ends of bronchovascular branchings and in centrilobular regions.

Akira et al. (29) classified the radiographic findings of HR-CT into four types, as follows: type I, small nodules located around the ends of bronchovascular branchings; type II, small nodules located in a centrilobular area and connected to small linear opacities branching 1 mm apart; type III, nodules accompanied by ring-shaped or small ductal opacities connected to proximal bronchovascular bundles; and type IV, large cystic opacities accompanied by dilated proximal bronchi. They concluded that the classification based on CT findings reflected the clinical stages and pathological changes in the course of the disease.

Pulmonary Function Testing

Pulmonary function testing typically discloses marked obstructive impairment, which is characteristic of this disease. In some patients, especially those with progressive disease, a mixed obstructive–restrictive pattern may be seen. Hypoxemia, an early and common blood gas abnormality, is associated with hypercapnia in the late stage. The residual volume (RV) and the ratio of RV to total lung capacity (RV/TLC) usually increase. The patients finally succumb to chronic respiratory failure and pulmonary hypertension with right ventricular failure.

C. Pathological Findings

In the macroscopic view, the cut surface of the lungs is hyperinflated and many yellowish nodular lesions, 2 to 3 mm or larger in diameter, are seen scattered throughout the whole of the lung. Bronchiolectasis and bronchiectasis of various degrees are found. The typical pathological features are thickening of the walls of the respiratory bronchiole with infiltration of lymphocytes, plasma cells, and histiocytes (Fig. 4). These chronic inflammatory lesions are situated in the centrilobular regions. Extension of these inflammatory changes toward the peribronchiolar tissues also is common. In the advanced stage, narrowing and constriction of respiratory bronchioli by infiltration of these cells, proliferation of lymphoid follicles, accumulation of foamy cells within the wall and neighboring area, and secondary ectasis of proximal terminal bronchioli are found (20). Pathological changes other than overinflation are not seen in the alveoli of the distal lobules.

Sato et al. reported that DPB presents bronchus-associated lymphoid tissue hyperplasia more frequently than other respiratory diseases (30).

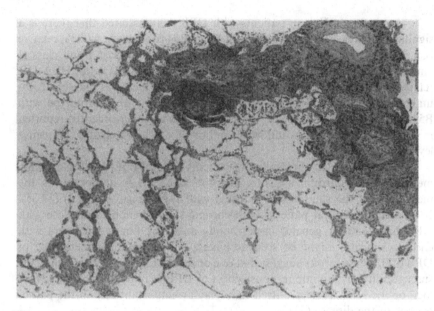

Figure 4 Thickening of the wall of the respiratory bronchiole with infiltration of lymphocytes, plasma cells, and histiocytes. (Hematoxylin and eosin stain; original magnification × 10.)

D. Pathogenesis and Genetic Background

The cause of diffuse panbronchiolitis is unknown. The clinical features and course somewhat resemble those of cystic fibrosis, but there are no systemic abnormalities involving the endocrine system. The concentration of electrolytes in the patient's perspiration is normal, and ΔF508-1 mutation of the cystic fibrosis gene is not found in DPB (31). These results confirm that DPB is a different disease. Abnormalities associated with other sinobronchial syndromes, including immotile cilia syndrome, IgA deficiency, and IgG subclass deficiency, are not found in patients with DPB.

There are many cases of familial DPB in Japan. It is typical for some siblings of a patient with the disease to have only chronic sinopulmonary infection or chronic paranasal sinusitis. The frequency of chronic sinusitis among the family members of DPB patients as analyzed: in the DPB group ($n = 26$), 50% of the families had at least one family member who suffered from chronic sinusitis, in contrast to 18.9% of the families in the control group ($n = 127$) (32). These observations suggest that this disease may have a genetic basis.

Analysis of HLA in patients with DPB demonstrated that there is a significant increase in the frequency of HLA-B54 (frequency, 63.2%; relative risk, 13.30; corrected p value $< 1.08 \times 10^{-10}$) in HLA class I and class II antigens (33). In addition, the frequencies of Cw1 and MC1 (an HLA-DR related antigen) were slightly increased (33). These increases may be attributable to the formation by Cw1 and MC1 antigens of a haplotype with B54. The increased frequency of HLA B54 was independently reported in another recent study and was confirmed at the nucleotide sequence level (34).

Analysis of HLA in families of patients with DPB revealed that family members with chronic sinusitis had the same HLA haplotype as the member(s) of the same family affected with DPB (Figs. 5 and 6) (32,35). It was suggested that patients with chronic sinusitis alone and those with DPB have similar genetic backgrounds and that family members with chronic sinusitis might be seen as having a mild or incomplete type of DPB (32). These results suggest that one or some of the genes controlling the susceptibility or immune responsiveness of DPB may be located near HLA loci, or the HLA molecule itself may play an important role in the pathogenesis of the disease (33).

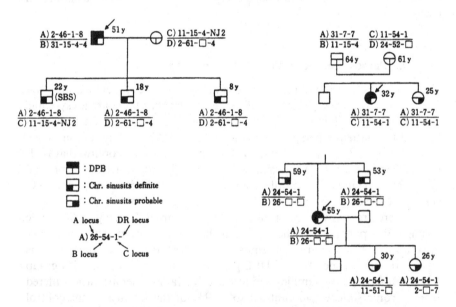

Figure 5 Genetic analysis of HLA in three families of patients with diffuse panbronchiolitis. The patients with chronic sinusitis alone and those with diffuse panbronchiolitis have similar HLA haplotypes. (From Ref. 30.)

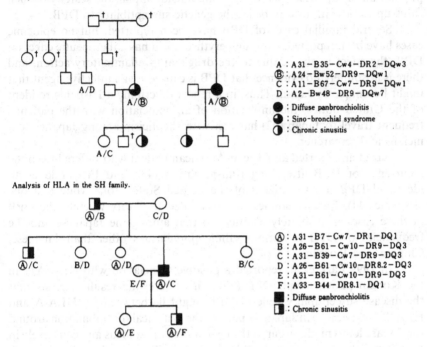

Figure 6 Genetic analysis of HLA in two families with DPB; as in Figure 5, the DPB haplotypes are similar to those for chronic sinusitis alone. (From Ref. 33.)

Another interesting feature of DPB is that this disease is prevalent primarily in Japan and is very rare in western countries. Interestingly, the incidence of HLA B54 antigen in the Japanese population is about 11%, whereas no whites, blacks, American Indians, or Mexicans have been found to have this antigen (33). Worldwide, only the Japanese, Chinese (10%), and Korean (2.8%) populations have demonstrated this unique antigen. These data suggest that DPB may be rare or nonexistent in races without the B54 or B54-related haplotype. After Sugiyama et al. reported a case of DPB in a second-generation Korean immigrant to Japan (36), some cases of Korean and Chinese were reported (37,38). Poletti et al. described the disease in an Italian man examined at autopsy, the first reported case of DPB in Europe (39). Randhawa et al. reported two cases occurring in white patients and one in a Japanese immigrant to North America (40). Another autopsied case, in an American of Japanese ancestry in Hawaii, was known (41). Since a more extensive survey would undoubtedly bring to light more cases of DPB in the population of Japanese ancestry residing outside Japan, the scarcity of such cases up to now in no way belies the genetic susceptibility to DPB.

Several familial cases of DPB have been reported, but no epidemic cases have been reported. Although erythromycin has a therapeutic effect on DPB, the effect might be due to the drug's anti-inflammatory action, and there is absolutely no evidence that DPB is caused by an infective agent that might be unique to Japan. Thus, in a report describing a Hispanic resident of the United States, the implication of an association with the patient's frequent travel to Japan (42) has met with skepticism among Japanese clinicians and researchers.

Baz et al. reported an African-American patient who suffered from the recurrence of DPB after lung transportation (43), and Fitzgerald et al. identified DPB in five citizens of the United States, four white and one Hispanic (44). Further studies will be needed to clarify whether the DPB in these cases is absolutely identical to that among the Japanese and the frequencies of DPB in various ethnic populations other than Japanese, Chinese, and Korean.

In 1999 Park et al. reported a positive association with HLA-A11 in the Korean patients with DPB (45). This interesting result suggests that the disease susceptibility gene of DPB might lie between the HLA-A and HLA-B loci because in Japanese people, the historical recombination around the disease locus might occur at the near side of the A locus and conversely in Koreans at the near side of the B locus (Fig. 7). Ten years later Keicho et al. analyzed genetic markers and predicted the most likely region for the disease susceptibility gene between these two HLA loci (46).

E. Diffuse Panbronchiolitis and Rheumatoid Arthritis

It is noted with interest that some cases of DPB are accompanied by rheumatoid arthritis. We have encountered five such cases including one autopsied case (47) and one case diagnosed after thoracoscopic lung biopsy. We reported two such cases together with HLA analysis (48). In our HLA analysis, both cases had the same HLA haplotype, A24-B54-Cw1-DR4 (48). As described earlier in the chapter, an increase of B54 is found upon HLA analysis of specimens from DPB patients. This antigen, B54, is known to form part of the characteristic Japanese haplotype A24/A11-B54-Cw1-DR4 (49). Consequently, the frequency of DR4 was also increased in the DPB patients in our study (60.0%) compared with the controls (37.9%) (33), and the increase in the frequency of HLA-DR4 was tentatively attributed to linkage disequilibrium with the HLA-B54. On the other hand, the association of rheumatoid arthritis with HLA-DR4 is well established in various ethnic groups including the Japanese (50–52). Because the frequency of

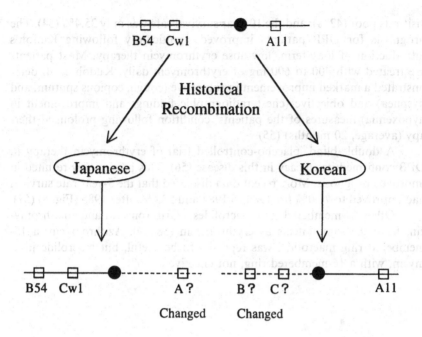

● ; Putative susceptibility gene
of diffuse panbronchiolitis

Figure 7 Hypothesis of difference of association in Japanese and Korean DPB patients.

HLA-B54 is significantly increased among patients with DPB and since B54 is correlated with DR4 as the extended haplotype, both DPB and rheumatoid arthritis have the same HLA haplotype correlation including B54 and DR4. Therefore, it is likely that more Japanese patients with DPB incidentally accompanied by rheumatoid arthritis will be encountered in the future (48). Hayakawa et al. reported the findings for the bronchiolar regions in rheumatoid arthritis (53). These conditions quite resemble DPB clinically and pathologically. Further studies will be needed to clarify these similarities.

F. Prognosis and Treatment

Diffuse panbronchiolitis was formerly a chronic and progressive illness with poor prognosis. Untreated, the 5-year survival rate from the patient's first visit was poor (42%); and the 10-year survival rate was only 25.4% (54). The prognosis for DPB patients improved significantly following Kudoh's introduction of long-term, low-dose erythromycin therapy. Most patients are treated with 400 to 600 mg of erythromycin daily. Kudoh et al. demonstrated a marked improvement in subjective (cough, copious sputum, and dyspnea) and objective (chest radiographic findings and improvement in hypoxemia) measures of the patients' condition following prolonged therapy (average, 20 months) (55).

A double-blind, placebo-controlled trial of erythromycin therapy in DPB confirmed its efficacy in this disease (56). This presumably resulted in improved prognosis. More recent data disclosed that the 5-year rate survival had improved to 71.0% for 1980 to 1984 and 93.4% after 1985 (Fig. 8) (57).

Other 14-membered ring macrolides, clarithromycin and roxithromycin, have the same effects as erythromycin (58–60). Azithromycin, a 15-membered ring macrolide, was reported to be useful, but macrolide josamycin, with a 16-membered ring, not effective (61,62).

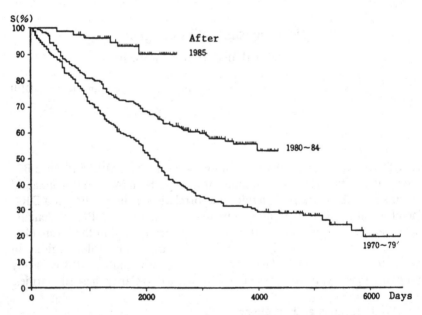

Figure 8 Survival curve of patients with diffuse panbronchiolitis: patients diagnosed after 1985 have better prognosis than those of 1970–1979 and 1980–1987. (From Ref. 53.)

III. Mechanisms of Erythromycin Therapy

Because serum and sputum erythromycin levels were below the minimum inhibitory concentrations for common superinfecting organisms (e.g., *H. influenzae, P. aeruginosa*), the improvement could not be attributed to the drug's antibacterial action (63). From this point of view, the mechanisms of long-term erythromycin therapy against DPB have been intensively studied.

Erythromycin interferes with neutrophil chemotaxis and decreases the number of neutrophils in bronchoalveolar lavage fluid (BALF) following challenge with gram-negative bacteria (64). It was demonstrated that marked neutrophilia was present in BALF from patients with DPB and that erythromycin reduced this neutrophilia (65). Hojo et al. reported that erythromycin does not directly affect neutrophil functions (66). Erythromycin may suppress neutrophil chemotactic activity such as that of interleukin 8 (IL-8) and/or leukotriene B4 (64) and thus indirectly reduce neutrophilia.

Another possible mechanism of action of erythromycin is suppression of hypersecretion in airways. Patients with DPB usually expectorate a huge amount of sputum. Erythromycin inhibits respiratory glycoconjugate secretion from human airways in vitro (67). Tamaoki et al. reported that erythromycin also inhibits chloride ion secretion across canine tracheal epithelial cells and noted that this action possibly reflects the clinical efficacy of this antibiotic in the treatment of airway hypersecretion (68). In view of these reports, Suga et al. administered erythromycin to a patient with bronchioalveolar carcinoma with bronchorrhea and obtained marked reduction in the volume of sputum (69).

Another possible mechanism of action of erythromycin is by way of an effect on lymphocytes. Sugiyama et al. reported that the percentage of activated T cells with the expression of HLA-DR decreased in the peripheral blood of DPB patients after erythromycin therapy (70). In vitro, erythromycin (71) and roxithromycin (72) had a suppressive effect on the proliferative response of human lymphocytes stimulated with mitogens and antigens. Keicho et al. reported that erythromycin promotes differentiation of human monocyte–macrophage lineage, altering the functions of these cells (73).

Additionally, erythromycin suppressed the mortality rate of mice with *P. aeruginosa* bacteremia (74) and inhibited the production of elastase by this bacterium without affecting its proliferation in vitro (75). Takizawa et al. reported that erythromycin suppressed the expression of IL-6 mRNA by human bronchial epithelial cells (76). Oishi et al. showed that levels of IL-8 in bronchoalveolar lavage fluid were decreased after erythromycin therapy (77,78), and Takizawa et al. reported that erythromycin suppressed the expression of IL-8 from airway epithelial cells (79). The latter condition was due to the inhibition of transcription factors, NF κB or activator protein-1

(80,81). Long-term administration of erythromycin also suppressed inflammatory cytokine production in rat alveolar macrophages (82). So, this drug might have a suppressive effect on cytokine expression in human cells, and this newly identified possible mode of action may have relevance to the antibiotic's clinical effectiveness in airway inflammatory diseases.

Acknowledgments

This work was supported by Health Science Research Grants for Surveys and Research on Specific Diseases from the Ministry of Health Labour and Welfare of Japan (2000–2002). Special thanks are given to Mitsugu Hironaka, M.D., Jichi Medical School, for the photograph used as Figure 4.

References

1. Thomson SC. Some of the syndromes and complications of sinusitis. Practitioner 1914; 92:74.
2. Wasson WW. Bronchosinusitis. J Am Med Assoc 1929; 93:2018–2021.
3. Clerf LH. Interrelationship of sinus disease and bronchiectasis with special reference to prognosis. Laryngoscope 1934; 44:568–571.
4. Farrell JT. The connection of bronchiectasis and sinusitis. J Am Med Assoc 1936; 106:92–96.
5. Greenberg SD, Ainsworth JZ. Comparative morphology of chronic bronchitis and chronic sinusitis, with discussion of "sinobronchial" syndrome. South Med J 1966; 59:64–74.
6. Quinn LH, Meyer OO. Relationship of sinusitis and bronchiectasis. Arch Otolaryngol 1929; 10:152–165.
7. Sasaki CT, Kirchner JA. A lymphatic pathway from the sinuses to the mediastinum. Arch Otolaryngol 1967; 85:432–444.
8. Chew W, Burnsed D. The sinobronchial syndrome. Ear Nose Throat J 1979; 58:446–450.
9. Mikami R. Relationship between upper and lower respiratory tract in the pathogenesis of chronic respiratory infection. Kishokukaihou 1975; 26:74–81.
10. Chipps BE, Talamo RC, Winkelstein JA. IgA deficiency, recurrent pneumonias and bronchiectasis. Chest 1978; 73:519–526.
11. Bjorkander J, Bake B, Oxelius VA, Hanson LA. Impaired lung function in patients with IgA deficiency and low levels of IgG2 or IgG3. N Engl J Med 1985; 313:720–724.
12. Beck CS, Heiner DC. Selective immunolobulin G4 deficiency and recurrent infections of the respiratory tract. Am Rev Respir Dis 1981; 124:94–96.
13. Umetsu DT, Ambrosino DM, Quinti I, Siber GR, Geha RS. Recurrent sinopulmonary infection and impaired antibody response to bacterial capsular

polysaccharide antigen in children with selective IgG-subclass deficiency. N Engl J Med 1985; 313:1247–1251.

14. Schoettler JJ, Schleissner LA, Heiner DC. Familial IgE deficiency associated with sinopulmonary disease. Chest 1989; 96:516–521.

15. Sugiyama Y, Maeda H, Okumura K, Takaku F. Progressive sinobronchiectasis associated with the "bare lymphocyte syndrome" in an adult. Chest 1986; 89:398–401.

16. Sugiyama Y, Kudoh S, Kitamura S. A case of the bare lymphocyte syndrome with clinical manifestations of diffuse panbronchiolitis. Jpn J Thorac Dis 1989; 27:980–983.

17. Azuma A, Keicho N, Furukawa H, Yabe T, Kudoh S. Prolonged survival of a bare lymphocyte syndrome type I patient with diffuse panbronchiolitis treated with erythromycin. Sarcoidosis Vasc Diffuse Lung Dis 2001; 18:312–313.

18. Yamanaka A. Histology of chronic bronchitis. Saishinigaku 1960; 15:2035–2044.

19. Yamanaka A, Saiki S, Tamura S, Saito K. The problems of chronic obstructive pulmonary disease: especially concerning diffuse panbronchiolitis. Naika 1969; 23:442–451.

20. Homma H, Yamanaka A, Tanimoto S, Tamura M, Chijimatsu Y, Kira S, Izumi T. Diffuse panbronchiolitis. A disease of the transitional zone of the lung. Chest 1983; 83:63–69.

21. Izumi T. A nation-wide survey of diffuse panbronchiolitis in Japan and the high incidence of diffuse panbronchiolitis seen in Japanese respiratory clinics. In: Grassi C, Rizzato G, Pozzi E, eds. Sarcoidosis and Other Granulomatous Disorders. Amsterdam: Elsevier Science Publishers, 1988:753.

22. Izumi, T. Annual report on the study of interstitial lung diseases. Ministry of Health and Welfare in Japan, 1983, p3.

23. Hirata T, Nishikawa S, Izumi T. An immunological study on diffuse panbronchiolitis. Jpn J Chest Dis 1979; 38:90–95.

24. Sugiyama Y, Izumi T, Kitamura S, Takaku F, Suzaki H. Levels of cold hemagglutinin in patients with diffuse panbronchiolitis and various respiratory diseases. Kokyu 1984; 3:694–699.

25. Takizawa H, Tadokoro K, Miyoshi Y, Horiuchi T, Ohta K, Shoji S, Miyamoto T. Serological characterization of cold agglutinin in patients with diffuse panbronchiolitis. Jpn J Thorac Dis 1986; 24:257–263.

26. Sugiyama Y, Sugama Y, Takeuchi K, Kudoh S, Kitamura S. Analysis of peripheral lymphocyte subsets and changes due to erythromycin therapy in patients with diffuse panbronchiolitis. Jpn J Thorac Dis 1990; 28:1574–1580.

27. Nakata K, Tanimoto H. Diffuse panbronchiolitis. Jpn J Clin Radiol 1981; 26:1133–1142.

28. Nishimura K, Kitaichi M, Izumi T, Itoh H. Diffuse panbronchiolitis: correlation of high-resolution CT and pathologic findings. Radiology 1992; 184:779–785.

29. Akira M, Kitatani F, Yong-Sik L, Kita N, Yamamoto S, Higashihara T, Morimoto S, Ikezoe J, Kozuka T. Diffuse panbronchiolitis: evaluation with high-resolution CT. Radiology 1988; 168:433–438.

30. Sato A, Chida K, Iwata M, Hayakawa H. Study of bronchus-associated lymphoid tissue in patients with diffuse panbronchiolitis. Am Rev Respir Dis 1992; 146:473–478.
31. Akai S, Okayama H, Shimura S, Tanno Y, Sasaki H, Takishima T. Delta F508 mutation of cystic fibrosis gene is not found in chronic bronchitis with severe obstruction in Japan. Am Rev Respir Dis 1992; 146:781–783.
32. Sugiyama Y, Kitamura S. Chronic sinusitis among family members of patients with diffuse panbronchiolitis. Jpn J Thorac Dis 1995; 33:140–143.
33. Sugiyama Y, Kudoh S, Maeda H, Suzaki H, Takaku F. Analysis of HLA antigens in patients with diffuse panbronchiolitis. Am Rev Respir Dis 1990; 141:1459–1462.
34. Keicho N, Tokunaga K, Nakata K, Taguchi Y, Azuma A, Bannai M, Emi M, Ohishi N, Yazaki Y, Kudoh S. Contribution of HLA genes to genetic predisposition in diffuse panbronchiolitis. Am J Respir Crit Care Med 1998; 158: 846–850.
35. Sugiyama Y, Kudoh S, Suzaki H, Maeda H. HLA antigens of four families with diffuse panbronchiolitis. Igaku no ayumi 1984; 129:537–538.
36. Sugiyama Y, Takeuchi K, Yotsumoto H, Takaku F, Maeda H. A case of diffuse panbronchiolitis in a second-generation Korean male. Jpn J Thorac Dis 1986; 24:183–187.
37. Kim YW, Han SK, Shim YS, Kim KY, Han YC, Seo JW, Im JG. The first report of diffuse panbronchiolitis in Korea: five case reports. Intern Med 1992; 31:695–701.
38. Chu YC, Yeh SZ, Chen CL, Chen CY, Chang CY, Chiang CD. Diffuse panbronchiolitis: report of a case. J Formosan Med Assoc 1992; 91:912–915.
39. Poletti V, Pateli M, Poletti G, Bertanti T, Spiga L. Diffuse panbronchiolitis observed in an Italian. Chest 1990; 98:515.
40. Randhawa P, Hoagland MH, Yousem SA. Diffuse panbronchiolitis in North America. Am J Surg Pathol 1991; 15:43–47.
41. Personal communication.
42. Homer RJ, Khoo L, Smith GJW. Diffuse panbronchiolitis in a Hispanic man with travel history to Japan. Chest 1995; 107:1176–1178.
43. Baz MA, Kussin PS, Van Trigt P, Davis RD, Roggli VL, Tapson VF. Recurrence of diffuse panbronchiolitis after lung transplantation. Am J Respir Crit Care Med 1995; 151:895–898.
44. Fitzgerald J, King T, Lynch D, Tuder R, Schwarz M. Diffuse panbronchiolitis in the United States. Am J Respir Crit Care Med 1996; 154:497–503.
45. Park MH, Kim YW, Yoon HI, Yoo CG, Han SK, Shim YS, Kim WD. Association of HLA class I antigens with diffuse panbronchiolitis in Korean patients. Am J Respir Crit Care Med 1999; 159:526–529.
46. Keicho N, Ohashi J, Tamiya G, Nakata K, Taguchi Y, Azuma A, Ohishi N, Emi M, Park MH, Inoko H, Tokunaga K, Kudoh S. Fine localization of a major disease-susceptibility locus for diffuse panbronchiolitis. Am J Hum Genet 2000; 66:501–507.

47. Sugiyama Y, Saitoh K, Kano S, Kitamura S. An autopsy case of diffuse panbronchiolitis accompanying rheumatoid arthritis. Respir Med 1996; 90:175–177.
48. Sugiyama Y, Ohno S, Kano S, Maeda H, Kitamura S. Diffuse panbronchiolitis and rheumatoid arthritis: a possible correlation with HLA-B54. Intern Med 1994; 33:612–614.
49. Tokunaga K, Omoto K, Akaza T, Akiyama N, Amemiya H, Naito S, Sasazuki T, Satoh H, Juji T. Haplotype study on C4 polymorphism in Japanese. Association with MHC alleles, complotypes, and HLA-complement haplotypes. Immunogenetics 1985; 22:359–365.
50. Maeda H, Juji T, Mitsui H, Sonozaki H, Okitsu K. HLA DR4 and rheumatoid arthritis in Japanese people. Ann Rheum Dis 1981; 40:299–302.
51. Stastny P. Association of the B-cell alloantigen DRw4 with rheumatoid arthritis. N Engl J Med 1978; 298:869–871.
52. Karr RW, Rodey GE, Lee T, Schwartz BD. Association of HLA-DRw4 with rheumatoid arthritis in black and white patients. Arthritis Rheum 1980; 23: 1241–1245.
53. Hayakawa H, Sato A, Imokawa S, Toyoshima M, Chida K, Iwata M. Bronchiolar disease in rheumatoid arthritis. Am J Respir Crit Care Med 1996; 154:1531–1536.
54. Nakada K, Inatomi K. Prognosis and treatment. Annual report on the study of diffuse interstitial lung disease. Ministry of Health and Welfare in Japan. 1981, p21.
55. Kudoh S, Uetake T, Hagiwara K, Hirayama M, Kyo E, Kimura J, Sugiyama Y. Clinical effect of low-dose long-term erythromycin chemotherapy on diffuse panbronchiolitis. Jpn J Thorac Dis 1987; 25:632–642.
56. Yamamoto M. Therapeutic effect of erythromycin on diffuse panbronchiolitis. Double-blind, placebo-controlled study. Annual Report on the Study of Diffuse Interstitial Lung Disease. Ministry of Health and Welfare in Japan 1991, p18–20.
57. Kudoh S, Azuma A, Yamamoto M, Izumi T, Ando M. Improvement of survival in patients with diffuse panbronchiolitis treated with low-dose erythromycin. Am J Respir Crit Care Med 1998; 157:1829–1832.
58. Tamaoki J, Takeyama K, Tagaya E, Konno K. Effect of clarithromycin on sputum production and its rheological properties in chronic respiratory tract infections. Antimicrob Agents Chemother 1995; 39:1688–1690.
59. Sugiyama Y, Yamanaka K, Kitamura S. The effect of 14-membered ring macrolide, roxithromycin, on diffuse panbronchiolitis. Shindan To Chiryou 1993; 81:1293–1296.
60. Nakamura H, Fujishima S, Inoue T, Ohkubo Y, Soejima K, Waki Y, Mori M, Urano T, Sakamaki F, Tasaka S, Ishizaka A, Kanazawa M, Yamaguchi K. Clinical and immunoregulatory effects of roxithromycin therapy for chronic respiratory tract infection. Eur Respir J 1999; 13:1371–1379.
61. Kobayashi H, Takeda H, Sakayori S, Kawakami Y, Otsuka Y, Tamura M, Konishi K, Tanimoto S, Fukakusa M, Shimada K, et al. Study on azithromycin

in treatment of diffuse panbronchiolitis. Kansenshogaku Zasshi 1995; 69:711–722.

62. Oritsu M. Effectiveness of macrolide antibiotics other than erythromycin. Therapeutic Research 1990; 11:545–546.

63. Nagai H, Shishido H, Yoneda R, Yamaguchi E, Tamura A, Kurashima A. Long-term low-dose administration of erythromycin to patients with diffuse panbronchiolitis. Respiration 1991; 58:145–149.

64. Kadota J, Sakito O, Kohno S, Sawa H, Mukae H, Oda H, Kawakami K, Fukushima K, Hiratani K, Hara K. A mechanism of erythromycin treatment in patients with diffuse panbronchiolitis. Am Rev Respir Dis 1993; 147:153–159.

65. Ichikawa Y, Koga H, Tanaka M, Nakamura M, Tokunaga N, Kaji M. Neutrophilia in bronchoalveolar lavage fluid of diffuse panbronchiolitis. Chest 1990; 98:917–923.

66. Hojo M, Fujita I, Hamasaki Y, Miyazaki M, Miyazaki S. Erythromycin does not directly affect neutrophil functions. Chest 1994; 105:520–523.

67. Goswami SK, Kivity S, Marom Z. Erythromycin inhibits respiratory glyco-conjugate secretion from human airways in vitro. Am Rev Respir Dis 1990; 141:72-B.

68. Tamaoki J, Isono K, Sakai N, Kanemura T, Konno K. Erythromycin inhibits Cl secretion across canine tracheal epithelial cells. Eur Respir J 1992; 5:234–238.

69. Suga T, Sugiyama Y, Fujii T, Kitamura S. Bronchioloalveolar carcinoma with bronchorrhoea treated with erythromycin. Eur Respir J 1994; 7:2249–2251.

70. Sugiyama Y, Sugama Y, Takeuchi K, Kudoh S, Kitamura S. Analysis of peripheral lymphocyte subsets and changes due to erythromycin therapy in patients with diffuse panbronchiolitis. Jpn J Thorac Dis 1990; 28:1574–1580.

71. Keicho N, Kudoh S, Yotsumoto H, Akagawa KS. Antilymphocytic activity of erythromycin distinct from that of FK506 or cyclosporin A. J Antibiot 1993; 46:1406–1413.

72. Konno S, Adachi M, Asano K, Okamoto K, Takahashi T. Inhibition of human T-lymphocyte activation by macrolide antibiotic, roxithromycin. Life Sci 1992; 51:PL231–PL236.

73. Keicho N, Kudoh S, Yotsumoto H, Akagawa KS. Erythromycin promotes monocyte to macrophage differentiation. J Antibiot 1994; 47:80–89.

74. Hirakata Y, Kaku M, Tomono K, Tateda K, Furuya N, Matsumoto T, Araki R, Yamaguchi K. Efficacy of erythromycin lactobionate for treating *Pseudomonas aeruginosa* bacteremia in mice. Antimicrob Agents Chemother 1992; 36:1198–1203.

75. Sakata K, Yajima H, Tanaka K, Sakamoto Y, Yamamoto K, Yoshida A, Dohi Y. Erythromycin inhibits the production of elastase by *Pseudomonas aeruginosa* without affecting its proliferation in vitro. Am Rev Respir Dis 1993; 148:1061–1065.

76. Takizawa H, Desaki M, Ohtoshi T, Kikutani T, Okazaki H, Sato M, Akiyama N, Shoji S, Hiramatsu K, Ito K. Erythromycin suppresses interleukin 6

expression by human bronchial epithelial cells: a potential mechanism of its anti-inflammatory action. Biochem Biophys Res Commun 1995; 210:781–786.

77. Oishi K, Sonoda F, Kobayashi S, Iwagaki A, Nagatake T, Matsushima K, Matsumoto K. Role of interleukin-8 (IL-8) and an inhibitory effect of erythromycin on IL-8 release in the airways of patients with chronic airway disease. Infect Immun 1994; 62:4145–4152.

78. Sakito O, Kadota J, Kohno S, Abe K, Shirai R, Hara K. Interleukin 1-beta, tumor necrosis factor alpha, and interleukin 8 in bronchoalveolar lavage fluid of patients with diffuse panbronchiolitis: a potential mechanism of macrolide therapy. Respiration 1996; 63:42–48.

79. Takizawa H, Desaki M, Ohtoshi T, Kawasaki S, Kohyama T, Sato M, Tanaka M, Kasama T, Kobayashi K, Nakajima J, Ito K. Erythromycin modulates IL-8 expression in normal and inflamed human bronchial epithelial cells. Am J Respir Crit Care Med 1997; 156:266–271.

80. Desaki M, Takizawa H, Ohtoshi T, Kasama T, Kobayashi K, Sunazuka T, Omura S, Yamamoto K, Ito K. Erythromycin suppresses nuclear factor-kappaB and activator protein-1 activation in human bronchial epithelial cells. Biochem Biophys Res Commun 2000; 267:124–128.

81. Abe S, Nakamura H, Inoue S, Takeda H, Saito H, Kato S, Mukaida N, Matsuhima K, Tomoike H. Interleukin-8 gene repression by clarithromycin is mediated by the activator protein-1 binding site in human bronchial epithelial cells. Am J Respir Cell Mol Biol 2000; 22:51–60.

82. Sugiyama Y, Yanagisawa K, Tominaga S-I, Kitamura S. Effects of long-term administration of erythromycin on cytokine production in rat alveolar macrophages. Eur Respir J 1999; 14:1113–1116.

18

Manifestations of Wegener's Granulomatosis in the Upper and Lower Airways

DAVID B. HELLMANN

The Johns Hopkins University School of Medicine
Baltimore, Maryland, U.S.A.

Introduction

Wegener's granulomatosis is an inflammatory condition of unknown cause that can affect any organ system but most frequently involves the upper respiratory tract, the lower respiratory tract, and the kidneys (1–5). Although Wegener's is often classified as a form of vasculitis, the inflammatory lesions can include not only arteritis but also granulomas with acute and chronic inflammation and large areas of tissue necrosis (3–5). Indeed, biopsy specimen from the upper airways show granulomatous inflammation and necrosis occuring much more often than vasculitis (5). Respiraory tract involvement is important because it usually causes the initial symptoms, it frequently provides sites for biopsy to confirm the diagnosis, and it can result in serious morbidity or death (5). Treatment with immunosuppressive agents and prednisone has transformed the course of Wegener's from a rapidly fatal disease to a chronic disease that may remit and relapse (5).

In the United States, the annual incidence of Wegener's is 4 per million persons, and the prevalence is 3 per 100,000 (6). Men and women are affected equally (5,7). The average age of patients with Wegener's is approximately 41 years, but onset may occur as early as 8 or as late as 80 (5). Seasonal variance in onset of the disease has been noted, with the highest incidence in winter and the lowest in summer (8). No racial or occupational risk factor has been identified (5,7).

I. Upper Respiratory Tract Manifestations

More than 70% of patients with Wegener's present with symptoms of the ears, nose, sinuses, or throat, and nearly all patients develop upper respiratory symptoms eventually (Table 1) (5,9–12). Sinusitis is the most common upper tract manifestation, ultimately occuring in about 85% of patients (5). Maxillary sinusitis occurs most frequently (Fig. 1), but all sinuses can be involved (10,11). Initially, the sinusitis of Wegener's is often difficult to distinguish from routine sinusitis. Only when the sinusitis proves refractory to therapy or becomes associated with other features (e.g., saddle nose deformity, hemoptysis, or hematuria) does the possibility of Wegener's become evident (5).

Nasal disease develops in about 70% of patients. Disease of the nose develops insidiously and is usually bilateral (13). Serosanguinous nasal drainage is complicated by development of nasal crusting (13). Wegener himself emphasized the extensive crusting that is present on examination (1,2). Patients may also describe removing prodigiously large nasal crusts. The crusting is frequently associated with obstruction of the nasal passages, pain, and mucosal ulceration and epistaxis (5,13). Upon removal of crusts under cocaine anesthesia, friable mucosa is revealed (13). Perforation of the nasal septum or destruction of the bridge of the nose (resulting in the classic "saddle nose" deformity) may develop (13).

Table 1 Frequency of Upper Respiratory Tract Symptoms in Wegener's Granulomatosis

Manifestation	Onset	Ever
Sinusitis	50	85
Nasal involvement	35	70
Otitis media	25	45
Hearing loss	15	40
Subglottic stenosis	1	15
Oral lesions	2	10

Source: Reprinted with permission from Hoffman et al. Wegener granulomatosis: an analysis of 158 patients. Ann Intern Med 1992; 116: 488–498.

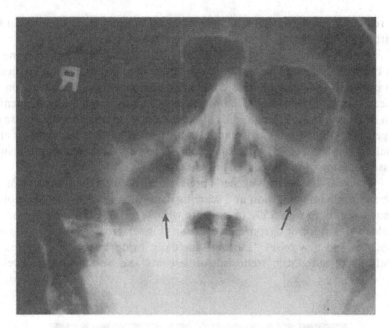

Figure 1 X-ray showing opacification of maxillary sinuses (arrows) in Wegener's granulomatosis.

Ear involvement (Table 2) occurs in 19 to 61% of patients (14,15). Serous otitis media, the commonest otological manifestation of Wegener's, is caused by blockage of the eustachian tube (15). The ear disease, like the sinusitis, may precede by months recognition of Wegener's involving other organs. Indeed, rarely is Wegener's diagnosed in patients with ear disease alone. Wegener's is one of the few systemic diseases, outside of relapsing polychondritis, that can cause a red, painful ear from chondritis. That chondritis spares the ear lobe (where cartilage is absent) helps distinguish

Table 2 Otological Manifestations of Wegener's Granulomatosis

External ear	Chondritis, otitis externa, tympanic membrane granulomata
Middle ear	Serous otitis media, suppurative otitis media
Inner ear	Sensorineural deafness, vertigo
Facial nerve palsy	

Source: Reproduced with permission from Murty GI. Wegener's granulomatosis: otorhinolaryngological manifestations. Clin Otolaryngol 1990;15:385–393.

the red ear of Wegener's (or relapsing polychondritis) from the red ear of frostbite or diabetic infection.

Otitis externa may be caused by otitis media or from Wegener's involvement. Hearing loss eventually develops in almost half of the patients and is usually associated with a conductive component (e.g., obstruction of the ear canal, otitis media) (5,15). Vertigo occurs, but much less frequently than hearing loss (15). Mastoiditis also frequently complicates the course of Wegener's. Other otological manifestations of Wegener's are vertigo and facial nerve palsy (14,15). Mastoidectomy is less effective than immunosuppressive treatment of the underlying disease.

Tracheal disease in Wegener's preferentially affects the subglottic area, where chronic inflammation and scarring cause stenosis (16–34). Subglottic stenosis occurs in 6 to 25% of patients with Wegener's (14) and is usually heralded by stridor or dyspnea on exertion (Fig. 2). Hoarseness, throat pain, dysplasia, and new-onset "snoring" (actually stridor) may be other manifestations of subglottic stenosis. Adolescents and young adults develop

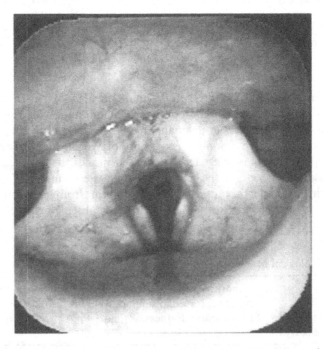

Figure 2 Laryngoscopic appearance of subglottic stenosis in Wegener's granulomatosis. (Image courtesy of Dr. Bernard Marsh.)

subglottic stenosis more commonly than older adults (5,25). Subglottic stenosis may be the very first feature of Wegener's, preceding by months or years other signs of the disease (25). Biopsies of the subglottic area rarely show vasculitis (5,25). Management of subglottic stenosis is challenging, since stenosis may worsen or occur at a time when disease is inactive in other organs (13,33). Tracheotomy is frequently required (14,25,35). Experience indicates that local corticosteroid injections help (14,35).

Wegener's may also diffusely involve the endobronchial tube, producing a cobblestone appearance on bronchoscopy. Endobronchial Wegener's may cause persistent cough. Extensive endobronchial disease may result in collapse of a portion of the lung.

Wegener's in the oral pharynx can cause gingival hyperplasia that originates in the interdental papilla areas and may lead to tooth mobility or tooth loss (14,36). Ulcerative stomatitis may also occur. Rarely, patients with Wegener's present with palatal ulceration or striking enlargement of the submandibular glands (37). Destructive oral ulcers may be mistaken for malignancy (14). Wegener's may also cause parotid gland enlargement, mimicking Sjögren's syndrome (37–39).

II. Lower Respiratory Tract Manifestations

Almost half of patients present with pulmonary symptoms or signs, and ultimately 85% develop lower respiratory tract abnormalities (Table 3) (3,5). The most common symptoms are cough, hemoptysis, and pleurisy (3,5,27,40,41). Hemoptysis may rarely be massive. Breathlessness may be aggravated by anemia.

Table 3 Frequency of Lower Respiratory Tract Abnormalities in Wegener's Granulomatosis

Feature	Onset	Eventual
Infiltrates	25	65
Nodules	25	55
Cough	20	45
Hemoptysis	15	30
Pleuritis	10	30

Source: Reprinted with permission from Hoffman et al. Wegener granulomatosis: an analysis of 158 patients. Ann Intern Med 1992; 116:488–498.

Radiological abnormalities occur even more commonly than chest symptoms. Indeed, one-third of patients with no lower respiratory tract symptoms have chest image abnormalities (3,5,41); the most common such abnormality is multiple nodular infiltrates that tend to cavitate (Figs. 3–5) (3). Densities usually predominate in the lower lobes, are discrete and 1 cm or more in diameter, and are multiple and bilateral in two-thirds of cases (24,42). In contrast to tuberculosis, Wegener's usually spares the apical or posterior segments of the upper lobes (27). Hemoptysis may lead to dramatically appearing alveolar infiltrates. Pleural effusions occur in less than 10% of patients, and interstitial lung disease (in the absence of super-imposed opportunistic infection) is rare (3,14). In one series of 225 patients, only 2 developed interstitial lung disease (14). Hilar adenopathy is so unusual in Wegener's that its presence should suggest another diagnosis (3,13).

Computed tomographic (CT) chest images are more sensitive than chest x-rays and may show abnormal results when the chest x-ray is negative (43). The most common finding is multiple nodules or masses ranging in size from 0.3 to 5.0 cm (43–45). The nodules in Wegener's in some ways resemble those seen with septic emboli, pulmonary infarcts, and tumor emboli of hematogenous metastases—that is, the nodules in each of these conditions have "feeding vessels" and are associated with wedge-shaped lesions abut-

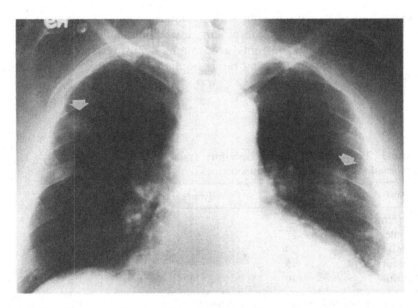

Figure 3 Chest x-ray showing bilateral nodular infiltrates (arrowheads) in a patient with Wegener's granulomatosis.

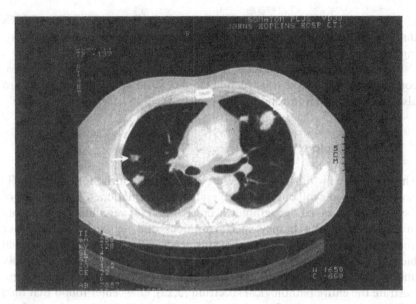

Figure 4 Chest CT image showing multiple nodules (arrows) in a patient with Wegener's granulomatosis.

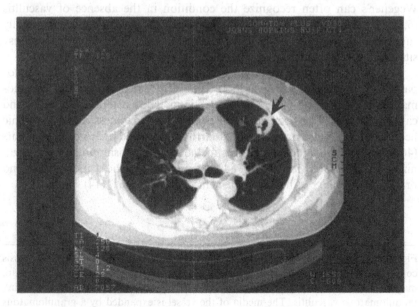

Figure 5 Chest CT image showing cavitary nodule (arrow) in a patient with Wegener's granulomatosis.

ting the pleura (43). One CT feature that may help distinguish these entities is that the nodules in Wegener's show spiculation and linear scarring emanating from the pulmonary nodules (43).

Pulmonary infarction tests are abnormal in most patients. The most common abnormality is obstruction, found in 55% (3). About one-third also show reduction in total lung capacity (3).

III. Pathology

The distinctive histological changes in Wegener's comprise four findings: (1) acute and chronic inflammation, (2) granuloma formation, (3) large areas of tissue necrosis, called "geographic necrosis," and (4) vasculitis (1–3,5). Only in large, open-lung biopsy specimens does one regularly find all four abnormalities (Fig. 6) (5). Percutaneous needle biopsies and transbronchial biopsies produce results showing vasculitis less than 10% of time (3). Biopsy and surgical materials from upper respiratory tract specimens rarely demonstrate the entire pathological spectrum (5,25). One center found that only 16% of biopsy samples from the upper respiratory tract demonstrated the triad of necrosis, vasculitis, and granulomatous inflammation (5). However, pathologists who are familiar with the distinctive pattern of necrosis seen in Wegener's can often recognize the condition in the absence of vasculitis (5,25). The presence of geographic necrosis and granuloma are especially suggestive of Wegener's (3,5). The most useful upper respiratory tract biopsy sites are, in decreasing order, the sinuses, nose, and subglottic region (5).

In a series of 87 open-lung biopsies from 67 patients, the major pathological findings were vasculitis, parenchymal necrosis, and granulomatous inflammation (46). The vasculitis included arteritis, venulitis, and capillaritis (46). The necrosis manifested as microabscess and geographic necrosis (46). Diffuse pulmonary hemorrhage occurred in 3% of the patients (46). Minor nondiagnostic changes included tissue eosinophilia (47), organizing intraluminal fibrosis, lipoid pneumonia, lymphoid aggregates, and bronchiolar changes (including bronchiolitis obliterans) (14).

Figure 6 (A) Lung tissue in Wegener's granulomatosis showing necrobiosis consisting of fibrinoid necrosis and giant cells. (Hematoxylin and eosin stain; magnification × 100.) (B) Lung tissue in Wegener's granulomatosis showing granulomatous vasculitis. The media of the vessel is expanded by a granulomatous process with necrosis. Elastic tissue stain shows the destruction of elastica in the involved area. (Verhoff, van Gieson stain, magnification × 100.) (Photomicrographs courtesy of Dr. Frederic Askin.)

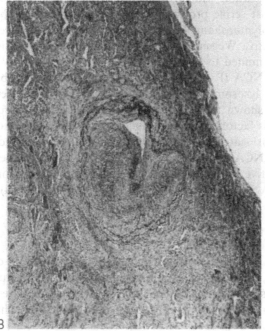

The most common renal biopsy finding in Wegener's is a focal, segmental, necrotizing glomerulonephritis (5). Vasculitis outside the glomerulus or granuloma appears in less than 10% of specimens (5).

IV. Etiology and Pathogenesis

The cause of Wegener's is not known. Infections or autoimmunity or both are thought to participate in the pathogenesis (3,5). The observations that Wegener's occurs most commonly in the winter (8) and that some patients, especially those with disease limited to the respiratory tract appear to improve with trimethoprim–sulfamethoxazole therapy (5,48) have suggested an infectious etiology. However, no specific infectious disease agent has been identified. Other observations—the multisystem nature of the disease, the response to immunosuppressive therapy, and the presence of a novel auto-antibody (the antineutrophil cytoplasmic antibody)—have suggested that Wegener's is an autoimmune disease (15,49–55). It is also possible that the pathogenesis of Wegener's is due to an interplay of infections and autoimmune mechanisms.

Most recently work has focused on the putative role of antineutrophilic cytoplasmic antibody (ANCA) in the pathogenesis of Wegener's (55–58). There are two main types of ANCA that differ in their antigenic targets and their association with Wegener's. Cytoplasmic ANCA (C-ANCA) is directed against serine protease, an enzyme contained in the cytoplasmic granules of polymorphonuclear cells and macrophages. The sensitivity of C-ANCA for active Wegener's correlates with the extent of disease, ranging from 70% in limited to Wegener's to 96% in multisystem Wegener's. The perinuclear ANCA (P-ANCA) pattern is produced by antibodies directed against other lysosomal enzymes, most frequently myeloperoxidase (59). Studies have shown that when polymorphonuclear cells are primed with tumor necrosis factor, small amounts of serine proteinase and myeloperoxidase are translocated from the cytoplasm to the cell surface (55). In the presence of ANCA, these primed polymorphonuclear cells degranulate and relase destructive superoxide products (55). These observations invite speculation that ANCA may be pathogenic in Wegener's (60–64).

V. Diagnosis

The diagnosis of Wegener's can be made confidently when the clinical picture is compatible, the pathology is consistent, and stains and cultures have ruled out other causes (infections, tumor) (5). The triad of upper respiratory tract disease, lower respiratory tract disease, and glomerulonephritis gives the classic clinical picture. However, many patients present with disease limited to one or two regions. While the classic clinical triad is not required for diagnosis, pathological confirmation is needed. As noted, small upper respiratory biopsy samples rarely show the entire range of pathological changes, but in the hands of a skilled pathologist, changes very suggestive of Wegener's can often be identified.

The C-ANCA pattern is 90 to 98% specific and 60 to 90% sensitive for the diagnosis of Wegener's (49). The P-ANCA pattern occurs in 5 to 30% of Wegener's patients but is not specific: P-ANCA occurs in a wide variety of disease including polyarthritis, systemic lupus erythematosus, and inflammatory bowel disease (49,56).

The high specificity of the C-ANCA raises the question of whether the traditional practice of always seeking biopsy confirmation should still be followed. However, the seriousness of Wegener's, the toxicity of the treatment, and the reports of false-positive C-ANCAs should continue to make biopsy confirmation desirable in almost all cases.

VI. Differential Diagnosis

With upper respiratory tract symptoms, the chief diagnostic dilemma is distinguishing Wegener's from common self-limited infectious diseases. The possibility of Wegener's should be considered when symptoms fail to respond to antibiotics·or are associated with unusual features (e.g., saddle nose, stridor, proptosis, scleritis, weight loss, hematuria).

Other chronic diseases of upper and lower airways must be distinguished from Wegener's. Sarcoidosis can affect the nose, sinuses, and lung. Chest CT images may help with the distinction: hilar adenopathy is classic in sarcoidosis but very rare in Wegener's. Lung cancer can resemble Wegener's in causing pulmonary nodules and masses. Tracheal involvement can be seen with many diseases but few of these regularly involve the subglottic region as Wegener's does (25). Lymphoma may involve any site, inclding the nose, and must be differentiated from Wegener's. Syphilis, tuberculosis, fungal infections (e.g., histoplasmosis), lymphomatoid granulomatosis, and Churg–Strauss vasculitis and metastatic carcinoma can all mimic upper and lower respiratory tract signs of Wegener's. Thus, biopsy specimens are useful not only for what they show but also for what they help exclude.

VII. Treatment

The treatment of Wegener's has become dramatically more effective over the last 50 years. In the precorticosteroid era, more than 80% of patients with generalized Wegener's died within 2 years (3,65). The use of corticosteroids in the 1950s had little effect on outcome. However, in the 1970s, the National Institutes of Health revolutionized the treatment with the demonstration of the efficacy of using both prednisone (begun at 1 mg/kg/day for 1 month then tapered) and oral, daily cyclophosphamide (at 2 mg/kg/day). Of the patients so treated with prednisone and cyclophosphamide, 91% improved and 75% achieved remission (5). Similar regimens have resulted in a 10-year survival rate of 90% (66). Gradually, however, the limits of the efficacy and the sobering toxicity of chronic, daily cyclophosphamide became evident. For example, 25% of patients never achieved remission, and half of those who remitted later relapsed (5). In addition, patients treated with daily, chronic cyclophosphamide demonstrated a staggering accumulation of side effects, including a 2.4-fold increased risk of developing cancer, a 40% chance of developing hemorrhagic cystitis, and a 60% chance of ovarian failure (5). These data prompted trials of intravenous monthly, pulse cyclophosphamide, which had been shown to be as effective but less toxic in treating lupus nephritis. Unfortunately, most of the studies suggest that intravenous, pulse cyclophosphamide is less effective in treating Wegener's (65).

Over the last 15 years, two other strategies for reducing toxicity have emerged. The first is to use immunosuppressive agents other than cyclophosphamide. The best tested regimen has been the combination of prednisone and methotrexate (65). Methotrexate is usually taken orally, once a week, in doses of 15 to 25 mg. Several studies have shown that prednisone and methotrexate can effectively treat some patients with Wegener's (65–70). There are at least three important caveats: (1) methotrexate and prednisone have been shown to be effective only for patients who do not have "immediately life-threatening" disease, since methotrexate and prednisone have not been shown to be effective for treating life-threatening disease; (2) methotrexate is contraindicated in patients who have renal insufficiency (e.g., serum creatinine > 2.0 mg/dL) or liver disease or are pregnant; and (3) while most patients treated with methotrexate improve, virtually all relapse if methotrexate is stopped.

The second strategy for treating Wegener's has been to use daily, oral cyclophosphamide for a brief "induction phase" (e.g., 3–6 months) and then stop cyclophosphamide while starting another, more benign immunosuppressive drug such as methotrexate or azathioprine for maintenance (65,71). Although little experience with this approach has accumulated, it appears to be effective for patients with either generalized or limited disease, and it appears to be less toxic than the standard regimen of chronic cyclophosphamide therapy (71).

Trimethoprim–sulfamethoxazole (TMP-S) has three possible roles in Wegener's: preventing relapse, preventing *Pneumocystis carinii* pneumonia and treating active Wegener's. The first two roles of TMP-S have been proven

(48,65). The efficacy of using TMP-S to treat Wegener's is controversial, and the drug has never been formally tested in a randomized, controlled trial (5,65). TMP-S appears unlikely to be effective for patients with severe disease.

The toxicity of daily oral cyclophosphamide can be reduced by following several guidelines. The dose of cyclophosphamide should be adjusted for the patient's age and renal function. The duration of therapy should be as brief as possible. Patients should be instructed to drink at least 6 glasses of fluid daily to decrease the risk of hemorrhagic cystitis (65). Patients on cyclophosphamide should also receive prophylactic treatment against *Pneumocystis carinii* pneumonia and should have complete blood counts often (e.g., every 15 days). The dose of cyclophosphamide should be adjusted to prevent or minimize leukopenia; it is not necessary to achieve leukopenia with cyclophosphamide to achieve remission (65).

Studies indicate that C-ANCA titers do not correlate well enough with disease activity to allow serial changes to dictate therapy. For example, Kerr et al., in a study of 106 patients, found that serial titers correlated with a change in activity of disease in only 64% of patients (72). Moreover, a rise in C-ANCA titer preceded flare-up of disease in only 24% of cases (72).

Local care is also important in upper respiratory tract disease (65). Saline nasal spray helps reduce nasal crusting. Antibiotics are often needed to treat superinfection of sinuses or ears (5). Local corticosteroid injections may help patients with subglottic involvement to avoid tracheotomy (35,54,56). For patients with significant stenosis, carbon dioxide laser surgery is usually ineffective (14). Some physicians favor endoscopic dilation when possible (14). Others approach the problem with aggressive surgical management, with splitting of the anterior ring and posterior body of the cricoid cartilage followed by costal cartilage and skin grafting (35).

References

1. Wegener F. Über generalisierte, septische Fäberkrankungen. Verh Dtsch Pathol Ges 1936; 29:202–210.
2. Wegener F. Über eine eigenartige Rhinogene granulomatose mit besonderer Beteiligung des arterien Systems und der Nieren. Beitr Pathol Anat Allg Pathol 1939; 36–68.
3. Fauci AS, Haynes BF, Katz P, Wolff SM. Wegener's granulomatosis: prospective clinical and therapeutic experience with 85 patients for 21 years. Ann Intern Med 1983; 98:76–85.
4. Fahey JL, Leonard E, Churg J, Godman G. Wegener's granulomatosis. Am J Med 1954; 17:168–179.
5. Hoffman GS, Kerr GS, Leavitt RY, Hallahan CW, Lebovics RS, Travis WD, Rottem M, Fauci AS. Wegener granulomatosis: an analysis of 158 patients. Ann Intern Med 1992; 116:488–498.

6. González-Gay MA, Garcia-Porrua C. Epidemiology of the vasculitides. In: Stone J, Hellmann DB, eds. Rheumatic Disease Clinics of North America. Philadelphia: WB Saunders, 2001:729–749.

7. Cotch MF, Hoffman GS, Yerg DE, Kaufman GI, Targonski P, Kaslow RA. The epidemiology of Wegener's granulomatosis. Estimates of the five-year period prevalence, annual mortality, and geographic disease distribution from population-based data sources. Arthritis Rheum 1996; 39:87–92.

8. Raynauld J-P, Bloch DA, Fries JF. Seasonal variation in the onset of Wegener's granulomatosis, polyarteritis nodosa and giant cell arteritis. J Rheumatol 1993; 20:1524–1526.

9. Brown HA, Woolner LB. Findings referable to the upper part of the respiratory tract in Wegener's granulomatosis. Ann Otol Rhinol Laryngol 1960; 69:810–829.

10. Kornblut AD, Wolff SM, DeFries HO, Fauci AS. Wegener's granulomatosis. Laryngoscope 1980; 90:1453–1465.

11. Fauci AS, Wolff SM. Wegener's granulomatosis: studies in eighteen patients and a review of the literature. Medicine 1973; 52:535–561.

12. Kornblut AD, Wolff SM, DeFries HO, Fauci AS. Wegener's granulomatosis. Otolaryngol Clin North Am 1982; 15:673–683.

13. McDonald TJ, DeRemee RA. Wegener's granulomatosis. Laryngoscope 1983; 93:220–231.

14. Leavitt RY, Fauci AS. Less common manifestations and presentations of Wegener's granulomatosis. Curr Opin Rheumatol 1992; 4:16–22.

15. Murty GE. Wegener's granulomatosis. otorhinolaryngological manifestations. Clin Otolaryngol 1990; 15:385–393.

16. Thomas K. Laryngeal manifestations of Wegener's granuloma. J Laryngol Otol 1970; 84:101–106.

17. Atkins JP, Eisman SH. Wegener's granulomatosis. Ann Otol Rhinol Laryngol 1959; 68:524–547.

18. Kurita S, Hirano M. Wegener's granuloma localized in the larynx: report of a case. Auris Nasus Larynx 1983; 10:S97–S104.

19. Terent A, Wibell L, Lindholm CE, Wilbrand H. Laryngeal granuloma in the early stages of Wegener's granulomatosis. J Otorhinolaryngol Relat Spec 1980; 42:258–265.

20. Hirsch MM, Houssiau FA, Collard P, Devegelaer J-P, deDeuxchaisnes CN. A rare case of bronchial stenosis in Wegener's granulomatosis. Dramatic response to intravenous cyclophosphamide and oral cotrimoxazolle. J Rheumatol 1992; 19:821–824.

21. Arauz JC, Fonseca R. Wegener's granulomatosis appearing initially in the trachea. Ann Otol Rhinol Laryngol 1982; 91:593–594.

22. Kulis JC, Nequin ND. Tracheo-esophageal fistula due to Wegener's granulomatosis. J Am Med Assoc 1965; 191:148–149.

23. Talerman A, Wright D. Laryngeal obstruction due to Wegener's granulomatosis. Arch Otolaryngol 1972; 96:376–379.

24. Lampman JH, Querubin R, Kondapalli P. Subglottic stenosis in Wegener's granulomatosis. Chest 1981; 79:230–232.

25. Hellmann D, Laing T, Petri M, Jacobs D, Crumley R, Stulbarg M. Wegener's granulomatosis: isolated involvement of the trachea and larynx. Ann Rheum Dis 1987; 46:628–631.

26. Waxman J, Bose WJ. Laryngeal manifestations of Wegener's granulomatosis. case reports and review of the literature. J Rheumatol 1986; 13:408–411.

27. Carrington CB, Liebow AA. Limited forms of angiitis and granulomatosis of Wegener's type. Am J Med 1969; 41:497–527.

28. Cohen SR, Landing BH, King KK, Isaacs H. Wegener's granulomatosis causing laryngeal and tracheobronchial obstruction in an adolescent girl. Ann Otol Rhinol Laryngol 1978; S87:15–19.

29. Thomas K. Laryngeal manifestations of Wegener's granuloma. J Laryngol Otol 1970; 84:101–106.

30. Bohlman ME, Ensor RE, Goldman SM. Primary Wegener's granulomatosis of the trachea: radiologic manifestations. South Med J 1984; 77:1318–1319.

31. Cohen MI, Gore RM, August CZ, Ossoff RH. Tracheal and bronchial stenosis associated with mediastinal adenopathy in Wegener's granulomatosis: CT findings. J Comput Assist Tomogr 1984; 8:327–329.

32. McDonald TJ III, Neel HB, DeRemee RA. Wegener's granulomatosis of the subglottis and the upper portion of the trachea. Ann Otol Rhinol Laryngol 1982; 91:588–592.

33. Shah IA, Holstege A, Riede UN. Bioptic diagnosis of Wegener's granulomatosis in the absence of vasculitis and granulomas. Pathol Res Pract 1984; 178:407–412.

34. Walton EW. Giant-cell granuloma of the respiratory tract (Wegener's granulomatosis). Br Med J 1958; 265–270.

35. McCaffrey TV. Management of subglottic stenosis in the adult. Ann Otol Rhinol Laryngol 1991; 100:90–94.

36. Handlers JP, Waterman J, Abrams AM, Melrose RJ. Oral features of Wegener's granulomatosis. Arch Otolaryngol 1985; 111:267–270.

37. Specks U, Colby TV, Olsen KD, DeRemee RA. Salivary gland involvement in Wegener's granulomatosis. Arch Otolaryngol Head Neck Surg 1991; 117:218–223.

38. Murty GE, Mains BT, Bennett MK. Salivary gland involvement in Wegener's granulomatosis. J Laryngol Otol 1990; 104:259–261.

39. Stuckey SL, Smart PJ. Wegener's granulomatosis: parotid involvement and associated pancreatitis with CT findings. Australas Radiol 1992; 36:343–346.

40. Brandwein S, Esdaile J, Danoff D, Tannenbaum H. Wegener's granulomatosis. Clinical features and outcome in 13 patients. Arch Intern Med 1983; 143:476–479.

41. Flye MW, Mundinger GH, Fauci AS. Diagnostic and therapeutic aspects of the surgical approach to Wegener's granulomatosis. J Thorac Cardiovasc Surg 1979; 77:331–337.

42. Grotz W, Mundinger A, Wurtemberger G, Peter HH, Schollmeyer P. Radiographic course of pulmonary manifestations of Wegener's granulomatosis under immunosuppressive therapy. Chest 1994; 105:509–513.

43. Kuhlman JE, Hruban RH, Fishman EK. Wegener granulomatosis: CT features of parenchymal lung disease. J Comput Assist Tomogr 1991; 15:948–952.

44. Papiris SA, Manoussakis MN, Drosos AA, Kontogiannis D, Constantopoulos SH, Moutsopoulos HM. Imaging of thoracic Wegener's granulomatosis: the computed tomographic appearance. Am J Med 1992; 93:529–536.

45. Pretorius ES, Stone JH, Hellmann DB, Fishman EK. Wegener's granulomatosis: spectrum of CT findings in diagnosis, disease progression and response to therapy. Crit Rev Diagn Imaging 2000; 41:279–313.

46. Travis WD, Hoffman GS, Leavitt RY, Pass HI, Fauci AS. Surgical pathology of the lung in Wegener's granulomatosis. Review of 87 open lung biopsies from 67 patients. Am J Surg Pathol 1991; 15(4):315–333.

47. Yousem SA, Lombard CM. The eosinophilic variant of Wegener's granulomatosis. Hum Pathol 1988; 19:682–688.

48. Stegeman CA, Tervaert JWC, DeJong PE, Kallenberg CGM. Trimethoprim–sulfamethoxazole (Co-trimoxazole) for the prevention of relapses of Wegener's granulomatosis. N Engl J Med 1996; 335:16–20.

49. Rao JK, Weinberger M, Oddone EZ, Allen NB, Landsman P, Feussner JR. The role of antineutrophil cytoplasmic antibody (c-ANCA) testing in the diagnosis of Wegener granulomatosis. Ann Intern Med 1995; 123:925–932.

50. Reinhold-Keller E, Kekow J, Schnabel A, Schmitt WH, Heller M, Beigel A, Duncker G, Gross WL. Influence of disease manifestation and antineutrophil cytoplasmic antibody titer on the response to pulse cyclophosphamide therapy in patients with Wegener's granulomatosis. Arthritis Rheum 1994; 37:919–924.

51. Hollander D, Manning RT. The use of ankylating agents in the treatment of Wegener's granulomatosis. Ann Intern Med 1967; 67:393–398.

52. Hoffman GS, Leavitt RY, Fleisher TA, Minor JR, Fauci AS. Treatment of Wegener's granulomatosis with intermittent high-dose intravenous cyclophosphamide. Am J Med 1990; 89:403–410.

53. Hoffman GS, Leavitt RY, Kerr GS, Fauci AS. The treatment of Wegener's granulomatosis with glucocorticoids and methotrexate. Arthritis Rheum 1992; 35:1322–1329.

54. Sneller MC, Hoffman GS, Talar-Williams C, Kerr GS, Hallahan CW, Fauci AS. An analysis of forty-two Wegener's granulomatosis patients treated with methotrexate and prednisone. Arthritis Rheum 1995; 38:608–613.

55. Falk RJ, Terrell RS, Charles LA, Jennette JC. Anti-neutrophil cytoplasmic autoantibodies induce neutrophils to degranulate and produce oxygen radicals in vitro. Proc Natl Acad Sci U S A 1990; 87:4115–4119.

56. Lebovics RS, Hoffman GS, Leavitt RY, Kerr GS, Travis WD, Kammerer W, Hallahan C, Rottem M, Fauci AS. The management of subglottic stenosis in patients with Wegener's granulomatosis. Laryngoscope 1992; 102:1341–1345.

57. Jinnah HA, Dixon A, Brat DJ, Hellmann DB. Chronic meningitis with cranial neuropathies in Wegener's granulomatosis: case report and review of the literature. Arthritis Rheum 1997; 40:573–577.

58. Ludeman J, Utecht B, Gross WL. Antineutrophil cytoplasm antibodies in

Wegener granulomatosis recognize an elastinolytic enzyme. J Exp Med 1990; 171:357–367.

59. Falk RJ, Jeannette JC. Anti-neutrophil cytoplasmic autoantibodies with specificity for myeloperoxidase in patients with systemic vasculitis and idiopathic necrotizing and crescentic glomerulonephritis. N Engl J Med 1988; 318: 1651–1657.

60. Nolle B, Specks U, Ludemann J, Rohrbach MS, DeRemee RA, Gross WL. Anticytoplasmic autoantibodies: their immunodiagnostic value in Wegener granulomatosis. Ann Intern Med 1989; 111:28–40.

61. Jeannette JC. Antineutrophil cytoplasmic autoantibody-associated diseases: a pathologist's perspective. Am J Kidney Dis 1991; 18:164–170.

62. Gross WL, Schmitt WH, Csernock E. Antineutrophil cytoplasmic autoantibody-associated diseases: a rheumatologist's perspective. Am J Kidney Dis 1991; 18:175–179.

63. Gross WL, Csernok E, Helmchen U. Antineutrophil cytoplasmic autoantibodies, autoantigens, and systemic vasculitis. APMIS 1995; 103:81–97.

64. Russell KA, Specks U. Are antineutrophil cytoplasmic antibodies pathogenic? Experimental approaches to understand the antineutrophil cytoplasmic antibody phenomenon. In: Stone J, Hellmann DB, eds. Rheumatic Disease Clinics of North America. Philadelphia: WB Saunders, 2001:815–832.

65. Regan MJ, Hellmann DB, Stone JH. The Treatment of Wegener's Granulomatosis. In: Stone J, Hellmann DB, eds. Rheumatic Disease Clinics of North America. Philadelphia: WB Saunders, 2001:863–886.

66. Reinhold-Keller E, Beuge N, Latza U, et al. An interdisciplinary approach to the care of patients with Wegener's granulomatosis. Long-term outcome in 155 patients. Arthritis Rheum 2000; 43:1021–1032.

67. Stone J, Tun W, Hellmann D. Treatment of non–life threatening Wegener's granulomatosis with methotrexate and daily prednisone as the initial therapy of choice. J Rheumatol 1999; 26:1134–1139.

68. Langford CA, Talar-Williams C, Sneller MC. Use of methotrexate and glucocorticoids in the treatment of Wegener's granulomatosis. Long-term renal outcome in patients with glomerulonephritis. Arthritis Rheum 2000; 43:1836–1840.

69. Hoffman GS, Leavitt RY, Kerr GS, et al. The treatment of Wegener's granulomatosis with glucocorticoids and methotrexate. Arthritis Rheum 1992; 35:1322–1329.

70. DeGroot K, Muhler M, Reinhold-Keiler E, et al. Induction of remission in Wegener's granulomatosis with low dose methotrexate. J Rheumatol 1998; 25:492–495.

71. Langford CA, Talar-Williams C, Barron KS, et al. A staged approach to the treatment of Wegener's granulomatosis. Arthritis Rheum 1999; 42:2666–2673.

72. Kerr GS, Fleisher TA, Hallahan CW, Leavitt RY, Fauci AS, Hoffman GS. Limited prognostic value of changes in antineutrophil cytoplasmic antibody titer in patients with Wegener's granulomatosis. Arthritis Rheum 1993; 36:365–371.

19

Manifestation of Sarcoidosis in the Upper and the Lower Airways

DAVID R. MOLLER and IRINA PETRACHE

The Johns Hopkins University
Baltimore, Maryland, U.S.A.

Introduction

Sarcoidosis is recognized as a multisystem granulomatous disease of unknown origin characterized by noncaseating granulomas and infiltration by activated, cytokine-producing T cells and macrophages at sites of inflammation. Although the disease most commonly affects the lower respiratory tract and intrathoracic lymph nodes, symptomatic involvement of the upper respiratory tract including the nose, sinuses, larynx, or trachea is seen in approximately 10% of patients and is responsible for considerable morbidity. Involvement of the intrathoracic airways in sarcoidosis is common and typically presents with dyspnea, cough, and airflow limitation. This chapter reviews the spectrum of manifestations of sarcoidosis of the upper respiratory tract and lower airways, as well as the state of our knowledge regarding the immunopathogenesis of sarcoidosis and new therapeutic strategies for the treatment of this disease.

I. General Features

Sarcoidosis is a disease characterized by noncaseating epithelioid granulomas in multiple organ systems (90). Granulomas are typically accompanied by activated T cells, macrophages, and giant cells. Although any organ of the body can be affected, the lungs or intrathoracic lymph nodes are involved in over 90% of patients with sarcoidosis. Eye and skin involvement is seen in approximately 20% of patients, and symptomatic involvement of other organ systems occurs less frequently. Sarcoidosis of the upper respiratory tract is found in approximately 10% of patients, often in patients with pulmonary involvement (75,84).

There are considerable geographic and racial differences in the frequency of the disease. The prevalence of sarcoidosis ranges from 10 to 40 cases per 100,000 population in North America, Britain, and southern Europe, but fewer than 10 per 100,000 in Japan (50). Higher prevalence rates have been noted in Scandinavian countries, among Irish women in London, and among African Americans in southeastern United States. In the United States, the age-adjusted annual incidence rate has been estimated at 35.5 per 100,000 for blacks (46) and 10.9 for whites (19). Women appear to be more frequently affected than men in almost all studies. The usual age of onset of sarcoidosis is from 20 to 40 years, with a second peak after age 50 in women from Japan and Scandinavia (50).

The clinical presentations of sarcoidosis vary greatly (102,129). Approximately 35 to 50% of individuals are asymptomatic but have sarcoidosis diagnosed after an incidental radiographic finding of bilateral hilar adenopathy. In other patients, sarcoidosis presents in an acute or subacute form. Löfgren's syndrome is characterized by an abrupt onset of erythema nodosum, fevers, and often polyarthritis and uveitis in association with bilateral hilar adenopathy (74). Subacute, symptomatic presentations of sarcoidosis most frequently involve the respiratory system and are typically associated with pulmonary infiltrates. Extrapulmonary sarcoidosis dominates the clinical picture in 10 to 20% of patients, who may have no clinically significant pulmonary disease. There is heterogeneity in the clinical presentation and severity of disease among different populations. Several studies suggest sarcoidosis is more severe and chronic in black populations (55,60,102,129). Erythema nodosum is more commonly seen among Caucasian and Scandinavian populations than in blacks. In Japan, cardiac sarcoidosis accounts for as many as 50% of cases of sarcoidosis, at least 5 to 10 times the reported prevalence found in North American or European studies of sarcoidosis (56).

The etiology of sarcoidosis remains unknown (24,92). Genetic susceptibility to sarcoidosis is likely, given that familial clustering of the diseases occurs in 5 to 17% of patients, with monozygotic twins more frequently affected than dizygotic twins (21,119). Studies of HLA phenotyping and genotyping among different ethnic groups have demonstrated specific HLA types with disease presentations such as DR17 and bilateral hilar adenopathy or erythema nodosum in Swedish patients, DR15 and DR5 in chronic disease, and DRw52 and limited disease in Japanese patients (120). One study reported an association between sarcoidosis and major histocompatibility complex (MHC) haplotypes containing glutamine at position 69 of the $DP\beta_1$-chain that are known to be risk factors for susceptibility to chronic beryllium disease (78,114). These results have not been confirmed in larger studies (80).

Recently, a multicenter case–control study of the etiology of sarcoidosis (ACCESS), funded by the National Heart, Lung, and Blood Institute, was established to develop clues to the cause of sarcoidosis. Preliminary analysis of the study results, presented at the American Thoracic Society International Conference in 2000, demonstrated positive associations between sarcoidosis and agricultural employment, and exposures to insecticides or mold or mildew at work. The odds ratios for these associations were modest, around 1.5, but statistically significant. Perhaps the most notable result was the lack of evidence for sarcoidosis association and previously hypothesized environmental factors such as exposure to metals, wood dusts, and pine pollens, and the lack of one or more dominant exposures positively associated with sarcoidosis risk. A strong familial association with sarcoidosis was confirmed by this study, as was a negative association with cigarette smoking (121).

An infectious cause of sarcoidosis has been postulated since the early delineation of the disease. The search for infectious causes of sarcoidosis has utilized a variety of culture techniques and more recently, polymerase chain reaction methods to identify microbial DNA in patients with sarcoidosis. Traces of mycobacterial DNA or RNA have been reported in 0 to 75% of tissues from patients with sarcoidosis but have also been found in significant numbers of control specimens (81). Japanese investigators have found high numbers of *Proprionibacterium acnes* or *P. granulosum* DNA genomes in over 90% of lymph node samples from patients with sarcoidosis, with only low levels of these bacterial DNA from control samples (53). Preliminary reports suggest that these findings have been confirmed in European and North American patients with sarcoidosis by these workers in collaborative studies (Sixth World Association of Sarcoidosis and Other Granulomatous Diseases, Kumamoto, Japan). However, the role of *P. acnes* in sarcoidosis remains uncertain, given the presence of these organisms in normal tissues and the lack of specificity in the immune responses to these organisms in patients with sarcoidosis. High antibody titers to viruses [e.g., Epstein–Barr virus (EBV), type 6 human T-cell leukemia virus (HTLV-1)], and bacteria (*Borrelia burgdorferi, Chlamydia,* others) are likely the result of nonspecific hypergammaglobulinemia and not representative of specific infectious agents in sarcoidosis. Despite these

inconclusive reports, observations that transplant recipients with sarcoidosis develop granulomas in their allografts and that disseminated granulomatous inflammation has developed in nonsarcoidosis patients transplanted
with organs from donors with sarcoidosis support the possibility that sarcoidosis is caused by a transmissible agent (9,48).

Reports of time–space clustering, seasonal variation, and occupational
associations (e.g., health care workers, firefighters) suggest that environmental exposures could trigger the onset of sarcoidosis (24,50). Chronic
beryllium disease, a granulomatous lung disease found in a minority of
workers exposed to beryllium dusts, is histologically identical to pulmonary
sarcoidosis, supporting the possibility that noninfectious, environmental
factors may play a causal role in sarcoidosis (26). The lack of systemic
features typical of sarcoidosis in chronic beryllium disease suggests that
beryllium is not a direct cause of sarcoidosis throughout the world.

Without a clearly defined environmental or infectious etiology of sarcoidosis, other investigators have suggested that sarcoidosis is a form of
autoimmune disease. Consistent with this possibility, sarcoidosis is associated with hypergammaglobulinemia, immune complex formation, abnor-
mally high antibody titers to a variety of infectious agents, and cytokine
dysregulation (62,92).

A diagnosis of sarcoidosis is established on the basis of a compatible
clinical picture, evidence of noncaseating granulomas on biopsy of involved
tissues, and exclusion of malignancy, infectious granulomatous disorders
such as tuberculosis or fungal disease, and environmental granulomatous
disorders. A biopsy sample of a skin nodule, a superficial lymph node, a
lacrimal gland, nasal mucosae, or conjunctivae may provide histological
confirmation of a diagnosis of sarcoidosis when these tissues are inflamed.
Commonly, bronchoscopic biopsy is employed to confirm a diagnosis of
pulmonary sarcoidosis.

The clinical course is highly variable in sarcoidosis (102,129). Overall,
50 to 65% of patients will undergo spontaneous remission, usually (>85%)
within the first 2 years. Over 80% of patients with Löfgren's syndrome have
spontaneous remissions, usually within several months. Other patients have
persistent pulmonary inflammation that results in progressive fibrocystic
changes and respiratory insufficiency. Estimates of patients with clinically
apparent sarcoidosis who die as a result of their disease, usually from
pulmonary or cardiac involvement, range from under 1% to 6% (38,102,
129). An analysis of mortality data from U.S. hospitals from 1979 to 1991
found that 0.02% of the total deaths in the United States were caused by
sarcoidosis (38). In the United States, age-adjusted mortality rates were
found to be consistently higher in blacks than in whites, supporting the
clinical impression of more serious disease in the former group, although

the results may also reflect a higher incidence of the disease in this population (38,112).

The standard treatment for sarcoidosis is corticosteroid therapy for patients with progressive organ dysfunction. Although there is general agreement that corticosteroids can improve organ function in most patients, controversy continues over whether steroid treatment alters the long-term course of the disease (24). Alternative therapies are available for selected clinical presentations including upper respiratory tract sarcoidosis (see Sec. II). For example, hydroxychloroquine, chloroquine, or methotrexate may be useful in mucocutaneous disease (130). Limited data on the effectiveness of other nonsteroidal alternatives in pulmonary and visceral sarcoidosis have led to controversies over the roles of these agents in the management of sarcoidosis.

II. Sarcoidosis of the Upper Respiratory Tract (SURT)

Sarcoidosis of the upper respiratory tract has been described in 5 to 17% of patients, usually in those with long-standing disease (57,58,100,148). In children, sarcoidosis of the upper respiratory tract is rare, with only anecdotal case reports in the literature (117). The nasal mucosa and overlying skin, nasal bone, nasopharyngeal and sinusal mucosa, and laryngeal structures may be involved with granulomatous inflammation. Lupus pernio, a particularly disfiguring form of cutaneous sarcoidosis of the face, in which violaceous plaques and nodules cover the nasal alae, nose, cheeks, eyelids, ears, and neckline, is a common accompaniment of nasal sarcoidosis (57,58,100). In 1889, Besnier coined the term "lupus pernio" in one of the earliest known patients with sarcoidosis who had cutaneous facial nodules and nasal mucosal lesions (15).

A. Sinonasal Manifestations

SURT commonly affects the nasal mucosa of the septum and inferior turbinates and sinus tissues. Presenting symptoms of nasal sarcoidosis include nasal congestion, dizziness, crusting, epistaxis, anosmia, rhinorrhea, or sinusitis (67,100). Nasal congestion may be severe and is often unresponsive to decongestants and inhaled nasal steroids. Granulomatous inflammation may cause destruction of contiguous bone, leading to nasal septal perforation and a "saddle nose" deformity, particularly in patients who have undergone submucous resection (66,67,87). The authors have also treated two patients with orbital bone destruction secondary to the effects of granulomatous inflammation in the maxillary sinus. Palatal perforation has also been described. Granulomatous inflammation of the maxillary, ethmoid, and sphenoid sinuses in sarcoidosis manifests with congestion, pain, and swelling, and often, recurrent infectious sinusitis. One report documented a case of mucormycosis in a patient with nasal sarcoidosis who presented with necrotic nasal discharge, proptosis, or periorbital edema (4).

B. Oropharyngeal Manifestations

Granulomatous inflammation of salivary, parotid, and lacrimal glands may result in enlarged, tender glands in less than 5% of patients with sarcoidosis (75,84). Involvement of these tissues may result in a sicca syndrome (i.e., dry mouth and dry eyes). Occasionally, parotid enlargement is massive, mimicking mumps. A presentation of fever, parotid enlargement, facial palsy, and uveitis with bilateral hilar adenopathy, known as uveoparotid fever, or Hëërfordt's syndrome, is an uncommon manifestation of sarcoidosis. Gallium-67 scan uptake in the parotid, lacrimal, and salivary glands may result in a "panda" sign in patients with significant involvement of these glands. When seen in conjuction with bilateral uptake in the hilar region and right paratracheal region (i.e., a "lambda" sign) the combination (lambda–panda) sign is reported to be highly suggestive of sarcoidosis (137). In one case report oropharyngeal sarcoidosis, involving primarily the base of the tongue, presented as obstructive sleep apnea associated with dysphagia for solids (36).

C. Laryngeal Manifestations

Laryngeal sarcoidosis is an uncommon manifestation of sarcoidosis, occurring in less than 1% to 5% of patients, and rarely as the sole manifestation of sarcoidosis (17,84,99). Presenting symptoms include hoarseness, dysphonia, dysphagia, or dyspnea. Rarely, stridor, vocal cord paralysis, or acute respiratory failure secondary to upper airway obstruction requiring emergent tracheostomy has been reported (17,145). The most common physical findings of laryngeal sarcoidosis are supraglottic edema with paleness and diffuse thickening with infiltration of the epiglottis, subglottis, aryepiglottic folds, and false cords. Nodules are occasionally seen. Biopsy of the laryngeal tissues reveals submucosal noncaseating granulomas. As with nasal sarcoidosis, laryngeal involvement is frequently associated with chronic skin lesions, particularly lupus pernio.

D. Tracheal Manifestations

Rare examples of tracheal stenosis have been reported in sarcoidosis (18,47,67,73,111). In several cases, stenosis of the major bronchi either alone or accompanied by tracheal stenosis has been found (18,47). Tracheal stenosis secondary to sarcoidosis may lead to dyspnea, stridor, wheezing, or high-pitched inspiratory squeaks. Physical signs of major airway stenosis include chest tightness, wheezing, and stridor. Pulmonary function tests demonstrating fixed or variable extrathoracic airflow obstruction have been described.

III. Pulmonary Sarcoidosis and Intrathoracic Airway Disease

The most common symptoms of pulmonary sarcoidosis are cough and shortness of breath, usually of a progressive, insidious nature (75,84,90). These symptoms may be a manifestation of predominantly interstitial lung involvement, obstructive airway disease, or both. The cough is typically nonproductive and may be severe. Dyspnea is characteristically worse with exertion. Sputum production and hemoptysis are frequent in patients with chronic fibrocystic sarcoidosis, a condition that can be associated with bronchiectasis and recurrent respiratory infections. Chest tightness and wheezing are not uncommon, particularly with endobronchial disease or fibrocystic changes, but are rarely the only manifestations. Physical findings of pulmonary sarcoidosis are usually minimal. Crackles are found in less than 20% of patients with sarcoidosis in the absence of obvious heart failure. Wheezes are found in a small minority of patients, generally in those with bronchial hyperreactivity. Clubbing is rare, even in advanced fibrocystic sarcoidosis.

A. Chest Radiography

By international convention, the chest roentenogram in patients with sarcoidosis is divided into stages or types (79,90,102,129). A normal chest radiograph, or stage 0, is found in 5 to 10% of patients with sarcoidosis, frequently in those with extrapulmonary manifestations of sarcoidosis. A stage I chest radiograph, seen in 40 to 50% of patients on initial presentation, is characterized by bilateral hilar adenopathy with clear lung fields. Right-sided paratracheal adenopathy often accompanies the bilateral adenopathy. A stage II chest radiograph, characterized by bilateral hilar adenopathy and pulmonary infiltrates, is seen in 30 to 50% of patients. Commonly, the infiltrates demonstrate fine, linear markings and small reticulonodules. When interstitial infiltrates are seen without evidence of hilar adenopathy, the chest radiograph is designated as stage III. This radiographic pattern is recognized in 15 to 20% of patients on initial presentation. Patients with evidence of fibrosis on chest radiographs are often designated as stage IV. Radiographic findings include cephalad hilar retraction, volume loss, coarse fibrous strands, small and large bullae, cystic changes and honeycombing from destructive inflammation, and distortion of lung tissue by fibrosis.

Computed tomography (CT) may detect enlarged mediastinal nodes or parenchymal infiltrates that are not visualized on plain chest radiograph (14,97). As might be expected, CT findings of fibrocystic changes, honeycombing, and bronchiectasis indicate a poor response to therapy. In contrast, more diffuse ground-glass opacities, thought to represent inflammation of the interstitium, often demonstrate improvement upon follow-up CT scanning. High resolution, thin-section CT images (1.0–1.5 mm slices) provide radiographic evidence that nodular parenchymal infiltrates tend to follow bronchovascular structures, an observation that helps explain the frequent involvement of airways in sarcoidosis (14). CT scanning may also demonstrate small-airway obstruction in sarcoidosis (40,68,97). For example, Lenique and colleagues found that in 65% of patients, CT scans showed bronchial abnormalities that closely correlated with mucosal thickening and/ or bronchial granulomas (68). CT imaging may also help delineate less common manifestations of sarcoidosis in the chest including mycetomas, major airway stenoses, or superimposed malignancy.

B. Pulmonary Function Tests

Pulmonary function tests have only a modest correlation with chest radiographs (14,79,97,101,129). In patients with type I chest radiographs, pulmonary function tests are normal in about 80% of patients; some have an isolated reduction in diffusing capacity. However, forced vital capacity (FVC), forced expiratory volume in one second (FEV_1), and the lung's diffusing capacity for carbon monoxide (DLCO) may be normal even when the chest radiograph shows pulmonary infiltrates. When pulmonary infiltrates are present on chest radiograph, restrictive impairment with reduction in lung volumes, FVC, and FEV_1 is found in 40 to 70% of patients. Reduction in diffusing capacity can be seen in association with restrictive impairment or as an isolated deficit. Gas exchange is usually preserved until extensive fibrocystic changes are evident, in contrast to idiopathic pulmonary fibrosis, where hypoxemia is found early in the course of the disease. Carbon dioxide retention is unusual except in advanced pulmonary disease.

Airflow obstruction assessed by spirometry or flow–volume curves is present in 30 to 70% of patients with pulmonary sarcoidosis depending on the stage of chest radiograph (6,30,44,61,88,107,124,136). When more sensitive techniques are used, the frequency of airway abnormalities increases even more (32,69). For example, Levinson and coworkers reported that airway function was abnormal in all 18 patients (11 smokers) with restrictive pulmonary sarcoidosis by at least one of a battery of tests (69). Reduced FEV_1/FVC ratios were found in 6 of 18 patients, all of whom had reduced lung volumes or DLCO. Increased upstream airway resistance was found in 16 of 18 patients, though 11 of these patients were smokers. Dutton and coworkers found that 12 of 24 patients with sarcoidosis had small-airway disease determined by the frequency dependence of compliance or the ratio of closing volume to vital capacity; 6 of 24 patients had evidence of large-airway disease by either reduced FEV_1/FVC ratios or airways resistance (R_{aw}) measurement (32). They suggested synergism between sarcoidosis and smoking and airways disease that could lead to significant hyperinflation of the lung. Harrison and coworkers found that a decrease in FEV_1/FVC ratio was the most common physiological abnormality in 107 patients with recently diagnosed sarcoidosis, with 57% having airflow obstruction and only 27% with reduced DLCO and 7% restrictive impairment (44). Overall, pulmonary function tests results suggestive of small-airways obstruction were found in 30 to 50% of patients with stage I chest radiographs and 44 to 73% in those with stage II chest radiographs. Sharma and Johnson studied 123 black American nonsmoking patients with sarcoidosis and found airway obstruction in 78 (63%), a frequency that was considerably higher than the historical frequency reported for white European and American patients and Japanese patients (124). In this study, the degree of airways obstruction did not correlate with the radiological staging of the disease, since significant obstructive impairment was present even in patients with stage 1 disease or a normal roentgenogram. Other studies have shown that obstructive impairment is found in essentially all patients with more advanced fibrocystic disease, no doubt as a result of bullous and fibrocystic changes and associated bronchiectasis (88). In addition to severe airflow limitation, reductions in lung volumes, hypoxemia, and reduced exercise capacity are typically seen in these patients.

C. Pathological Correlates of Intrathoracic Airway Disease

Obstructive airways disease has multiple pathological correlates in sarcoidosis (68,70,75,118). First, sarcoidosis may result in airways dysfunction by compressing or narrowing the lumina of large airways by extrinsic compression by enlarged lymph nodes or confluent neighboring granulomatous lesions (75). Second, noncaseating granulomatous inflammation involving the endobronchial mucosa may result in narrowing or occlusion of the airway lumen. Bronchial or bronchiolar granulomas are seen over 50% of open-lung biopsy specimens (118). Bjermer and coworkers found that nearly half of all endobronchial biopsy specimens were positive for granulomatous inflammation in sarcoidosis (16). Third, airways may be narrowed by granulomatous inflammation of parenchymal bronchovascular structures (68). The resultant scarring of supporting airways structures frequently leads to distortion of airways with traction emphysema, bronchitis, and bronchiectasis. Finally, bronchial hyperresponsiveness, which may have its origin in the narrowing of the airways from endobronchial granulomatous inflammation, edema, or effects on neuromuscular function, may contribute to the symptomatic presentation of airflow obstruction (12,88).

D. Bronchostenosis

Bronchoscopic studies suggest that partial obstruction of bronchial airways may be seen in 2 to 26% of patients undergoing this procedure (107,142). Symptomatic bronchostenosis occurs in less than 10% of patients but can cause wheezing, stridor, high-pitched inspiratory squeaks, and mild to severe respiratory distress (43,58,142). Bronchostenosis may result from extrinsic compression from enlarged hilar nodes or distortion of airways from scarring of supporting airways structures, or granulomatous inflammation of endobronchial mucosa. Often, the stenotic lesions are multiple, involving lobar, segmental, or subsegmental bronchi (58,107). Lobar atelectasis secondary to compression of bronchi by enlarged hilar nodes has been described in sarcoidosis (20,86,98,107,135). The right middle lobe is most frequently affected, likely because of its often small size, fishmouth opening, and the presence of nearby lymph nodes (98,135). Atelectasis of the upper lobe segments in the absence of fibrocystic changes is less common. The rarity of lobar atelectasis in sarcoidosis should always lead to consideration of alternative diagnoses such as mediastinal fibrosis, tuberculosis, or malignancy.

Bronchography has documented single or multiple segmental tracheal or bronchial stenoses, sometimes associated with stenotic webs, bronchiectasis, and poststenotic dilatation in sarcoidosis (107,142). More recently, computed tomography and magnetic resonance imaging have been found useful in delineating anatomical structures in tracheal and bronchial stenosis and have largely replaced bronchography (68,86).

E. Bronchial Hyperresponsiveness

A factor that may contribute to airflow limitation in sarcoidosis is the presence of bronchial hyperresponsiveness, found in about 20% of patients (12,105,106,128). Bechtel and colleagues found that 10 of 20 patients with sarcoidosis demonstrated increased methacholine responsiveness (12). These responders tended to be more symptomatic and to have more airway obstruction, smaller vital capacities, and lower single-breath diffusion capacities for carbon monoxide, although the differences did not reach statistical significance. The results suggested that hyperresponsiveness could contribute to airway obstruction and respiratory symptoms in sarcoidosis. Manresa Presas and coworkers also reported that 50% of patients with stage I sarcoidosis demonstrated bronchial hyperresponsiveness to methacholine, though there were no differences between responders and nonresponders (82). In contrast, Olafsson and coworkers found no increase in the frequency of bronchial hyperreactivity in stage I and II sarcoidosis with normal spirometry (106).

F. Smoking and Sarcoidosis

The influence of smoking on sarcoidosis appears to be complex. The frequency of small-airways disease in smokers with sarcoidosis was noted to be significantly higher than in smokers without sarcoidosis (32). On the other hand, Valeyre and coworkers found that patients with sarcoidosis were less likely to smoke than an aged-matched group in the general population (30 vs 46% smokers) (143). Furthermore, they found that the severity of sarcoidosis appeared to be the same in these two groups, suggesting that the reason for this negative association was not related to reduction in the severity of their disease. These findings have been confirmed more recently by the ACCESS study, which found a highly significant negative association between active and passive smoking and the risk of developing sarcoidosis (presented in 2000 at the American Thoracic Society International Conference). Valeyre et al. suggested that smoking might reduce the likelihood of developing sarcoidosis by enhancing the accumulation of alveolar macrophages in the lower respiratory tract. Although the mechanisms underlying these observations are unclear and may differ, the frequency and degree of small-airways obstruction in patients with sarcoidosis who smoke suggest that smoking may be an important contributor to respiratory symptoms in active pulmonary sarcoidosis.

IV. Diagnosis

A diagnosis of SURT is frequently based on a compatible clinical presentation and biopsy of non–upper respiratory tract tissues (e.g., skin, cervical lymph node, or transbronchial biopsy when there is associated pulmonary involvement). Biopsy of the nasal mucosa, sinus tissue, or laryngeal tissue may confirm a diagnosis of SURT when the diagnosis is in question or when the clinical manifestations are dominated by upper respiratory tract findings. Differential diagnoses include Wegener's granulomatosis, mycobacterial or fungal infections, malignancy, Milkerson–Rosenthal syndrome, Sjögren's syndrome, or Crohn's disease (101). The presence of SURT may be suggested by abnormal flow–volume curves consistent with variable extrathoracic upper airway obstruction (17).

Fiberoptic bronchoscopy is frequently used to confirm a diagnosis of pulmonary sarcoidosis because of the high yield and relative safety of the procedure. The yield ranges from 40% to over 90% when pulmonary infiltrates are seen radiographically, and at least four to six transbronchial biopsy specimens are taken (39,79). When hilar adenopathy alone is present on routine chest radiography, the yield of transbronchial biopsy may approach 50%, indicating that subclinical granulomatous inflammation is present despite an absence of radiographic infiltrates. Extensive fibrocystic sarcoidosis has a low yield owing to extensive parenchyma fibrosis and distorted airways.

Widespread endobronchial nodules (cobblestoning of the airways) are highly suggestive of sarcoidosis and when biopsied, demonstrate granulomas in 40 to 55% of cases (7,16,139). A recent study found endobronchial abnormalities in 55% of 154 patients with biopsy-proven sarcoidosis undergoing diagnostic bronchoscopy (139). Abnormalities included erythema, nodules, plaques, and cobblestoning. Endobronchial biopsies were positive in 71% of patients (85% of black and 38% white patients) regardless of the visual abnormalities; 2 of 4 patients with normal appearing mucosa also had positive biopsy results. A prospective study of 34 patients (65% African American) found that the addition of samples from endobronchial biopsies increased the yield of transbronchial biopsy results by 20%, with no added complications (127). These results confirm that endobronchial abnormalities are common in sarcoidosis and that bronchial biopsies may enhance the yield of bronchoscopic biopsy procedures even in the absence of visual abnormalities.

A. Nonhistological Approaches to Diagnosis

Landmark studies in the early 1980s established that active pulmonary sarcoidosis is characterized by an increase in the proportion of lymphocytes recovered by bronchoalveolar lavage (20–50%) compared with normal (< 10% lymphocytes) (51,146). Furthermore, in approximately 90% of cases, BAL lymphocytes are typified by a dominance of $CD4^+$ T cells in contrast to the $CD8^+$ BAL lymphocytosis seen in hypersensitivity pneumonitis, viral infections, and many drug reactions (51). Although elevated $CD4^+$ BAL lymphocytosis may support a diagnosis of sarcoidosis, studies from around the world have led to the generally held view that neither BAL lymphocytosis nor elevated $CD4^+/CD8^+$ ratios findings are sufficiently predictive to establish a diagnosis of sarcoidosis in absence of biopsy evidence of granulomatous inflammation (24).

Levels of serum angiotensin-converting enzyme (ACE) are elevated in 30 to 80% of patients with clinically active disease but are also seen in many conditions, including tuberculosis, chronic beryllium disease, hyperthyroidism, and fungal infections (25,72). Given the low specificity of this test, with positive and negative predictive values of less than 70 to 80%, a consensus view is that ACE levels are of limited utility in the diagnosis and management of sarcoidosis (25).Total-body gallium-67 scans are nonspecific with the possible exception of a panda plus lambda pattern, which may support a diagnosis of sarcoidosis (137). Occasionally, gallium scans are useful to identify potential sites for biopsy in patients with neurosarcoidosis and no easily accessible sites of inflammatory involvement.

V. Immunopathogenesis

The pathological hallmark of sarcoidosis is the presence of compact epithelioid cell granulomas (75,90). The dominant cell in the central core is the epithelioid cell, thought to be a differentiated form of a mononuclear phagocyte. Typically, $CD4^+$ lymphocytes and mature macrophages are interspersed throughout the epithelioid core, while both $CD4^+$ and $CD8^+$ lymphocytes are found around the periphery of the granuloma. Giant cells, occasionally with cytoplasmic inclusions such as asteroid bodies and Schaumann bodies, are scattered within the inflammatory locus. Granulomas may resolve leaving little evidence of their prior presence, or they may develop fibrotic changes that usually begin in the periphery and travel centrally. Hyalinized granulomas and fibrosis are often characteristic of chronic, long-standing sarcoidosis.

Immunohistochemical studies of sarcoid tissue and analyses of bronchoalveolar lavage specimens have shown that T cells at sites of sarcoid inflammation express high levels of class II MHC molecules (DR, DQ, DP), receptors for interleukin 2 (IL-2), CD45R0, (very late activation antigen 1) (VLA-1), and members of tumor necrosis factor–ligand and TNF–receptor superfamilies (2,123). These activated T cells at sites of inflammation express lymphokines known to be involved in granuloma formation (e.g., IL-2, IFN-γ, TFN-α), and molecules that function in monocyte chemotaxis and migration inhibition (1,2,65,91,94,110,116).

Most circulating T cells and T cells recovered by bronchoalveolar lavage recognize specific antigenic peptide–MHC complexes by the $\alpha\beta^+$ T-cell antigen receptor (TCR), whereas a minority express a $\gamma\delta^+$ TCR (27). The hypervariable regions of these receptors is derived from imprecisely rearranged variable (V), diversity (D) (β and δ only), and joining (J) segments of the TCR chains that contact specific peptide fragments displayed between the α helices of an MHC molecule. Importantly, BAL studies have revealed that BAL T cells of patients with sarcoidosis have a reduced density of the antigen-specific T-cell receptor compared with healthy controls, in keeping with recent activation through this surface receptor (31). Consistent with antigen-specific T-cell activation in sarcoidosis, subgroups of patients have been identified with biased expression of specific Vβ, Vα, or γδ$^+$ TCR genes in the lung or blood (33,34,42,93,95,140). For example, Swedish investigators have found preferential expansion of Vα2.3$^+$ T cells in the lungs of Swedish patients expressing HLA-DR17(3) haplotypes (42). Preferential expression of specific TCR Vβ genes has also been seen among T cells at sites of granulomatous inflammation of Kveim–Siltzbach skin reactions (64). Sequence analyses of TCR genes from expanded αβ$^+$ and γδ$^+$ T cells among lung and skin T-cell populations in sarcoidosis have shown that these subsets are oligoclonal, strongly supportive of the concept that sarcoidosis is driven by T cells stimulated by conventional antigens (93). The discovery of the chemical nature of the peptides or compounds that stimulate these specific T-cell subsets may provide insight into the etiology of sarcoidosis.

Alveolar macrophages and monocytes from patients with sarcoidosis demonstrate features of activated, proinflammatory cells. Alveolar macrophages from patients with sarcoidosis express higher levels of transferrin receptors and IL-2 receptors and contain increased amounts of and produce higher levels of reactive oxygen species, lysozyme, ACE, and 1,25-dihydroxy vitamin D than normal alveolar macrophages (138). A high level of MHC class II (DR, DQ) molecules, adhesion molecules (CD49a, CD54, CD102), and accessory molecules CD86 (B7.2), CD80 (B7.1), and CD40 on these cells likely contributes to the enhanced ability of these cells to present antigen compared with alveolar macrophages from healthy controls (80,103, 149). Alveolar macrophages from patients with sarcoidosis demonstrate enhanced production of the proinflammatory cytokines TNF-α, IL-6, IL-8, IL-15, granulocyte-macrophage colony-stimulating factor (GM-CSF), and possibly IL-1 (1,138). Chemotactic cytokines (chemokines) such as macrophage chemotactic protein 1 (MCP-1), RANTES, monocyte inhibitory protein 1 (MIP-1), and IL-16 have been described in BAL or tissue specimens in sarcoidosis that likely play an important role in recruiting CD4$^+$ T cells and activated mononuclear cells to sites of inflammation (133). Importantly, alveolar macrophages from patients with active pulmonary sarcoidosis have also been shown to produce excess amounts of IL-12 and IL-18, cytokines critical to T helper 1 (TH1) cell development and important in the production of IFN-γ by T cells and natural killer (NK) cells (41,94,126).

A conceptual framework for understanding the mechanisms of granulomatous inflammation in sarcoidosis is provided by the TH1/TH2 paradigm in which the pattern of cytokines expressed by activated CD4$^+$ (and CD8$^+$) T cells largely determines the nature of an immune response (96,125). Differentiated TH1 cells express IFN-γ, IL-2, and lymphotoxin, which are important in macrophage activation, lymphocyte proliferation, and cell-mediated immune responses. TH2 cells express IL-4, IL-5, IL-9, and IL-13, cytokines that are important in antibody-mediated responses, macrophage suppression, and antihelminthic and allergic responses. TH1 and TH2 subsets show cross-regulation, with IFN-γ from TH1 cells downregulating cytokine production and proliferation by TH2 cells, and IL-4 downregulating IFN-γ production by TH1 cells (96,141). Polarization toward either type 1 or type 2 cytokine patterns is seen in the evolution of immune responses in many infectious and autoimmune processes, including leprosy, tuberculosis, and schistosomiasis (125,141).

Recent studies of TCR and cytokine gene expression in sarcoidosis support the concept that sarcoidosis is an antigen-driven, TH1-mediated granulomatous disorder, dominated by enhanced expression of IFN-γ, IL-12, and IL-18 with little or no expression of type 2 cytokines, IL-4 or IL-5 (41,91,94,126,144). IFN-γ is a potent costimulator of IL-12, and IL-12 potently enhances IFN-γ production, allowing a positive feedback loop that can perpetuate a TH1-dependent granulomatous response in sarcoidosis. Our group has speculated that any etiological agent of sarcoidosis has the ability to both nonspecifically induce IL-12 production from mononuclear phagocytes and induce a disease-specific, adaptive T-cell immune response (91,94). Consistent with this hypothesis, Zissel and coworkers found that spontaneous BAL cell production of T-cell growth factor β (TGF-β), a potent inhibitor of IL-12 and TH1 cytokine production, was greater in patients with active disease who underwent spontaneous remission than in patients who required therapy or had progressive disease (150). The determinants of the chronic, fibrotic outcome in 10 to 20% of patients with sarcoidosis are not known, but profibrotic cytokines are known to be produced in the lungs of patients with pulmonary sarcoidosis. TGF-β, insulin-like growth factor 1 (IGF-1), and fibronectin are present in lung biopsy specimens from patients with pulmonary sarcoidosis, suggesting that the persistent production of these and other profibrotic mediators is critical in the development of pulmonary fibrosis in patients who do not undergo remission of their inflammatory response (91,138). Whether this fibrosis occurs in the context of tissue damage from unremitting TH1-mediated inflammation or results from a switch to a more fibrosis-prone TH2-mediated cytokine milieu has not yet been established.

VI. Clinical Course and Treatment

Several studies have demonstrated that radiographic staging provides prognostic information in sarcoidosis (102,129). Patients presenting with a type I chest radiograph have the best overall prognosis, with 60 to 90% having spontaneous remissions. In contrast, only 40 to 70% of patients with a stage II chest radiograph and 10 to 20% of patients with a stage III chest radiograph undergo spontaneous remission. Spontaneous remission is rare with stage IV disease. Remission occurs within 2 years in over 85% of patients who eventually undergo remission. Severe pulmonary sarcoidosis, nasal sarcoidosis, and lupus pernio rarely undergo spontaneous remission, and treatment should not be delayed in the presence of significant symptoms (59,75, 84,90).

Patients who present with Löfgren's syndrome or a type I chest radiograph (in the absence of significant extrapulmonary disease) usually do not need to be treated with corticosteroids because most of them will undergo spontaneous remission. Threatened organ failure such as severe ocular, central nervous system, or cardiac disease should always be promptly treated with high doses of corticosteroids (24).

A. Treatment of Sarcoidosis of the Upper Respiratory Tract

Inhaled nasal steroids are often tried in nasal sarcoidosis with occasionally positive responses. However, severe nasal and sinus sarcoidosis require systemic therapy (Table 1). The antimalarial drugs chloroquine and hydroxychloroquine have been used as first-line drugs for lupus pernio, other disfiguring sarcoidosis skin disease, and nasal sarcoidosis when there are no specific indications for corticosteroid therapy because of pulmonary or systemic sarcoidosis (58,75,84,130). Beneficial effects may not be evident for 2 to 3 months, with overall response rates approximating 35 to 50%. Chloroquine may be useful in chronic laryngeal sarcoidosis, though steroids are usually used initially to prevent acute airway obstruction. Because of the potential for irreversible ocular toxicity with chloroquine, low doses of the drug (250 mg/day) are usually prescribed for 6-months interval followed by a 6-month drug-free period (59). Serial ophthalmological evaluations should be performed every 3 to 4 months during therapy. Hydroxycholorquine appears to be less efficacious, but this drug may be used for prolonged periods without causing retinal toxicity. For this reason, hydroxychloroquine is often tried before chloroquine. Corticosteroids alone are usually effective in the treatment of symptomatic sarcoidosis of the nasal, sinus, and laryngeal structures, though frequently moderate daily doses of corticosteroids (e.g., 10–20 mg/day) are required for significant symptomatic control. Methotrexate has also been used for severe upper respiratory tract

Table 1 Treatment of Sarcoidosis of the Upper Respiratory Tract

Drug	Effectiveness	Usual dose	Major side effects
Initial therapy			
Topical nasal steroids	< 10%	Product dependent	Irritation
Hydroxychloroquine sulfate	< 35–50%	200 mg every 24 h to every 12 h	Gastrointestinal symptoms, retinopathy (rare)
Chloroquine phosphate	< 50%	500 mg every 24 h for 2 weeks 500 mg every 48 h for 5 1/2 months 6 months drug free	Retinopathy, gastrointestinal symptoms
Oral corticosteroids	> 75%	30–40 mg every 24 h for 2 weeks Taper by 5 mg every 2 weeks Maintenance dose 5–10 mg every 24 h for chronic disease	Cushingoid habitus, weight gain, hypertension, hyperglycemia, osteoporosis
Recalcitrant disease			
Methotrexate	< 50%	5–15 mg/week	Hepatic toxicity, pulmonary toxicity, bone marrow suppression, gastrointestinal toxicity

sarcoidosis and lupus pernio with anecdotal successes (45,58). The potential effectiveness of pentoxifylline or thalidomide (see later) in SURT is not known. The role of surgery in the management of severe sinonasal disease with significant anatomical blockage is controversial, with anecdotal reports of postsurgical worsening of symptoms due to increased disease activity, and one small retrospective study reporting symptomatic improvement when surgery was used in conjunction with nasal steroids (63).

B. Treatment of Tracheobronchial Stenosis

Steroid therapy is indicated for symptomatic tracheobronchial stenosis related to granulomatous inflammation in sarcoidosis. Improvements in physiological function and resolution in stenosis have been reported in response to corticosteroid therapy (23,113). However, response to therapy is often poor, particularly in the presence of fixed stenosis (107). Mechanical dilatation has been attempted in selected cases with some successes reported (35,135). For example, Fouty and coworkers described six patients with symptomatic and refractory airway stenosis who were symptomatically improved following dilatation with a Fogarty embolectomy catheter of the stenotic areas under direct bronchoscopic vision (35).

C. Treatment of Pulmonary Sarcoidosis

Indications for corticosteroid therapy in pulmonary sarcoidosis remain controversial (24,60). Asymptomatic patients with normal lung function or patients with minimal symptoms and mild functional abnormalities are usually observed without treatment until there is disease progression. Progressive, disabling dyspnea and cough with progressive radiographic findings or pulmonary impairment is considered to be an indication for a course of therapy. Low dose corticosteroid therapy also is usually prescribed for patients with advanced fibrocystic disease, with the goal of preventing or slowing further progression of respiratory insufficiency.

Corticosteroids remain the cornerstone of therapy for pulmonary (and organ-threatening extrapulmonary) sarcoidosis. Although controversy exists regarding their overall effectiveness in altering the long-term course of pulmonary disease, there is no disagreement that corticosteroids acutely provide symptomatic relief and reverse organ dysfunction in more than 90% of patients with symptomatic disease. One recent review of controlled clinical trials concluded that oral corticosteroids improved the chest x-ray scores, symptoms, and spirometry over 6 to 24 months but found a lack of data beyond this treatment duration (108). The optimal doses and duration of corticosteroid treatment have not been established by rigorous clinical studies. Initial treatment of pulmonary and systemic sarcoidosis usually begins with 30 to 40 mg/day of prednisone (59). After several months of gradual tapering, a maintenance dose of 5 to 15 mg/day of prednisone can be achieved, which is usually sufficient to suppress progressive lung disease. Alternate-day therapy (e.g., 10–30 mg every other day) can be considered following an initial course of daily-dose corticosteroid therapy to establish the extent of clinical response. Treatment is ordinarily continued for a minimum of 10 to 12 months, since premature tapering is likely to result in relapse of disease. Overall, 16 to 74% of patients experience relapse when steroid therapy is tapered (52,60,84,102,129). Patients who have progressive disease while tapering usually respond to a small increase in daily dose of corticosteroids. Intermittent attempts to taper steroids are appropriate in the first several years of treatment, but patients with repetitive relapses usually require indefinite suppressive therapy.

The long-term benefits of corticosteroid therapy in pulmonary sarcoidosis are not proven by rigorous studies. Some prospective studies of patient groups with a high likelihood of spontaneous remission failed to find any long-term benefit of steroid therapy in altering outcomes in pulmonary sarcoidosis (52,54). A recent multicenter, randomized, double-blind, placebo-controlled trial evaluated the effect of early treatment in 189 patients with stage I and II sarcoidosis presenting with normal pulmonary function tests (109). Patients with stage II sarcoidosis who received 3 months of oral steroid therapy followed by 15 months of inhaled steroids experienced an improvement in FVC and DLCO at 5 years compared with placebo-treated patients. No benefit was seen for the early treatment of stage I sarcoidosis (109). Retrospective studies from centers treating patients with chronic disease suggest that corticosteroids prevent or delay organ dysfunction, though at a cost of drug toxicity (24,60). Importantly, a recent prospective study by the British Thoracic Society Sarcoidosis Study found that chronic maintenance corticosteroid therapy in patients with stage II or III sarcoidosis significantly improved long-term pulmonary function compared with a group treated with intermittent corticosteroid therapy for symptomatic disease (37). This study supports the view that chronic corticosteroid therapy may prevent or delay progressive pulmonary fibrosis in patients with chronic active pulmonary sarcoidosis.

Several studies have investigated the effect of corticosteroid therapy on airflow obstruction, with variable results. Some studies suggest that obstructive disease may improve with institution of corticosteroid therapy (13,85,131). Other studies suggest that corticosteroid therapy may not be helpful in improving small-airways disease (28,29,113). For example, Renzi and colleagues reported that small-airways disease did not improve after 4 months of corticosteroid treatment in patients with stage II or III chest radiographs, though significant improvements were found in diffusion and alveolar–arterial oxygen tension gradients (113). DeRemee and Anderson studied 107 patients with sarcoidosis and found that dyspnea was most frequently associated with expiratory slowing and often distorted, fibrotic changes on chest radiograph (29). This expiratory slowing rarely improved with corticosteroid therapy, and the authors, recommendation was to begin treatment before the onset of dyspnea. Anecdotal experience suggests that a few patients with pulmonary sarcoidosis have progressively severe obstructive lung disease despite moderate doses of daily corticosteroid therapy, with a clinical picture suggestive of bronchiolitis obliterans.

D. Inhaled Corticosteroids

Inhaled corticosteroids may be helpful in reducing symptoms of endobronchial sarcoidosis such as cough or airway irritability. Patients with abnormal bronchial hyperresponsiveness to methacholine and obstructive impairment may have some symptomatic relief with bronchodilators and inhaled steroids. A role for inhaled corticosteroids in the treatment of parenchymal pulmonary sarcoidosis is uncertain. Early studies using beclomethasone failed to show benefit, perhaps because of low drug doses. More recently, several studies have reported some effectiveness of budesonide, a more potent inhaled steroid, in improving symptoms or lung function in pulmonary sarcoidosis (122,132,151). Zych and coworkers found that following 6 weeks of systemic steroids, inhaled budesonide (1.6 mg/day) was comparable to prednisone (10 mg/day) with no difference in pulmonary function tests (151). Selroos also reported that inhaled budesonide 2.4 mg/day was effective in the long-term maintenance of patients with pulmonary sarcoidosis following initial treatment with oral methylprednisolone (122). The overall benefits were modest, dose dependent, and involved patients with mild disease and good prognoses. Other studies failed to demonstrate benefit of inhaled topical steroids, particularly in patients with more advanced disease (3,89). For example, Milman and coworkers found that inhaled budesonide in doses of 1.2 to 2.0 mg/day for one year had no discernible clinical or biochemical effect on pulmonary sarcoidosis in 21 patients with biopsy-proven sarcoidosis (89). Dysphonia and oral thrush are common with budesonide; systemic side effects have also been documented (132). Overall, these studies and anecdotal experiences suggest that inhaled corticosteroids should not be routinely prescribed, except possibly for mild disease, and perhaps in patients who mainly have cough and in whom a short-term (< 6 months) course of inhaled steroids may improve symptoms (108).

E. Methotrexate

Case reports have documented that methotrexate (10–20 mg/week) is useful in treating some patients with severe nasal, sinus, laryngeal, and skin sarcoidosis (58,101). More recently, methotrexate has been proposed as an alternative therapy for pulmonary sarcoidosis that is refractory to low doses of corticosteroid therapy or as a steroid-sparing treatment (11,77). One clinical study found that methotrexate allowed 70% of patients to reduce or eliminate their corticosteroid dose, though improvement in some patients was not noted until after 6 to 12 months of methotrexate therapy (76). Other experiences have not been as favorable, and randomized or comparison clinical trials have not yet been reported. Risks of methotrexate include hepatic toxicity, opportunistic infections, and bone marrow suppression.

F. Azathioprine

Anecdotal experience and several small clinical studies have shown that azathioprine in a dose of 100 to 200 mg/day may be useful in chronic corticosteroid-refractory pulmonary sarcoidosis (24) or as a steroid-sparing therapy (49,71). Bone marrow toxicities, gastrointestinal symptoms, skin rashes and arthralgias, and possibly a slightly increased risk of malignancy are potential drawbacks, but overall the drug is often well tolerated and is used by many clinicians as second-line therapy for severe or progressive pulmonary and extrapulmonary disease. Azathioprine does not appear to be effective in many cases of severe nasal/sinus or skin sarcoidosis.

G. Other Nonsteroidal Agents

Pentoxifylline was found to be beneficial when used alone or with corticosteroids in the initial treatment of pulmonary sarcoidosis in a clinical study from Germany (147). Our anecdotal experience suggests that the drug is effective in only a small minority of patients with mild pulmonary or hepatic disease, and possibly as a steroid-sparing drug. Gastrointestinal side effects and headache may limit dosage to subtherapeutic levels, but given the relative safety of the drug, further studies seem merited. The antimalarial drugs (see earlier) have also been used in the treatment of pulmonary sarcoidosis with varying degrees of success. In a recent randomized trial comparing a prolonged versus short chloroquine course in 18 patients (17 of the initial 21 were white), maintenance treatment was successful in attenuating the decline in lung function observed in the patients off therapy, but at the expense of a high incidence of side effects (8). Anecdotal case reports suggest that thalidomide may be beneficial in pulmonary or cutaneous sarcoidosis (22). Peripheral neurotoxicity and the well-known teratogenicity of the drug limit its attractiveness as a therapeutic agent to carefully selected patients with refractory sarcoidosis. Another single case study reported success with the antileprosy drug clofazimine in laryngeal sarcoidosis (115). Chlorambucil and cyclophosphamide have had anecdotal successes in treating progressive sarcoidosis refractory to corticosteroids, though the oncogenic potential suggests the use of these agents should be extremely limited. Clinical experience has shown that cyclosporine A is ineffective and toxic in pulmonary sarcoidosis; a potential role in severe neurosarcoidosis remains uncertain (134). More recently, there has been an increased interest in evaluating specific TNF-α inhibitory treatment in sarcoidosis. Among the few cases reported, one patient with pulmonary sarcoidosis deemed refractory to more traditional immunosuppressive therapy experienced improvement in the vital capacity with no serious side effects at 16 weeks after initiation of Infliximab therapy (10). However, concerns about the drugs' safety and limited experience with its use prohibit routine treatment with these agents, until more ample studies are performed.

H. Transplantation

Organ transplantation has been performed successfully in patients with end-stage lung, heart, liver, and kidney sarcoidosis. Recurrent granulomas often occur in allografts, but they are usually of little clinical relevance and respond to an increase in immunosuppression (83,104). Despite reoccurrence of granulomas in some patients, survival rates for lung transplantation are comparable to other indications, with 3- and 5-year survival rates of approximately 70 and 56%, respectively (9), although more recent reports give more pessimistic outcomes with 3-year mortality rates of 50% (5). Thus, there is increasing consensus that lung or other organ transplantation should be considered in patients with end-stage sarcoidosis.

Acknowledgments

This work was supported in part by Grant No. HL54658 from the National Heart, Lung, and Blood Institute and the Hospital for the Consumptives of Maryland (Eudowood).

References

1. Agostini C, Trentin L, Facco M, Sancetta R, Cerutti A, Tassinari C, Cimarosto L, Adami F, Cipriani A, Zambello R, Semenzato G. Role of IL-15, IL-2, and their receptors in the development of T cell alveolitis in pulmonary sarcoidosis. J Immunol 1996; 157:910–918.
2. Agostini C, Zambello R, Sancetta R, Cerutti A, Milani A, Tassinari C, Facco M, Cipriani A, Trentin L, Semenzato G. Expression of tumor necrosis factor receptor superfamily members by lung T lymphocytes in interstitial lung disease. Am J Respir Crit Care Med 1996; 153:1359–1367.
3. Alberts C, van der Mark TW, Jansen HM. Inhaled budesonide in pulmonary sarcoidosis: a double-blind, placebo-controlled study. Dutch Study Group on Pulmonary Sarcoidosis. Eur Respir J 1995; 8:682–688.
4. Alloway JA, Buchsbaum RM, Filipov PT, Reynolds BN, Day JA. Mucormycosis in a patient with sarcoidosis. Sarcoidosis 1995; 12:143–146.
5. Arcasoy SM, Christie JD, Pochettino A, Rosengard BR, Blumenthal NP, Bavaria JE, Kotloff RM. Characteristics and outcomes of patients with sarcoidosis listed for lung transplantation. Chest 2001; 120:873–880.
6. Argyropoulou PK, Patakas DA, Louridas GE. Airway function in stage I and stage II pulmonary sarcoidosis. Respiration 1984; 46:17–25.
7. Armstrong JR, Radke JR, Kvale PA, Eichenhorn MS, Popovich J Jr. Endoscopic findings in sarcoidosis. Characteristics and correlations with radiographic staging and bronchial mucosal biopsy yield. Ann Otol Rhinol Laryngol 1981; 90:339–343.
8. Baltzan M, Mehta S, Kirkham TH, Cosio MG. Randomized trial of prolonged chloroquine therapy in advanced pulmonary sarcoidosis. Am J Respir Crit Care Med 1999; 160:192–197.
9. Barbers RG. Role of transplantation (lung, liver, and heart) in sarcoidosis. Clin Chest Med 1997; 18:865–874.

10. Baughman RP, Lower EE. Infliximab for refractory sarcoidosis. Sarcoidosis Vasc Diffuse Lung Dis 2001; 18:70–74.

11. Baughman RP, Winget DB, Lower EE. Methotrexate is steroid sparing in acute sarcoidosis: results of a double blind, randomized trial. Sarcoidosis Vasc Diffuse Lung Dis 2000; 17:60–66.

12. Bechtel JJ, Starr T 3rd, Dantzker DR, Bower JS. Airway hyperreactivity in patients with sarcoidosis. Am Rev Respir Dis 1981; 124:759–761.

13. Benatar SR, Clark TJ. Pulmonary function in a case of endobronchial sarcoidosis. Am Rev Respir Dis 1974; 110:490–496.

14. Bergin CJ, Bell DY, Coblentz CL, Chiles C, Gamsu G, MacIntyre NR, Coleman RE, Putman CE. Sarcoidosis: correlation of pulmonary parenchymal pattern at CT with results of pulmonary function tests. Radiology 1989; 171:619–624.

15. Besnier E. Lupus pernio de la face: sinovites fangeuses (*Scrofulo tuberculensis*) symmetriques des extrémities supérieures. Ann Dermat Syph 1889; 10:333.

16. Bjermer L, Thunell M, Rosenhall L, Stjernberg N. Endobronchial biopsy positive sarcoidosis: relation to bronchoalveolar lavage and course of disease. Respir Med 1991; 85:229–234.

17. Bower JS, Belen JE, Weg JG, Dantzker DR. Manifestations and treatment of laryngeal sarcoidosis. Am Rev Respir Dis 1980; 122:325–332.

18. Brandstetter RD, Messina MS, Sprince NL, Grillo HC. Tracheal stenosis due to sarcoidosis. Chest 1981; 80:656.

19. Bresnitz EA, Strom BL. Epidemiology of sarcoidosis. Epidemiol Rev 1983; 5:124–156.

20. Brown KT, Yeoh CB, Saddekni S. Balloon dilatation of the left main bronchus in sarcoidosis. AJR Am J Roentgenol 1988; 150:553–554.

21. Buck A. Epidemiologic investigations of sarcoidosis. IV$_4$ Discussion and summary. Am J Hyg 1961; 74:189–202.

22. Carlesimo M, Giustini S, Rossi A, Bonaccorsi P, Calvieri S. Treatment of cutaneous and pulmonary sarcoidosis with thalidomide. J Am Acad Dermatol 1995; 32:866–869.

23. Corsello BF, Lohaus GH, Funahashi A. Endobronchial mass lesion due to sarcoidosis: complete resolution with corticosteroids. Thorax 1983; 38:157–158.

24. Costabel U, Hunninghake GW. ATS/ERS/WASOG statement on sarcoidosis. Sarcoidosis Statement Committee. American Thoracic Society. European Respiratory Society. World Association for Sarcoidosis and Other Granulomatous Disorders. Eur Respir J 1999; 14:735–737.

25. Costabel U, Teschler H. Biochemical changes in sarcoidosis. Clin Chest Med 1997; 18:827–842.

26. Cullen MR, Kominsky JR, Rossman MD, Cherniack MG, Rankin JA, Balmes JR, Kern JA, Daniele RP, Palmer L, Naegel GP, et al. Chronic beryllium disease in a precious metal refinery. Clinical epidemiologic and immunologic evidence for continuing risk from exposure to low level beryllium fumes. Am Rev Respir Dis 1987; 135:201–208.

27. Davis MM, Boniface JJ, Reich Z, Lyons D, Hampl J, Arden B, Chien Y.

Ligand recognition by alpha beta T cell receptors. Annu Rev Immunol 1998; 16:523–544.

28. DeRemee RA. The present status of treatment of pulmonary sarcoidosis: a house divided. Chest 1977; 71:388–393.

29. DeRemee RA, Andersen HA. Sarcoidosis: a correlation of dyspnea with roentgenographic stage and pulmonary function changes. Mayo Clin Proc 1974; 49:742–745.

30. Dines DE, Stubbs SE, McDougall JC. Obstructive disease of the airways associated with stage I sarcoidosis. Mayo Clin Proc 1978; 53:788–791.

31. Du Bois RM, Kirby M, Balbi B, Saltini C, Crystal RG. T-lymphocytes that accumulate in the lung in sarcoidosis have evidence of recent stimulation of the T-cell antigen receptor. Am Rev Respir Dis 1992; 145:1205–1211.

32. Dutton RE, Renzi PM, Lopez-Majano V, Renzi GD. Airway function in sarcoidosis: smokers versus nonsmokers. Respiration 1982; 43:164–173.

33. Forman JD, Klein JT, Silver RF, Liu MC, Greenlee BM, Moller DR. Selective activation and accumulation of oligoclonal V beta-specific T cells in active pulmonary sarcoidosis. J Clin Invest 1994; 94:1533–1542.

34. Forrester JM, Wang Y, Ricalton N, Fitzgerald JE, Loveless J, Newman LS, King TE, Kotzin BL. TCR expression of activated T-cell clones in the lungs of patients with pulmonary sarcoidosis. J Immunol 1994; 153:4291–4302.

35. Fouty BW, Pomeranz M, Thigpen TP, Martin RJ. Dilatation of bronchial stenoses due to sarcoidosis using a flexible fiberoptic bronchoscope. Chest 1994; 106:677–680.

36. Fuso L, Maiolo C, Tramaglino LM, Benedetto RT, Russo AR, Spadaro S, Pagliari G. Orolaryngeal sarcoidosis presenting as obstructive sleep apnoea. Sarcoidosis Vasc Diffuse Lung Dis 2001; 18:85–90.

37. Gibson GJ, Prescott RJ, Muers MF, Middleton WG, Mitchell DN, Connolly CK, Harrison BD. British Thoracic Society Sarcoidosis study: effects of long term corticosteroid treatment. Thorax 1996; 51:238–247.

38. Gideon NM, Mannino DM. Sarcoidosis mortality in the United States 1979–1991: an analysis of multiple-cause mortality data. Am J Med 1996; 100:423–427.

39. Gilman MJ. Transbronchial biopsy in sarcoidosis. Chest 1983; 83:159.

40. Gleeson FV, Traill ZC, Hansell DM. Evidence of expiratory CT scans of small-airway obstruction in sarcoidosis. AJR Am J Roentgenol 1996; 166:1052–1054.

41. Greene CM, Meachery G, Taggart CC, Rooney CP, Coakley R, O'Neill SJ, McElvaney NG. Role of IL-18 in CD4[+] T-lymphocyte activation in sarcoidosis. J Immunol 2000; 165:4718–4724.

42. Grunewald J, Janson CH, Eklund A, Ohrn M, Olerup O, Persson U, Wigzell H. Restricted V alpha 2.3 gene usage by CD4[+] T lymphocytes in bronchoalveolar lavage fluid from sarcoidosis patients correlates with HLA-DR3. Eur J Immunol 1992; 22:129–135.

43. Hadfield JW, Page RL, Flower CD, Stark JE. Localised airway narrowing in sarcoidosis. Thorax 1982; 37:443–447.

44. Harrison BD, Shaylor JM, Stokes TC, Wilkes AR. Airflow limitation in sarcoidosis—a study of pulmonary function in 107 patients with newly diagnosed disease. Respir Med 1991; 85:59–64.

45. Henderson CA, Ilchyshyn A, Curry AR. Laryngeal and cutaneous sarcoidosis treated with methotrexate. J R Soc Med 1994; 87:632–633.

46. Henke CE, Henke G, Elveback LR, Beard CM, Ballard DJ, Kurland LT. The epidemiology of sarcoidosis in Rochester, Minnesota: a population-based study of incidence and survival. Am J Epidemiol 1986; 123:840–845.

47. Henry DA, Cho SR. Tracheal stenosis in sarcoidosis. South Med J 1983; 76: 1323–1324.

48. Heyll A, Meckenstock G, Aul C, Sohngen D, Borchard F, Hadding U, Modder U, Leschke M, Schneider W. Possible transmission of sarcoidosis via allogeneic bone marrow transplantation. Bone Marrow Transplant 1994; 14: 161–164.

49. Hof DG HP, Godfrey WA. Long-term use of azathioprine as a steroid sparing treatment for chronic sarcoidosis. Am J Respir Crit Care Med 1996; 153:A870.

50. Hosoda Y, Yamaguchi M, Hiraga Y. Global epidemiology of sarcoidosis. What story do prevalence and incidence tell us? Clin Chest Med 1997; 18:681–694.

51. Hunninghake GW, Crystal RG. Pulmonary sarcoidosis: a disorder mediated by excess helper T-lymphocyte activity at sites of disease activity. N Engl J Med 1981; 305:429–434.

52. Hunninghake GW, Gilbert S, Pueringer R, Dayton C, Floerchinger C, Helmers R, Merchant R, Wilson J, Galvin J, Schwartz D. Outcome of the treatment for sarcoidosis. Am J Respir Crit Care Med 1994; 149:893–898.

53. Ishige I, Usui Y, Takemura T, Eishi Y. Quantitative PCR of mycobacterial and propionibacterial DNA in lymph nodes of Japanese patients with sarcoidosis. Lancet 1999; 354:120–123.

54. Israel HL, Fouts DW, Beggs RA. A controlled trial of prednisone treatment of sarcoidosis. Am Rev Respir Dis 1973; 107:609–614.

55. Israel HL, Karlin P, Menduke H, DeLisser OG. Factors affecting outcome of sarcoidosis. Influence of race, extrathoracic involvement, and initial radiologic lung lesions. Ann N Y Acad Sci 1986; 465:609–618.

56. Iwai K, Tachibana T, Takemura T, Matsui Y, Kitaichi M, Kawabata Y. Pathological studies on sarcoidosis autopsy. I. Epidemiological features of 320 cases in Japan. Acta Pathol Jpn 1993; 43:372–376.

57. James DG. Lupus pernio. Lupus 1992; 1:129–131.

58. James DG, Barter S, Jash D, MacKinnon DM, Carstairs LS. Sarcoidosis of the upper respiratory tract (SURT). J Laryngol Otol 1982; 96:711–718.

59. Johns CJ, Michele TM. The clinical management of sarcoidosis. A 50-year experience at the Johns Hopkins Hospital. Medicine (Baltimore) 1999; 78:65–111.

60. Johns CJ, Zachary JB, Ball WC Jr. A ten-year study of corticosteroid treatment of pulmonary sarcoidosis. Johns Hopkins Med J 1974; 134:271–283.

61. Kaneko K, Sharma OP. Airway obstruction in pulmonary sarcoidosis. Bull Eur Physiopathol Respir 1977; 13:231–240.

62. Kataria YP, Holter JF. Immunology of sarcoidosis. Clin Chest Med 1997; 18:719–739.

63. Kay DJ, Har-El G. The role of endoscopic sinus surgery in chronic sinonasal sarcoidosis. Am J Rhinol 2001; 15:249–254.

64. Klein JT, Horn TD, Forman JD, Silver RF, Teirstein AS, Moller DR. Selection of oligoclonal V beta-specific T cells in the intradermal response to Kveim–Siltzbach reagent in individuals with sarcoidosis. J Immunol 1995; 154:1450–1460.

65. Konishi K, Moller DR, Saltini C, Kirby M, Crystal RG. Spontaneous expression of the interleukin 2 receptor gene and presence of functional interleukin 2 receptors on T lymphocytes in the blood of individuals with active pulmonary sarcoidosis. J Clin Invest 1988; 82:775–781.

66. Krespi YP, Kuriloff DB, Aner M. Sarcoidosis of the sinonasal tract: a new staging system. Otolaryngol Head Neck Surg 1995; 112:221–227.

67. Lefrak S, Di Benedetto R. Systematic sarcoidosis with severe involvement of the upper respiratory tract. Am Rev Respir Dis 1970; 102:801–807.

68. Lenique F, Brauner MW, Grenier P, Battesti JP, Loiseau A, Valeyre D. CT assessment of bronchi in sarcoidosis: endoscopic and pathologic correlations. Radiology 1995; 194:419–423.

69. Levinson RS, Metzger LF, Stanley NN, Kelsen SG, Altose MD, Cherniack NS, Brody JS. Airway function in sarcoidosis. Am J Med 1977; 62:51–59.

70. Lewis MI, Horak DA. Airflow obstruction in sarcoidosis. Chest 1987; 92:582–584.

71. Lewis SJ, Ainslie GM, Bateman ED. Efficacy of azathioprine as second-line treatment in pulmonary sarcoidosis. Sarcoidosis Vasc Diffuse Lung Dis 1999; 16:87–92.

72. Lieberman J. Elevation of serum angiotensin-converting-enzyme (ACE) level in sarcoidosis. Am J Med 1975; 59:365–372.

73. Lindsey JR PH. Sarcoidosis of the upper respiratory tract. Ann Otol 1951; 60:549.

74. Löfgren S. Acta Med Scand 1946; 124:1–197.

75. Longcope WT FD. A study of sarcoidosis based on a combined investigation of 160 cases including 30 autopsies from the Johns Hopkins Hospital and the Massachusetts General Hospital. Medicine 1952; 31:1.

76. Lower EE, Baughman RP. Prolonged use of methotrexate for sarcoidosis. Arch Intern Med 1995; 155:846–851.

77. Lower EE, Baughman RP. The use of low dose methotrexate in refractory sarcoidosis. Am J Med Sci 1990; 299:153–157.

78. Lympany PA, Petrek M, Southcott AM, Newman Taylor AJ, Welsh KI, du Bois RM. HLA-DPB polymorphisms: Glu 69 association with sarcoidosis. Eur J Immunogenet 1996; 23:353–359.

79. Lynch JP 3rd, Kazerooni EA, Gay SE. Pulmonary sarcoidosis. Clin Chest Med 1997; 18:755–785.

80. Maliarik MJ, Chen KM, Major ML, Sheffer RG, Popovich J Jr, Rybicki BA, Iannuzzi MC. Analysis of HLA-DPB1 polymorphisms in African-Americans with sarcoidosis. Am J Respir Crit Care Med 1998; 158:111–114.
81. Mangiapan G, Hance AJ. Mycobacteria and sarcoidosis: an overview and summary of recent molecular biological data. Sarcoidosis 1995; 12:20–37.
82. Manresa Presas F, Romero Colomer P, Rodriguez Sanchon B. Bronchial hyperreactivity in fresh stage I sarcoidosis. Ann N Y Acad Sci 1986; 465:523–529.
83. Martinez FJ, Orens JB, Deeb M, Brunsting LA, Flint A, Lynch JP 3rd. Recurrence of sarcoidosis following bilateral allogeneic lung transplantation. Chest 1994; 106:1597–1599.
84. Mayock RL BP, Morrison CE. Manifestations of sarcoidosis. Am J Med 1963; 35:67–89.
85. Meier-Sydow J, Rust MG, Kappos A, Kronenberger H, Nerger K, Schultze-Werninghaus G. The long-term course of airflow obstruction in obstructive variants of the fibrotic stage of sarcoidosis and of idiopathic pulmonary fibrosis. Ann N Y Acad Sci 1986; 465:515–522.
86. Mendelson DS, Norton K, Cohen BA, Brown LK, Rabinowitz JG. Bronchial compression: an unusual manifestation of sarcoidosis. J Comput Assit Tomogr 1983; 7:892–894.
87. Miglets AW, Viall JH, Kataria YP. Sarcoidosis of the head and neck. Laryngoscope 1977; 87:2038–2048.
88. Miller A, Teirstein AS, Jackler I, Chuang M, Siltzbach LE. Airway function in chronic pulmonary sarcoidosis with fibrosis. Am Rev Respir Dis 1974; 109:179–189.
89. Milman N, Graudal N, Grode G, Munch E. No effect of high-dose inhaled steroids in pulmonary sarcoidosis: a double-blind, placebo-controlled study. J Intern Med 1994; 236:285–290.
90. Mitchell DN, Scadding JG. Sarcoidosis. Am Rev Respir Dis 1974; 110:774–802.
91. Moller DR. Cells and cytokines involved in the pathogenesis of sarcoidosis. Sarcoidosis Vasc Diffuse Lung Dis 1999; 16:24–31.
92. Moller DR. Etiology of sarcoidosis. Clin Chest Med 1997; 18:695–706.
93. Moller DR. Involvement of T cells and alterations in T-cell receptors in sarcoidosis. Semin Respir Infect 1998; 13:174–183.
94. Moller DR, Forman JD, Liu MC, Noble PW, Greenlee BM, Vyas P, Holden DA, Forrester JM, Lazarus A, Wysocka M, Trinchieri G, Karp C. Enhanced expression of IL-12 associated with Th1 cytokine profiles in active pulmonary sarcoidosis. J Immunol 1996; 156:4952–4960.
95. Moller DR, Konishi K, Kirby M, Balbi B, Crystal RG. Bias toward use of a specific T-cell receptor beta-chain variable region in a subgroup of individuals with sarcoidosis. J Clin Invest 1988; 82:1183–1191.
96. Mosmann TR, Coffman RL. TH1 and TH2 cells: different patterns of lymphokine secretion lead to different functional properties. Annu Rev Immunol 1989; 7:145–173.

97. Muller NL, Mawson JB, Mathieson JR, Abboud R, Ostrow DN, Champion P. Sarcoidosis: correlation of extent of disease at CT with clinical, functional, and radiographic findings. Radiology 1989; 171:613–618.

98. Munt PW. Middle lobe atelectasis in sarcoidosis. Report of a case with prompt resolution concomitant with corticosteroid administration. Am Rev Respir Dis 1973; 108:357–360.

99. Neel HB 3rd, McDonald TJ. Laryngeal sarcoidosis: report of 13 patients. Ann Otol Rhinol Laryngol 1982; 91:359–362.

100. Neville E, Mills RG, James DG. Sarcoidosis of the upper respiratory tract and its relation to lupus pernio. Ann N Y Acad Sci 1976; 278:416–426.

101. Neville E, Mills RG, Jash DK, Mackinnon DM, Carstairs LS, James DG. Sarcoidosis of the upper respiratory tract and its association with lupus pernio. Thorax 1976; 31:660–664.

102. Neville E, Walker AN, James DG. Prognostic factors predicting the outcome of sarcoidosis: an analysis of 818 patients. Q J Med 1983; 52:525–533.

103. Nicod LP, Isler P. Alveolar macrophages in sarcoidosis coexpress high levels of CD86 (B7.2), CD40, and CD30L. Am J Respir Cell Mol Biol 1997; 17:91–96.

104. Nunley DR, Hattler B, Keenan RJ, Iacono AT, Yousem S, Ohori NP, Dauber JH. Lung transplantation for end-stage pulmonary sarcoidosis. Sarcoidosis Vasc Diffuse Lung Dis 1999; 16:93–100.

105. Ohrn MB, Skold CM, van Hage-Hamsten M, Sigurdardottir O, Zetterstrom O, Eklund A. Sarcoidosis patients have bronchial hyperreactivity and signs of mast cell activation in their bronchoalveolar lavage. Respiration 1995; 62:136–142.

106. Olafsson M, Simonsson BG, Hansson SB. Bronchial reactivity in patients with recent pulmonary sarcoidosis. Thorax 1985; 40:51–53.

107. Olsson T, Bjornstad-Pettersen H, Stjernberg NL. Bronchostenosis due to sarcoidosis: a cause of atelectasis and airway obstruction simulating pulmonary neoplasm and chronic obstructive pulmonary disease. Chest 1979; 75:663–666.

108. Paramothayan NS, Jones PW. Corticosteroids for pulmonary sarcoidosis. Cochrane Database Syst Rev 2000; 4.

109. Pietinalho A, Tukiainen P, Haahtela T, Persson T, Selroos O. Early treatment of stage II sarcoidosis improves 5-year pulmonary function. Chest 2002; 121:24–31.

110. Pinkston P, Bitterman PB, Crystal RG. Spontaneous release of interleukin-2 by lung T lymphocytes in active pulmonary sarcoidosis. N Engl J Med 1983; 308:793–800.

111. Poe DL SP. Sarcoidosis of the upper respiratory tract. Arch Otolaryngol 1950; 51:414.

112. Reich JM. Course and prognosis of sarcoidosis in African-Americans versus Caucasians. Eur Respir J 2001; 17:833.

113. Renzi GD, Renzi PM, Lopez-Majano V, Dutton RE. Airway function in sarcoidosis: effect of short-term steroid therapy. Respiration 1981; 42:98–104.

114. Richeldi L, Sorrentino R, Saltini C. HLA-DPB1 glutamate 69: a genetic marker of beryllium disease. Science 1993; 262:242–244.
115. Ridder GJ, Strohhacker H, Lohle E, Golz A, Fradis M. Laryngeal sarcoidosis: treatment with the antileprosy drug clofazimine. Ann Otol Rhinol Laryngol 2000; 109:1146–1149.
116. Robinson BW, McLemore TL, Crystal RG. Gamma interferon is spontaneously released by alveolar macrophages and lung T lymphocytes in patients with pulmonary sarcoidosis. J Clin Invest 1985; 75:1488–1495.
117. Roger G, Gallas D, Tashjian G, Baculard A, Tournier G, Garabedian EN. Sarcoidosis of the upper respiratory tract in children. Int J Pediatr Otorhinolaryngol 1994; 30:233–240.
118. Rosen Y, Vuletin JC, Pertschuk LP, Silverstein E. Sarcoidosis: from the pathologist's vantage point. Pathol Annu 1979; 14:405–439.
119. Rybicki BA, Harrington D, Major M, Simoff M, Popovich J Jr, Maliarik M, Iannuzzi MC. Heterogeneity of familial risk in sarcoidosis. Genet Epidemiol 1996; 13:23–33.
120. Rybicki BA, Maliarik MJ, Major M, Popovich J Jr, Iannuzzi MC. Genetics of sarcoidosis. Clin Chest Med 1997; 18:707–717.
121. Rybicki BA IM, Frederick MM, Thompson BW, Rossman MD, Bresnitz EA, Terrin ML, Moller DR, Barnard J, Baughman RP, DePalo L, Hunninghake G, Johns C, Judson MA, Knatterud GL, McLennan G, Newman LS, Rabin DL, Rose C, Teirstein AS, Weinberger SE, Yeager H, Cherniack R. The A. Familial aggregation of sarcoidosis. A case-control etiologic study of sarcoidosis (ACCESS). Am J Respir Crit Care Med 2001; 164:2085–2091.
122. Selroos OB. Use of budesonide in the treatment of pulmonary sarcoidosis. Ann N Y Acad Sci 1986; 465:713–721.
123. Semenzato G, Agostini C, Trentin L, Zambello R, Chilosi M, Cipriani A, Ossi E, Angi MR, Morittu L, Pizzolo G. Evidence of cells bearing interleukin-2 receptor at sites of disease activity in sarcoid patients. Clin Exp Immunol 1984; 57:331–337.
124. Sharma OP, Johnson R. Airway obstruction in sarcoidosis. A study of 123 nonsmoking black American patients with sarcoidosis. Chest 1988; 94:343–346.
125. Sher A, Coffman RL. Regulation of immunity to parasites by T cells and T cell–derived cytokines. Annu Rev Immunol 1992; 10:385–409.
126. Shigehara K, Shijubo N, Ohmichi M, Takahashi R, Kon S, Okamura H, Kurimoto M, Hiraga Y, Tatsuno T, Abe S, Sato N. IL-12 and IL-18 are increased and stimulate IFN-gamma production in sarcoid lungs. J Immunol 2001; 166:642–649.
127. Shorr AF, Torrington KG, Hnatiuk OW. Endobronchial biopsy for sarcoidosis: a prospective study. Chest 2001; 120:109–114.
128. Shorr AF, Torrington KG, Hnatiuk OW. Endobronchial involvement and airway hyperreactivity in patients with sarcoidosis. Chest 2001; 120:881–886.
129. Siltzbach LE, James DG, Neville E, Turiaf J, Battesti JP, Sharma OP, Hosoda Y, Mikami R, Odaka M. Course and prognosis of sarcoidosis around the world. Am J Med 1974; 57:847–852.

130. Siltzbach LE, Teirstein AS. Chloroquine therapy in 43 patients with intra-thoracic and cutaneous sarcoidosis. Acta Med Scand Suppl 1964; 425:302–308.
131. Smellie HAG, Marshall R. The effect of corticosteroid treatment on pulmonary function in sarcoidosis. Thorax 1961; 16:87–91.
132. Spiteri MA. Inhaled corticosteroids in pulmonary sarcoidosis. Postgrad Med J 1991; 67:327–329.
133. Standiford TJ, Rolfe MW, Kunkel SL, Lynch JP 3rd, Burdick MD, Gilbert AR, Orringer MB, Whyte RI, Strieter RM. Macrophage inflammatory protein-1 alpha expression in interstitial lung disease. J Immunol 1993; 151:2852–2863.
134. Stern BJ, Schonfeld SA, Sewell C, Krumholz A, Scott P, Belendiuk G. The treatment of neurosarcoidosis with cyclosporine. Arch Neurol 1992; 49:1065–1072.
135. Stinson JM, Hargett D. Prolonged lobar atelectasis in sarcoidosis. J Natl Med Assoc 1981; 73:669–671.
136. Stjernberg N, Thunell M. Pulmonary function in patients with endobronchial sarcoidosis. Acta Med Scand 1984; 215:121–126.
137. Sulavik SB, Spencer RP, Weed DA, Shapiro HR, Shiue ST, Castriotta RJ. Recognition of distinctive patterns of gallium-67 distribution in sarcoidosis. J Nucl Med 1990; 31:1909–1914.
138. Thomas PD, Hunninghake GW. Current concepts of the pathogenesis of sarcoidosis. Am Rev Respir Dis 1987; 135:747–760.
139. Torrington KG, Shorr AF, Parker JW. Endobronchial disease and racial differences in pulmonary sarcoidosis. Chest 1997; 111:619–622.
140. Trentin L, Zambello R, Facco M, Tassinari C, Sancetta R, Siviero M, Cerutti A, Cipriani A, Marcer G, Majori M, Pesci A, Agostini C, Semenzato G. Selection of T lymphocytes bearing limited TCR-V beta regions in the lung of hypersensitivity pneumonitis and sarcoidosis. Am J Respir Crit Care Med 1997; 155:587–596.
141. Trinchieri G, Scott P. Interleukin-12: a proinflammatory cytokine with immunoregulatory functions. Res Immunol 1995; 146:423–431.
142. Udwadia ZF, Pilling JR, Jenkins PF, Harrison BD. Bronchoscopic and bronchographic findings in 12 patients with sarcoidosis and severe or progressive airways obstruction. Thorax 1990; 45:272–275.
143. Valeyre D, Soler P, Clerici C, Pre J, Battesti JP, Georges R, Hance AJ. Smoking and pulmonary sarcoidosis: effect of cigarette smoking on prevalence, clinical manifestations, alveolitis, and evolution of the disease. Thorax 1988; 43:516–524.
144. Walker C, Bauer W, Braun RK, Menz G, Braun P, Schwarz F, Hansel TT, Villiger B. Activated T cells and cytokines in bronchoalveolar lavages from patients with various lung diseases associated with eosinophilia. Am J Respir Crit Care Med 1994; 150:1038–1048.
145. Weisman RA, Canalis RF, Powell WJ. Laryngeal sarcoidosis with airway obstruction. Ann Otol Rhinol Laryngol 1980; 89:58–61.

146. Yeager H Jr, Williams MC, Beekman JF, Bayly TC, Beaman BL. Sarcoidosis: analysis of cells obtained by bronchial lavage. Am Rev Respir Dis 1977; 116:951–954.
147. Zabel P, Entzian P, Dalhoff K, Schlaak M. Pentoxifylline in treatment of sarcoidosis. Am J Respir Crit Care Med 1997; 155:1665–1669.
148. Zeitlin JF, Tami TA, Baughman R, Winget D. Nasal and sinus manifestations of sarcoidosis. Am J Rhinol 2000; 14:157–161.
149. Zissel G, Ernst M, Schlaak M, Muller-Quernheim J. Accessory function of alveolar macrophages from patients with sarcoidosis and other granulomatous and nongranulomatous lung diseases. J Investig Med 1997; 45:75–86.
150. Zissel G, Homolka J, Schlaak J, Schlaak M, Muller-Quernheim J. Anti-inflammatory cytokine release by alveolar macrophages in pulmonary sarcoidosis. Am J Respir Crit Care Med 1996; 154:713–719.
151. Zych D, Pawlicka L, Zielinski J. Inhaled budesonide vs prednisone in the maintenance treatment of pulmonary sarcoidosis. Sarcoidosis 1993; 10:56–61.

20

Manifestations of Immune Deficiency Syndromes in the Upper and Lower Airways

JEFFREY L. KISHIYAMA and **DANIEL C. ADELMAN**

University of California
San Francisco, California, U.S.A.

Introduction

Upper and lower respiratory infections are among the most commonly encountered illnesses seen by primary care physicians and subspecialists including allergy/immunologists, pulmonologists, and otolaryngologists. While treatment of uncomplicated sinusitis, otitis media, bronchitis, and pneumonia is straightforward, recurrent or refractory infection challenges the physician to recognize and identify underlying conditions predisposing to infection. A broad range of risk factors may contribute to recurrent or relapsing infection, including anatomical derangements, aeroallergen hypersensitivity, cigarette smoke exposure, cystic fibrosis, antibiotic resistance, and immunodeficiency disorders. Numerous underlying systemic disorders such as sickle cell disease, viral infections, splenectomy, malnutrition, cirrhosis, diabetes mellitus, renal failure, and alcoholism can cause variable degrees of secondary immune impairment. In addition to classic immunosuppressive medications, drugs such as parenteral gold, prednisone, and phenytoin can cause immunoglobulin abnormalities (see Table 1).

This chapter focuses on primary immunodeficiency disorders and their contribution to upper and lower airway infection. Particular attention is

Table 1 Causes of Hypogammaglobulinemia in Adults

Primary	Secondary or acquired
Common variable immunodeficiency	Diminished synthesis
Selective IgA or IgM deficiency	Uremia
IgG subclass deficiency	Infections with cytomegalovirus
Kappa/Lambda light chain deficiency	or Epstein–Barr virus
Congenital hypogammaglobulinemia	Immunosuppressive chemotherapy
surviving to adulthood (e.g., X-linked	Hypercatabolic states
agammaglobulinemia, autosomal	Myotonic dystrophy
recessive agammaglobulinemia,	Severe malnutrition
hyper-IgM immunodeficiency)	Hyperthyroidism
	Protein-losing states
	Protein-losing enteropathy
	Nephrosis
	Lymphoproliferative malignancies

directed to humoral immunodeficiency, including common variable immunodeficiency (CVI or acquired hypogammaglobulinemia), X-linked agammaglobulinemia (XLA), selective IgA deficiency, and IgG subclass deficiency. There is also a brief discussion of hyper-IgE syndrome, a primary immunodeficiency disorder characterized by immune dysregulation.

I. Host Defense

Human airways contain both nonspecific and specific host defense mechanisms to ward off foreign invasion. Nonimmune defenses include physical barriers, mucociliary clearance, and secretions. The secretory blanket consists of two separable layers, the surface mucus (gel) layer and a deeper aqueous (serous, periciliary) layer. The mucus blanket contributes to the protective barrier function by entrapping microorganisms and particles, ultimately moving toward the posterior pharynx through mucociliary transport. The mucus layer floats on a periciliary or serous layer, which mechanically couples to the ciliary movement. The periciliary layer also contains aqueous proteins including enzymes, antioxidants, and plasma proteins. The enzymes lysozyme and lactoferrin are nonspecific, broad-spectrum antimicrobial proteins found in considerable concentration in airways secretions.

Other nonspecific immunological systems include cellular responses by phagocytes, neutrophils, and natural killer cells, as well as serum complement cascades, and the generation of inflammatory eicosanoids, cytokines, and mediators. Phylogenetically more sophisticated defense systems rely on specific immunological memory and include T-cell-mediated cellular immunity and antibody-mediated humoral immunity. Mechanisms of lymphocyte trafficking promote homing to specialized lymphoid sites in the lamina propria of mucosl surfaces. Although lymphocytes continue to migrate, patterns demonstrate preferred regional patterns of circulation. Surface marker analysis and in vitro tests of lymphocyte function suggest that these mucosa-associated lymphocytes differ phenotypically from other circulating T cells and may primarily provide support for local immunoglobulin-producing B cells (1).

In immunocompetent individuals, humoral immune function plays a fundamental role in mucosal immunity. Progenitor- and pre-B lymphocytes are found in the bone marrow. Progenitor-B cells undergo immunoglobulin heavy chain gene rearrangement and pre-B cells express μ heavy chain in the cytoplasm. Once the cells have expressed IgM on their surfaces, they are termed early B lymphocytes and will migrate to the peripheral lymph nodes. When mature, resting B lymphocytes are activated by antigen exposure and enter the proliferative phase. There is an increase in the expression of HLA class II antigens and cytokine receptors on the cell surface, with subsequent clonal expansion. After several rounds of cell division, the B cells enter the fully differentiated stages of development to begin producing immunoglobulin plasma cells at a high rate.

Although serum antibodies can neutralize some viruses and microbial toxins, the physiological relevance of humoral immunity appears to be primarily related to its ability to recognize and bind microbial pathogens, thereby activating complement, enhancing opsonization, and mediating antibody-dependent, cell-mediated cytotoxicity. Activation of the classical complement pathway depends on the specificity of antigen–antibody interaction, resulting in immunoglobulin conformational changes and increased binding affinity for circulating C1. As part of a recurring theme, this initial immunologically specific reaction is able to recruit nonspecific immune effector mechanisms. The consequences of an activated complement cascade are increased opsonizatin of antibody-C3b-coated pathogens, generation of chemotactic and inflammatry mediators C5a and C3a, and osmotic cytolysis by the terminal complement components.

Aside from its interaction with the complement system, antigen–antibody complexes can interact with a variety of cells through specific immunoglobulin receptors (FcRs). Several classes of FcR, each characterized by its binding affinity, are expressed on surface membranes of macrophages, mononuclear cells, neutrophils, and lymphocytes. When antigen–antibody complexes bind, these FcRs are capable of signal transduction, leading to intracellular events and immune cell activation. Furthermore, there is now evidence that FcRs and immunoglobulin may modulate antibody production through immunoregulatory feedback mechanisms.

II. Humoral Immunodeficiency

A. General Considerations

Immunoglobulin isotype deficiencies are the most common of the primary immunodeficiency disorders. Selective IgA deficiency has a prevalence of approximately 1 in 400 to 1 in 700 among western Europeans and North Americans but is found much less often among patients of African-American and Asian background. Common variable immunodeficiency, a most serious and potentially life-threatening humoral immune disorder, is characterized by deficiency of all immunoglobulin isotypes (panhypogammaglobulinemia) and has a prevalence of 1 in 50,000 to 75,000. The prevalence of XLA, a congenital deficiency of antibody production presenting in infancy and early childhood, is less than 1 in 100,000 (2–6).

The clinical manifestations of humoral immunodeficiency range from minimal to severe, typically presenting with recurrent sinopulmonary bacterial infections including sinusitis, otitis media, pneumonia, bronchitis, and mastoiditis. Infections may be prolonged or may be associated with unusual complications, such as bacteremia, osteomyelitis, and meningitis. Infections by high grade encapsulated organisms such as *Streptococcus pneumoniae* and *Hemophilus influenzae* occur as a direct result of impaired antigen-specific antibody production (Table 2). Accurate diagnosis of primary immunodeficiency is important because of the prognostic implications that accompany these diseases. Early and aggressive treatment of infections is necessary to prevent recurrent and chronic pulmonary infections from leading to irreversible tissue destruction, bronchiectasis, and obstructive lung disease. Previous sinus surgery, bronchiectasis, and excessive useof antibiotics predispose patients to development of infections with more virulent pathogens, such as *Staphylococcus aureus* and *Pseudomonas aeruginosa*. Exposure to cigarette smoke may be particularly deleterious in patients with hypogammaglobulinemia, since smoking can lead to chronic obstructive bronchitis (7).

B. Selective IgA Deficiency

Selective IgA deficiency is the most common primary immunodeficiency disorder affecting humans and is defined as serum IgA below 5 mg/dL. Immunoglobulin A is the antibody isotype produced in the largest quantity, however, serum levels are low (50–200 mg/dL) because most of this

Table 2 Infectious Organisms Found in Hypogammaglobulinemia

Organism	Common infection site	Relative frequency
Bacterial		
Streptococcus pneumoniae	Sinopulmonary, otitis	Common
Hemophilus influenzae	Sinopulmonary, otitis	Common
Staphylococcus aureus	Sinopulmonary, otitis	Less common
Pseudomonas aeruginosa	Bronchopulmonary	Less common
Salmonella spp.	Gastrointestinal	Less common
Shigella spp.	Gastrointestinal	Less common
Campylobacter spp.	Gastrointestinal	Less common
Mycoplasma pneumoniae	Respiratory, joints	Uncommon
Viral		
Herpes zoster	Shingles	Common
Herpes simplex	Recurrent, severe	Less common
Cytomegalovirus	Systemic, severe	Rare
Enteroviral infections	Meningoencephalitis	Rare in common variable
(e.g., ECHO virus,		immunodeficiency, more
Coxsackie virus)		common in X-linked
		agammaglobulinemia
Mycobacterial	Various	Uncommon
Fungal	Various	Less common
Protozoan		
Giardia lamblia	Gastrointestinal	Common
Pneumocystis carinii	Respiratory, systemic	Rare

immunoglobulin is found in saliva, tears, mucus, milk, prostatic fluid, and other secretions. Since secreted, dimeric IgA constitutes the first line of mucosal defense, the most frequent manifestation of low to absent IgA levels is recurrent mucosal infection, especially involving the upper and lower airways. Significantly, most patients have minimal or no clinical symptoms, and only a minority develop a multitude of associated problems. Some asymptomatic patients with selective IgA deficiency have been found to have higher compensatory levels of secreted monomeric IgM (8); however, mucosal IgM may be less efficient at neutralization or clearance of viruses (9).

The prevalence of selective IgA deficiency is two to four times higher in patients with atopic disease than the general population. Allergic symptoms in these patients tend to be more difficult to control, although the reasons for this have not been fully elucidated. Two theories to explain this phenomenon are (1) that the absence of secretory IgA decreases the "competition" of antigen for preformed IgE molecules at the mucosal surfaces and (2) that the lack of secretory IgA permits the absorption of antigen across the mucosal surface, which in turn promotes the formation of antigen-specific IgE antibody.

There is an increased prevalence of gastrointestinal disorders in patients with selective IgA deficiency. Celiac disease is found with increased frequency, and other associated gastrointestinal complications include diarrhea with intestinal lymphoid nodular hyperplasia, giardiasis, inflammatory bowel disease, and pernicious anemia associated with anti–parietal cell and anti–intrinsic factor antibodies. Other clinical syndromes associated with selective IgA deficiency are a variety of autoimmune disorders, including systemic lupus erythematosus, rheumatoid arthritis, pernicious anemia, immune endocrinopathies, thyroiditis, myasthenia gravis, and autoimmune hemolytic anemia.

The etiology of the selective deficiency of IgA is not known. There appear to be normal or only slightly decreased numbers of circulating B cells expressing membrane-bound IgA; however, many coexpress membrane IgM and IgD. This is consistent with a less mature phenotype and implies a pathogenetic defect impairing terminal B-lymphocyte differentiation. Whether the maturational defect is due to an intrinsic B-cell defect or a regulatory T-cell defect has not been clearly established. Nevertheless, in vitro studies have corroborated these observations, demonstrating that lymphocytes from IgA-deficient patients will synthesize IgA but not secrete it.

Overall, the prognosis for these patients is generally good when infections are promptly and appropriately managed. Clinical management of selective IgA deficiency is primarily supportive, with agrressive treatment of infectious complications as the mainstay of therapy. Patients with selective IgA deficiency should not receive replacement immunoglobulin, since these preparations contain only scant quantities of IgA, insufficient amounts to increase mucosal secretory levels. In addition, the absence of IgA in some patients leads to the generation of high titers of anti-IgA antibodies. These patients are at high risk of experiencing anaphylactoid reactions to any infussed blood product containing trace IgA. The risk of transfusion reactions can be minimized by thorough washing of packed erythrocytes or by transfusing blood products obtained from IgA-deficient patients.

C. Hyper-IgE Syndrome

Hyper-IgE syndrome is an immunodeficiency disorder characterized by very high IgE levels, but its clinical manifestations do not suggest a primary humoral immunodeficiency. Instead, affected individuals suffer from recurrent staphylococcal abscesses especially involving the skin, lungs, and other sites. In affected patients, *S. aureus* is a ubiquitous pathogen, but *Candida* and *Aspergillus* spp. and other fungal species are not infrequent. These patients demonstrate a plethora of immunological abnormalities including very high IgE levels, eosinophilia, impaired cell-mediated and humoral responses to neoantigens, and variable neutrophil chemotactic defects (7,8). All patients suffer from recurrent, severe abscesses involving skin and viscera, with airway involvement being extremely common. This may be manifested in the form of sinusitis, otitis, and mastoiditis. In most all patients, deep-seated lung abscesses often result in pneumatocele formation. The clinical presentation of hyper-IgE syndrome can be mistaken for chronic granulomatous disease, a granulocyte disorder of impaired neutrophil oxidative burst and bacterial killing.

The elevated serum IgE levels are pronounced, ranging as high as 40,000 IU/mL. There are very few conditions with total IgE levels of this magnitude, but atopic dermatitis, allergic bronchopulmonary aspergillosis, and the very rare IgE myeloma are among them. Indeed, hyper-IgE syndrome and atopic dermatitis can be difficult to distinguish because both conditions are associated with severe eczematoid dermatitis, lichenification, eosinophilia, and wheal and flare reactions to multiple foods and aeroallergens (12). The presence of multiple abscesses and the distribution of dermatitis can differentiate between the two clinical diagnoses. Moreover, a variety of anthropomorphic abnormalities have been associated with hyper-IgE syndrome, including characteristic facies, delayed dental shedding, and skeletal abnormalities. Clinical allergic syndromes of allergic rhinitis and asthma were also not common in one series of more than 30 patients (12). Although there have been inconsistent reports of abnormal neutrophil chemotaxis, granulocyte function is otherwise normal, and immunological assays of phagocytosis, oxidative burst, and bacterial killing are unremarkable.

The pathophysiology of the disease is not well understood, and the various immunological abnormalities could represent primary defects or secondary markers of immune dysregulation. No specific immune reconstitution is available, but prophylactic antibiotics, as well as prompt aggressive management of infections, abscesses, and pneumatoceles, can lead to improved clinical prognosis.

D. IgG Subclass Deficiency

The IgG immunoglobulin isotype consists of four IgG subclasses, IgG1 (70%), IgG2 (20%), IgG3 (7%), and IgG4 (3%). These isotype subclasses are defined by antigenic differences foundin the Fc portion of the immunoglobulin molecule and differ in their ability to fix complement and bind monocytes and macrophages. An equally important functional difference lies in their ability to respond to antigens of different types. The IgG1 and IgG3 subclasses give the best functional antibody responses to protein antigens; the IgG2 subclass gives a humoral response primarily to polysaccharide antigens.

Deficiencies of each subclass have been described and appear to be of variable clinical significance. Some patients with isolated IgG subclass deficiencies can have recurrent sinopulmonary infections with *Streptococcus pneumoniae, Hemophilus influenzae,* and *Staphylococcus aureus.* Isolated IgG2 deficiency is associated with recurrent infections with organisms expressing polysaccharide/carbohydrate antigens in their bacterial capsule. These patients have impaired antibody responses to polysaccharide vaccines including Pneumovax or unconjugated HiB (*Hemophilus influenzae* B) but apparently normal antibody responses to protein or such protein-conjugated vaccines as tetanus or diphtheria toxoids (dT).

Patients with IgG3 deficiency are proported to have an increase incidence of certain bacterial infections. IgG3 may also play a key role in virus neutralization (13). Other patients with documented IgG subclass deficiencies have no significant clinical manifestations. It has been hypothesized that compensatory increases in other subclasses accounts for the lack of symptoms.

The observed association of IgG2, IgG4, IgE, and IgA deficiencies provided early insight to the pathogenesis of IgG subclass deficiencies. The immunoglobulin heavy chain genes are all located in a single region on chromosome 14. The exons coding for the constant region sequences are arranged linearly as follows: μ, δ, $\gamma 3$, $\gamma 1$, $\alpha 1$, $\gamma 2$, $\gamma 4$, ϵ and $\alpha 2$. Deletion of any of the constant heavy chain genes (single or adjacent) or any aberrations in isotype switching can lead to deficiencies of one or more of the IgG isotypes. This makes it easier to understand why combined IgG2 and IgG4 or IgG1 and IgG3 deficiencies are frequently observed. Similarly, IgG subclass deficiency is found in approximately 15% of IgA-deficient patients.

It can be difficult to determine the appropriate indication for treatment of patients with isolated IgG subclass deficiency with replacement immunoglobulin. The decision should not be made on the basis of low quantitative levels of the subclass alone; the clinical condition and the patient's response to immunization must be the basis for the decision to treat. It can be quite useful to follow patients closely for a period of several months, sequentially on, then off replacement immunoglobulin therapy, monitoring objective clinical signs (e.g., number of days of school or work missed, number of unscheduled physician visits for infections, number of days of fever), before committing the patient to life-long therapy with gammaglobulin.

III. Common Variable Immunodeficiency

The most common cause of panhypogammaglobulinemia in adults is common variable immunodeficiency (CVI); a heterogeneous immunodeficiency disorder clinically characterized by an increased incidence of recurrent infections, autoimmune phenomena, and neoplastic diseases. The onset of CVI generally is during adolescence or early adulthood, but it can occur at any age. Males and females are affected equally.

The observed increased susceptibility to infection in CVI is directly related to the low levels of serum immunoglobulin and the inability to produce specific antibodies following antigenic challenge. The pattern of immunoglobulin isotype deficiency is variable. Most patients present with significantly depressed IgG levels, but over time all antibody classes (IgG, IgA, and IgM) may be affected. The most common infections are sinusitis, otitis media, bronchitis, and pneumonia, with bronchiectasis seen in as many as 28% of affected patients (14,15). The common organisms found in recurrent infections in CVI patients are listed in Table 2.

In addition to the humoral immunodeficiency, most CVI patients also exhibit at least partial impairment of cellular immunity. Consequently, there is an increased incidence of opportunistic infections with mycobacterium, fungi, and *Pneumocystis carinii* compared with the general population (although these infections still remain quite rare). Patients with CVI appear to tolerate most viral infections well, although approximately 20% develop reactivated herpes zoster (shingles). Similarly, severe and recurrent infections with herpes simplex and cytomegalovirus have been reported (16,17).

Gastrointestinal disorders are common in patients with CVI. Chronic infections and malabsorption, chronic inflammatory bowel disease, atrophic gastritis, achlorhydria, and gastrointestinal malignancies are frequent problems for these patients. *Giardia lamblia* is a common cause of diarrhea in CVI patients and if left untreated, significant malabsorption, weight loss and related morbidity can result. Common variable immunodeficiency patients are also at greater risk for the development of infections by species of *Salmonella*, *Shigella*, and *Campylobacter*. Clinically, all diarrheal illnesses lasting more than a few days in these patients should be aggressively evaluated and treated. Malabsorption frequently develops secondary to bacterial overgrowth and can lead to hypoalbuminemia, hypocalcemia, and deficiency of the fat-soluble vitamins. In affected patients, fecal fat determinations are frequently abnormal, and small-bowel biopsy specimens reveal flattened villi and lymphocytic infiltrates in the lamina propria, similar to what is seen histologically in gluten-sensitive (celiac) enteropathies. In contrast to patients with celiac disease, however, CVI patients with malabsorption do not respond to gluten-free diets or empiric therapy with broad-spectrum antibiotics. CVI patients also frequently develop achlorhydria and atrophic gastritis.

Autoimmune phenomena develop in one in five patients with CVI, including inflammatory bowel disease, autoimmune cytopenias (e.g., hemolytic anemia, pernicious anemia, immune thrombocytopenic purpura neutropenia), hypo- or hyperthyroidism, rheumatoid arthritis, systemic lupus erythematosus, and Sjögren's syndrome. In contrast to that found in immunocompetent patients, most CVI patients clinically manifesting autoimmune phenomena do not produce the common serological markers of disease (i.e., seronegative ANA, rheumatoid factor, etc.). The higher incidence of autoimmune syndromes observed in these patients suggests that the immunodeficiency of CVI is also associated with immune dysregulation. In general, treatment of the autoimmune disorders of CVI is similar to that in nonimmunocompromised patients except that cytotoxic, immunosuppressive agents are to be avoided whenever possible to minimize further compromise of immune function.

Thirty percent of CVI patients clinically exhibit splenomegaly and/or lymphadenopathy. Biopsy samples of lymphoid tissue typically reveal reactive follicular hyperplasia and a paucity of plasma cells. Neoplastic disorders, especially lymphoproliferative malignancies, develop at a higher frequency in patients with CVI. The incidence of lymphoma in CVI patients is between 50- and 400-fold higher than the age-adjusted rates in the general population, and the vast majorities are of B-cell origin. There also appears to be a higher incidence of gastric carcinoma, basal cell carcinoma, and other skin cancers (18).

The inability to produce normal quantitative and functional antibody responses in CVI can be due to a wide variety of immunological abnormalities. The most common defect seen in CVI appears to be a failure of B lymphocytes to normally differentiate into cells able to secrete immunoglobulin in vivo.

Coculture mixing studies combining B cells from CVI patients and normal allergenic T cells demonstrated impaired in vitro immunoglobulin production, while T cells from CVI patients supported immunoglobulin production by normal B cells. These simple mixing studies suggested that most CVI patients had intrinsic B-cell defects. Saxon and colleagues analyzed B cells in vitro from CVI patients to determine the stage(s) of defective development (19). In 2 of 15 patients, B cells failed to respond to in vitro activation signals; in 1 of 15 patients, B cells responded normally to the activation signals but failed to proliferate normally in response to mitogens; and in 12 of 15 patients, B cells responded to activation and proliferation signals but did not fully differentiate into immunoglobulin-secreting plasma cells. The data suggest that a defect in response to late-acting signals of differentiation might play a significant role in the pathophysiology of the disease.

Other potential mechanisms have been proposed to explain the B-cell abnormalities and impaired humoral function. Although circulating B-lymphocyte numbers are typically low-normal to normal, they differ phenotypically from normal control CD19$^+$ B cells by expressing less surface L-selectin and bright CD20 (20). In a subset of patients with low-normal numbers of B cells, CD95 and CD38, two surface molecules involved in induction and protection from apoptosis, respectively, showed differential expression in CVI patients compared with controls (21). These studies suggest that failure to overcome physiological apoptosis, a normal event in immune cell developmental regulation, may block their normal maturation processes.

Other mechanisms of antibody deficiency include impaired T-cell helper function, excessive T-cell suppressor activity, or abnormal antigen processing and presentation. Few patients demonstrate overt cell-mediated immunodeficiency, yet delayed hypersensitivity skin responses are abnormal in 50% of patients with CVI. A variety of in vitro abnormalities of T-cell function have also been observed, including deficient secretion of the cytokines interferon gamma (IFN-γ), interleukins 2, 4, and 5 (IL-2, -4, -5), inefficient signaling via CD40–CD154 (gp39 or CD40 ligand) cell-to-cell interactions, and decreased proliferative responses to T-cell receptor-mediated activation signals (22,23).

Sneller and Strober performed in vitro stimulation of CVI B cells, with supernatants from T-cell hybridomas to promote immunoglobulin production, suggesting that T-cell-derived soluble factors were missing in these patients (24). Cytokines play important roles in the maturation and differentiation of B cells. For example, IL-4 is involved in both the coactivation of resting B cells (with antigen) to proliferation and isotype commitment; IL-2 promotes proliferation of *Staphylococcus aureus* Cowan I-activated B cells; and IL-5 influences maturation and immunoglobulin production of activated B cells. Interleukin 6 drives differentiation of B cells into high rate immunoglobulin-secreting cells, induces proliferation of Epstein-Barr virus transformed cell lines and hybridoma cells in vitro, functions as an autocrine growth factor for human myeloma cells, and has a multitude of systemic effects similar to those of IL-1 and tumor necrosis factor (TNF). This interleukin may also provide a potent stimulus for the induction of autoimmunity.

In view of the potentially important role played by cytokines in both B-cell differentiation and autoimmune phenomena, Adelman and colleagues postulated that some CVI patients would exhibit elevated serum levels of IL-6 as a consequence of the inability of their B cells to terminally differentiate into high rate immunoglobulin-secreting cells despite having the ability to undergo activation and proliferation (25). These investigators measured IL-6 in the sera of 17 CVI patients, and in 13 they found IL-6 levels to be 3- to 18-fold higher than in unaffected subjects, including patients with selective IgA deficiency, hyper-IgM immunodeficiency, X-linked agammaglobuline-mia, or cystic fibrosis. Serum IL-6 binding activity was normal in all subjects, but spontaneous IL-6 production by blood mononuclear cells was substantially greater than from normal subjects. Interestingly, lipo-polysaccharide-stimulated IL-6 production by blood mononuclear cells from normal subjects raised serum IL-6 levels to the unstimulated levels seen in the patients with CVI, demonstrating that IL-6 in CVI patients' blood monuclear cells is being maximally produced. Subsequent research has confirmed that the IL-6 produced by CVI patients is functionally normal, and the level of IL-6 receptor (IL-6R) expression on mitogen-stimulated B cells from CVI patients was no different from that in normal cells. These observations may explain the clinical manifestations of auto-immunity and lymphoproliferation characteristic of CVI.

Recognizing that IL-2 is a critical factor in many immunological cascades and promotes T-cell growth, differentiation, and activation and B-lymphocyte immunoglobulin secretion, Cunningham-Rundles and col-leagues administered weekly subcutaneous IL-2 conjugated by polyethylene glycol to a small cohort of patients with hypogammaglobulinemia. There were measurable increases in several parameters of immune function, including increased T-cell proliferation to mitogens and antigen, increased cytokine production, and an increase in vivo antibody production (26–30).

In summary, multiple immunological derangements have been noted in patients with CVI, including impaired B-cell differentiation, abnormal T-cell regulation, and accessory cell function. The clinical significance of in vitro aberrant responses, however, is not entirely clear. CVI is truly a heterogeneous disease, and many different mechanisms potentially leading to the low serum immunoglobulin levels are observed in these patients.

IV. X-Linked Agammaglobulinemia

Unlike CVI, X-linked agammaglobulinemia results from a single defective gene product-mutation in the gene encoding for a cytoplasmic tyrosine kinase, an enzyme found in B-lineage lymphocytes. Two independent groups found the molecular defect in 1993 (31,32), and the affected gene product is a cytoplasmic tyrosine kinase enzyme, *Btk* (Bruton agammaglo-bulinemia tyrosine kinase). Although XLA is characterized primarily by a maturational block in between pro-/pre-B and B-cell development, resulting in normal numbers of bone marrow pro-/pre-B cells but no circulating mature B cells, *Btk* is actually found throughout each stage of B-lymphocyte develoment. The tyrosine kinase is not present in T-lineage cells. As a consequence, T lymphocytes are quantitatively and functionally normal (33). Many different mutations of the *Btk* gene have been identified, and mutation analysis can be used to identify carriers in affected families.

Although the immunoglobulin levels drop as maternally derived antibodies fall, the average age of diagnosis is 2.5 to 3.5 years. All major classes of antibodies are affected, so patients have markedly reduced or absent IgG, IgA, IgM, and IgE, and undetectable serum isohemaglutinins (i.e., naturally occurring IgM directed against major blood group antigens). Increases in specific antibody titer after vaccination are not seen, and similar to CVI, bacterial infections with pyogenic encapsulated bacteria are the most common manifestation. Upper and lower respiratory, skin, and gastrointestinal infections predominate where antibody-mediated opsonization contributes substantially to host defense.

Unlike CVI, patients with XLA demonstrate unusual susceptibility to certain disseminated enteroviral infections. These disseminated enteroviral infections can be insidious and progressive and difficult to diagnose (34–36). Symptomatic polomyelitis occurs secondary to live attenuated viral inoculation with oral polio vaccine (OPV), or chronic meningoencephalitis can lead to mental status changes, cognitive impairment, paresis, and death. Biopsy samples of affected tissue may show inflammation, and cerebral spinal fluid often demonstrates nonspecific mononuclear cell pleocytosis with elevated protein levels. Serologial testing is not applicable in patients with hypogammaglobulinemia, and viral cultures lack sensitivity. Polymerase chain reaction (PCR) techniques are promising diagnostic assays; however, prognosis remains grim for patients with disseminated infections.

V. Laboratory Evaluation

The clinical immunology laboratory can assist the clinician in diagnosing these various humoral immunodeficiency syndromes. Laboratory evaluation of patients suspected of having a humoral immunodeficiency should include quantitative serum immunoglobulins (IgG, IgA, IgM, IgE) and especially, assessment of specific antibody responses to immunonizations with protein and carbohydrate antigens. This is most easily accomplished by measuring antitetanus, antidiphtheria, and antipneumococcal antibody titers before and 3 to 4 weeks after vaccination with diphtheria-tetanus (DT) and Pneumovax. In this context, a fourfold increase in antibody titer is considered to be normal. In selected patients, quantification of IgG subclasses may be appropriate, particularly when total IgG immunoglobulins are at the low end of the normal range. The ultimate decision to treat patients with replacement immunoglobulin should be made on the basis of clinical condition, quantitative levels of immunoglobulin isotypes, and the lack of response to vaccine immunization.

Lymphocyte enumeration and phenotyping by flow cytometry can sometimes be indicated in hypogammaglobulinemia. With multicolor flow cytometry, lymphocyte subsets, activation markers, and other phenotypic features can be accurately delineated. In vivo delayed hypersensitivity skin tests to recall antigens such as tetanus toxoid, purified protein derivative, *Candida*, mumps, *Coccidiodes*, and *Trichophyton* antigen offer complementary and inexpensive screening of cell-mediated immune function.

In the setting of primary humoral immunodeficiency, serological testing is insensitive and unreliable. For accurate detection of viral infections, including but not limited to hepatitis virus, herpes virus, and human immunodeficiency virus, culture or PCR assays must be obtained.

VI. Treatment

The treatment of primary humoral immunodeficiency centers around the management of both the acute and chronic problems associated with the syndrome. Acutely, infections need to be treated with the appropriate antibiotics; more chronically, replacement of antibody is essential for infection prophylaxis. Prompt and aggressive treatment of all acute infections is the most important part of the acute management of these patients. Sometimes antibiotic therapy must be empirically initiated without the luxury of adequate cultures and sensitivities to guide the choice of antimicrobial agents. Under these circumstances, empirical therapy with activity against encapsulated organisms, such as *Streptococcus pneumoniae* and *Hemophilus influenzae*, should be employed. Many patients are predisposed to chronic infections with *Staphylococcus aureus* by reason of previous sinus surgeries. For chronic sinusitis, adequate coverage for anaerobic pathogens is recommended. The duration of antibiotic treatment may need to be longer than in the immunocompetent patient, and occasionally, intravenous antibiotics are required for adequate control of infection. Sinus infections refractory to antibiotics may require surgical drainage, with bacterial and fungal cultures obtained on the contents of the sinuses.

Central to the long-term management of patients with CVI, XLA, and selected cases of IgG subclass deficiency is antibody replacement therapy. Subsequent to the introduction of intravenous immunoglobulin (IVIg) for human use in the early 1980s, clinical studies were performed that established that IVIg administerd at doses of 300 to 600 mg/kg every 3 to 4 weeks was the preferred therapy for infection prophylaxis. Although there is some individual variation in catabolic rate for IgG, in general the half-life of infused immunoglobulin is approximately 21 days. Most practitioners administer 300 to 500 mg/kg every 3 to 4 weeks to maintain trough IgG levels above 5.0 g/L. This level correlates well with clinical efficacy.

There appears to be no difference in efficacy between specific IVIg preparations, but there are distinct safety advantages of new products containing multiple viral inactivation steps, such as solvent–detergent treatment or pasteurization. While there have been no reports of hepatitis B or HIV transmission through IVIg treatment, there have been sporadic instances of hepatitis C infection developing in IVIg-treated patients receiving products that were not subjected to viral inactivation measures.

Some products have markedly lower trace IgA content and would be better choices in patients with concomitant IgA deficiency and measurable titers of anti-IgA antibodies. This therapy is generally well tolerated, but some patients can experience infusion-rate-dependent fevers, myalgias, cephalgia, chills, and abdominal pain with nausea and vomiting. These symptoms, as well as fatigue, are more commonly observed in newly treated patients. Premedication with diphenhydramine and acetaminophen can ameliorate many of the infusion-related symptoms. Alternatively, some patients tolerate certain preparations better than others.

VII. Summary

Recurrent upper and lower respiratory infections challenge the physician to recognize when underlying primary immunodeficiency may be responsible for their frequency, refractory nature, or associated complications. Accurate diagnosis is important because of the prognostic implications of chronic pulmonary infections leading to tissue destruction, bronchiectasis, and irreversible obstructive lung disease. Most of these patients will initially present to their internists and family practitioners. A high index of suspicion, documentation of infection by radiography or culture, and consideration of more common causes of secondary immunodeficiency are the initial steps in identifying appropriate candidates for an immunological workup.

References

1. Goldblum RM, Hanson LA, Brandtzaeg P. The mucosal defense system. In: Stiehm ER, ed. Immunologic Disorders in Infants and Children. 4th ed. Philadelphia: WB Saunders Co, 1996:174.

2. Lederman HM, Winkelstein JA. X-linked agammaglobulinemia: an analysis of 96 patients. Medicine 1985; 64:145.

3. Conley ME, Stiehm ER. Immunodeficiency disorders: general considerations. In: Stiehm ER, ed. Immunologic Disorders in Infants & Children. 4th ed. Philadelphia: WB Saunders Co, 1996:205.

4. Waldmann TA. Immunodeficiency diseases: primary and acquired. In: Samter M, Talmage DW, Frank MM, Austen KF, Claman HN, eds. Immunological Diseases. 4th ed. Boston: Little, Brown, 1988:411–465.

5. McCluskey DR, Boyd NAM. Prevalence of primary hypogammaglobulinaemia in Northern Ireland. Proc R Coll Physicians (Edinb) 1989; 19:191–194.

6. Fasth A. Primary immunodeficiency disorders in Sweden: cases among children, 1974–1979. J Clin Immunol 1982; 86–92.

7. Popa V. Airway obstruction in adults with recurrent respiratory infections and IgG deficiency. Chest 1994; 105:1066–1072.

8. Cunningham-Rundles C. Physiology of IgA and IgA deficiency. J Clin Immunol 2001; 21:303–309.

9. Savilahti E, Klemola T, Carlsson B, Mellander L, Stenvik M, Hovi T. Inadequacy of mucosal IgM antibodies in selective IgA deficiency: excretion of attenuated polio viruses is prolonged. J Clin Immunol 1988; 8:89–94.

10. Buckley RH, Wray BB, Belmaker EZ. Extreme hyperimmunoglubulin E syndrome and undue susceptibility to infection. Pediatrics 1972; 49:59–70.

11. Buckley RH. The hyper-IgE syndrome. Clin Rev Allergy Immunol 2001; 20:139–154.

12. Grimbacker B, et al. Hyper-IgE syndrome with recurrent infections—an autosomal dominant multisystem disorder. N Engl J Med 1999; 340:692–302.

13. Hanson LA, Soderstrom R, Avanzini A, Bengtsson U, Bjorkander J, Soderstrom T. Immunoglobulin subclass deficiency. Pediatr Infect Dis J 1988; 7:S17–S21.

14. Cunningham-Rundles C, Bodian C. Common variable immunodeficiency: clinical and immunological features of 248 patients. Clin Immunol 1999; 92:34–48.

15. Hermans PE, Diaz-Buxo JA, Stobo JD. Idiopathic late-onset immunoglobulin deficiency; clinical observations in 50 patients. Am J Med 1976; 61:221–237.

16. Freeman HJ, Shnitka TK, Piercey JRA, Weinstein WM. Cytomegalovirus infection of the gastrointestinal tract in a patient with late onset immunodeficiency syndrome. Gastroenterology 1977; 73:1397–1403.

17. Straus SE, Seidlin M, Takiff H, Jacobs D, Bowen D, Smith HA. Oral acyclovir to suppress recurring herpes simplex virus infections in immunodeficient patients. Ann Intern Med 1984; 100:522–524.

18. Cunningham-Rundles C, Siegal FP, Cunningham-Rundles S, Lieberman P. Incidence of cancer in 98 patients with common varied immunodeficiency. J Clin Immunol 1987; 7:294–299.

19. Saxon A, Giorgi JV, Sherr EH, Kagan JM. Failure of B cells in common variable immunodeficiency to transit from proliferation to differentiation is associated with altered B cell surface molecule display. J Allergy Clin Immunol 1989; 84:44–55.

20. Saxon A, Keld B, Braun J, Dotson A, Sidell N. Long-term administration of 13-*cis*-retinoic acid in common variable immunodeficiency: circulating interleukin-6 levels, B-cell surface molecule display, and in vitro and in vivo B-cell antibody production. Immunology 1993; 80:477–487.

21. Saxon A, Keld B, Diaz-Sanchez D, Guo BC, Sidell N. B cells from a distinct subset of patients with common variable immunodeficiency (CVID) have increased CD95 (apo-1/fas), diminished CD38 expression, and undergo enhanced apoptosis. Clin Exp Immunol 1995; 102:17–25.

22. Sneller MC, Strober W. Abnormalities of lymphokine gene expression in patients with common variable immunodeficiency. J Immunol 1990; 144:3762–3769.

23. Farrington M, Grosmaire LS, Nonoyama S, Fischer SH, Hollenbaugh D, Ledbetter JA, Noelle RJ, Aruffo A, Ochs HD. CD40 ligand expression is defective in a subset of patients with common variable immunodeficiency. Proc Natl Acad Sci U S A 1994; 91:1099–1103.

24. Sneller MC, Strober W. Abnormalities of lymphokine gene expression in patients with common variable immunodeficiency. J Immunol 1990; 144:3762–3769.

25. Adelman DC, Matsuda T, Hirano T, Kishimoto T, Saxon A. Elevated seruminterleukin-6 in patients with common variable immunodeficiency associated with a failure in B cell differentiation. J Allergy Clin Immunol 1990; 86:512–521.

26. Cunningham-Rundles C, Mayer L, Spira E, Mendelsohn L. Restoration of immunoglobulin secretion in vitro in common variable immunodeficiency by in vivo treatment with polyethylene glycol–conjugated human recombinant interleukin-2. Clin Immunol Immunopathol 1992; 64:46–56.

27. Robb RJ. Interleukin 2: the molecule and its function. Immunol Today 1981; 5:203–209.

28. Cunningham-Rundles C, Bodian C, Ochs HD, Martin S, Reiter-Wong M, Zhuo Z. Long-term low-dose of IL-2 enhances immune function in common variable immunodeficiency. Clin Immunol 2001; 100:181–190.

29. Cunningham-Rundles C, Kazbay K, Hassett J, Zhou Z, Mayer L. Brief report: enhanced humoral immunity in common variable immunodeficiency after long-term treatment with polyethylene glycol–conjugated interleukin-2. N Engl J Med 1994; 331:918–921.

30. Cunnungham-Rundles C, Mayer L, Sapira E, Mendelsohn L. Restoration of immunoglobulin secretion in vitro in common variable immunodeficiency by in vivo treatment with polyethylene glycol–conjugated human recombinant interleukin-2. Clin Immunol Immunopathol 1992; 64:46–56.

31. Tsukada S, Saffran DC, Rawlings DJ, Parolini O, Allen RC, Klisak I, Cooper MD, Conley ME, Witte ON. Deficient expression of a B-cell cytoplasmic tyrosine kinase in human X-linked agammaglobulinemia. Cell 1993; 72:279–290.

32. Vetrie D, Vorechovsky I, Sideras P, Holland J, Davies A, Flinter F, Hammarstrom L, Kinnon C, Levinsky R, Bobrow M, Smith CI, Bentley DR. The gene involved in X-linked agammaglobulinaemia is a member of the src family of protein-tyrosine kinases. Nature 1993; 361:226–233.

33. Conley ME. B cells in patients with X-linked agammaglobulinemia. J Immunol 1985; 134:3070–3074.

34. McKinney RE, Katz SL, Wilfert CM. Chronic enteroviral meningoencephalitis in agammaglobulinemic patients. Rev Infect Dis 1987; 9:334–356.

35. Wilfert CM, Buckley RH, Mohanakumar T, Griffith JF, Katz SL, Whisnant JK, Eggleston PA, Moore M, Treadwell E, Oxman MN, Rosen FS. Persistent and fatal central-nervous-system ECHO virus infections in patients with agammaglobulinemia. N Engl J Med 1977; 296:1485–1489.

36. Bardelas JA, Winkelstein JA, Seto DS, Tsai T, Roger AD. Fatal ECHO 24 infection in a patient with hypogammaglobulinemia: relationship to dermato-myositis-like syndrome. J Pediatr 1977; 90:396–398.

37. Stiehm ER, ed. Immunologic Disorders in Infants and Children. 4th ed. Philadelphia: WB Saunders, 1996.

Index